ANATOMY SIMPLIFIED

ANATOMY SIMPLIFIED

Lalita Kulkarni

MBBS MS (Anatomy) DNB (Anatomy) MS (ENT) DNB (ENT)
Ex-Lecturer
Department of Anatomy
Smt. Kashibai Navale Medical College and General Hospital
Sinhgad, Pune, Maharashtra, India

Foreword

MN Koti

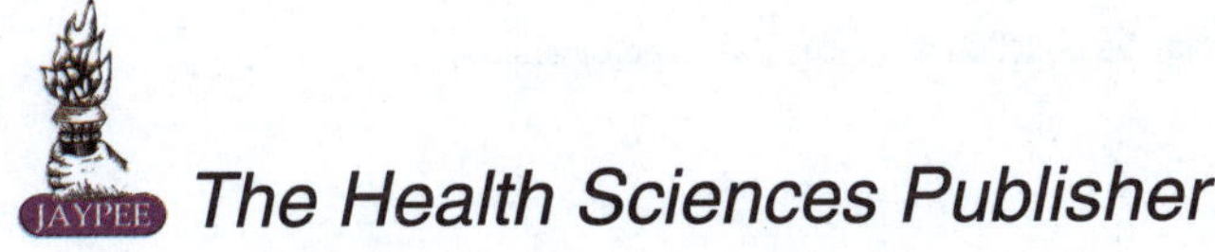

The Health Sciences Publisher

New Delhi | London | Philadelphia | Panama

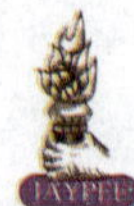

Jaypee Brothers Medical Publishers (P) Ltd

Headquarters

Jaypee Brothers Medical Publishers (P) Ltd
4838/24, Ansari Road, Daryaganj
New Delhi 110 002, India
Phone: +91-11-43574357
Fax: +91-11-43574314
Email: jaypee@jaypeebrothers.com

Overseas Offices

J.P. Medical Ltd
83 Victoria Street, London
SW1H 0HW (UK)
Phone: +44 20 3170 8910
Fax: +44 (0)20 3008 6180
Email: info@jpmedpub.com

Jaypee-Highlights Medical Publishers Inc
City of Knowledge, Bld. 237, Clayton
Panama City, Panama
Phone: +1 507-301-0496
Fax: +1 507-301-0499
Email: cservice@jphmedical.com

Jaypee Medical Inc.
The Bourse
111 South Independence Mall East
Suite 835, Philadelphia, PA 19106, USA
Phone: +1 267-519-9789
Email: jpmed.us@gmail.com

Jaypee Brothers Medical Publishers (P) Ltd
17/1-B Babar Road, Block-B, Shaymali
Mohammadpur, Dhaka-1207
Bangladesh
Mobile: +08801912003485
Email: jaypeedhaka@gmail.com

Jaypee Brothers Medical Publishers (P) Ltd
Bhotahity, Kathmandu, Nepal
Phone: +977-9741283608
Email: kathmandu@jaypeebrothers.com

Website: www.jaypeebrothers.com
Website: www.jaypeedigital.com

Inquiries for bulk sales may be solicited at: jaypee@jaypeebrothers.com

Anatomy Simplified

First Edition: **2015**

ISBN 978-93-5025-108-9

Printed at: Nova Publications & Printers Pvt. Ltd.

Dedicated to

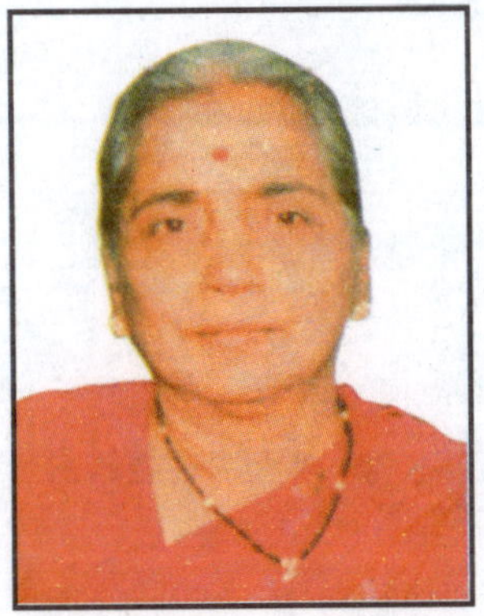

My Mother Late Mrs Usha Arvind Kulkarni
who believed 'Education' is the most precious
'Ornament' a daughter should possess

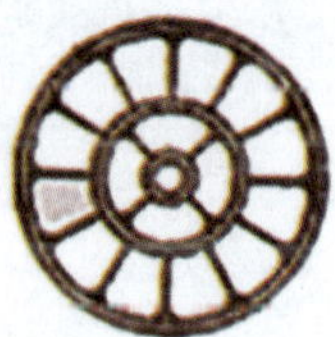

Foreword

Anatomy is a very vast and difficult subject to understand. It is also difficult to remember and to answer the questions in examination. I hereby introduce this book, *Anatomy Simplified,* to students and recommend them to follow the same to gain knowledge in anatomy in simple and easy way due to its following features:

- This book is designed like a *Made Easy* book, which is really simple and concise, but informative
- The diagrams and illustrations are attractive, easy to understand, easy to draw and self-explanatory
- The MCQs, short notes, long questions, etc. are very useful for the students
- Special importance given for Neuroanatomy, Embryology and Histology.

  Hence the book is definitely useful in all respects.

MN Koti MBBS MS

Professor

Department of Anatomy

Shridevi Institute of Medical Sciences and Research Hospital

Tumkur, Karnataka, India

Preface

Anatomy Simplified is a book meant for students of 1st year MBBS, dental, ayurvedic, homeopathic and students preparing for entrance examinations. Since the book also deals with surgical anatomy, it will be useful for students doing postgraduation in surgical discipline.

The book covers examination-oriented topics in Socratic method, in the form of 'questions and answers'. The book prepares the students even for 'viva voce' and makes students feel confident to appear for the examinations.

Certain topics like, neurobiotaxis, humeral torsion, surgical anatomy, and hearsay topics dealt in dissection hall are also covered up in the book. Key diagrams, which form the basis of the book, will make it simple to remember 'anatomy'.

Most of the sections are arranged into five chapters namely Key Questions, Short Notes, Long Questions, Key Diagrams with MCQ Tips and MCQs, which will enable the students to prepare for all types of examinations including viva voce and to acquire knowledge in a simple and systematic way. Separate Glossary for Neuroanatomy section is given considering its importance. Sections VII and VIII deal with Embryology and Histology. Section IX deals with the meanings of few Greek and Latin words used in anatomy.

Always a subject studied in own language is easy, similarly an attempt is made to make 'anatomy language, easy. It is difficult to make subject easy, but if the student adopts right methods of learning, it becomes Anatomy Simplified.

Lalita Kulkarni

Acknowledgments

At the outset, I owe every part of my success in all endeavors of my life to my father Shri Arvind G Kulkarni whose blessings are always upon me. I also thank my sisters who have directly and indirectly contributed to my education by inculcating right approach towards my studies and prayed for my success. I am immensely grateful to all my teachers who believed in my honest efforts. I especially want to mention about Dr MN Koti, who encouraged me to write this book.

I thank my typists Ms Archana and Ms Meenal, who in spite of being nonmedical staff understood the significance of my project. I also thank my other staff members.

I would like to express my gratitude to my husband, Mr Hemant, who has been supportive all throughout my venture and who believed in my efforts. I also thank my in-laws. I am immensely grateful to all my friends, throughout my medical career, who helped me to achieve my goals.

My thanks are also due to Shri Jitendar P Vij (Group Chairman), Mr Ankit Vij (Group President), Mr Tarun Duneja (Director–Publishing) and all staff of Bengaluru Branch of M/s Jaypee Brothers Medical Publishers (P) Ltd, whose efforts made this book possible.

Last but not least, the inspiration behind this book is indeed due to my students whom I taught and who made me feel the necessity to make 'Anatomy' a student-friendly subject and write the book titled *Anatomy Simplified*.

Contents

Instructions for Students

Dear Students,

- This is an examination-oriented book; for the detailed understanding of the subject you must read the standard textbooks
- Only important topics are covered in this book, to make it **simplified**
- To remember anatomy, you must draw diagrams repeatedly; a **diagram speaks more than 1000 words**!
- Form of the questions in the examination may differ than given in this book; so read the questions carefully in the examination.

Lalita Kulkarni

Key to Anatomy

A building has iron beams, bricks and cement; this is gross anatomy of building. Similarly, a human body is made up of bone (foundation of body), muscles, artery, veins and a drainage system of lymphatics.

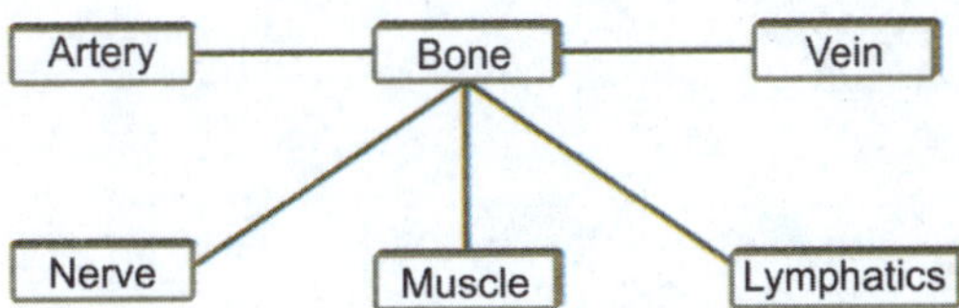

There is an architectural plan to any house; similarly body design is planned:

1. Skin is followed by subcutaneous tissue (superficial fascia), deep fascia, muscles, bone.
2. Artery is always in a deeper plane to be well protected, since it provides nutrition to the various parts of body.
3. An artery is always accompanied by vein.
4. Veins are accompanied by lymphatics.
5. If you are discussing artery automatically, other relations are the remaining structures of body, i.e. vein, nerve, lymph; if lymph is discussed, other structures form the relations.
6. Names of the arteries are given by and large by the organs it supplies. For example, artery going to uterus—uterine artery, artery going to thyroid—thyroid artery, etc.
7. Ligament connecting radius to ulna is known as radioulnar ligament; ligament connecting tibia to fibula is known as tibiofibular ligament.
8. Names given to any neurovascular bundle is according to the region it is present, e.g. femoral region—femoral artery, femoral vein, femoral nerve; axillary region—axillary artery, axillary vein, axillary nerve.

Introduction

Key points

- Anatomy classification
- Key general topics
  - Bone
- Joints
- Epiphysis
- Cartilages

Anatomy is a Greek word. The literal meaning of the word is:

- ANA—through
- TOMY—cutting.

It means by cutting through the cadaver, i.e. doing dissections one can acquire the knowledge of anatomy.

ANATOMY CLASSIFICATION

Anatomy can be studied under following subdivisions:

1. Gross anatomy—as seen by naked eyes (grossly, as in dissection hall).
2. Microscopic anatomy (histology)—as seen under microscope.
3. Developmental anatomy (embryology)—study of growing embryo.
4. Surface anatomy—marking deep structures on skin.

KEY GENERAL TOPICS

Bones

Types of Bone

1. According to the shape:
   a. Irregular bone, e.g. hip bone.

b. Long bone, e.g. femur, humerus.

c. Long short bone, e.g. metacarpals, metatarsals.

d. Flat bones, e.g. skull bones.

Sesamoid bone is a unique type of bone, which develops in a tendon, e.g. patella—in quadriceps tendon.

2. According to histology:

a. Cancellous bone.

b. Compact bone.

Every long bone has these structures.

3. According to location:

a. Appendicular skeleton, e.g. limb bones.

b. Axial skeleton, e.g. skull bones.

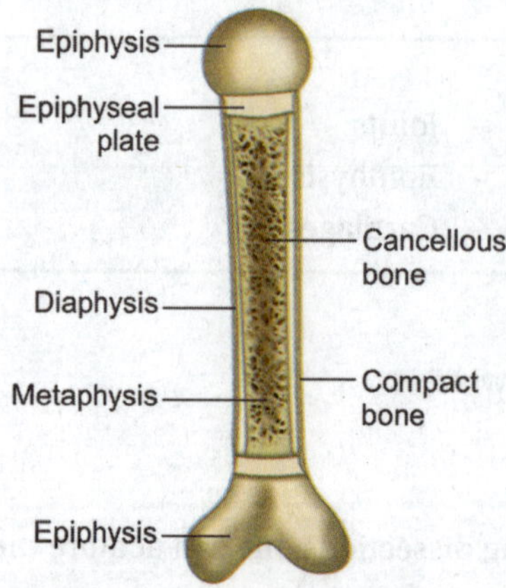

Parts of developing long bone

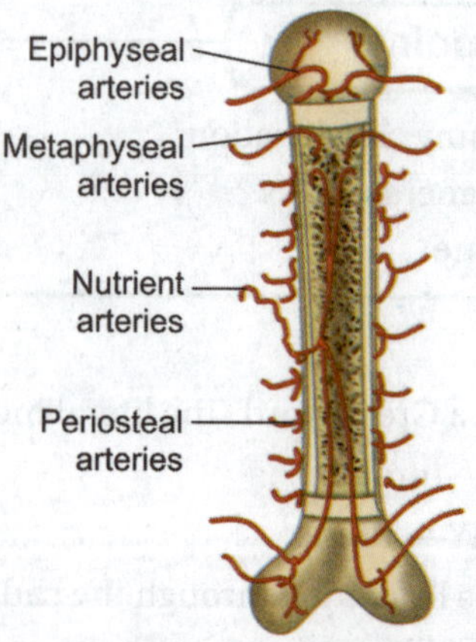

Blood supply of long bone

Parts of Long Bone

1. Upper end.

2. Shaft.

3. Lower end.

Joints

Junction between two or more bones is known as joint.

Classification of Joints

1. Depending on number of bones:

a. Simple joint—only two bones articulating, e.g. shoulder joint.

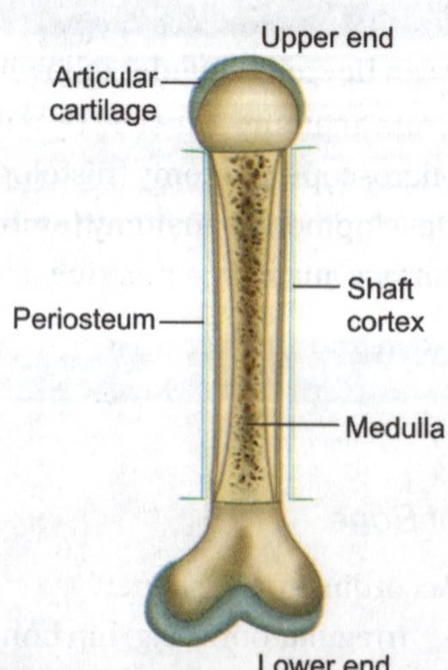

   b. Compound joint—two or more bones articulating, e.g. knee joint.

   c. Complex joint—joint cavity divided by articular disk, e.g. temporomandibular joint.

2. Depending upon mobility:

   a. Diarthrosis—freely movable, e.g. all appendicular joints.

   b. Amphiarthrosis—partially movable, e.g. manubriosternal joint, pubic symphysis.

   c. Synarthrosis—immovable, e.g. sutures of skull.

3. Depending on structure:

   a. Synovial joints—all freely movable joints.

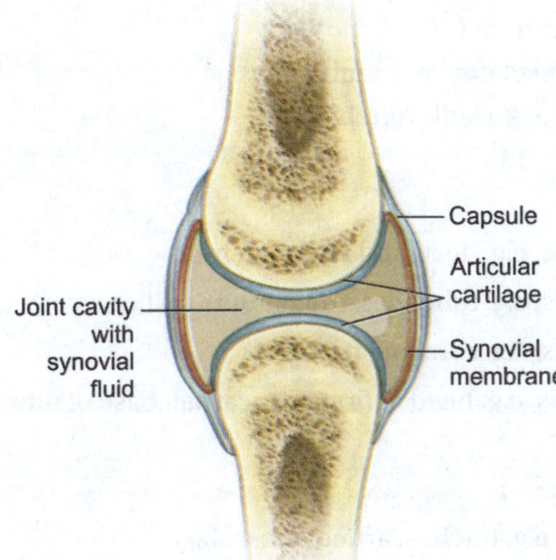

   b. Fibrocartilaginous—partially movable.

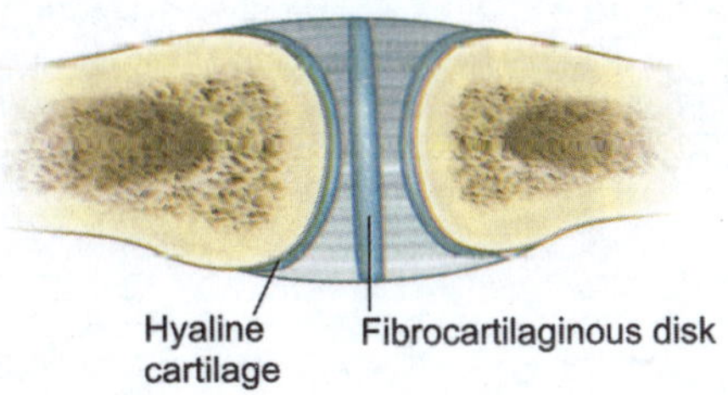

    c. Fibrous—immovable joints.

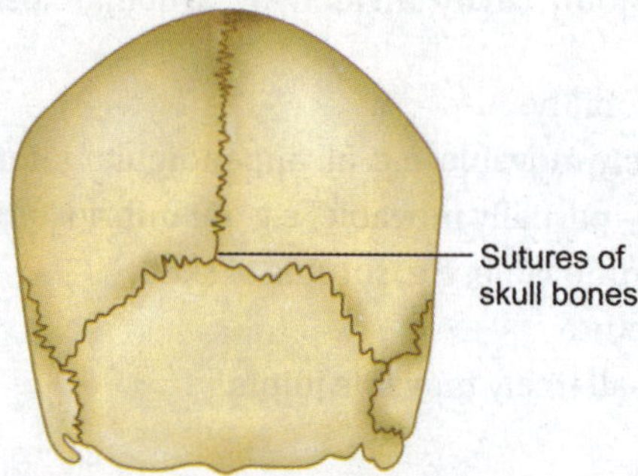

  4. Depending on location:
     a. Appendicular skeleton, e.g. limb bones.
     b. Axial skeleton, e.g. skull, vertebra.

Types of Epiphysis

  1. Pressure epiphysis, e.g. head and neck of femur.

  2. Traction epiphysis, e.g. tubercles, trochanters on bones.

  3. Atavistic epiphysis, e.g. coracoid process.

  4. Aberrant epiphysis, e.g. head of first metacarpal, base of other metacarpal bones.

Types of Cartilages

  1. Hyaline cartilage, e.g. trachea, articular cartilage.

  2. Elastic cartilage, e.g. pinna.

  3. Fibrocartilage, e.g. intervertebral disk.

SECTION - I

UPPER LIMB

Key Questions

Key questions

- Clavicle
- Scapula
- Humerus
- Radius
- Ulna
- Carpal bones
- Wrist complex
- Humeral torsion

Q. Surfaces of clavicle

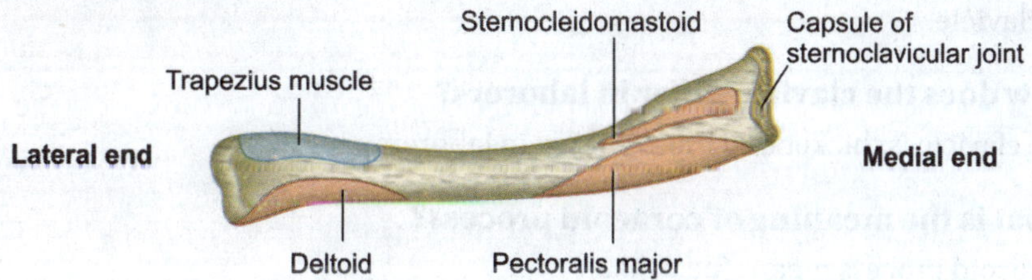

Superior surface of clavicle

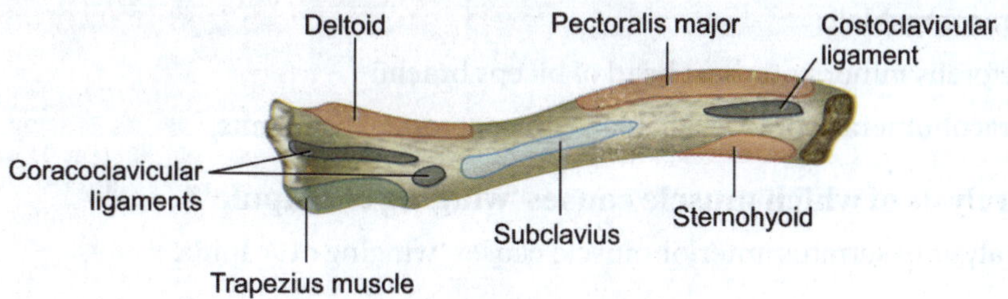

Inferior surface of clavicle

Q. Which long bone in the body is placed horizontally?

Ans. Clavicle is the long bone placed horizontally.

Q. What is the literal meaning of clavicle?

Ans. Clavicle means 'key'.

Q. What are the peculiarities of clavicle?

Ans.

- Clavicle is the only long bone that lies horizontally
- It is subcutaneous
- It is the first bone to ossify
- Most of it ossifies in the membrane
- It has two primary centers of ossification
- It usually has no medullary cavity
- It is the only bone pierced by a nerve (supraclavicular nerve).

Q. How does the clavicle differ in females?

Ans. The female clavicle is shorter, thinner, less curved and smoother, and its acromial end is lower than the sternal end.

Q. How does one determine the sex of clavicle?

Ans. Midshaft circumference is the most reliable single indicator of determining the sex of clavicle.

Q. How does the clavicle differ in laborers?

Ans. The clavicle is thicker and more curved in laborers.

Q. What is the meaning of coracoid process?

Ans. Coracoid process means 'beak like'.

Q. What are the attachments on coracoid process?

Ans. Following structures are attached on coracoid process:

- Coracobrachialis
- Pectoralis minor and short head of biceps brachii
- Coracohumeral, coracoclavicular, coracoacromial ligaments.

Q. Paralysis of which muscle causes 'winging of scapula'?

Ans. Paralysis of serratus anterior muscle causes 'winging of scapula.'

Q. What is the literal meaning of scapula?

Ans. Scapula means 'to dig'.

Q. Surfaces of scapula

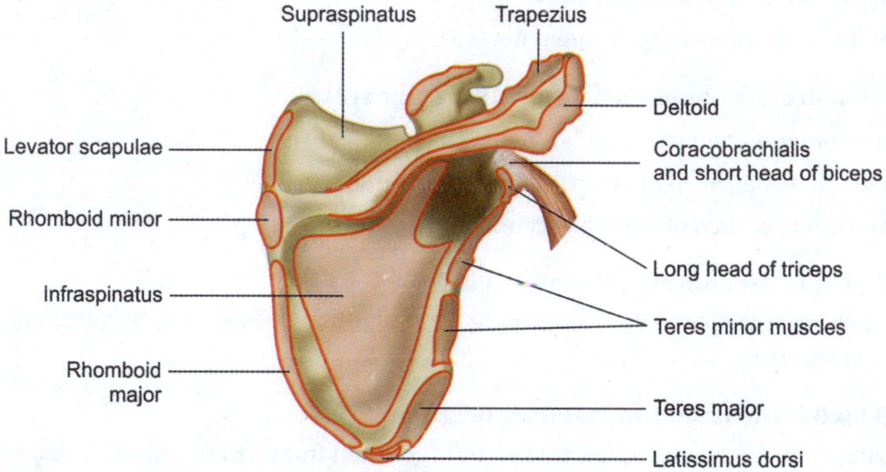

Dorsal surface of scapula

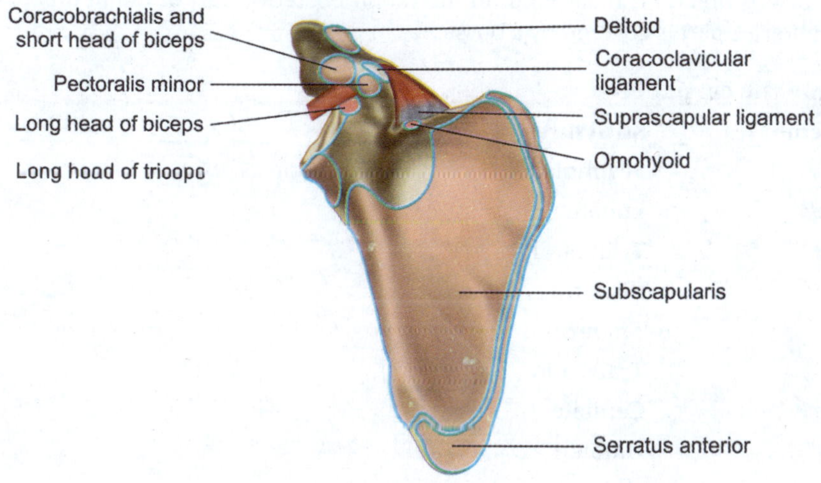

Costal surface of scapula

Q. Which group of muscles constitute the 'rotator cuff'?

Ans. Supraspinatus, infraspinatus, teres minor, subscapularis constitute the 'rotator cuff'.

Q. Which nerves are directly related to humerus?

Ans.

- At the surgical neck—axillary nerve
- At the radial groove—radial nerve
- At the medial epicondyle—ulnar nerve.

Q. What are the contents of intertubercular sulcus?

Ans. The contents of intertubercular sulcus are:

- Tendon of long head of biceps with its synovial sheath
- Ascending branch of anterior circumflex humeral artery.

Q. Which is the common flexor origin?

Ans. Medial epicondyle is the common flexor origin from where superficial flexors of the forearm arise.

Q. Which is the common extensor origin?

Ans. Lateral epicondyle is the common extensor origin from where superficial extensors of the forearm arise.

Q. What is attached to the radial tuberosity?

Ans. The biceps brachii is inserted onto the rough posterior part of radial tuberosity, while the anterior part is covered by a bursa.

Q. Name the carpal bones.

Ans.

Mnemonics	Structure
"She	Scaphoid
Looks	Lunate
Too	Triquetral
Pretty	Pisiform
Try	Trapezium
To	Trapezoid
Catch	Capitate
Her"	Hamate

Q. Which of the carpal bone is a sesamoid bone?

Ans. Pisiform bone is a sesamoid carpal bone, which develops in the tendon of flexor carpi ulnaris.

Q. When does the pisiform bone ossify?

Ans. Pisiform bone ossifies at the age of 12 years.

Q. Which is the key carpal bone?

Ans. Capitate is the key carpal bone.

Q. What is attached to the hook of hamate?

Ans. Flexor retinaculum is attached to the hook of hamate.

Q. What is wrist complex?

Ans. Wrist complex comprises of radiocarpal joint and midcarpal joint.

Q. What is angle of humeral torsion?

Ans. In lower mammals, the longest axes of proximal and distal humeral articular sur-faces make an angle of approximately 90°. But in human beings, the head end has rotated laterally for above 164°. This is humeral torsion.

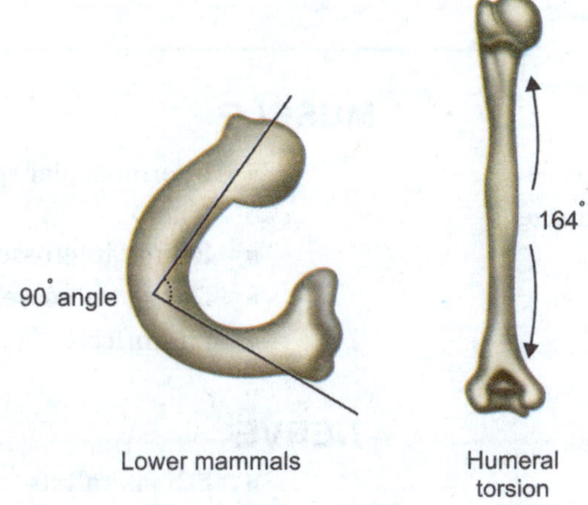

Angle of humeral torsion

Q. Which carpal bone gets fractured commonly on an outstretched hand?

Ans. Scaphoid bone gets fractured commonly on an outstretched hand.

Q. Where do you look for tenderness in cases of scaphoid bone fracture?

Ans. One looks for tenderness in anatomical snuffbox for scaphoid bone fracture.

Short Notes

Key short notes

MUSCLE

- Pectoralis major muscle
- Serratus anterior muscle
- Deltoid
- Coracobrachialis
- Biceps brachii
- Rotator cuff

- Intermuscular spaces in scapular region
- Palmar interossei
- Dorsal interossei
- Lumbricals

NERVE

- Axillary nerve
- Musculocutaneous nerve
- Ulnar nerve
- Median nerve
- Cutaneous nerve supply of upper limb

- Erb's paralysis
- Klumpke's paralysis
- Wrist drop
- Claw hand
- Carpal tunnel syndrome

ARTERY

- Scapular anastomosis
- Anastomosis around elbow joint

- Superficial and deep palmar arch

VEIN

- Cephalic vein

- Basilic vein

LYMPH NODES

- Axillary lymph nodes

- Lymphatic drainage of breast

Contd...

Contd...

JOINT

- Radioulnar joint
- Sternoclavicular joint
- Abduction at shoulder joint
- First carpometacarpal joint

MISCELLANEOUS

- Clavipectoral fascia
- Coracoid process
- Cubital fossa
- Flexor retinaculum
- Palmar aponeurosis
- Interosseous membrane
- Anatomical snuffbox
- Carrying angle
- Extensor retinaculum
- Fibrous flexor sheath
- Digital synovial sheath
- Dorsal digital expansion
- Space of whitlow

▶ MUSCLES

Q. PECTORALIS MAJOR MUSCLE

Pectoralis major muscle is the chief muscle in front of the chest.

Attachments

From

- Anterior surface of medial half of clavicle
- Half side of the anterior surface of sternum
- Second to sixth costal cartilage
- Few fibers from aponeurosis of external oblique muscle.

To

- Lateral lip of bicipital groove.

Nerve Supply

Medial and lateral pectoral nerves.

Action

Mainly adduction, medial rotation and flexion of arm.

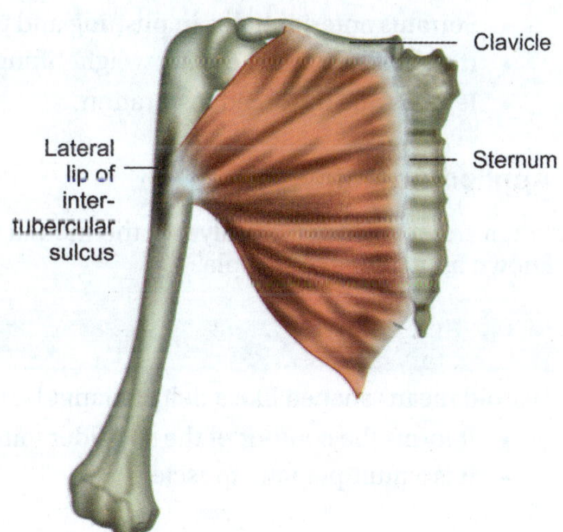

Pectoralis major attachment

Q. SERRATUS ANTERIOR

Serratus anterior is a large muscular sheet extending from ribs to scapula.

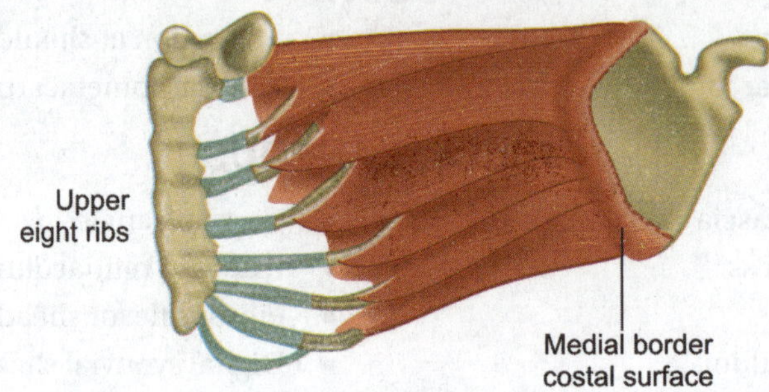

Serratus anterior muscle attachment

Attachments

From

- Upper eight ribs and intervening intercostal fascia.

To

- Costal surface of scapula along its medial border.

Nerve Supply

Long thoracic nerve (of Bell).

Action

- Serratus anterior helps in pushing and punching movements
- It stabilizes scapula during weight lifting
- It helps during forced inspiration.

Applied Anatomy

When the muscle gets paralyzed, the medial margin of scapula becomes prominent. This is known as 'winging of scapula.'

Q. DELTOID

Deltoid means shaped like a delta (triangular):

- It forms the contour of the shoulder joint
- It is a multipennate muscle.

Attachments

From

- Anterior border of lateral one third of clavicle
- Lateral border of acromion
- Crest of spine of scapula.

To

- Deltoid tuberosity on humerus.

Nerve Supply

Axillary nerve.

Action

- Acromial fibers are powerful abductors of the arm
- Anterior fibers are flexors and medial rotators of the arm.

Applied Anatomy

- Injury to axillary nerve leads to atrophy of deltoid muscle giving rise to bony prominences in shoulder region resembling shoulder dislocation
- Intramuscular injections are given in the lower half of muscle to avoid injury to the axillary nerve.

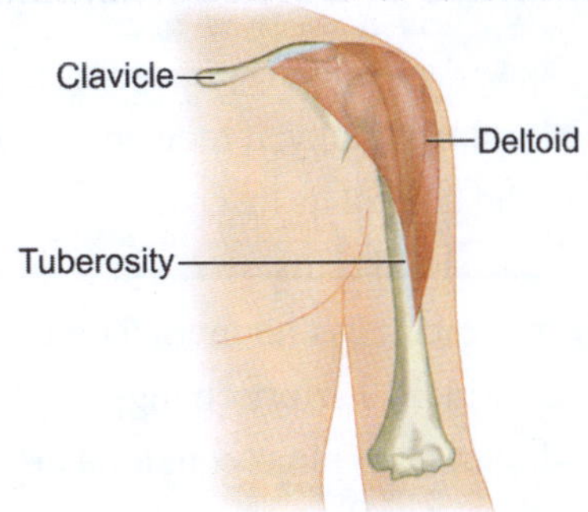

Deltoid attachments

Q. CORACOBRACHIALIS

Coracobrachialis is the key muscle of anterior compartment of arm.

Attachments

From

- Tip of coracoid process.

To

- Middle third of humerus medially.

Nerve Supply

Musculocutaneous nerve.

Action

Flexes the arm.

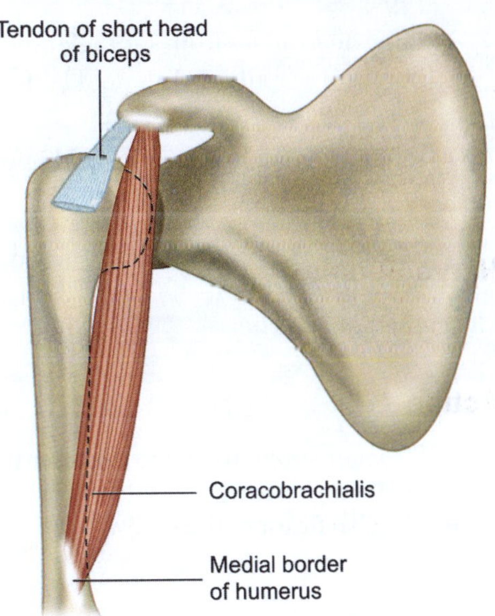

Coracobrachialis attachments

Peculiarities of Coracobrachialis

1. Coracobrachialis is pierced by musculocutaneous nerve.
2. Morphologically, it represents the medial compartment of arm.
3. At the level of its insertion:
   a. Deltoid is inserted.
   b. Brachialis and medial head of triceps begins.
   c. Brachial artery changes its course.
   d. Superior ulnar collateral artery originates.
   e. Median nerve crosses the brachial artery.
   f. Ulnar nerve pierces the medial intermuscular septum.
   g. Radial nerve pierces the lateral intermuscular septum.
   h. Nutrient artery enters.

Q. BICEPS BRACHII

Biceps brachii is the muscle of anterior compartment of arm.

Attachments

From

Biceps brachii has two heads of origin:

- Short head arises from tip of coracoid process
- Long head arises from supraglenoid tubercle of scapula and glenoid labrum.

To

- Radial tuberosity (it gives off bicipital aponeurosis at this point).

Nerve Supply

Musculocutaneous nerve.

Action

- Stronger supinator when the forearm is flexed
- It is also flexor of the elbow.

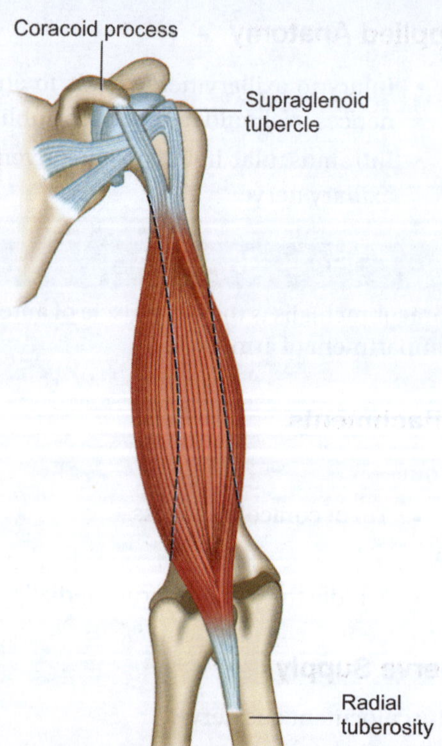

Attachments of biceps brachii

Applied Anatomy

When the arm gets fixed in abduction due to biceps tendon dislocation, it can be replaced by flexing the forearm and rotating the limb.

Q. ROTATOR CUFF

Rotator cuff is a fibrous sheath formed by four flattened tendons, which merge with the capsule of shoulder joint and strengthen it (like muscles around shoulder joint).

The tendons of muscles, which form the cuff, are:

- Supraspinatus
- Infraspinatus
- Teres minor
- Subscapularis.

The muscles forming the cuff arise from scapula and get inserted on to the greater and lesser tubercles of humerus. The cuff strengthens the shoulder joint all around except inferiorly.

Applied Anatomy

Inferior dislocations of shoulder joint are common, since:

- Capsule is lax (loose) inferiorly
- Cuff strengthens the joint all around except inferiorly.

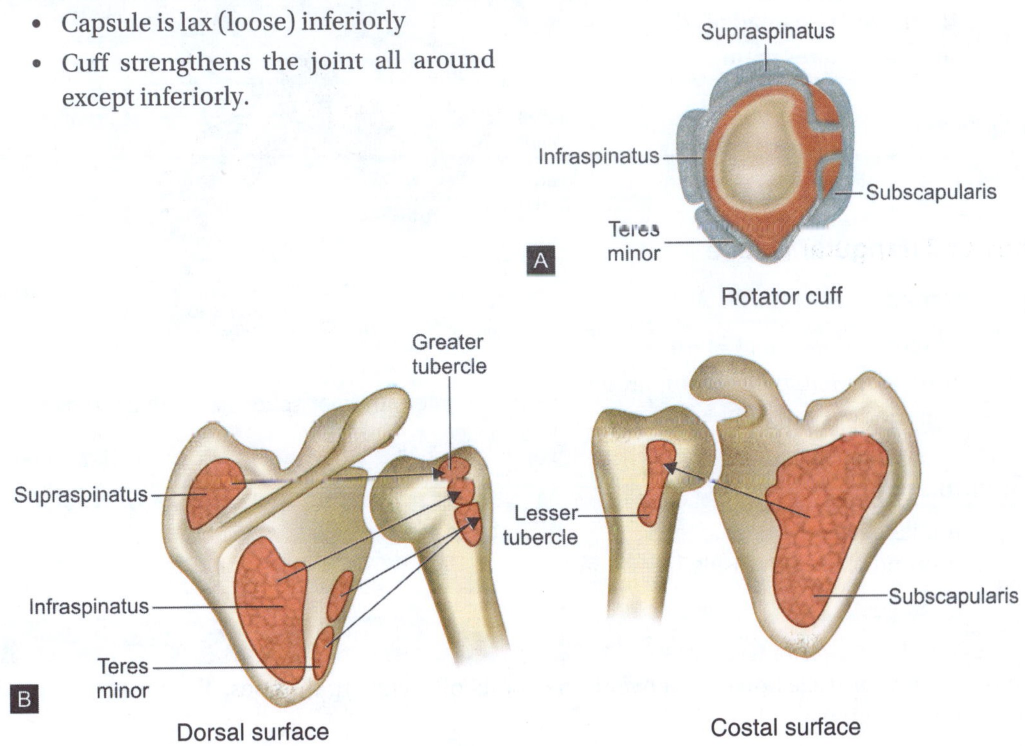

Q. INTERMUSCULAR SPACES

There are three intermuscular spaces in the scapular region. They are given below.

Quadrangular Space

Boundaries

- Superiorly: Teres minor
- Inferiorly: Teres major
- Medially: Long head of triceps
- Laterally: Surgical neck of humerus.

Contents

- Axillary nerve
- Posterior circumflex humeral vessels.

Upper Triangular Space

Boundaries

- Medially: Teres minor
- Laterally: Long head of triceps
- Inferiorly: Teres major.

Contents

Circumflex scapular vessels.

Lower Triangular Space

Boundaries

- Medially: Long head of triceps
- Laterally: Medial border of humerus
- Superiorly: Teres major.

Contents

- Radial nerve
- Profunda brachii vessels.

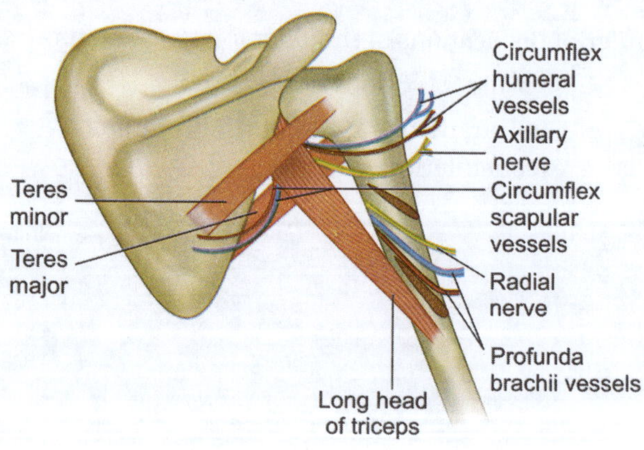

Intermuscular spaces in scapular region

Q. PALMAR INTEROSSEI

There are four muscles placed between the shafts of metacarpal bones. They are numbered from lateral to medial side.

Attachments

From

- I medial side of base of first metacarpal bone
- II medial half of the palmar aspect of the shaft of second metacarpal bone
- III lateral part of the palmar aspect of fourth metacarpal
- IV lateral part of the palmar aspect of the shaft of the fifth metacarpal.

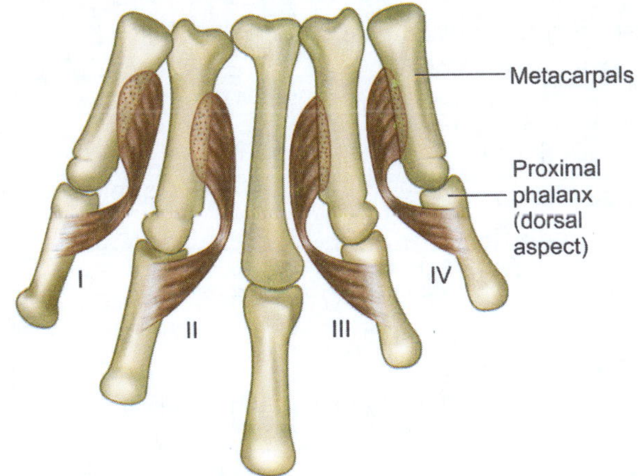

Palmar interossei attachments

To

- I medial side of the thumb
- II medial side of index finger
- III lateral side of fourth digit
- IV lateral side of fifth digit
- Middle finger has no insertion of any palmar interossei
- Each muscle is also inserted into dorsal digital expansion.

Nerve Supply

All palmar interossei are supplied by deep branch of ulnar nerve.

Action

All palmar interossei adduct the digits to the midline.

Q. DORSAL INTEROSSEI

Dorsal interossei are four small muscles placed between the metacarpal bones.

Attachments

From

- I shafts of first and second metacarpal
- II shafts of second and third metacarpal
- III shafts of third and fourth metacarpal
- IV shafts of fourth and fifth metacarpal.

Each muscle is inserted into dorsal digital expansion and the base of proximal phalanx.

To

- I lateral side of index finger
- II lateral side of middle finger
- III medial side of middle finger
- IV medial side of fourth digit.

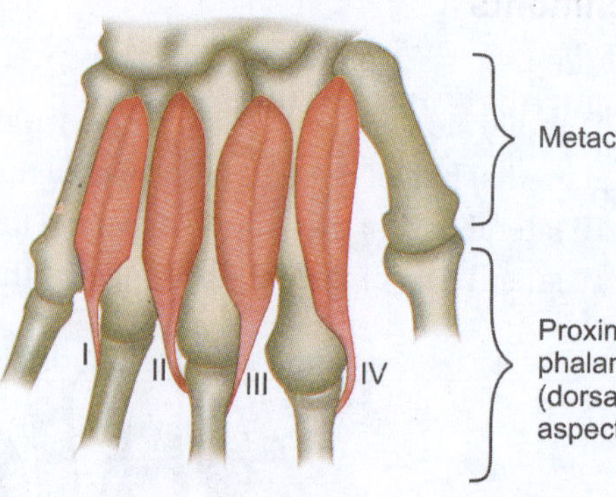

Dorsal interossei attachments

Nerve Supply

All dorsal interossei are supplied by deep branch of ulnar nerve.

Action

All dorsal interossei abduct the digits.

Applied Anatomy

- Paralysis of intrinsic muscles of the hand causes 'claw hand', in which there is hyperextension of metacarpophalangeal joints and flexion at interphalangeal joints
- Dorsal interossei are tested by asking the patient to spread out the fingers against resistance
- Palmar interossei are tested by placing a piece of paper in between the fingers (paper test).

Q. LUMBRICALS

Lumbricals are four small muscles, which take origin from the tendons of flexor digitorum profundus.

Attachments

From

- I lateral side of tendon of index finger
- II lateral side of tendon of middle finger
- III and IV adjacent sides of tendon of ring and little finger.

To

The tendons pass backwards on the lateral side of II, III, IV and V metacarpophalangeal joint to get inserted on the dorsal digital expansion.

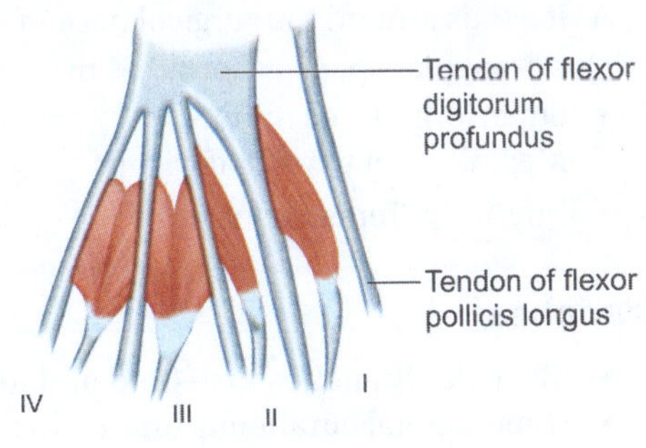

Lumbrical attachment

Nerve Supply

- First and second supplied by median nerve
- Third and fourth supplied by deep branch of ulnar nerve.

Action

The lumbricals flex the metacarpophalangeal joint and extend the interphalangeal joint (lumbricals connect the flexors to the extensors).

▶ NERVES

Q. AXILLARY NERVE

Axillary nerve is also known as circumflex humeral nerve.

Origin

Axillary nerve is a branch of posterior cord of brachial plexus.

Root Value

C5 and C6

Course

Axillary nerve begins in the axilla and winds around the surgical neck of humerus. Thus the nerve has a short course and ends by giving muscular, vascular, cutaneous and articular branches.

Relations

In the axilla and upper arm, it is lateral to the radial nerve, posterior to the axillary artery and anterior to the subscapularis.

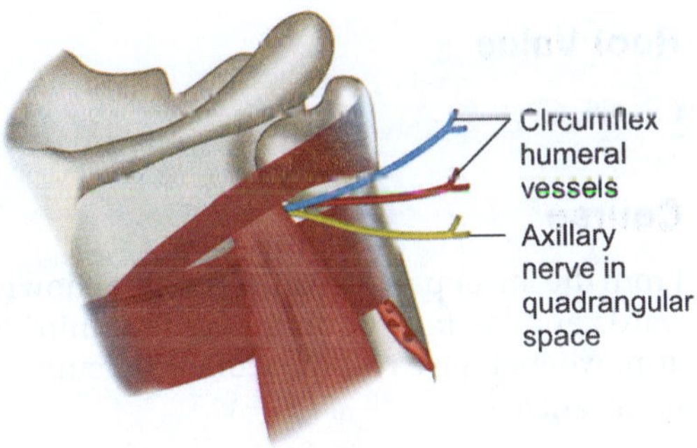

Axillary nerve in quadrangular scapular space

As it winds around the surgical neck of humerus, it passes through the quadrangular space. Quadrangular space is bounded by:

- Superiorly: Teres minor
- Medially: Long head of triceps
- Inferiorly: Teres major.

Branches

- Muscular branches to deltoid and teres minor
- Upper lateral cutaneous branch to the arm
- Articular branch to the shoulder joint
- Vascular branch to the posterior circumflex humeral artery.

Applied Anatomy

Axillary nerve may get injured by dislocation of the shoulder joint or by fracture of the surgical neck of the humerus.

Disability occurring due to axillary nerve injury is:

- Loss of abduction at the shoulder joint
- Loss of contour of the shoulder
- Sensory loss over upper part of the arm.

Q. MUSCULOCUTANEOUS NERVE

Musculocutaneous nerve is the key nerve of the front of the arm.

Origin

Musculocutaneous nerve is a branch of lateral cord of brachial plexus.

Root Value

C5, C6, C7.

Course

From the lower part of axilla, it courses downwards and laterally up to the middle third of arm, where it gives off muscular and cutaneous branches.

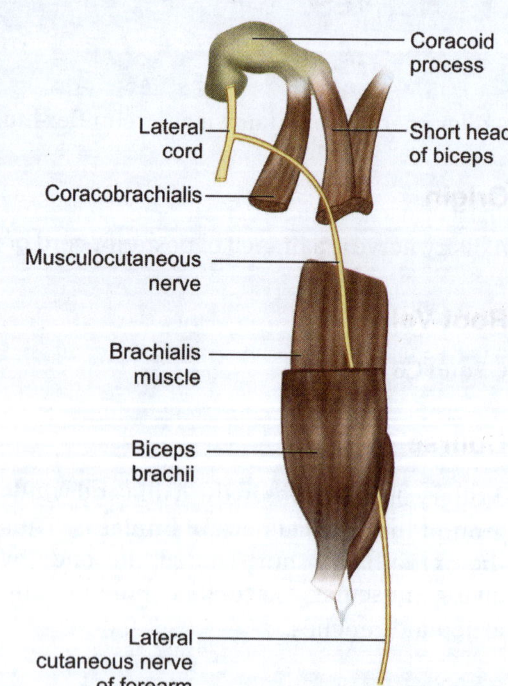

Musculocutaneous nerve course and origin

Relations

Musculocutaneous nerve accompanies axillary artery in the axilla and pierces coracobrachialis before entering the arm. Following are the relations in axilla:

- Anteriorly: Pectoralis major
- Posteriorly: Subscapularis
- Medially: Axillary artery; lateral root of median nerve
- Laterally: Coracobrachialis.

In the arm, it runs downwards and laterally between biceps and brachialis and then gets lateral to the tendon of biceps.

It terminates by piercing the deep fascia 2 cm above the bend of forearm by becoming lateral cutaneous nerve of forearm.

Branches

- Muscular branches to coracobrachialis, biceps and brachialis
- Cutaneous as the lateral cutaneous branch of the forearm
- Articular branch to the elbow joint
- A branch to the humerus, which enters along with the nutrient artery.

Q. ULNAR NERVE

Ulnar nerve is also described as 'musician nerve.'

Origin

Ulnar nerve originates from the medial cord of brachial plexus.

Root Value

C8, T1.

Course

Overall the nerve lies on the medial side of arm and forearm.

From its origin in the axilla, it lies on the medial side of arm then runs downwards to lie behind the medial epicondyle and again on the medial side of the forearm and hand.

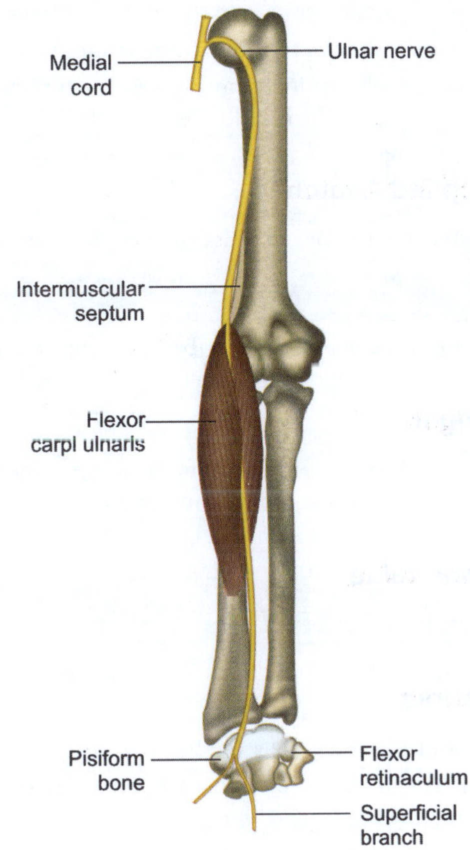

Course of ulnar nerve

Relations

In the axilla, the nerve lies medial to axillary artery and then medial to the brachial artery up to midarm, where the nerve pierces the medial intermuscular septum and runs distally to lie behind the medial epicondyle.

It enters the forearm between the two heads of flexor carpi ulnaris and descends on the medial side of the forearm on the flexor digitorum profundus; and 5 cm above the wrist, it gives off the dorsal cutaneous branch of hand.

It enters the hand by running superficial to flexor retinaculum and lateral to pisiform bone and terminates into superficial and deep branches.

Branches

- Muscular branches to flexor carpi ulnaris and medial half of flexor digitorum profundus
- Palmar cutaneous branch supplies the skin over the hypothenar eminence and medial 1½ finger
- Dorsal branch supplies ulnar 2½ fingers and adjoining area of dorsum of hand
- Articular branch to the elbow joint and wrist
- Superficial terminal branch supplies palmaris brevis and medial palmar skin
- Deep terminal branch, which supplies adductor pollicis, all interossei, third and fourth lumbricals muscle of the hand.

Applied Anatomy

Injury to ulnar nerve causes 'claw hand' involving mainly little and ring finger.

Q. MEDIAN NERVE

Median nerve is also described as 'laborer's nerve'.

Origin

Median nerve has two roots of origin—one from lateral cord and another from medial cord.

Root Value

C5, C6, C7, C8, T1.

Course

Overall the nerve lies in the middle of arm and forearm in close relation to brachial artery and then enters the hand by passing deep to the flexor retinaculum.

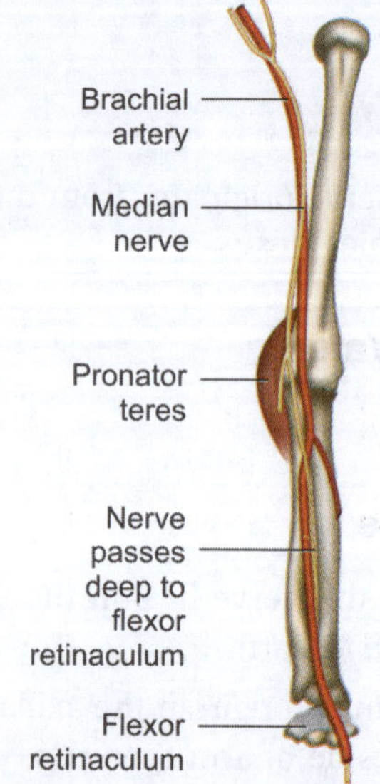

Median nerve origin and course

Relations

The two roots unite either anterior or lateral to third part of axillary artery:

1. In the arm it lies initially lateral to brachial artery then it crosses the artery and becomes medial to the artery.
2. It enters the forearm between the two heads of pronator teres it lies lateral to the ulnar artery and descends between flexor digitorum superficialis and flexor digitorum profundus.
3. About 5 cm proximal to flexor retinaculum, it becomes superficial projecting laterally from behind the tendon of palmaris longus. It runs deep to flexor retinaculum to enter the palm and immediately terminates into medial and lateral branches.

Branches

- Muscular branches to superficial flexors of the forearm (except flexor carpi ulnaris) and lateral half of flexor digitorum profundus
- Muscular branches to thenar muscles in the hand
- Anterior interosseous nerve
- Palmar cutaneous branch
- Articular branch supplying elbow joint and proximal radioulnar joint.

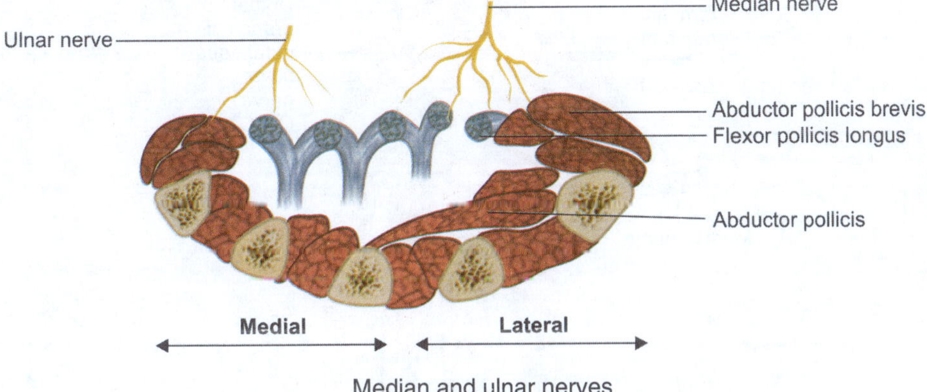

Median and ulnar nerves

Applied Anatomy

1. Ape thumb deformity: In this deformity, the thumb lies in line with the other metacarpals due to paralysis of opponens pollicis.
2. Pen test: In this test, the patient keeps the palm on the table. If the patient can not touch the pen kept above the palm it implies that abductor pollicis brevis is paralyzed.
3. It is mainly responsible for coarse movements of the hand and hence, it is known as 'laborer's nerve'.

Q. CUTANEOUS INNERVATION OF PALM

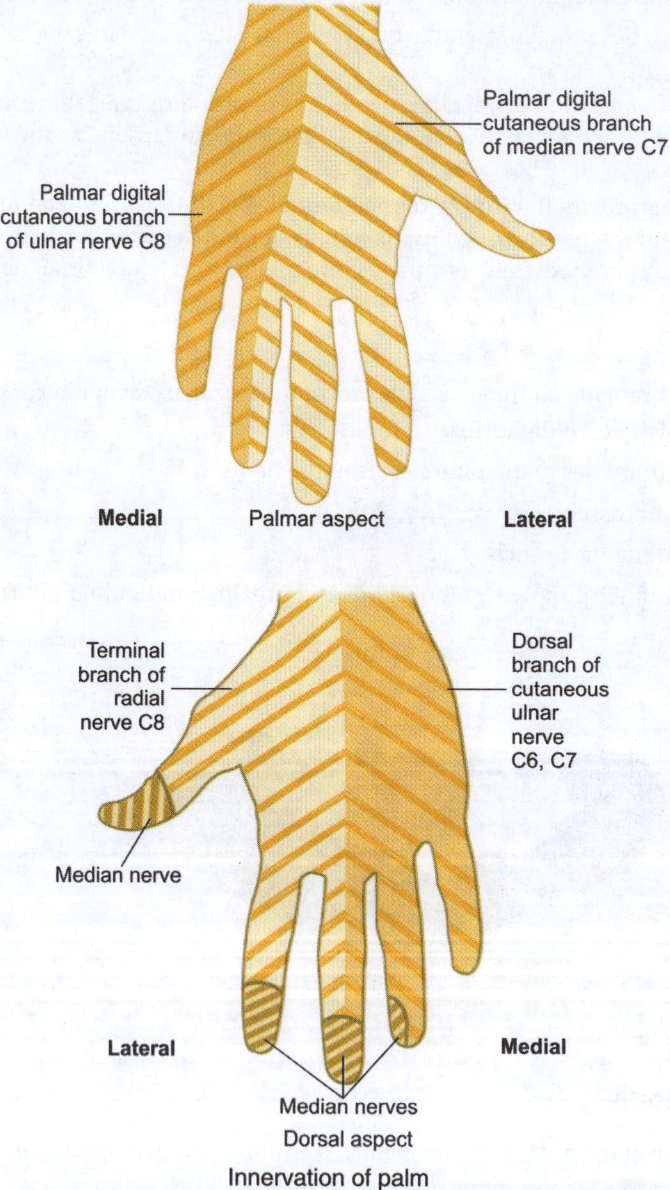

Innervation of palm

Q. ERB'S PARALYSIS

Erb's paralysis is an upper trunk brachial plexus injury:

- *Cause:* It is due to traction on arm at birth or fall on the shoulder
- *Roots:* Involved are C5, C6

- *Deformity:* Leads to typical 'porter tip' or 'policeman tip' deformity wherein arms hang by the side in adducted and medially rotated position (deltoid and lateral rotators are paralyzed):
  - Extension of elbow (flexor paralyzed)
  - Pronated forearm (supinator paralyzed).

Q. KLUMPKE'S PARALYSIS

Klumpke's paralysis is due to lower trunk brachial plexus injury:

- *Cause:* Due to hyperabduction of arm (fall from height or birth injury)
- *Roots:* Involved are C8, T1
- *Deformity:*
  - Clawing of the hand due to paralysis of flexors of fingers, wrist and intrinsic muscles of the hand
  - Cutaneous anesthesia along the ulnar border of the forearm and hand
  - Horner's syndrome.

Q. WRIST DROP

Wrist drop is due to injury to radial nerve in the radial groove of humerus.

- *Cause:* It is due to midfracture of humerus
- *Roots:* Involved are C5, C6, C7, C8, T1
- *Deformity:* Hand is flexed at the wrist and is flaccid due to paralysis of extensors of elbow, wrist and interphalangeal joints along with supinator and brachioradialis.

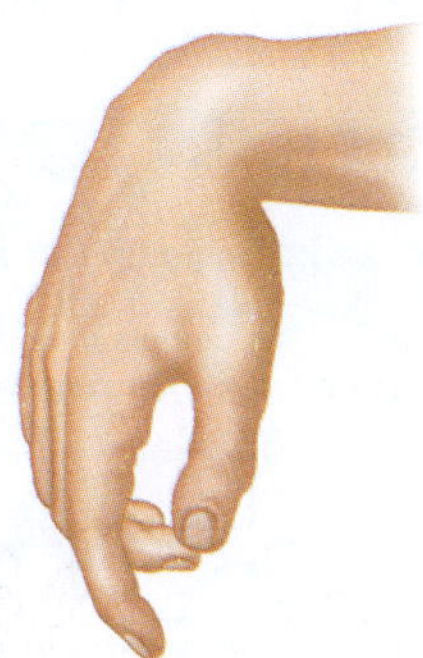

Wrist drop

Q. CLAW HAND

Claw hand is a posteffect of combined median and ulnar nerve lesion at elbow or lesion of medial cord of brachial plexus.

- *Deformity:* There is hyperextension at wrist and metacarpophalangeal joints, and flexion at interphalangeal joint.

This deformity is due to paralysis of interossei and lumbricals.

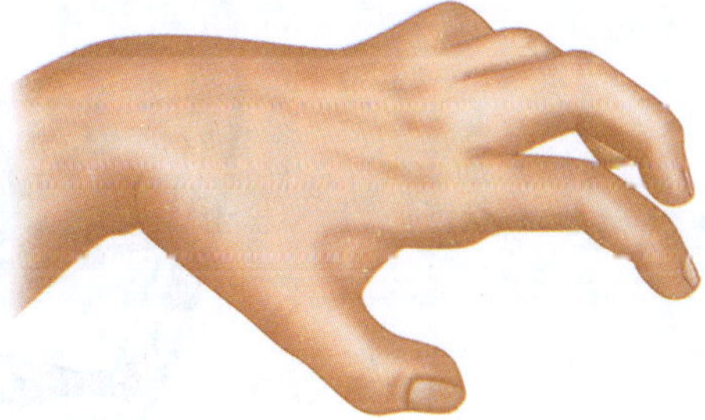

Claw hand

Q. CARPAL TUNNEL SYNDROME

Carpal tunnel syndrome is produced due to compression of median nerve in carpal tunnel.

Patient complains of painful paresthesia and numbness affecting the lateral 3½ fingers, which characteristically wakes up the patient at night because of tissue fluid accumulation. Patient also complains of inability to perform fine movements.

On examination, there is wasting of thenar eminence and hypoesthesia over radial 3½ fingers.

Skin over thenar eminence is not affected, since it is supplied by palmar cutaneous branch of median nerve, which takes origin proximal to carpal tunnel. Nerve conduction studies help to diagnose carpal tunnel syndrome.

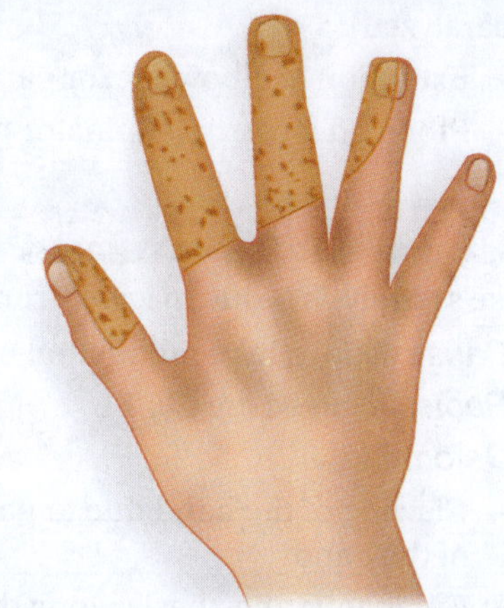

Area of sensory loss following division of median nerve

▶ ARTERIES

Q. SCAPULAR ANASTOMOSIS

Scapular anastomosis occurs between first part of subclavian artery and third part of axillary artery.

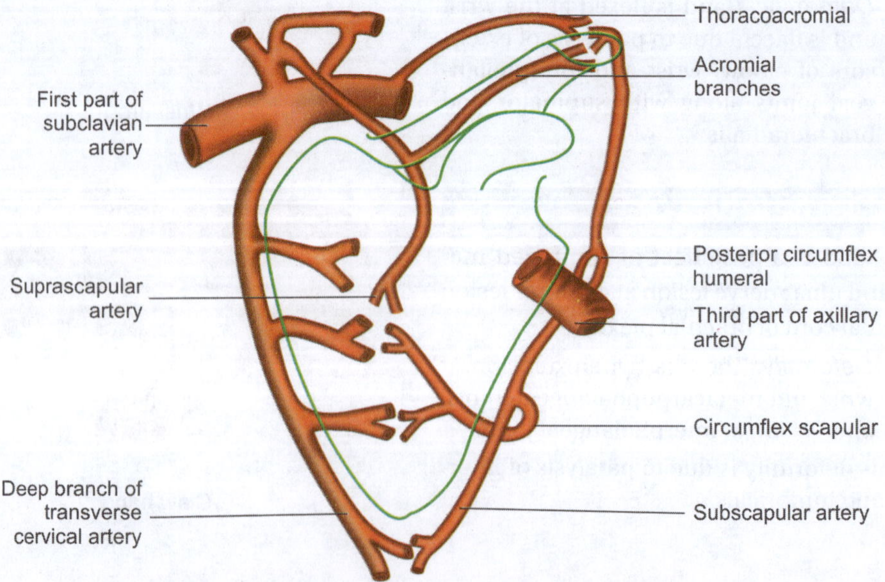

Anastomosis around scapula

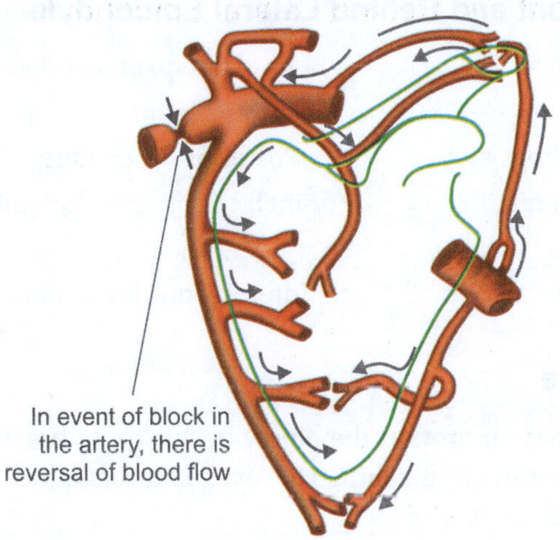

Functional anastomosis in event of block

Anastomosis over the scapula can be divided into anastomosis in two areas:

- Anastomosis around the body of scapula
- Anastomosis around the acromion process.

1. Anastomosis around body of scapula occurs between following branches:
   a. First part of subclavian artery   + Third part of axillary artery
      - Suprascapular   + Posterior circumflex humeral
      - Deep branch of transverse cervical   + Subscapular
2. Anastomosis around acromion process:
   a. Suprascapular   + Posterior circumflex humeral
   b. Thoracoacromial.

Surgical Importance

In event of blockage of any of the artery mentioned above in figure, blood can still flow to the upper limb through scapular anastomosis.

Q. ANASTOMOSIS AROUND ELBOW JOINT

Anastomosis around elbow joint occurs between brachial, radial and ulnar arteries.

Anastomosis around the elbow joint can be divided into anastomosis in three areas:

- Anastomosis in front and behind lateral epicondyle
- Anastomosis in front and behind medial epicondyle
- Above the olecranon process.

Anastomosis in Front and Behind Lateral Epicondyle

Front of lateral epicondyle	Behind lateral epicondyle
From	*From*
Above anterior descending branch of profunda brachii	Posterior descending branch of profunda brachii
+	+
Below radial recurrent	Interosseous recurrent

Surgical Importance

Due to rich collateral system around the elbow occlusion of brachial artery does not cause gangrene of the distal portion of the limb. However, laborers may experience forearm claudication (pain) during strenuous work.

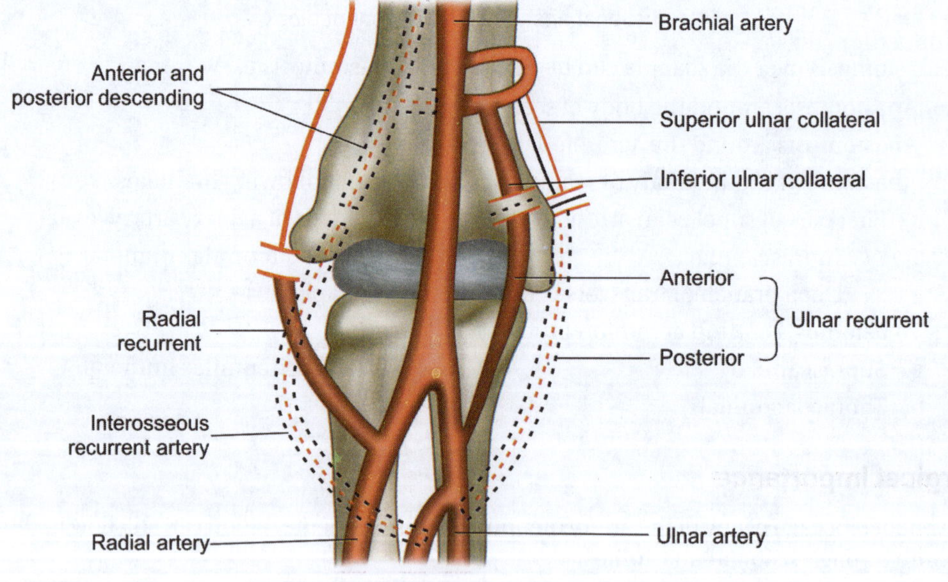

Elbow anastomosis

Q. SUPERFICIAL AND DEEP PALMAR ARCH

Superficial and deep palmar arch represents anastomosis between radial and ulnar arteries.

Superficial Palmar Arch

Formation

Superficial palmar arch is a direct continuation of ulnar artery beyond flexor retinaculum. On the lateral side, it is completed by one of the following branches of radial artery:

- Superficial palmar branch
- Radialis indicis
- Princeps pollicis.

Relations

Arch lies between palmaris brevis, palmar aponeurosis in front and flexor tendons behind.

Branches

Digital branches supply medial 3½ fingers.

Deep Palmar Arch

Formation

Deep palmar arch is a continuation of radial artery beyond the gap between the two heads of adductor pollicis. It is completed by deep branch of ulnar artery.

Relations

The arc lies at the level of proximal border of extended thumb. The deep branch of ulnar nerve lies within its concavity.

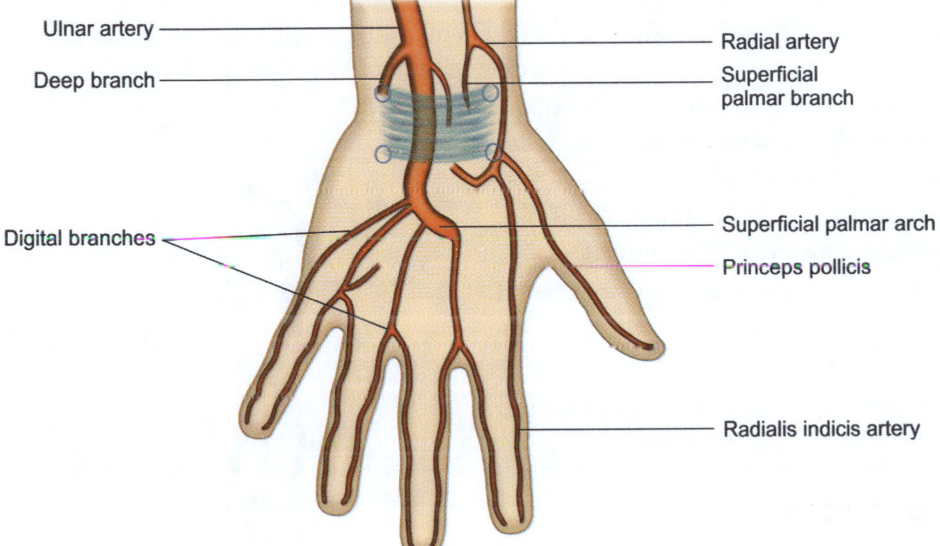

Superficial and deep palmar arch

Branches

- Three palmar metacarpal arteries
- Three perforating branches
- Recurrent branches.

Surgical Importance

In direct wounds of palmar arches, ligation of one of the forearm artery may be ineffective due to anastomosis between radial and ulnar arteries.

▶ VEINS

Q. CEPHALIC VEIN

Cephalic vein is preaxial vein of the upper limb.

Course

Cephalic vein begins from lateral end of dorsal venous arch and courses laterally upwards to end in axillary vein.

Relations

1. Cephalic vein runs upwards through the roof of anatomical snuffbox, winds around the lateral border of distal forearm to appear in front of elbow and lateral to biceps brachii.

2. After piercing the deep fascia at the lower border of pectoralis major, it lies in the deltopectoral groove.

3. It reaches the infraclavicular fossa, where it pierces clavipectoral fascia.

4. At the elbow, most of the venous blood is directed into the basilic vein via median cubital vein.

5. Lateral cutaneous nerve of forearm accompanies cephalic vein.

Applied Anatomy

Cephalic vein many times communicates with the external jugular vein by means of a small vein in front of clavicle. In radical surgeries, when axillary vein is sacrificed, this communicating vein enlarges and drains the complete upper limb.

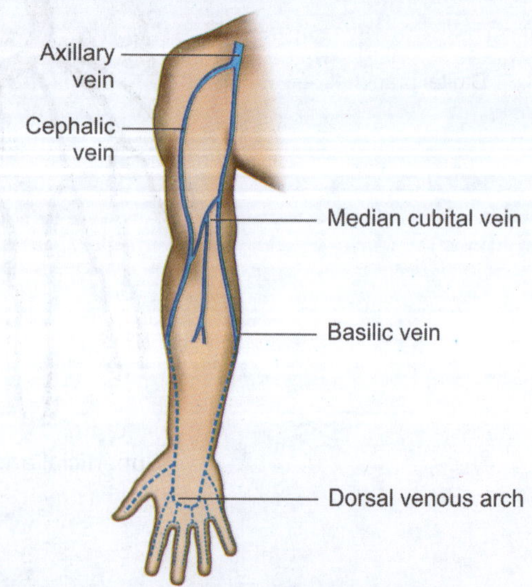

Veins of upper limb

Q. BASILIC VEIN

Basilic vein is the postaxial vein of upper limb.

Course

Basilic vein begins from the medial end of dorsal venous arch and runs along back of medial border of forearm to wind the elbow to continue in front till middle of the arm where it pierces the deep fascia to drain into axillary vein.

Relations

1. Basilic vein lies along the medial side of brachial artery up to the lower border of teres major.
2. Few centimeters above the elbow it is joined by the median cubital vein.
3. It is accompanied by posterior branch of medial cutaneous nerve of the forearm.

Applied Anatomy

1. Veins of the upper limb provide good access for intravenous supplementation.
2. Venous graft (reverse side) can be used in surgeries like stapedectomy for closing oval window.

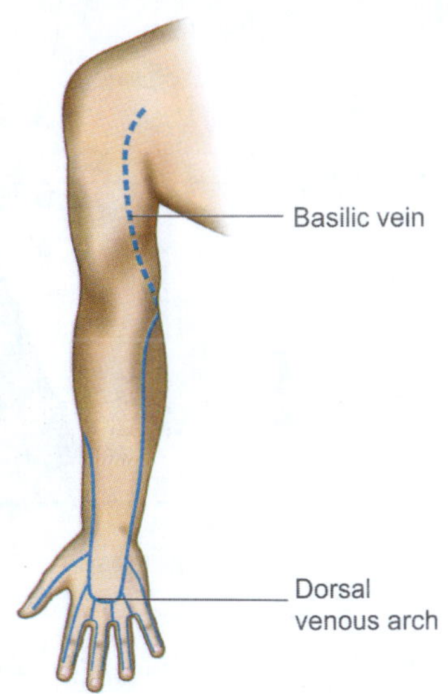

Basilic vein of upper limb

▶ LYMPH NODES

Q. AXILLARY LYMPH NODES

Axillary lymph nodes are divided into five groups:

- Anterior group (pectoral)
- Posterior group (scapular)
- Lateral group
- Central group
- Apical group (infraclavicular).

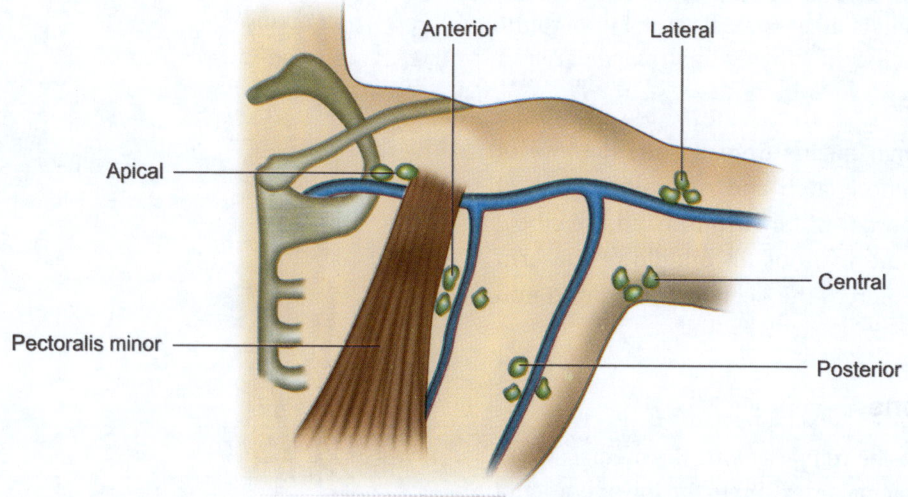

Axillary lymph nodes

Anterior Group

Anterior group lymph node lies along lateral thoracic vein and are in direct contact with the axillary tail of the breast. They drain upper half of the anterior wall of the trunk and major part of the breast.

Posterior Group

Posterior group lies along the subscapular vein and can be palpated along posterior fold of axilla. They drain upper half of the posterior wall of the trunk and axillary tail of breast.

Lateral Group

Lateral group lies along the axillary vein in the upper part of the arm. It receives lymph from the upper limb.

Central Group

Central group lies in the fat of axilla and is closely related to intercostobrachial nerve. They receive lymph from above mentioned nodes.

Apical Group

Apical group lies along the axillary vein and receives lymph from central group, upper part of breast and thumb.

Applied Anatomy

- Axillary abscess may arise due to suppuration of lymph nodes
- Malignancy involving drainage areas of axillary lymph nodes can give rise to enlargement of lymph nodes.

Q. LYMPHATIC DRAINAGE OF BREAST

Breast cancer is staged depending upon the number, size and fixity of axillary lymph nodes. Treatment of breast cancer is planned according to the stage of the disease. Lymph from the breast drains into following group of lymph nodes:

- 70% drains into axillary lymph nodes
- 20% drains into internal mammary lymph nodes
- 5% drains into posterior intercostal lymph nodes
- The axillary lymph nodes and the internal mammary lymph nodes are involved comparatively early; later, the supraclavicular lymph nodes, the opposite breast and the mediastinum are involved
- Some lymph reaches subdiaphragmatic and subperitoneal lymph plexus.

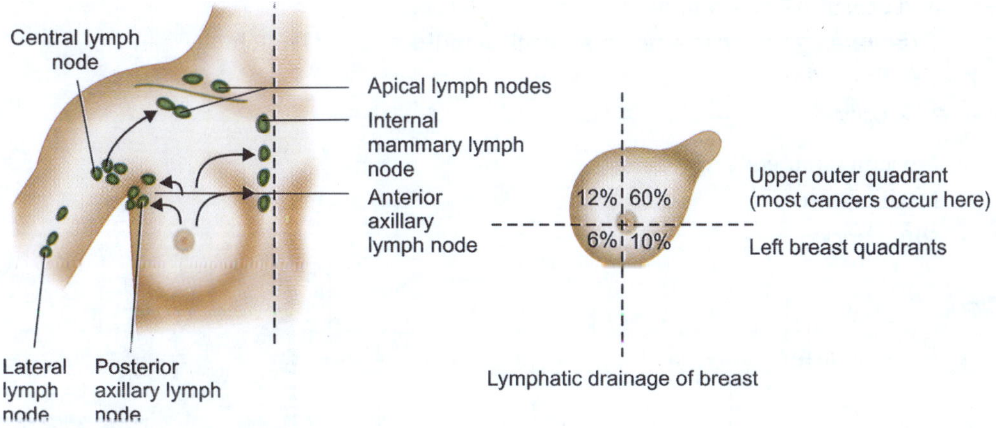

Lymphatic Vessels of the Breast

Superficial lymphatics drain the skin over the breast except the nipple and areola. Deep lymphatics drain the parenchyma of the breast, areola and nipple.

Virchow's Node

Virchow's node is an enlarged left supraclavicular node infiltrated with metastatic cancer from gastrointestinal tract (GIT) predominantly. Metastases to supraclavicular nodes also occurs from lung breast or genital cancers.

▶ JOINT

Q. RADIOULNAR JOINTS

Superior Radioulnar Joint

Type

- Pivot type of synovial joint.

Articular Surfaces

They are:

- Head of radius
- Radial notch on ulna and annular ligament.

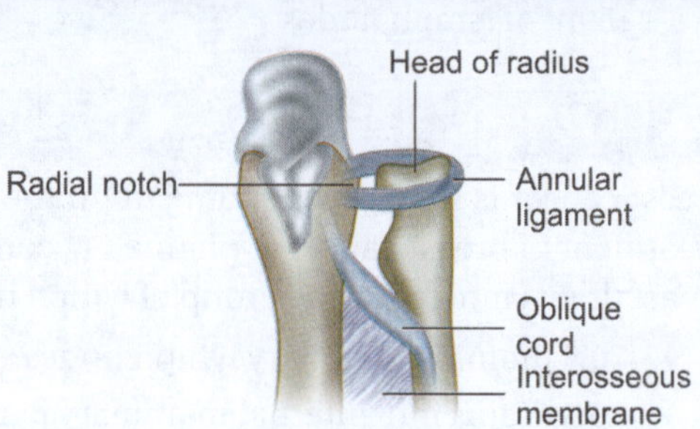

Superior radioulnar joint

Ligaments

Ligaments joining the articular surfaces are annular ligament and quadrate ligament.

- *Annular ligament:* It encircles the head of radius and is attached to radial notch of ulna and capsule of elbow joint
- *Quadrate ligament:* Extends from neck of radius to radial notch.

Nerve Supply

- Musculocutaneous nerve
- Median nerve
- Ulnar nerve.

Blood Supply

- Elbow anastomosis.

Action

The actions include:

- Pronation
- Supination.

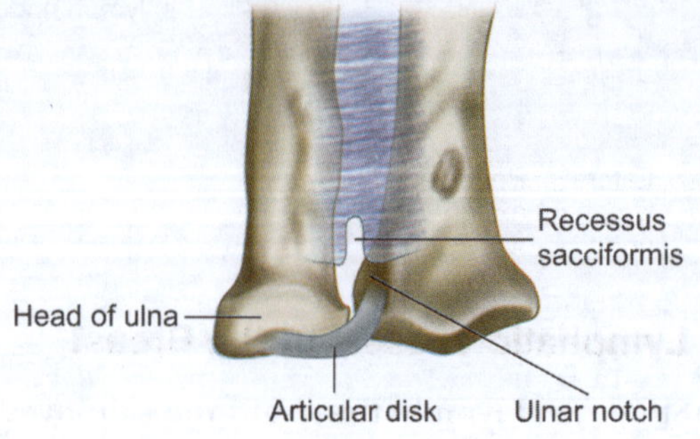

Inferior Radioulnar Joint

Type

Pivot type of synovial joint.

Articular Surfaces

They are:
- Head of ulna
- Ulnar notch on radius.

Ligaments

Ligaments joining the articular surfaces are given below.
- *Capsular ligament:* Surrounds the joint
- *Articular disk:* Extends from base of styloid process to ulnar notch.

Blood Supply

- Interosseous vessels.

Nerve Supply

- Interosseous nerve.

Actions

- Pronation
- Supination.

Q. STERNOCLAVICULAR JOINT

Type

- Synovial joint
- Compound joint
- Complex joint.

Articulating Bones

- Medial end of clavicle
- Clavicular notch of manubrium sterni
- Upper surface of first costal cartilage.

Ligaments

1. Capsule is attached laterally to the margins of medial end of clavicle. Medially to the margins of sternum and on first costal cartilage.
2. Articular disk is the key bond between articular surfaces.
3. Costoclavicular ligament is attached above to the medial end of clavicle and inferiorly to the first costal cartilage.

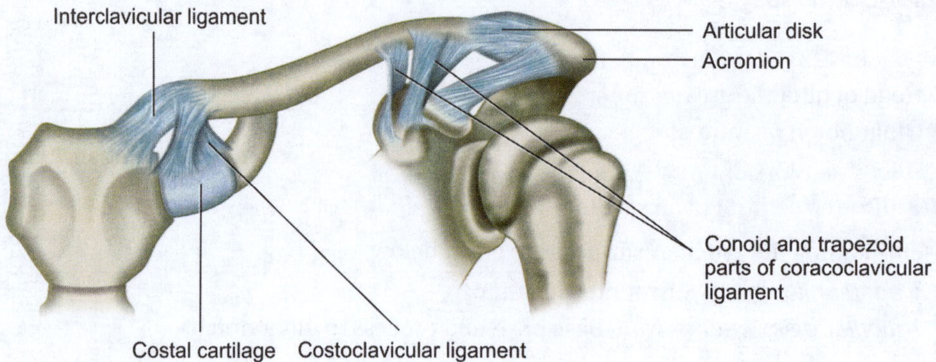

Nerve Supply

- Medial supraclavicular nerve.

Blood Supply

- Internal thoracic and suprascapular vessels.

Movements

1. Movements do not occur singularly at sternoclavicular joint, but collectively at the shoulder girdle.
2. Shrugging off shoulders, i.e. elevation of scapula is brought about by trapezius and levator scapula.
3. Depression of scapula is brought about by lower fibers of serratus anterior and pectoralis minor.
4. Pushing and punching movements are brought about by serratus anterior and pectoralis minor.
5. Retraction of scapula is brought about by rhomboids and trapezius.

Applied Anatomy

- Clavicle by and large gets dislocated at its medial end
- The weight of the upper limb is transmitted from scapula to clavicle through coracoclavicular ligament and from clavicle to the first rib by costoclavicular ligament. The clavicle fracture is often between these two ligaments.

Q. ABDUCTION AT SHOULDER JOINT

Abduction at shoulder joint is a complex movement, which can for convenience be separated into two coordinated movements.

$$[\text{Total}—120°(90° + 30°)]$$

1. Movement at Glenohumeral Joint

Allows about 120° of abduction being limited by impingement of the greater tubercle of the humerus on the acromion process.

Abduction at glenohumeral joint is a co-ordinated movement involving deltoid muscle and the rotator cuff:

- Rotator cuff holds the head in the socket
- Deltoid with supraspinatus brings about abduction
- Deltoid plus supraspinatus allows only 90° of abduction; further movement is restricted due to the impingement of greater tubercle of humerus on the acromion
- Further 30° abduction takes place only when the humerus rotates externally so that greater tubercle lies posterior acromion
- Infraspinatus and teres minor also act as short external rotators. While subscapularis as internal rotator.

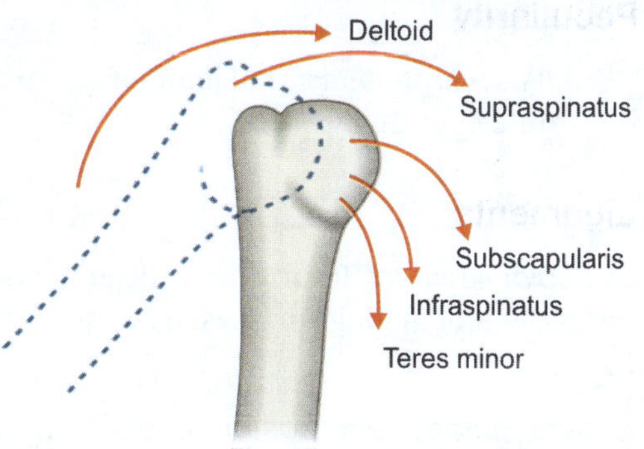

Muscle couple

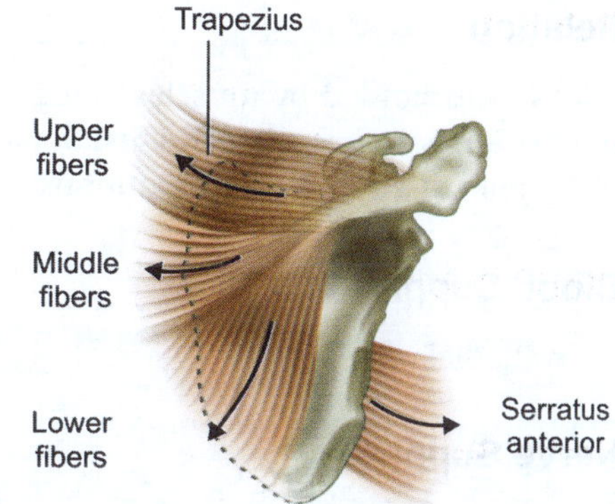

Muscles bringing about scapular rotation

2. Movement at Scapulothoracic Linkage

- Upward rotation of scapula is accomplished by synchronous action of two muscles—trapezius and serratus anterior.
- Basic action of trapezius is to rotate the scapula resulting in the glenoid fossa pointing upwards.
- This upward rotation of scapula brings about further abduction.

Q. FIRST CARPOMETACARPAL JOINT

Type

Synovial joint—saddle variety.

Articulating Surfaces

- Distal surface of trapezium
- Proximal surface of the base of first metacarpal bone.

Peculiarity

- First carpometacarpal joint has a separate joint cavity.

Ligaments

Capsular ligament: It surrounds the joint and binds the articulating surfaces. It is thick, but loose.

Lateral, anterior and posterior ligament: All these ligaments strengthen the joint capsule.

Relation

Joint is surrounded by muscles going to the thumb. Medially it is related to first dorsal interossei. Radial artery forms the posterior relation of the joint in the anatomical snuffbox.

Blood Supply

- Radial vessels.

Nerve Supply

- Median nerve.

Movement

1. Flexion and extension is brought about by the flexor pollicis tendons and extensor pollicis tendons respectively.
2. Adduction and abduction brought about by muscles supplying the pollex.
3. Opposition is brought about by mainly opponens muscle.
4. Circumduction is combination of above movements.

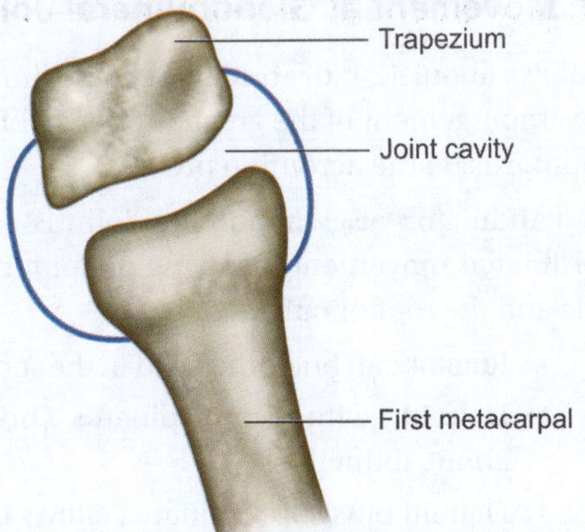

First carpometacarpal joint cavity

▶ MISCELLANEOUS

Q. CLAVIPECTORAL FASCIA

Clavipectoral fascia is a bilaminar fibrous sheath extending from clavicle to axillary fascia. It lies deep to the clavicular portion of pectoralis major muscle.

Attachments

- Medially it is attached to the first rib and costoclavicular ligament
- Laterally it is attached to the coracoid process and coracoclavicular ligament

- Above it splits to enclose subclavius muscle
- Below it splits to enclose pectoralis minor muscle
- Behind it merges with investing layer of deep cervical fascia.

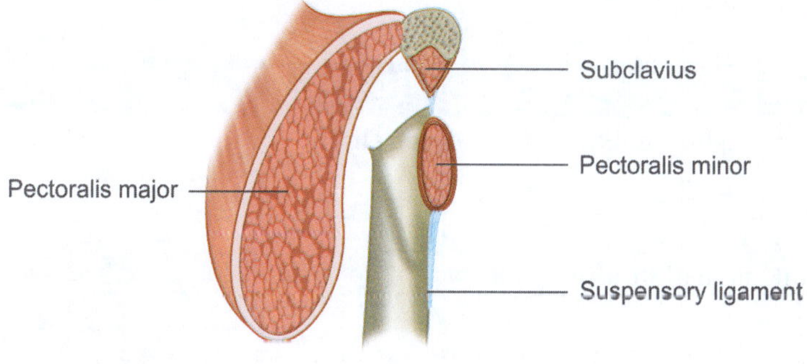

Clavipectoral fascia

Structures Piercing Clavipectoral Fascia

- Lateral pectoral nerve
- Cephalic vein
- Thoracoacromial vessels
- Lymphatics passing from the breast and pectoral region to the apical group of axillary lymph nodes.

Q. CORACOID PROCESS

Literal meaning of coracoid is 'bird's beak-like'. It is an atavistic type of epiphysis. It is a projection on costal surface of scapula.

Attachments

1. Muscles:
    - Pectoralis minor
    - Coracobrachialis.

Attachments on coracoid process

2. Ligaments:
   - Coracoclavicular
   - Coracoacromial
   - Coracohumeral.

Q. CUBITAL FOSSA

Cubital fossa is a triangular hollow in front of the elbow.

Boundaries

- Base: An imaginary line joining the two epicondyles
- Laterally: Medial border of the brachioradialis
- Medially: Lateral border of pronator teres
- Apex: Intersection of medial and lateral border.

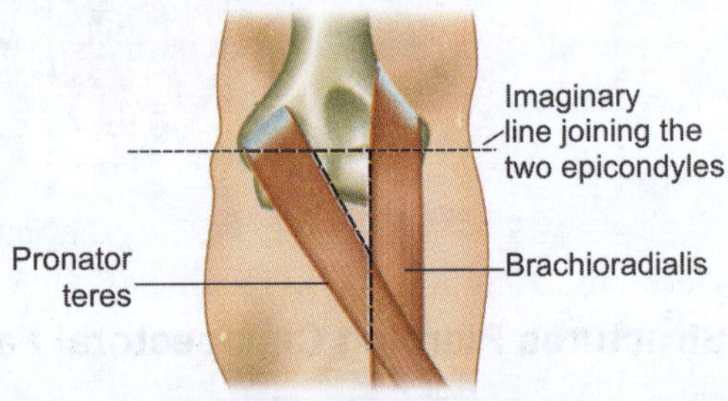

Cubital fossa boundaries

Roof

- Basilic vein
- Cephalic vein
- Median cubital vein
- Medial and lateral cutaneous nerve of forearm.

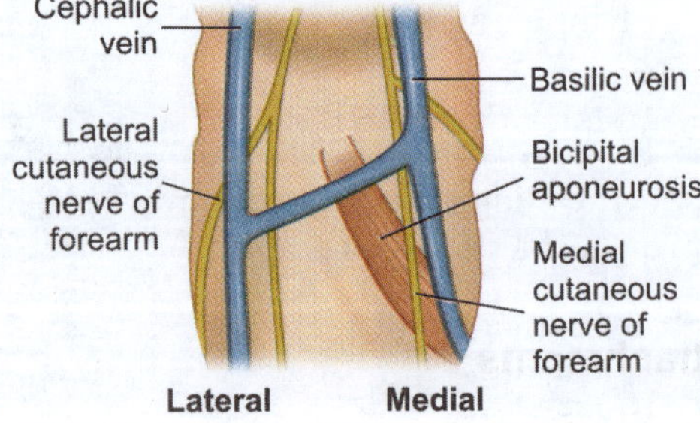

Floor

- Brachialis muscle
- Supinator muscle.

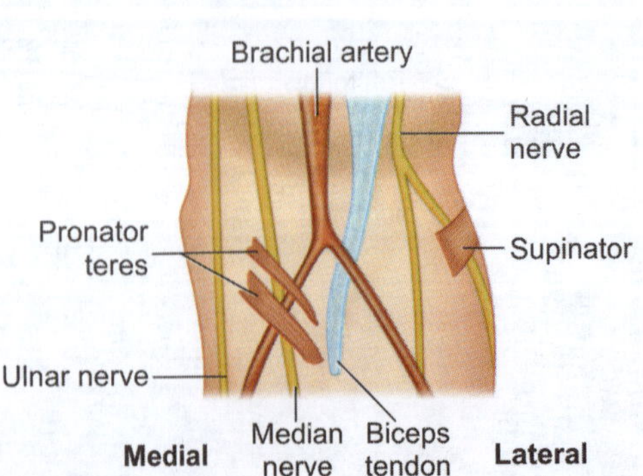

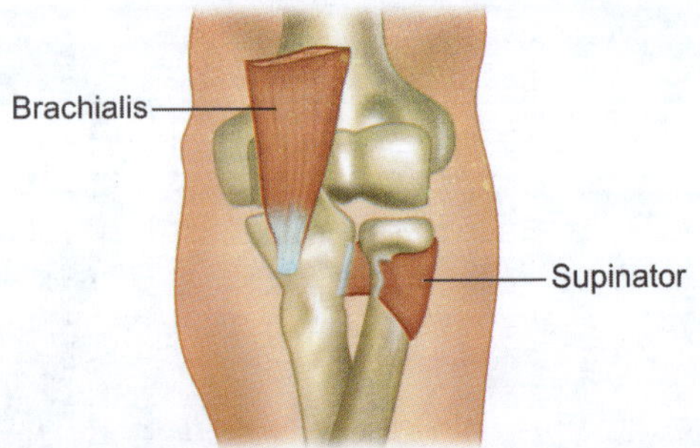

Contents

- Termination of brachial artery
- Origin of radial and ulnar arteries
- Tendon of biceps brachii muscle
- Radial nerve
- Median nerve.

Applied Anatomy

- Median cubital vein is an easily accessible vein for injecting intravenous fluids
- Blood pressure is recorded by auscultating brachial artery.

Q. FLEXOR RETINACULUM

Flexor retinaculum is fibrous sheath, which connects the corner carpal bones and converts the anterior concavity into a tunnel (when one holds a ball in the hand the depression in between the thenar and hypothenar eminence marks the flexor retinaculum).

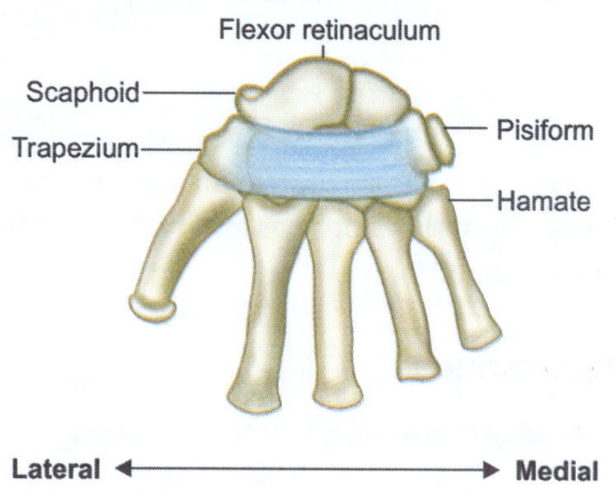

Attachments

- Medially: Pisiform bone and hook of hamate
- Laterally: Tubercle of scaphoid and crest of trapezium.

Relations

Structures passing superficial and deep to flexor retinaculum are:

Superficial	Deep
Tendon of palmaris longus	Median nerve
Palmar cutaneous branch of median and ulnar nerve	Tendon of flexor digitorum superficialis and profundus
Ulnar vessels	Tendon of flexor pollicis longus
	Radial and ulnar bursa

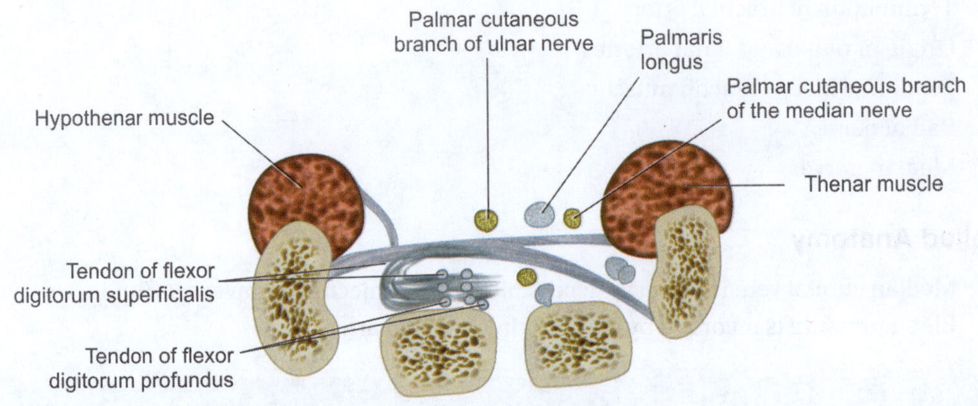

Relation of flexor retinaculum

Q. PALMAR APONEUROSIS

Palmar aponeurosis represents the deep fascia like in other part of the body and is superficial to vessels, nerves, muscles and tendons. It has central thick and strong portion and lateral thin and weak portion.

Peculiarities

1. It is derived from palmaris longus tendon.
2. Proximally it is attached to flexor retinaculum.
3. Distally, it divides opposite to the heads of metacarpals into four slips. Each slip has a superficial and deep part. The superficial part is attached to the skin of palm and fingers, and deep part divides into two processes, which are continuous with the fibrous flexor sheaths.
4. It sends slips to deep transverse metacarpal ligament
5. Digital vessels, nerves and tendons of lumbricals pass through the interval between the slips.

Function

Palmar aponeurosis improves the grip of the hand.

Applied Anatomy

Attachments of palmar aponeurosis are of surgical importance, in pathological contracture of palmar fascia (Dupuytren's contracture). In this condition, the proximal and intermediate phalanges of the fingers are acutely flexed because palmar fascia is attached to them. The distal phalanx remains extended as the fascia has no attachment to it.

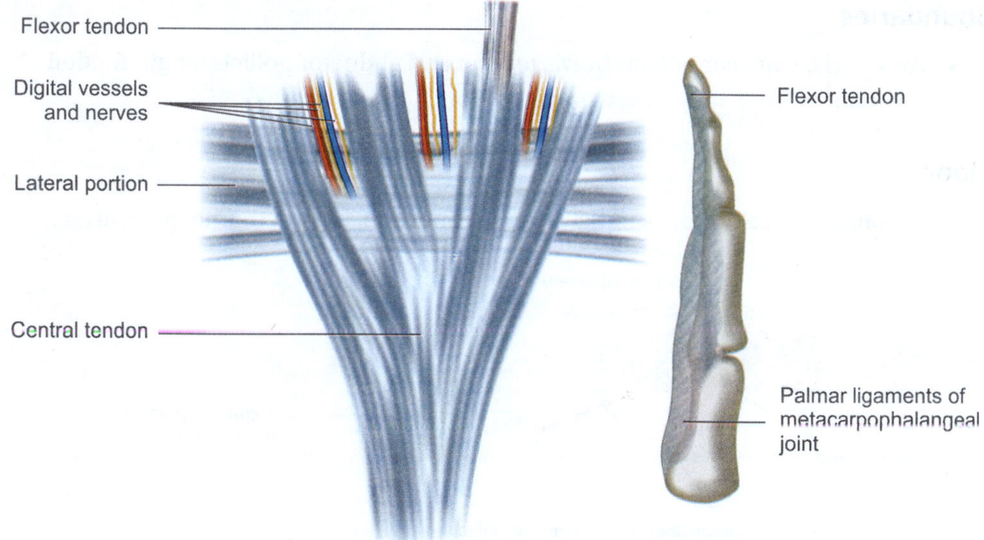

Palmar aponeurosis (parts and attachments)

Q. INTEROSSEOUS MEMBRANE

The interosseous membrane connects the shafts of the radius and ulna (appears very shiny in the cadaver).

- It is attached to the interosseous borders of radius and ulna
- The fibers run downwards, forward and medially (like hands in the pocket).

Functions

- It connects the radius to the ulna
- It provides base for attachments of muscles
- It transmits the force applied to the radius.

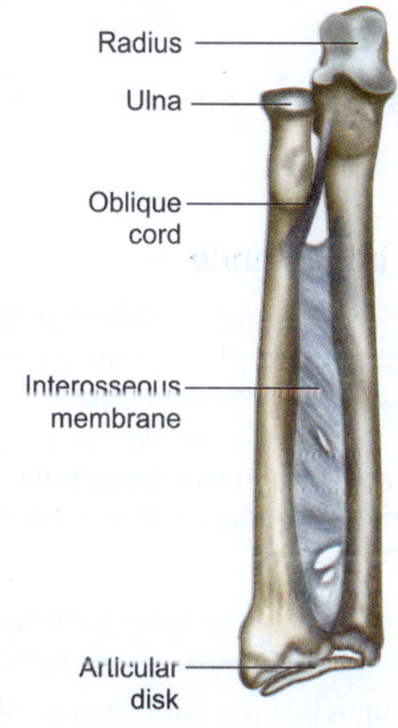

Interosseous membrane

Q. ANATOMICAL SNUFFBOX

Anatomical snuffbox can be appreciated in fully extended thumb. In earlier days, during dissections, anatomists would keep the snuff in this depression. Hence, it is known as anatomical snuff box.

Roof

Cephalic vein, cutaneous branches, skin, fascia of radial nerve.

Boundaries

- Anteriorly: Extensor pollicis brevis tendon and abductor pollicis longus tendon
- Posteriorly: Extensor pollicis longus tendon.

Floor

- Scaphoid bone: Tubercle, radial styloid, trapezium, base of thumb metacarpal.

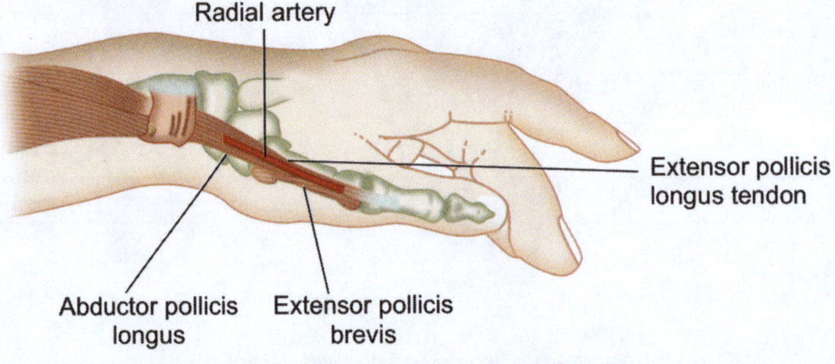

Anatomical snuffbox

Contents

- Radial artery.

Surgical Importance

- Tenderness can be elicited in this area in cases of scaphoid bone fracture due to out stretched hand injury
- One needs to retract the tendons in this area and incise the radial collateral ligament to approach wrist joint from lateral side.

Q. CARRYING ANGLE

Carrying angle is a peculiar feature of the elbow region. It is produced due to:

1. Projection of medial trochlear edge about 6 mm beyond it's lateral edge.
2. Obliquity of coronoid's superior articular surface.

When forearm is fully extended and supinated it diverges laterally forming the so called 'carrying angle' with the arm.

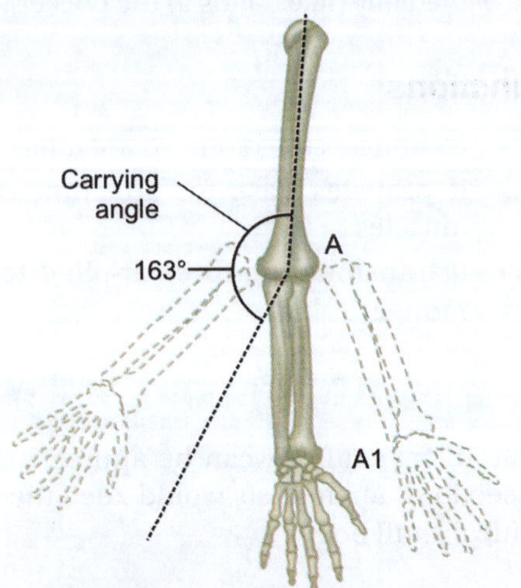

Formation of 'carrying angle'

Tilt of humeral and ulnar surface is almost the same thus the angle disappears in full flexion.

Applied Anatomy

- Carrying angle may vary in cases of fractures involving supracondylar area of humerus
- If the angle is increased it is known as cubitus valgus deformity
- Reversal of angle is known as cubitus varus deformity.

Q. EXTENSOR RETINACULUM

Extensor retinaculum is an oblique fibrous band on the back of wrist, which is nothing, but the modification of the deep fascia (like a friendship band). It holds the extensor tendons in position.

Attachments

- Laterally it is attached to lower 2–5 cm of the anterior border of radius
- Medially it is attached to the triquetrum and pisiform.

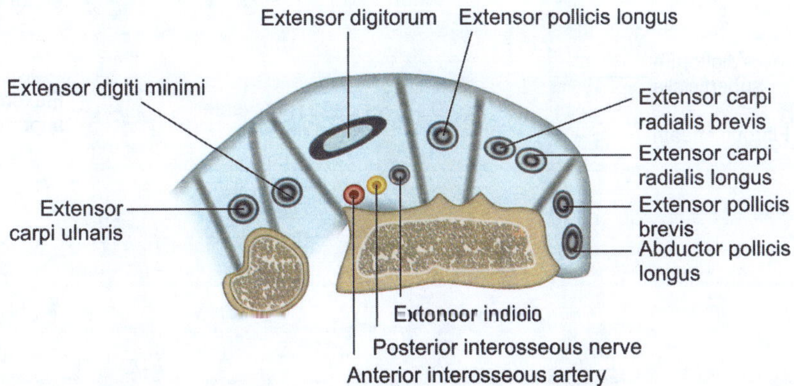

Abbreviation and its Expansion

- EPL: Extensor pollicis longus
- ECRL: Extensor carpi radialis longus
- EPB: Extensor pollicis brevis
- ECRB: Extensor carpi radialis brevis
- Abd PL: Abductor pollicis longus.

It is not attached to the lower end of ulna and thus it permits free movements of radius around ulna during pronation and supination.

Peculiarities

1. The retinacula send down septa, which are attached to the longitudinal ridges on the radius. Thus, the back of the wrist is divided into six osteofascial compartments.
2. Each compartment is lined by synovial sheath.

Q. FIBROUS FLEXOR SHEATH

Fibrous flexor sheath is the deep fascia of the digits. Proximally, it is continuous with the palmar aponeurosis.

Peculiarities

- The sheath is thin against the interphalangeal joints
- It is arranged transversely across the phalanges and cruciate against the joint.

Applied Anatomy

Tenosynovitis is an inflammatory condition of fibrous flexor sheath due to bacterial infection.

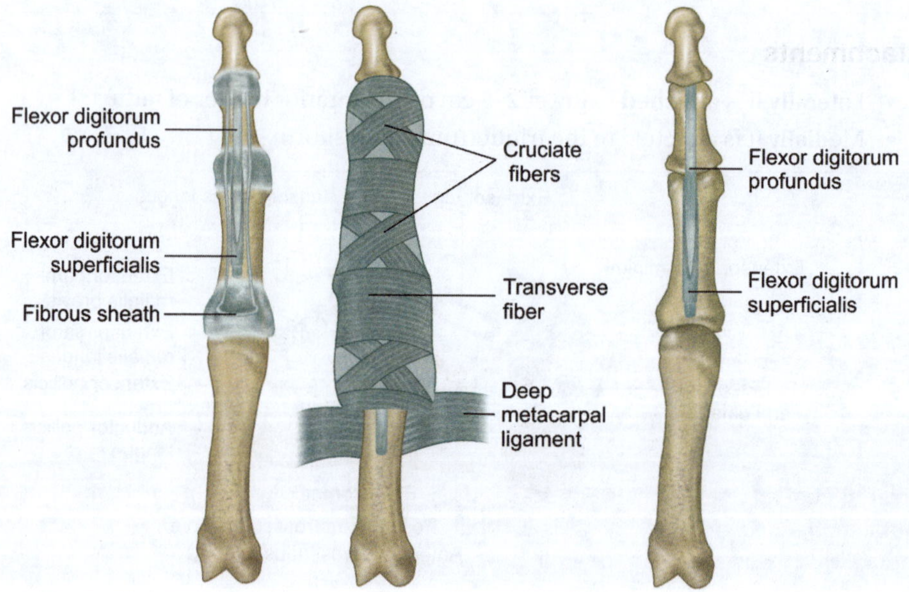

Arrangement of fibrous flexor sheath

Q. DIGITAL SYNOVIAL SHEATH

Synovial sheaths line the flexor tendons of the digits.

Arrangement

- Synovial sheaths of second, third and fourth digits are independent and terminate proximally at the level of head of the metacarpals
- Synovial sheath of little finger is continuous with the ulnar bursa
- Synovial sheath of thumb is continuous with the radial bursa.

Applied Anatomy

- Infections of little finger and thumb can spread to the palm and distal forearm
- Incision to drain digital synovial sheath is taken on the distal interphalangeal crease
- To drain the ulnar bursa, an incision is taken along the lateral margin of hypothenar eminence
- To drain the radial bursa, an incision is taken along the medial margin of thenar eminence.

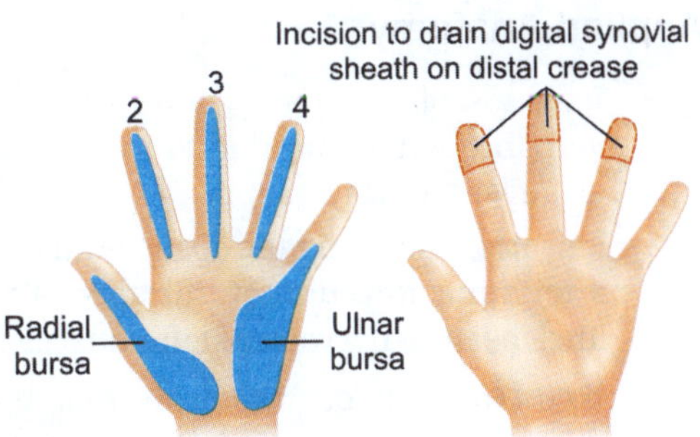

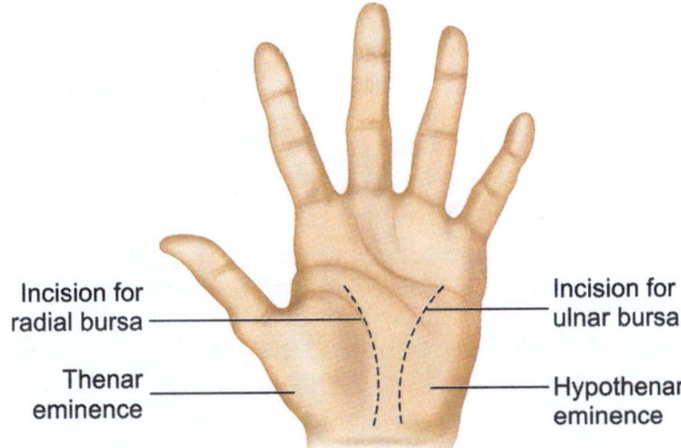

Q. DORSAL DIGITAL EXPANSION

Dorsal digital expansion is a hood-like fibrous expansion on the extensor aspect of the hand against the metacarpophalangeal joint. It receives insertion of dorsal interossei and lumbrical.

Q. SPACE OF WHITLOW

Space of whitlow is a space over the tip of the fingers and the thumb on its palmar aspect. The fat in this region is divided into compartments by virtue of septae (fibrous strands) going from the skin to the periosteum of terminal phalanx. Terminal branch of digital artery passes through this space.

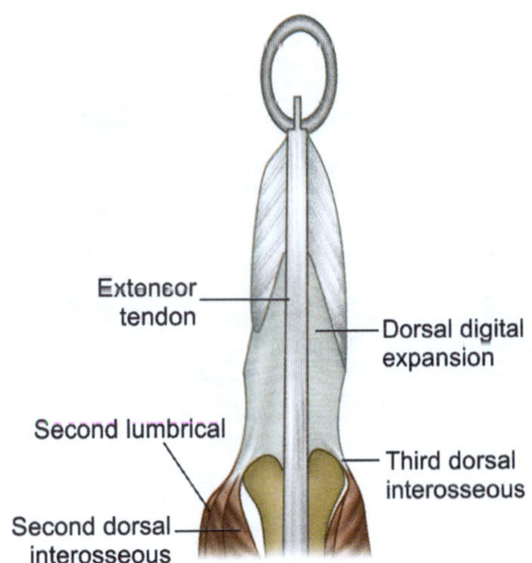

Applied Anatomy

- Infection of this space gives rise to severe throbbing pain due to the typical arrangement of the septa

- The artery reaching the space is an end artery thus infection of this space can lead to tissue necrosis, if left untreated

- To drain the infection in this area, the incision is given laterally.

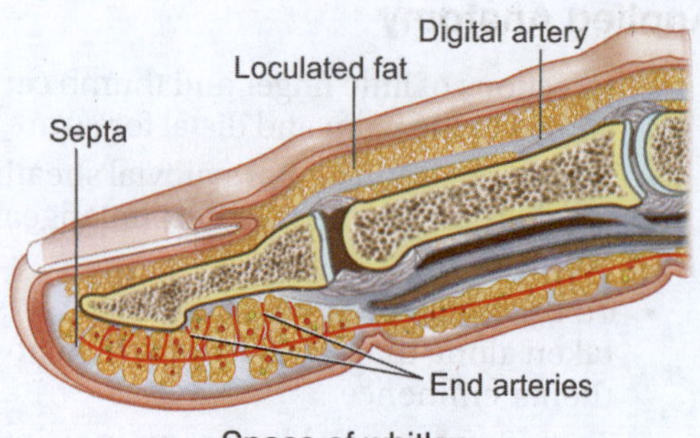

Long Questions

Q. DESCRIBE THE FORMATION AND BRANCHES OF BRACHIAL PLEXUS. ADD A NOTE ON ITS APPLIED ASPECT.

Brachial plexus is a network of nerves in the upper arm very close to the axillary artery. The parts of the brachial plexus can be compared to parts of the tree (namely—roots, trunk and branches).

Roots

Anterior primary rami of spinal nerves C5, C6, C7, C8, T1, contribute to the formation of brachial plexus (C4 and T2 may sometimes contribute in its formation).

Trunks

- C5, C6 join to form upper trunk
- C7 forms middle trunk
- C8, T1 join to form lower trunk.

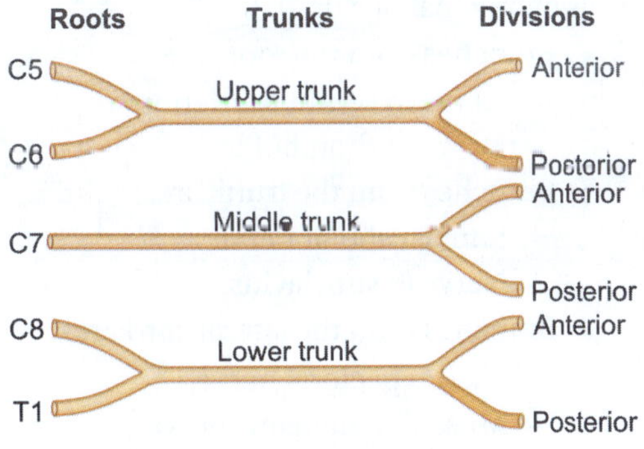

Framework of brachial plexus

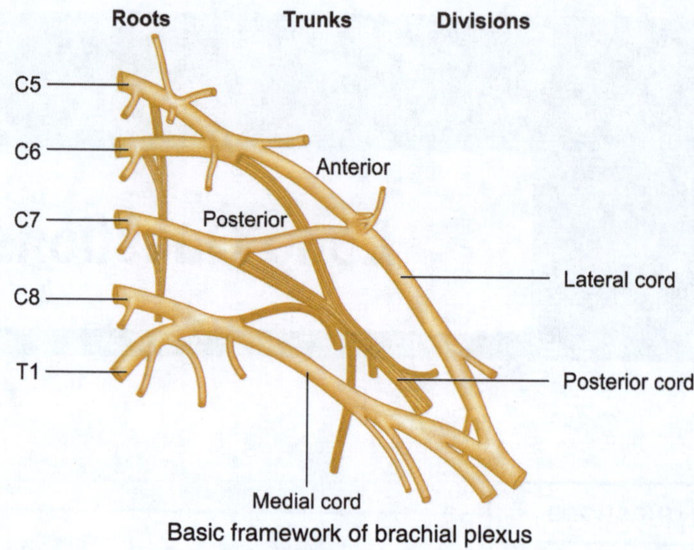

Basic framework of brachial plexus

Divisions

- Each trunk bifurcates into anterior and posterior divisions.

Cords

- Lateral cord is formed by the union of anterior division of upper and middle trunk
- Medial cord is continuation of anterior division of lower trunk
- Posterior divisions of all trunks form the posterior cord.

Branches

Branches arise from the roots, trunk and cords of brachial plexus.

- Branches from the roots are:
  - Nerve to serratus anterior
  - Nerve to rhomboids.
- Branches from the trunk are:
  - Suprascapular nerve
  - Nerve to subclavius.
- Branches from the lateral cord are:
  - Lateral pectoral nerve
  - Musculocutaneous nerve
  - Lateral root of median nerve.
- Branches from the medial cord are:
  - Medial pectoral nerve

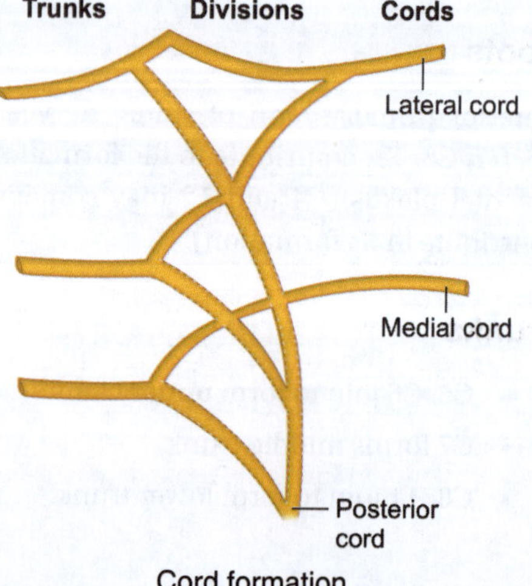

Cord formation

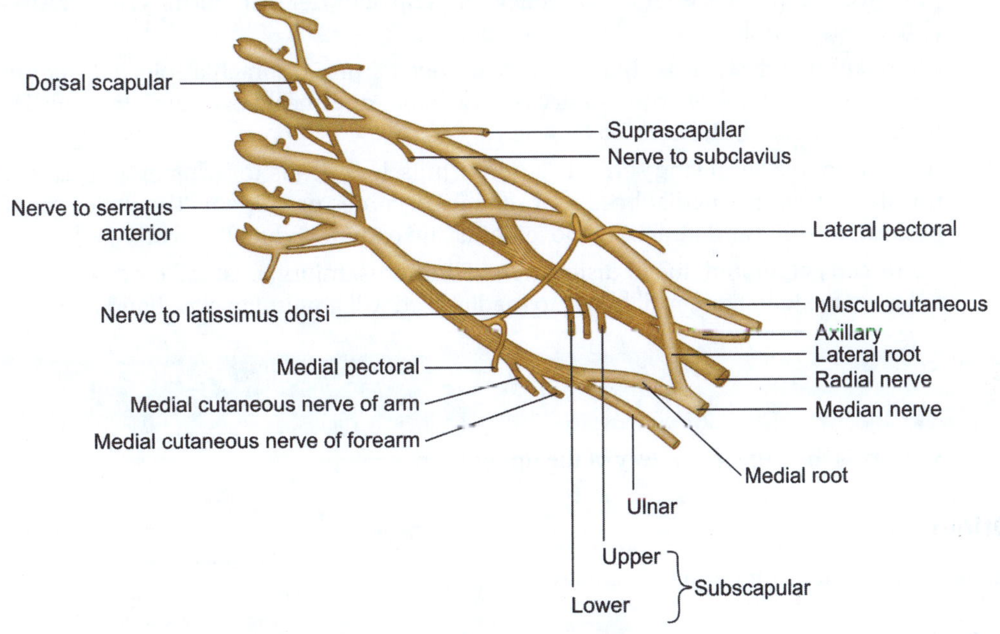

Branches of brachial plexus

- Medial cutaneous nerve of arm
- Medial cutaneous nerve of forearm
- Ulnar nerve
- Medial root of median nerve.

- Branches from the posterior cord are:
    - Upper subscapular
    - Nerve to latissimus dorsi
    - Lower subscapular
    - Axillary nerve
    - Radial nerve.

Relations

Axillary vessels lie entangled within the cords and branches of brachial plexus.

Brachial Plexus Injuries

1. Erb's paralysis: It is due to injury of upper trunk at Erb's point.

    Erb's point is a conglomeration of six nerves. It is here that the upper trunk usually stretches. In this deformity, the upper limb is adducted, extended and

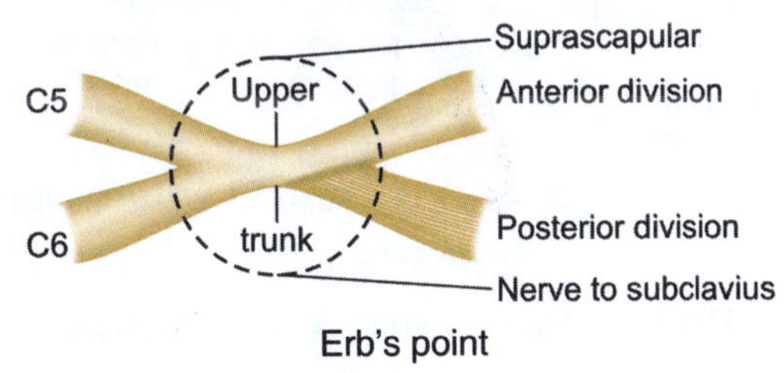

pronated. It is popularly known as policeman's tip or porter tip deformity (it is like trying to take tips secretly).

2. Klumpke's paralysis: It is due to injury of lower trunk of brachial plexus. Deformity produced due to lower trunk injury is claw hand, anesthesia over the ulnar border of forearm and hand, Horner's syndrome.

3. Injury to nerve supplying serratus anterior muscle: It leads to 'winging of scapula'. In this deformity, the medial border of scapula becomes prominent. The patient cannot perform pushing and punching movements and cannot abduct the arm.

4. Cords can get injured due to dislocation of humerus. Injury to lateral cord will amount to loss of flexion of forearm. Injury to medial cord will amount to claw hand mainly.

Q. DESCRIBE AXILLARY ARTERY IN DETAIL (ORIGIN, PARTS, RELATIONS AND BRANCHES).

Axillary artery is the principal artery of the upper limb.

Origin

Axillary artery is a continuation of subclavian artery.

Extent

Axillary artery extends from outer border of first rib to lower border of teres major.

Parts

For the sake of simplification, axillary artery is divided into three parts by 'pectoralis minor muscle'.

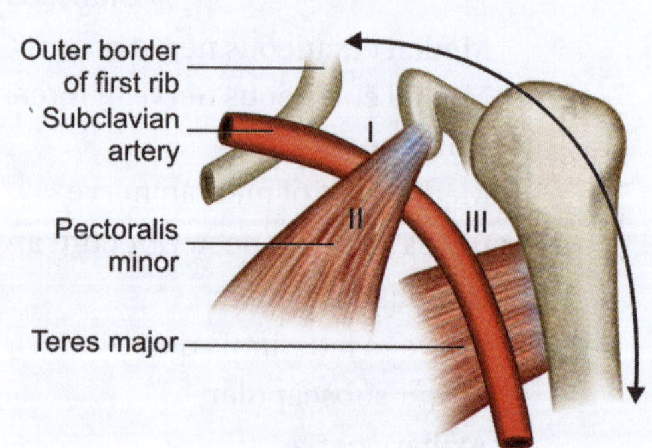

Parts of axillary artery

Relations

Axillary artery is closely related to cords and branches of brachial plexus (roots and

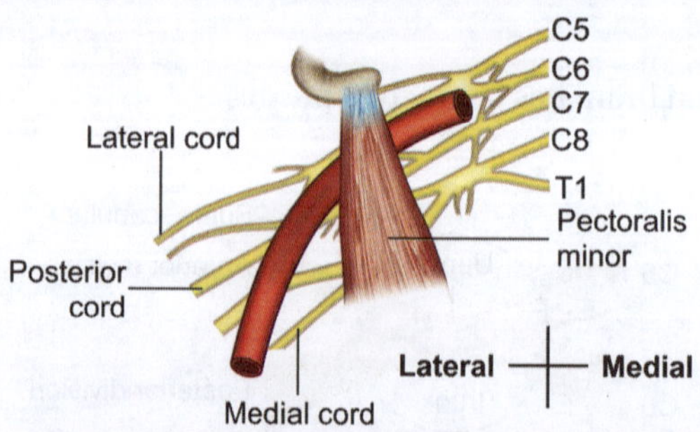

Relation of axillary artery to brachial plexus

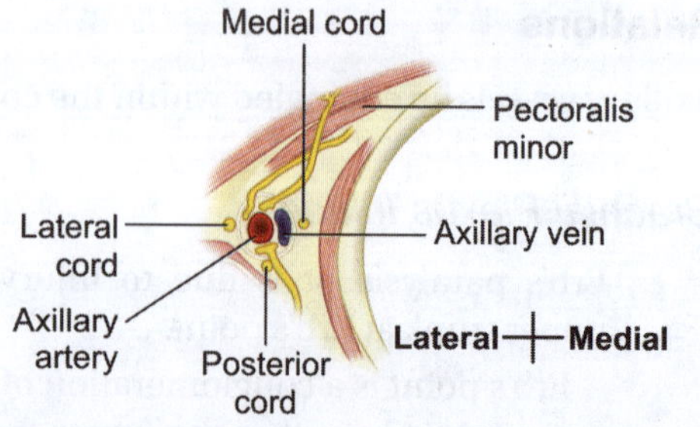

Transverse section of second part of axillary artery

trunks of brachial plexus are not related to the axillary artery). In fact, the cords and branches entangle the axillary artery.

All throughout, medial cord with its branches is related medially to the artery. While lateral cord with its branches is related laterally and posterior cord with it's branches is related posteriorly.

Branches

- First part has one branch:
  - Superior thoracic artery.
- Second part has two branches:
  - Acromiothoracic artery
  - Lateral thoracic artery.
- Third part has three branches:
  - Subscapular artery
  - Anterior circumflex humeral artery
  - Posterior circumflex humeral artery.

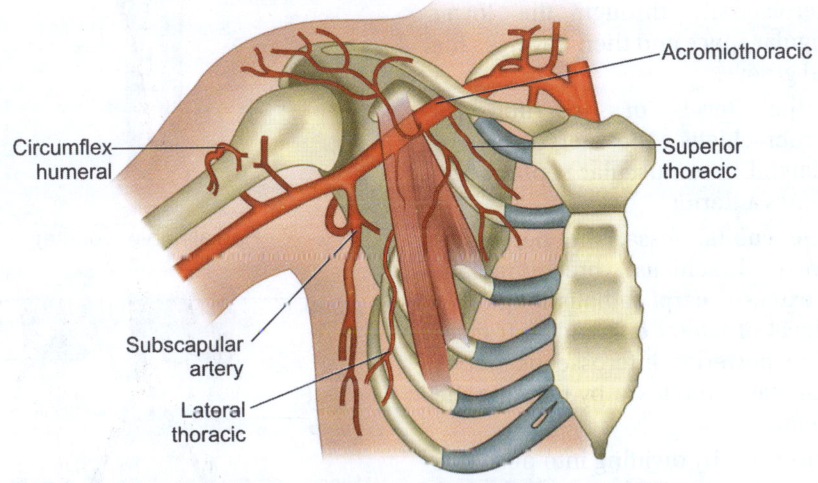

Branches of axillary artery

Applied Anatomy

1. When axillary artery gets blocked, a collateral circulation develops between subclavian and axillary artery through scapular anastomosis.
2. Hilton's method of drainage should be adopted in cases of axillary abscess (i.e. blunt dissection).

Radial nerve is the main nerve of the extensor compartment of the arm.

Origin

Posterior cord of brachial plexus.

Root Value

C5, C6, C7, C8, T1.

Course and Relations

1. In the axilla, it lies behind the third part of axillary artery and in front of subscapularis, latissimus dorsi and teres major.

2. In the upper arm, it lies behind the brachial artery and passes posterolaterally through the lower triangular space and then traverses the spiral groove.

3. At the level of insertion of coracobrachialis, the nerve pierces the lateral intermuscular septum and becomes anterior.

4. In the cubital fossa, the nerve lies between brachialis, brachioradialis and extensor carpi radialis longus. At the level of lateral epicondyle it gives off the posterior interosseous nerve, which leaves the fossa by piercing the supinator.

5. It terminates by dividing into posterior interosseous nerve (deep branch) and superficial cutaneous branch.

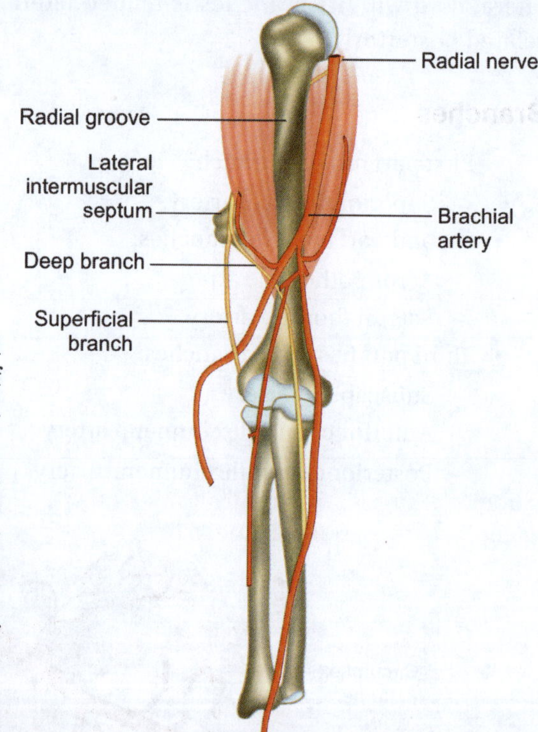

Radial nerve (course)

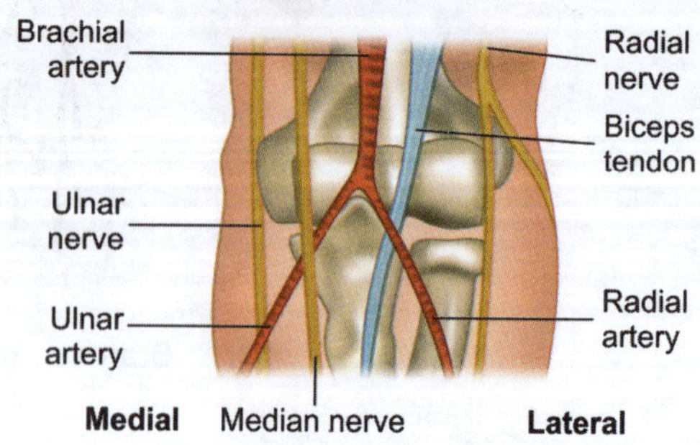

Radial nerve in cubital fossa

Branches

- *Muscular:* Triceps brachialis, brachioradialis and extensor carpi radialis longus
- *Cutaneous:* Posterior cutaneous nerve of arm and forearm, and lower lateral cutaneous nerve of arm
- *Articular:* Elbow joint.

Applied Anatomy

Radial nerve is commonly damaged in the radial groove due to intramuscular injections in the arm and sleeping in the armchair in a drunken state, i.e. crutch paralysis or Saturday night palsy. This leads to wrist drop and sensory loss on the back of forearm.

Q. DESCRIBE IN DETAIL SHOULDER JOINT.

Type

Synovial joint of ball and socket variety.

Articulating Surfaces

- Glenoid cavity of scapula
- Head of humerus.

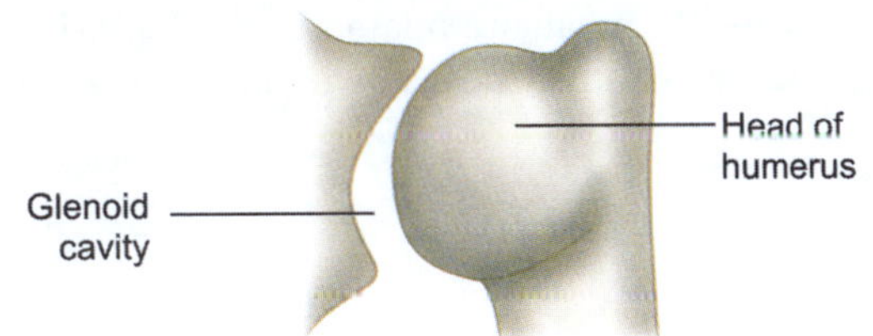

Articulating surfaces of shoulder joint

Nature

Shoulder joint is structurally a weak joint. The head of the humerus is four times the size of glenoid cavity. However, due to the disparity in size, the mobility of the joint is enhanced.

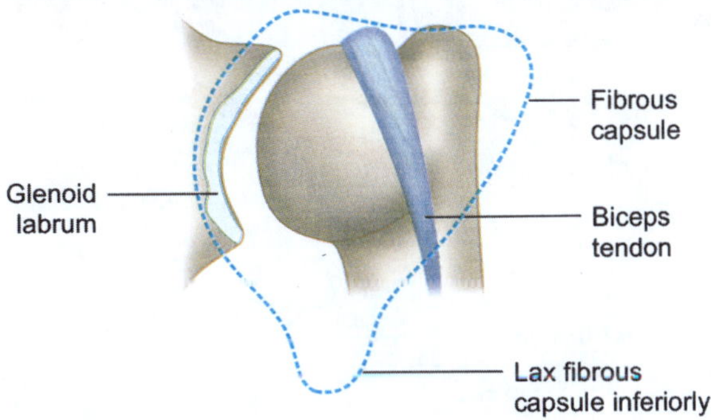

Fibrous capsule of shoulder joint

Ligaments

1. **Fibrous capsule:** It is attached along the margins of glenoid cavity of scapula. The supraglenoid tubercle is within the capsule:
   a. On the humerus it is attached to the anatomical neck. Attachment is deficient superiorly for the passage of tendon of biceps. While the capsule loosely hangs inferiorly up to the surgical neck of humerus.
   b. Anteriorly, the capsule is supplemented by glenohumeral ligament.
2. **Coracohumeral ligament:** It extends from root of the coracoid process to the neck of humerus, opposite the greater tubercle.

3. Transverse humeral ligament: It bridges the upper part of bicipital groove.
4. Glenoid labrum: It lines the glenoid cavity and deepens it.

Relations

Rotator cuff muscles, i.e. supraspinatus, infraspinatus, teres minor and subscapularis surround the shoulder joint. Rotator cuff muscles are covered by bulky deltoid muscle. Axillary neurovascular bundle gets related inferiorly.

Several bursae are related to the joint. Important bursae are subacromial, subscapularis and infraspinatus. The last two may communicate with the joint.

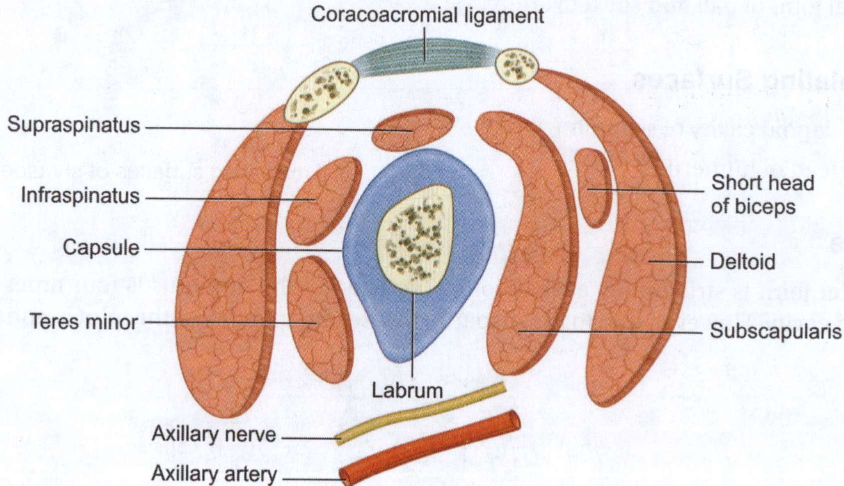

Blood Supply

- Circumflex humeral vessels
- Supra and subscapular vessels.

Nerve Supply

- Axillary nerve
- Musculocutaneous nerve
- Suprascapular nerve.

Action

The key muscles and action are mentioned below:

- Flexion—pectoralis major, deltoid
- Extension—deltoid, latissimus dorsi
- Adduction—pectoralis major, latissimus dorsi

- Abduction—deltoid, supraspinatus, serratus anterior, trapezius
- Medial rotation—pectoralis major, latissimus dorsi, deltoid, teres major
- Lateral rotation—deltoid, infraspinatus, teres minor.

Applied Anatomy

1. Inferior and recurrent dislocations are common due to the laxity of capsule.
2. Chronic tendonitis (painful arc syndrome): This syndrome is characterized by chronic thickening of the tendon of supraspinatus resulting in a typical impingement syndrome. The inflamed area is located by palpation of tender spot on the shoulder joint.
3. Frozen shoulder: Chronic inflammation of shoulder joint leads to adhesions between the rotator cuff muscles and humeral head.
4. Aspiration of shoulder joint is done by inserting a needle 1 cm inferior and lateral to the coracoid process.
5. Shoulder joint can be approached from front or behind, i.e. anterior exposure, posterior exposure, transacromial exposure.
6. Shoulder tip pain could be referred to pain from the diaphragm, since the phrenic nerve and supraclavicular nerve have the same root value (C3, C4).

Q. DESCRIBE IN DETAIL ELBOW JOINT.

Type

Synovial joint of hinge variety.

Articulating Surfaces

- Capitulum and trochlea of humerus
- Head of the radius and trochlear notch of ulna.

Nature

Elbow joint is in connection with the superior radioulnar joint. Humeroradial, humeroulnar and superior radioulnar joints are together known as cubital articulation.

Ligaments

1. **Fibrous capsule:** Superiorly it is attached to the lower end of humerus and includes radial fossa, coronoid fossa and olecranon fossa within it:
   a. Inferomedially it is attached to the rim of trochlear notch.

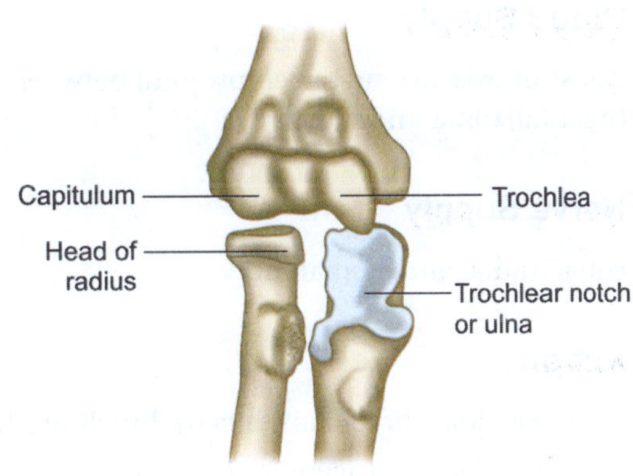

Articulating surfaces

b. Inferolaterally it is attached to the annular ligament of the superior radioulnar joint.

c. Capsule is reinforced anteriorly and posteriorly by ligaments carrying the same name (anterior ligament, posterior ligament).

2. **Ulnar collateral ligament:** It is a triangular ligament. Above, it is attached to the medial epicondyle and below it splits into anterior, posterior and oblique bands.

3. **Radial collateral ligament:** It extends from lateral epicondyle to the annular ligament.

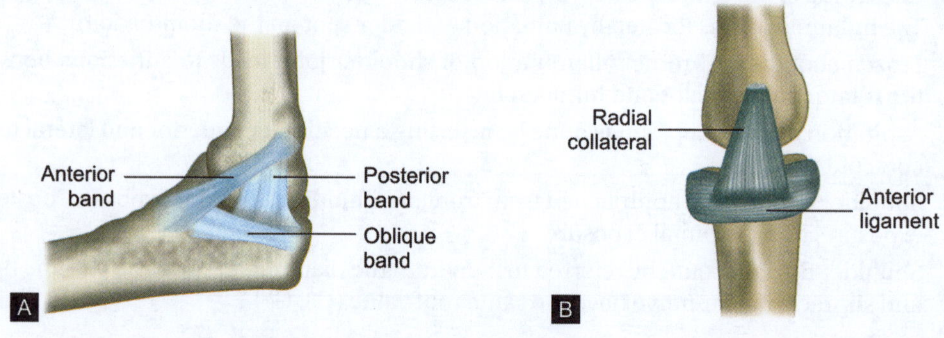

Ligaments of elbow joint

Relations

- Anteriorly—cubital fossa with its contents
- Medially—ulnar nerve and common flexor origin
- Laterally—supinator and common extensor origin.

Blood Supply

Anastomosis around the elbow joint between brachial, ulnar and radial.

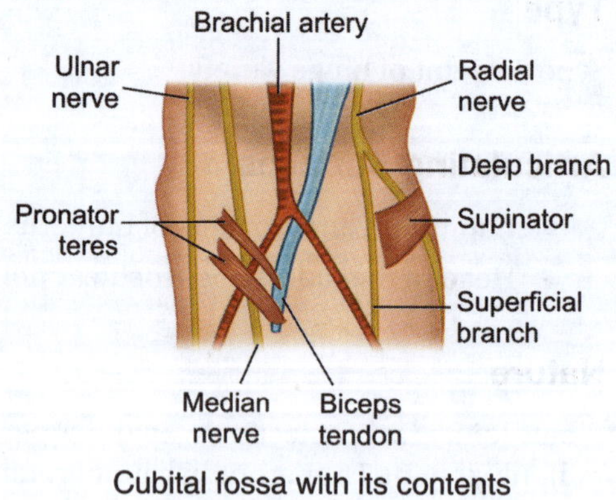

Cubital fossa with its contents

Nerve Supply

Ulnar, radial and median nerve.

Action

- Flexion—brachialis, biceps, brachioradialis
- Extension—triceps, anconeus.

Applied Anatomy

- Posterior dislocation of elbow joint is common and is accompanied by fracture of coronoid process
- Subluxation is common in children
- Tennis elbow—abrupt pronation may lead to pain and tenderness over the lateral epicondyle.

Q. DESCRIBE IN DETAIL WRIST JOINT.

Type

Synovial joint of ellipsoid variety.

Articulating Surfaces

- Inferior surface of lower end of radius and articular disk of radioulnar joint
- Scaphoid, lunate, triquetral bones.

Ligaments

- Fibrous capsule: It surrounds the articular surfaces
- Palmar radiocarpal ligament: It is a fibrous band extending from radius to lunate bone
- Dorsal radiocarpal ligament: It is the mirror image of palmar ligament on dorsal side
- Radial collateral ligament: It is attached above to the styloid process of radius and below to the lateral side of scaphoid bone
- Ulnar collateral ligament: It is attached above to the styloid process of ulna and below to the triquetral and pisiform bone.

Relations

Anteriorly, it is related to the flexor tendons and posteriorly it is related to the extensor tendons.

Blood Supply

Anterior and posterior carpal arch.

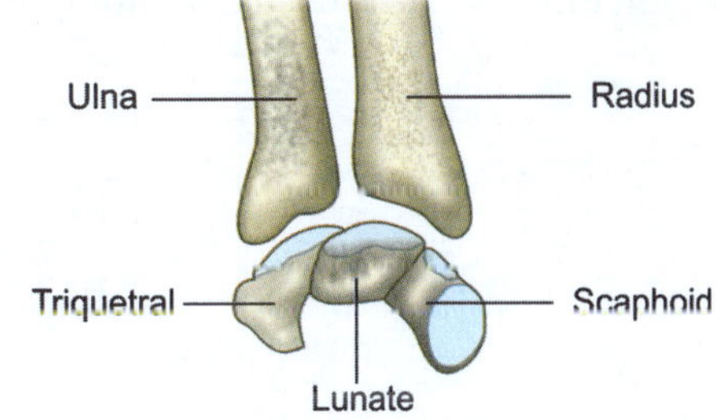

Articulating bones

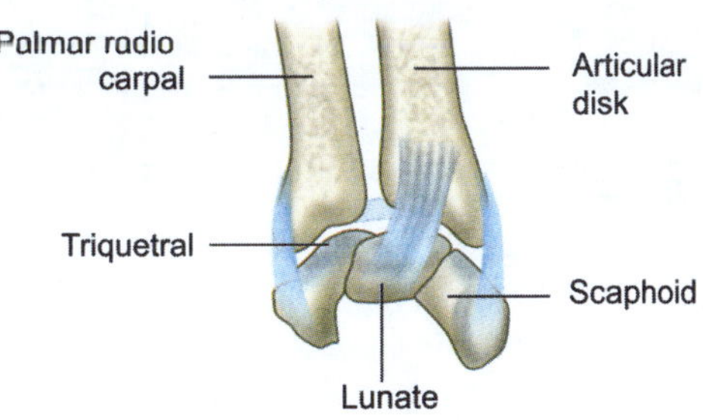

Ligaments of wrist joint

Nerve Supply

Anterior and posterior interosseous nerve.

Action

- Flexion and extension by the flexor and extensor tendons of the hand respectively.
- Abduction:
  - Flexor carpi radialis
  - Extensor carpi radialis longus
  - Abductor pollicis longus
  - Extensor pollicis brevis.
- Adduction:
  - Flexor carpi ulnaris
  - Extensor carpi ulnaris.

  Flexion is combined with adduction and extension with abduction.

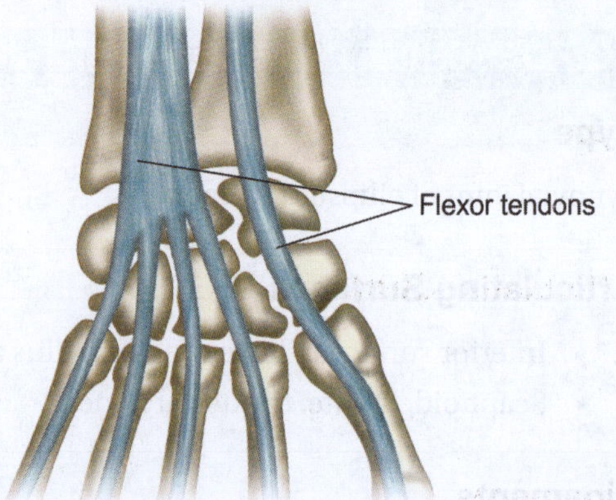

Anterior relations of wrist joint

Applied Anatomy

- Ganglion: It is a commonest cystic swelling on the back of the wrist
- Madelung's deformity: It is a congenital subluxation or dislocation of lower end of ulna
- Rheumatoid arthritis: It commonly affects the wrist joint.

Key Diagrams with MCQ Tips

Diagrams for

- Serratus anterior muscle
- Trapezius
- Dorsal interossei
- Palmar interossei
- Cubital fossa

- Flexor digitorum superficialis
- Flexor digitorum profundus
- Lymphatic drainage of breast
- Shoulder girdle

Q. Serratus anterior muscle

Ans.

- Inserted on costal surface of scapula along its medial border
- Long thoracic nerve of Bell (C5, C6, C7) supplies the muscle
- Injury to above nerve leads to 'winging of scapula'.

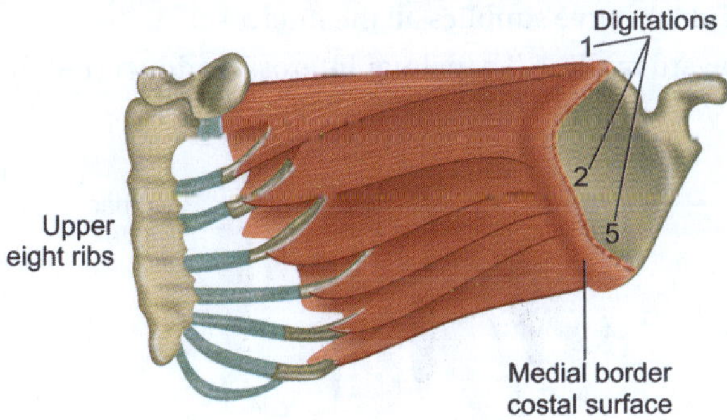

Q. Trapezius

Ans.

- Also known as shawl muscle
- Supplied by spinal part of accessory nerve
- Elevates and retracts the scapula.

Q. Dorsal interossei

Ans.

- Bipennate muscles taking origin from adjacent sides of metacarpal bones
- Deep branch of ulnar nerve supplies all the interossei
- Abducts digits away from midline [i.e. dorsal interossei abduct (DAB)].

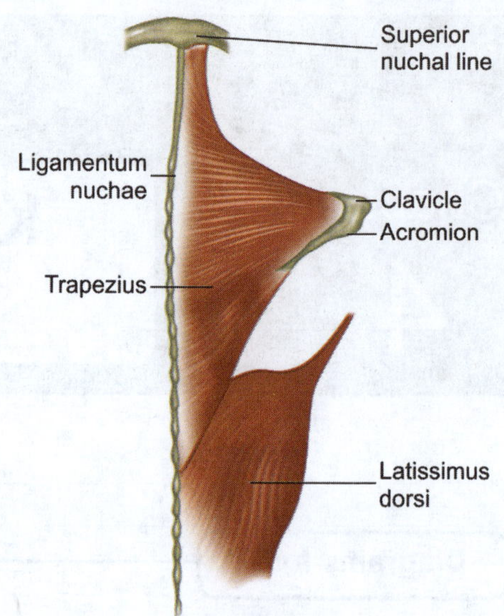

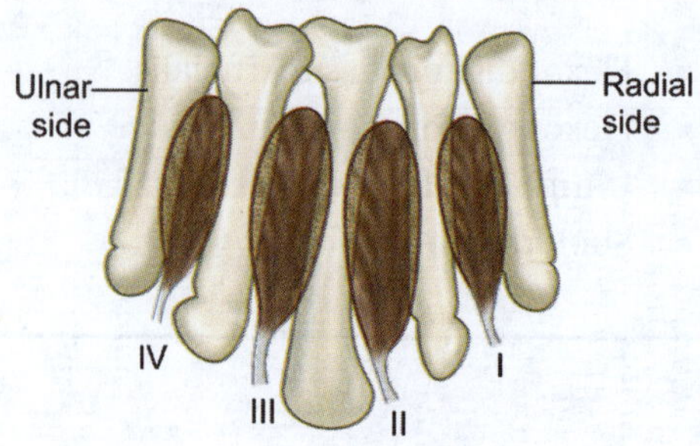

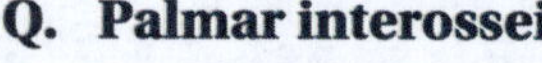
Dorsal interossei

Q. Palmar interossei

Ans.

- Unipennate muscles between the shafts of metacarpal
- Deep branch of ulnar nerve supplies all the interossei
- Adduct digits toward midline [i.e. palmar interossei adduct (PAD)].

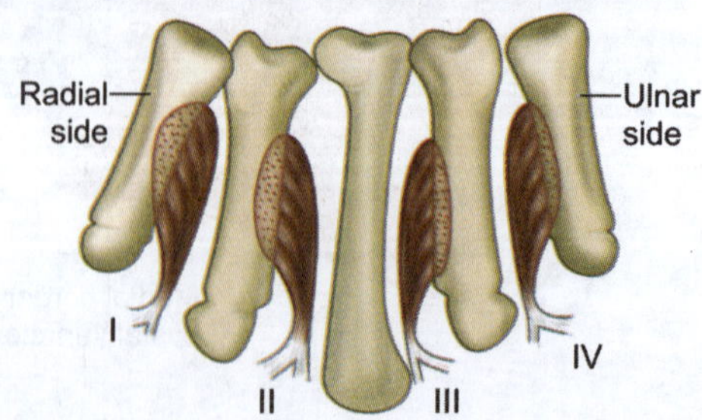

Palmar interossei

Q. Cubital fossa

Ans.

- Brachial artery lies medial to biceps tendon
- Ulnar nerve is posterior to medial epicondyle
- Median nerve passes between two heads of pronator teres
- Radial nerves divides into superficial and deep branches
- The deep branch goes below the upper border of supinator.

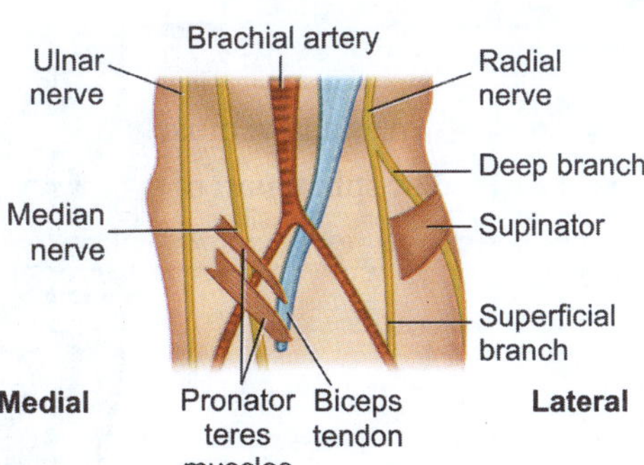

Q. Insertion of flexor digitorum superficialis

Ans.

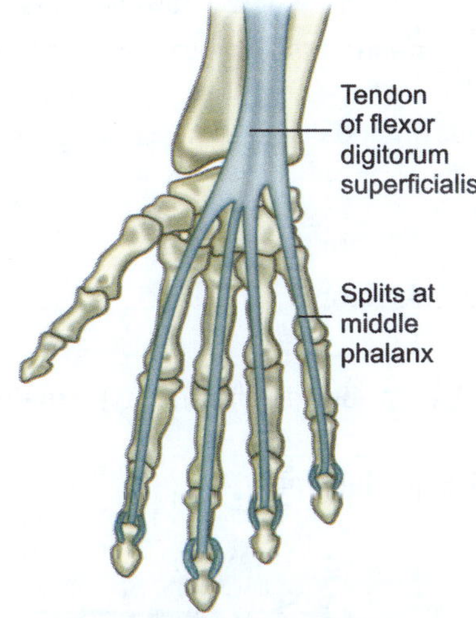

Flexor digitorum superficialis

Q. Flexor digitorum profundus

Ans.

- Flexor digitorum profundus is a hybrid muscle
- Medial half supplied by ulnar nerve
- Lateral half supplied by median nerve
- The tendon goes below the split end of flexor digitorum superficialis.

Q. Lymphatic drainage of breast

Ans.

- To axillary lymph nodes 75%
- To internal thoracic (mammary) nodes 20%

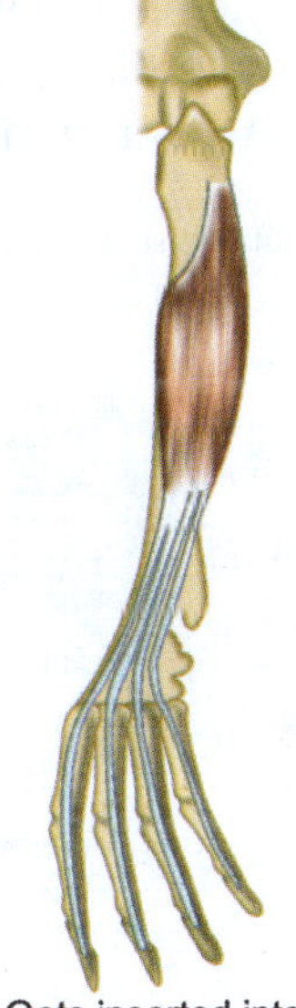

Flexor digitorum profundus

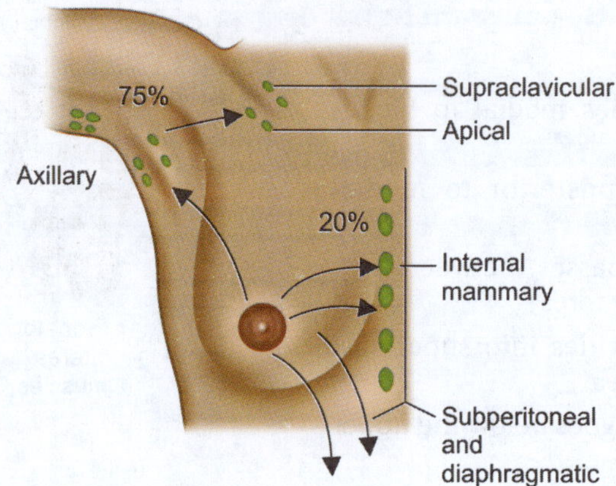

- To posterior intercostal nodes 5%
- Subareolar plexus of Sappey is present
- Radial incisions are taken to avoid cutting of lactiferous ducts
- Lymphatics from lower and inner quadrants of breast may communicate with subdiaphragmatic and subperitoneal plexus
- Staging of breast cancer depends on nodal status (size, number, fixity).

Q. Shoulder girdle

Ans.

- Connects upper limb with axial skeleton
- Two joints:
    - Sternoclavicular (synovial, compound, complex, type main bond of union is articular disk)
    - Acromioclavicular (plane synovial type).

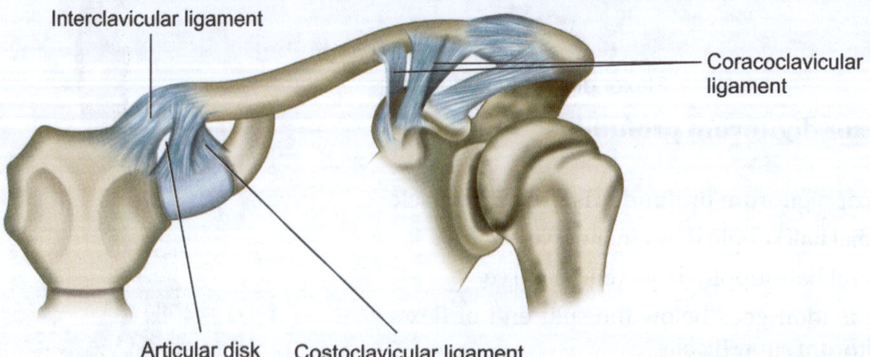

Q. Medial epicondyle—common flexor origin.

Q. Lateral epicondyle—common extensor origin.

Q. Capitate key carpal bone, first to ossify.

Q. Pisiform—sesamoid bone in tendon of flexor carpi ulnaris, last to ossify.

Q. Palmaris brevis—subcutaneous muscle of upper limb.

Q. Epiphyseal lines and capsular attachments

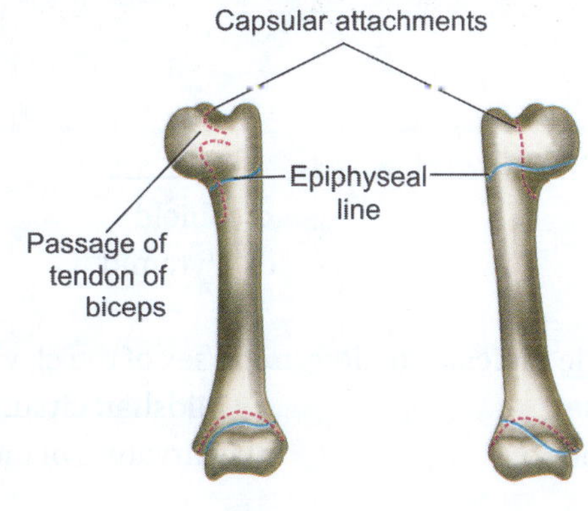

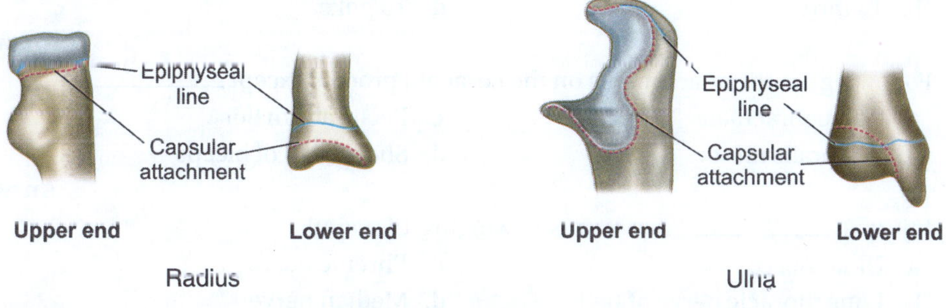

Multiple Choice Questions (MCQs)

1. The literal meaning of the word clavicle is ___________
   a. Lock
   b. Key
   c. Shield
   d. Pyramid

   Answer: b

2. The most reliable single indicator to determine sex of the clavicle is ___________
   a. Length of the bone
   b. Thickness of the bone
   c. Midshaft circumference of the bone
   d. Curvature of the bone

   Answer: c

3. Literal meaning of scapula is ___________
   a. To dig
   b. To throw
   c. To screw
   d. To poke

   Answer: a

4. Following are the attachments on the coracoid process except ___________
   a. Coracobrachialis
   b. Pectoralis minor
   c. Pectoralis major
   d. Short head of biceps

   Answer: c

5. Injury to ___________ nerve causes 'winging' of scapula.
   a. Ulnar nerve
   b. Long thoracic nerve of Bell
   c. Phrenic nerve
   d. Median nerve

   Answer: b

6. Following muscles constitute the 'rotator cuff' except ___________
   a. Supraspinatus
   b. Subscapularis
   c. Suprascapularis
   d. Infraspinatus

   Answer: c

7. The nerve related to the surgical neck of humerus is ___________
   a. Axillary nerve
   b. Radial nerve
   c. Ulnar nerve
   d. Median nerve

   Answer: a

8. Following nerve is related to the posterior aspect of medial epicondyle _____________
   a. Median
   b. Ulnar
   c. Radial
   d. Medial cutaneous nerve of arm

   Answer: b

9. Pisiform bone is a sesamoid bone, which develops in the tendon of _____________
   a. Flexor carpi radialis
   b. Flexor digitorum superficialis
   c. Flexor digitorum profundus
   d. Flexor carpi ulnaris

   Answer: d

10. Key carpal bone is _____________
    a. Pisiform
    b. Capitate
    c. Hamate
    d. Trapezium

    Answer: b

11. Coracobrachialis muscle is pierced by following nerve _____________
    a. Radial
    b. Ulnar
    c. Musculocutaneous
    d. Lateral cutaneous nerve of arm

    Answer: c

12. Middle finger receives insertion of which palmar interossei _____________
    a. I
    b. II
    c. III
    d. None

    Answer: d

13. All palmar interossei _____________ the digits.
    a. Abduct
    b. Adduct
    c. Flex
    d. Extend

    Answer: b

14. All dorsal interossei _____________ the digits.
    a. Abduct
    b. Adduct
    c. Flex
    d. Extend

    Answer: a

15. All interossei are supplied by _____________ nerve.
    a. Median
    b. Radial
    c. Ulnar
    d. Musculocutaneous

    Answer: c

16. Paper test is used to test the action of _____________
    a. Adductor pollicis
    b. Palmar interossei
    c. Dorsal interossei
    d. Opponens pollicis

    Answer: b

17. The lumbricals have the following action _____________
    a. Extend MP joint and flex IP joint
    b. Flex MP joint and extend IP joint
    c. Extend MP joint and extend IP joint
    d. Flex MP joint and also flex IP joint

    Answer: b

MP, metacarpophalangeal; IP, interphalangeal.

18. Musculocutaneous nerve descends in the arm between two muscles namely __________
    a. Coracobrachialis and brachialis
    c. Brachialis and biceps
    b. Pectoralis major and subscapularis
    d. Biceps and coracobrachialis

    Answer: c

19. The key nerve of the front of arm is __________
    a. Musculocutaneous
    c. Median
    b. Ulnar
    d. Radial

    Answer: a

20. The musculocutaneous nerve pierces __________ muscle.
    a. Biceps
    c. Coracobrachialis
    b. Pectoralis
    d. Brachialis

    Answer: c

21. Musculocutaneous nerve is the branch of __________ cord of brachial plexus.
    a. Medial
    c. Posterior
    b. Lateral
    d. Anterior

    Answer: b

22. Musician's nerve is __________
    a. Musculocutaneous nerve
    c. Radial nerve
    b. Ulnar nerve
    d. Median nerve

    Answer: b

23. Ulnar nerve enters the forearm between the two heads of __________
    a. Flexor digitorum superficialis
    c. Flexor carpi ulnaris
    b. Flexor carpi radialis
    d. Flexor digitorum profundus

    Answer: c

24. Median nerve lies between the two heads of __________
    a. Flexor carpi ulnaris
    c. Pronator teres
    b. Flexor carpi radialis
    d. Supinator

    Answer: c

25. Median nerve originates from two cords __________
    a. Medial cord and posterior cord
    c. Lateral cord and posterior cord
    b. Medial cord and lateral cord
    d. Medial, lateral and posterior cord

    Answer: b

26. Roots involved in Erb's paralysis are __________
    a. C5, C6
    c. C8, C9
    b. C6, C7
    d. C4, C5

    Answer: a

27. Central group of axillary lymph node is related to following nerve __________
    a. Axillary nerve
    c. Musculocutaneous nerve
    b. Radial nerve
    d. Intercostobrachial nerve

    Answer: d

28. Clavipectoral fascia encloses ____________ muscles.
    a. Subclavius and pectoralis major   c. Pectoralis major
    b. Pectoralis minor and subclavius   d. Coracobrachialis

    Answer: b

29. Coracoid process is ____________ type of epiphysis.
    a. Atavistic   c. Traction
    b. Pressure   d. Aberrant

    Answer: a

30. First carpometacarpal joint ____________ type of joint.
    a. Ball and socket   c. Saddle
    b. Condyloid   d. None of the above

    Answer: c

31. The upper trunk of brachial plexus is formed by union of ____________
    a. C4, C5   c. C6, C7
    b. C5, C6   d. C8, T1

    Answer: b

32. Extent of the axillary artery is between ____________
    a. Outer border of first rib to lower border of teres major
    b. First costal cartilage to upper border of teres major
    c. Outer border of first rib to upper border of teres major
    d. Inner border of first rib to lower border of teres major

    Answer. a

33. Axillary artery is divided into three parts by ____________ muscle.
    a. Pectoralis major   c. Teres major
    b. Pectoralis minor   d. Teres minor

    Answer. b

34. Shawl muscle is ____________
    a. Deltoid   c. Subscapularis
    b. Pectoralis major   d. Trapezius

    Answer: d

35. Brachial artery is ____________ to biceps tendon.
    a. Lateral   c. Medial
    b. Anterior   d. Posterior

    Answer: c

36. The last carpal bone to ossify is ____________
    a. Capitate   c. Hamate
    b. Pisiform   d. Scaphoid

    Answer: b

37. An alcoholic, who under the influence, slept with his arm on the chair and woke up in the morning with inability to move the arm. It is due to pressure on ______________
    a. Ulnar nerve
    b. Median nerve
    c. Radial nerve
    d. Interosseous nerve

    Answer: c

38. A porter carrying heavy weights on shoulder was unable to do pushing movements. The nerve likely to be injured is ________________
    a. Nerve to Latissimus dorsi
    b. Nerve to serratus anterior
    c. Nerve to subscapularis
    d. Nerve to subclavius

    Answer: b

39. Forceps were applied, while delivering a child. Later child develops 'claw hand'. This is due to injury to ____________ trunk of brachial plexus.
    a. Upper
    b. Middle
    c. Lower
    d. All

    Answer: c

40. Undue pressure was applied on head, while delivering the baby.
    Following which, a deformity, wherein abduction, flexion of arm was not possible (policeman's tip). This is due to injury to ____________
    a. C4, C5
    b. C5, C6
    c. C7, C8
    d. C8, T1

    Answer: b

41. A middle-aged woman wakes up in sleep with pain and tingling in hand. This is due to entrapment of ____________ nerve in hand.
    a. Median
    b. Ulnar
    c. Radial
    d. Musculocutaneous

    Answer: a

42. In a patient of leprosy, a thick cord-like structure was palpated behind medial epicondyle the nerve affected is ____________
    a. Ulnar
    b. Radial
    c. Musculocutaneous
    d. Median

    Answer: a

43. A 60-year-old female complains of swelling in breast. The area to be examined examined after breast examination is ____________
    a. Abdomen
    b. Pelvis
    c. Axilla
    d. Neck

    Answer: c

44. Axillary abscess should be drained by blunt dissection (Hilton's method) due to presence of ____________
    a. Axillary lymph nodes
    b. Axillary artery and vein
    c. Axillary nerve
    d. Axillary lymphatic vessels

    Answer: b

SECTION - II

LOWER LIMB

Key Questions

Key questions

- Hip bone
- Attachments on the iliac crest
- Location of iliac crest tubercle
- Summit and midpoint of the iliac crest
- Location of auricular surface
- Location of preauricular sulcus
- Preauricular sulcus attachment
- Pubic symphysis
- Divisions of ischial tuberosity
- Attachments on the ischial tuberosity
- Ischial spine attachments
- Ischial spine relations
- Pelvic brim index
- Classification of pelves
- Differences between male and female pelves
- Fovea of femoral head attachment
- Femoral head
- Neck shaft angle significance
- Trochanteric fossa attachment
- Attachments on lesser trochanter
- Attachments on the greater trochanter
- Angle of femoral torsion
- Quadrate tubercle attachment
- Third trochanter
- Adductor tubercle attachment
- Medicolegal importance of the lower end of femur
- Attachments on linea aspera
- Lateral condyle of femur
- Patella
- Proximal articular surface of tibia
- Tibial tuberosity attachment
- Nerve relation to the head of fibula
- Muscles attached to talus bone
- Tendon relation to sustentaculum tali
- Ligaments of sustentaculum tali
- Navicular tuberosity attachment
- Compare of carpal and tarsal bones
- Fabella

Q. What type of bone is hip bone?

Ans. Hip bone is a large irregular bone.

Q. Depict attachments on the iliac crest.

Ans.

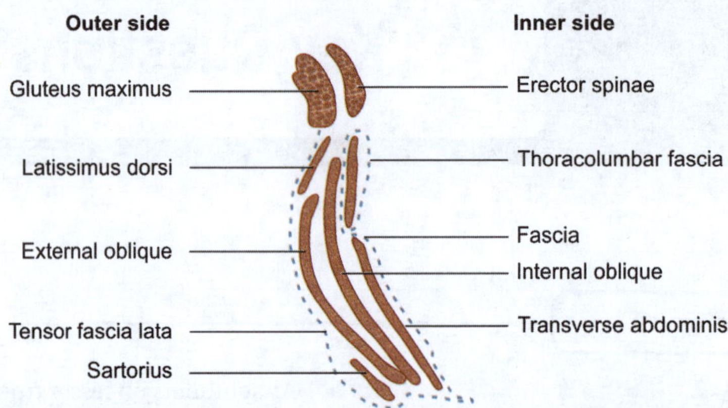

Q. Where is the tubercle of iliac crest located?

Ans. The tubercle of iliac crest is located on the outer lip, 5 cm dorsosuperior to anterior superior iliac spine.

Q. Is the summit of the iliac crest equivalent to the midpoint of the iliac crest?

Ans. No, the summit of the iliac crest is little behind the midpoint of the iliac crest and is between L3 and L4.

Q. Where is the auricular surface located? Why is it named so?

Ans. Auricular surface is immediately anteroinferior to the iliac tuberosity. It is shaped like an ear (wide above and narrow below).

Q. Where is the preauricular sulcus located?

Ans. As the name indicates it is located before auricular surface, i.e. between auricular surface and upper border of greater sciatic notch. It is prominent in females and is one of the feature for sex determination of the pelvis.

Q. What is attached to the preauricular sulcus?

Ans. Ventral sacroiliac ligament and few fibers of piriformis are attached to the preauricular sulcus.

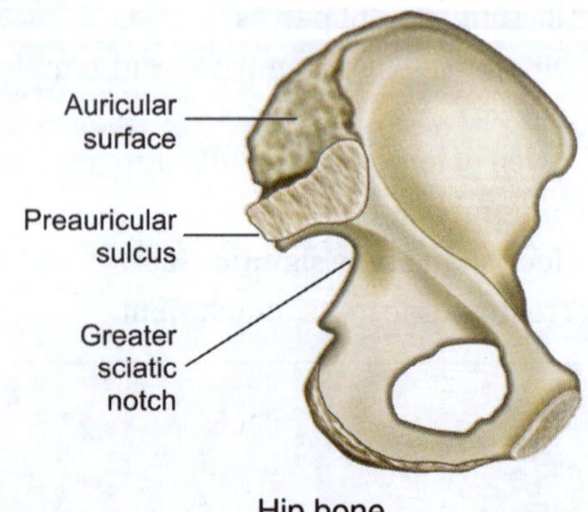

Q. What type of joint is pubic symphysis?

Ans. It is a fibrocartilaginous joint.

Q. Depict the divisions of ischial tuberosity.

Ans.

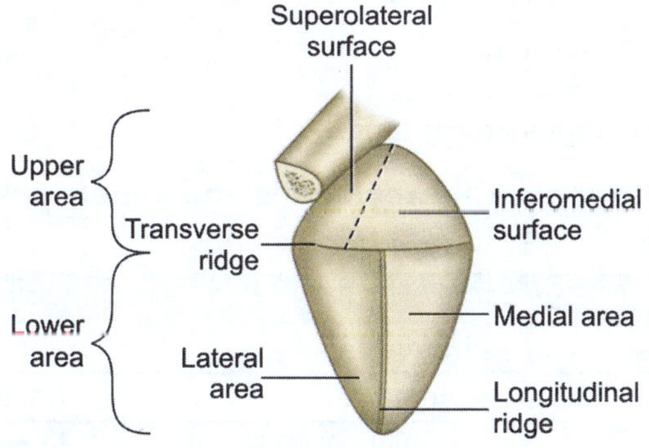

Q. Depict the attachments on the ischial tuberosity.

Ans.

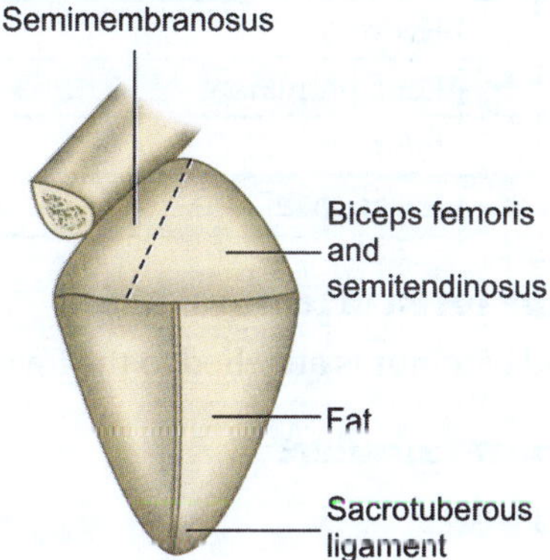

Q. What is attached to ischial spine?

Ans. Sacrospinous ligament is attached to the ischial spine.

Q. What are the relations of ischial spine?

Ans. Internal pudendal vessels and nerve to obturator internus are related posteriorly. Coccygeus muscle and posterior fibers of levator ani are related anteriorly.

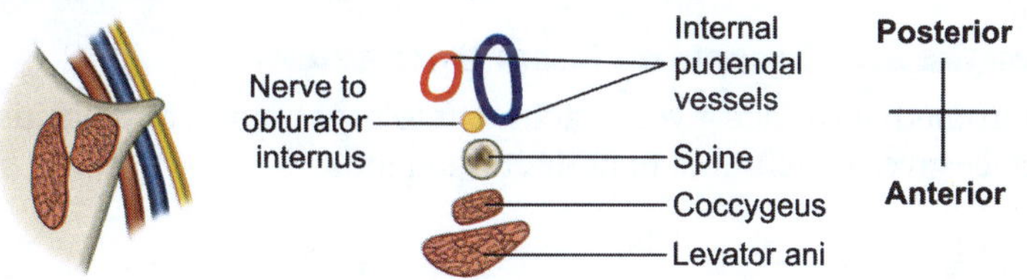

Q. What is pelvic brim index?

Ans. Pelvic brim index $= \dfrac{\text{Anteroposterior diameter}}{\text{Transverse diameter}} \times 100$

Q. How are the pelves classified depending on pelvic brim index?

Ans. The pelves are classified as follows:

- Platypellic—transversely long
- Mesatipellic—intermediate size
- Dolichopellic—anteroposteriorly long.

Q. What are the differences between male and female pelves?

Ans.

Criteria	Male	Female
Greater sciatic notch	Narrow	Wider
Acetabulum	Larger	Smaller
Iliac crest	More prominent	Less prominent
Iliac fossa	Shallow	Deeper
Pubic crest	Shorter	Longer
Ischiopubic rami	Everted	Not everted
Preauricular sulcus	Less prominent	More prominent
Ischial spine	Inturned	Straight, pointed
Obturator foramen	Large, oval	Small, triangular

Q. What is attached to the fovea of femoral head?

Ans. The ligament of the head of femur is attached to the fovea of femoral head.

Q. Is the femoral head intracapsular?

Ans. Femoral head is intracapsular.

Q. What is the neck shaft angle and mention its significance?

Ans. The femoral neck is at an angle with the shaft, this is the neck shaft angle. It is 125°. It facilitates the movement of hip joint thus helping the limb to swing freely away from the pelvis.

Q. What is attached to trochanteric fossa?

Ans. The tendon of obturator externus is attached to trochanteric fossa.

Q. Mention the attachments on lesser trochanter.

Ans. The anteromedial surface gives attachment to psoas major and iliacus, while the posterior surface gives attachment to adductor magnus.

Q. Depict the attachments on the greater trochanter.

Ans.

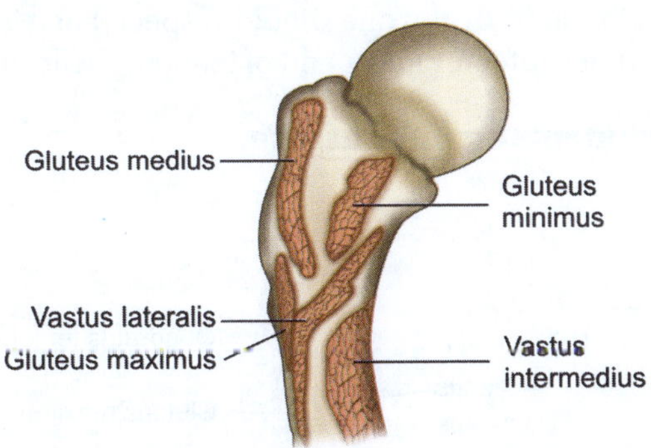

Q. What is angle of femoral torsion?

Ans. The transverse axis of the head of femur makes an angle with the transverse condylar axis. This is the angle of femoral torsion.

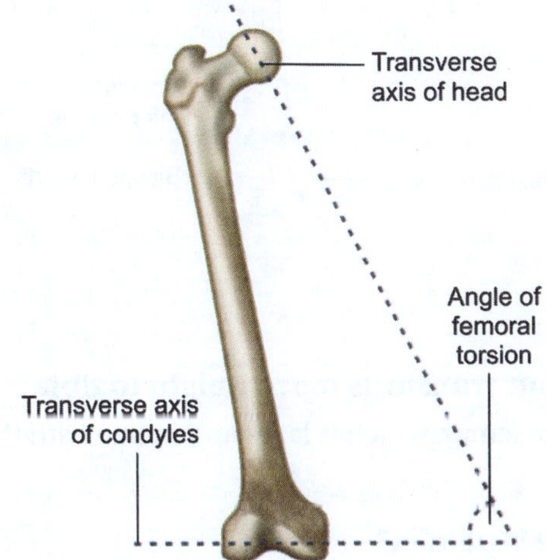

Q. What is attached to quadrate tubercle?

Ans. Quadratus femoris is attached to the quadrate tubercle.

Q. What is third trochanter?

Ans. Gluteal tuberosity when prominent is known as third trochanter.

Q. What is attached to adductor tubercle?

Ans. Adductor magnus is attached to adductor tubercle.

Q. What is the surgical importance of adductor tubercle?

Ans. The knee joint line passes through the adductor tubercle.

Q. What is the medicolegal importance of the lower end of femur?

Ans. In a dead fetus, if the ossification center is present on the lower end of femur it indicates that the child was alive at birth and one should suspect that it is an unnatural death. This is because ossification center for lower end of femur appears just before birth.

Q. Depict the attachments on linea aspera.

Ans.

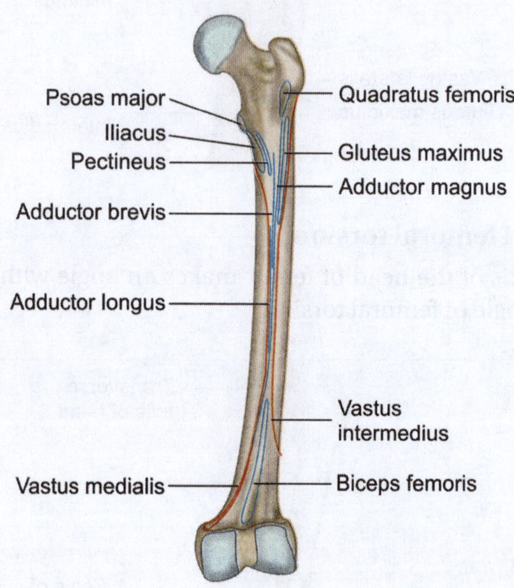

Q. Which part of femur transmits more weight to tibia?

Ans. The lateral condyle of femur, which is large and in line with the shaft of femur transmits more weight to tibia.

Q. What type of bone is patella?

Ans. Patella is a sesamoid bone, which develops in the tendon of quadriceps femoris.

Q. Depict the proximal articular surface of tibia.

Ans.

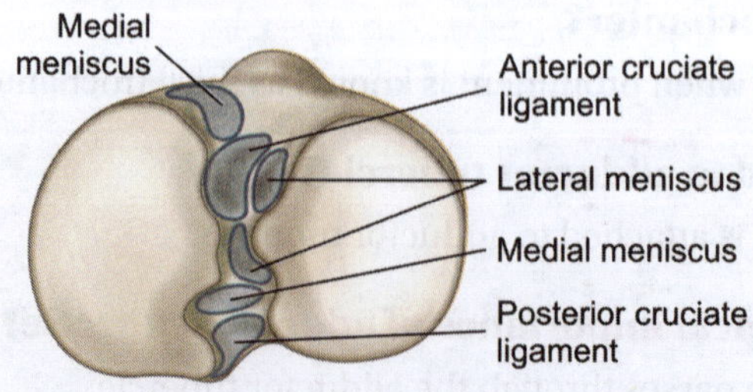

Mnemonic	Structure
"Medical	Medial meniscus anterior horn
College	Anterior **C**ruciate ligament
Lucknow	Anterior horn **L**ateral meniscus
Lucknow	Posterior horn **L**ateral meniscus
Medical	Posterior horn **M**edial meniscus
College"	Posterior **C**ruciate ligament.

Q. What is attached to the tibial tuberosity?

Ans. Proximally ligamentum patellae are attached to the smooth part and the distal rough part is related to the infrapatellar bursa.

Q. Which nerve is related to the head of fibula?

Ans. Common peroneal nerve winds around the head of fibula.

Q. What muscles are attached to talus bone?

Ans. No muscles are attached to the talus bone.

Q. Which tendon is related to sustentaculum tali?

Ans. The tendon of flexor hallucis longus is related to sustentaculum tali.

Q. What are the ligaments attached to sustentaculum tali?

Ans. Inferiorly the margins of the groove give attachment to the deep part of flexor retinaculum and to its medial margin plantar calcaneonavicular ligament, superficial fibers of deltoid ligament and talocalcaneal ligament are attached.

Q. What is attached to the navicular tuberosity?

Ans. The tibialis posterior muscle is attached to the navicular tuberosity.

Q. Compare carpal and tarsal bones.

Ans. Following are the differences between carpal and tarsal bones:

Criteria	Carpal	Tarsal
Size	Small	Large, bulky
Arrangement	Retained primitive pattern	Primitive pattern not maintained
Weight transmission	Function not present	Involved in weight transmission primarily
Rows	Proximal, distal	No defined rows Talus lies above Calcaneum behind

Q. What is fabella?

Ans. Fabella is a sesamoid bone developed in the lateral part of gastrocnemius tendon.

Short Notes

Contd...

Contd...

MISCELLANEOUS

- Femoral triangle
- Femoral sheath
- Adductor canal
- Foot drop
- Flexor retinaculum

- Popliteal fossa
- Deltoid ligament
- Spring ligament
- Cutaneous innervations
- Bursae around the knee joint

▶ MUSCLES

Q. PSOAS MAJOR

Psoas major is a long fusiform muscle extending from lumbar region to the upper thigh.

Attachments

Above

Anterior surfaces and lower border of all transverse process of lumbar vertebra and their adjacent bodies and intervertebral disks.

The muscle descends along the pelvic brim, behind the midpoint of inguinal ligament and in front of hip joint capsule.

Below

Along with iliacus gets attached to the lesser trochanter.

Relations in Lumbar Region

Above

Posterior to diaphragm, may be in contact with pleural sac.

Anteriorly

Kidney, psoas minor, renal vessels, ureter, gonadal vessels, genitofemoral nerve (right psoas related to inferior vena cava, left psoas to aorta).

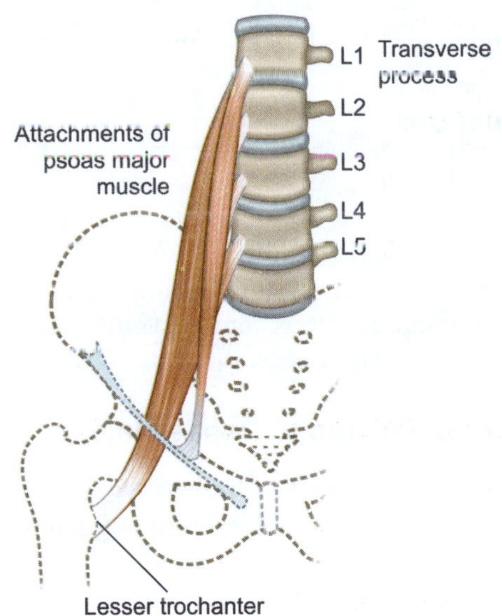

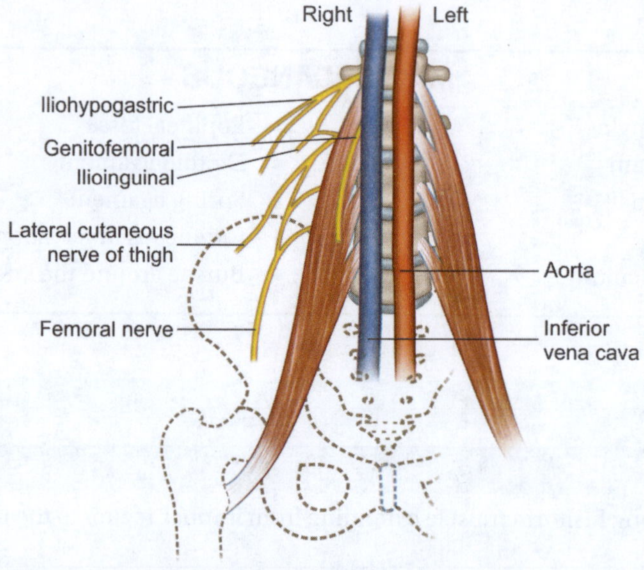

Lumbar plexus relation with psoas major

Posteriorly

Transverse process of lumbar vertebra and quadratus lumborum. The roots of lumbar plexus are within the muscle and branches emerge from its borders and surfaces.

Medial

Lumbar vertebral bodies, sympathetic chain.

Relations

In hip region:

- *Anteriorly:* Fascia lata, femoral artery
- *Posteriorly:* Hip joint
- *Medially:* Pectineus, medial circumflex femoral vessels, femoral vein
- *Laterally:* Iliacus.

Nerves Related to Psoas Major

- *Lateral border:* Iliohypogastric, ilio-inguinal, lateral femoral cutaneous, femoral
- *Anterolateral:* Genitofemoral nerve surface
- *Medial border:* Obturator, accessory obturator, upper root of lumbosacral trunk

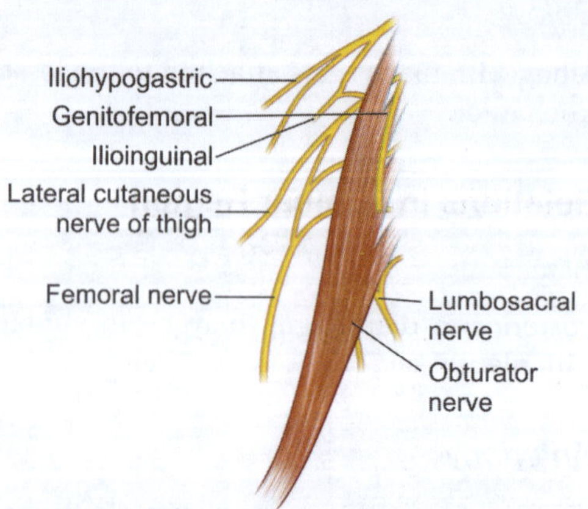

Nerves related to psoas major

Nerve Supply

Ventral rami of L1, L2, L3.

Action

Along with psoas it flexes the thigh on pelvis, helps in raising the trunk from lying position.

Applied Anatomy

In fracture neck of femur the limb is externally rotated and shortened, this is due to the action of psoas major, which acts as a lateral rotator.

Q. SARTORIUS

The muscle is also known as tailor's muscle. It extends in front of thigh diagonally.

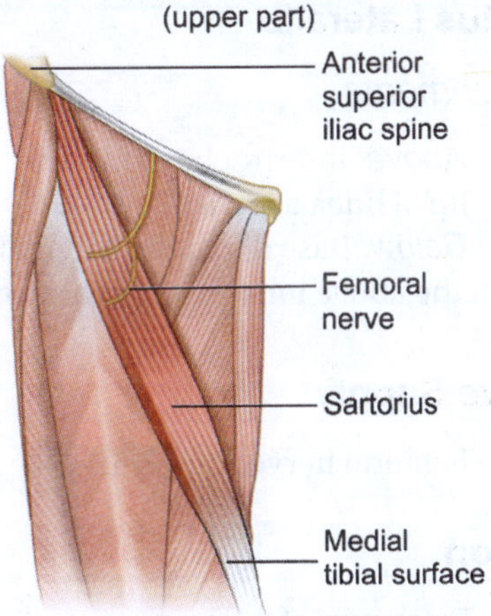

Sartorius muscle attachment

Attachments

- *Above:* Anterior superior iliac spine
- *Below:* Medial tibial surface.

Nerve Supply

Femoral nerve L2, L3.

Action

Flexing the leg at knee, flexing the thigh on pelvis (like sitting on the floor cross-legged).

Q. QUADRICEPS FEMORIS

As the name suggests it has four parts, rectus femoris, vastus medialis, vastus intermedius, vastus lateralis.

Rectus Femoris

Attachments

- *Above:* Anterior inferior iliac spine and few fibers from groove over acetabulum and fibrous capsule of hip joint
- *Below:* Base of patella.

Vastus Medialis

Attachments

- *Above:* Distal part of intertrochanteric line, spiral line, medial lip of linea aspera, medial supracondylar line, medial intermuscular septum
- *Below:* Medial border of patella.

Vastus Intermedius

Attachments

- *Above:* Most of the anterior and lateral surface of femoral shaft, lateral intermuscular septum
- *Below:* Lateral border of patella.

Vastus Lateralis

Attachments

- *Above:* Intertrochanteric line, greater trochanter, lateral lip of gluteal tuberosity, lateral lip of linea aspera
- *Below:* Base of patella, lateral border.

All the above muscles form a strong tendon and get attached to the patellar base.

Nerve Supply

- Femoral nerve, L2, L3, L4.

Action

- Extension of the knee.

Q. PECTINEUS

Pectineus is a hybrid muscle.

Attachments

- *Above:* Pecten pubis
- *Below:* Between lesser trochanter and linea aspera.

Nerve Supply

Femoral nerve, obturator nerve.

Action

Adduction of thigh assists in flexion of pelvis.

Q. GLUTEUS MAXIMUS

The bulk of buttock is formed by gluteus maximus.

Attachments

- *Above:* Posterior gluteal line and the area above it, few fibers from dorsal surface of sacrum, side of coccyx, sacrotuberous ligament, fascia over gluteus medius
- *Below:* Greater trochanter, gluteal tuberosity.

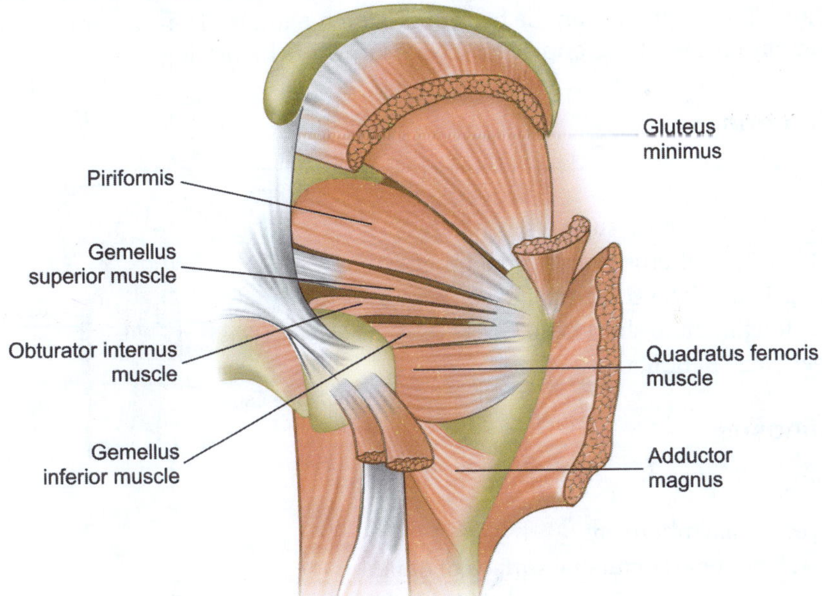

Muscles under the cover of gluteus maximus

Relations

Superficial

Adipose tissue.

Deep

- *Bones:* Ilium, sacrum, coccyx, ischial tuberosity, greater trochanter
- *Muscles:* Gluteus medius, piriformis, gemelli, obturator internus, quadratus femoris, biceps femoris, semitendinosus, semimembranosus, adductor magnus (all the muscles fan out below the cover of gluteus maximus)
- *Arteries:* Superior and inferior gluteal, internal pudendal, first perforating, medial circumflex femoral
- *Nerves:* Sciatic, pudendal, muscular branches from sacral plexus.

Nerve Supply

Inferior gluteal nerve L5, S1, S2.

Action

Extends the flexed thigh (helps in getting up from sitting position and while climbing stairs).

Q. HAMSTRINGS

String like muscles are present on the back of the thigh namely biceps femoris, semitendinosus, semimembranosus. This group of muscles is known as hamstrings.

Biceps Femoris

Attachments

- *Above:* As the name suggests it has two heads, ischial tuberosity gives attachment to long head, lateral lip of linea aspera gives attachment to short head
- *Below:* Head of fibula.

Semitendinosus

Attachments

- *Above:* Ischial tuberosity
- *Below:* Upper part of medial surface of tibia.

Semimembranosus

Attachments

- *Above:* Ischial tuberosity
- *Below:* Posteriorly in to the groove of medial condyle of tibia.

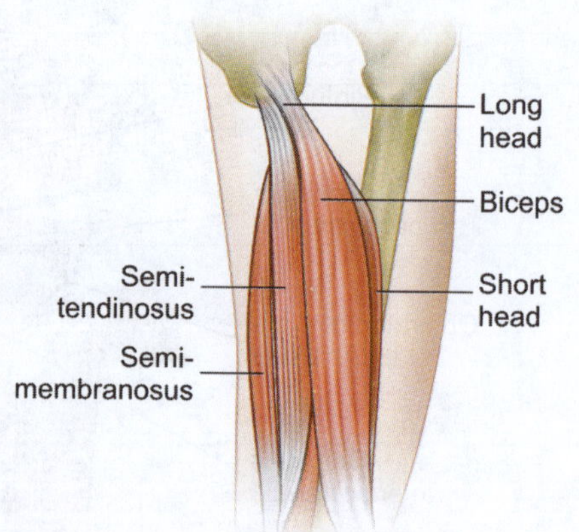

Nerve Supply

Tibial part of sciatic nerve. Short head of biceps supplied by common peroneal part of sciatic nerve.

Action

The group is the main flexor of the knee.

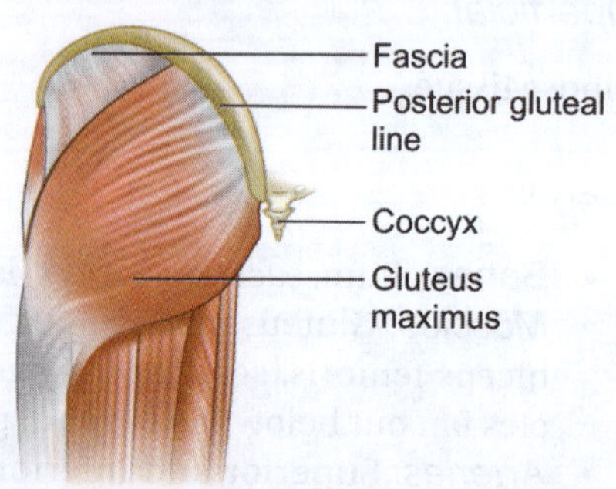

Q. TRICEPS SURAE

Gastrocnemius and soleus are together termed as triceps surae. They form the belly of the calf.

Gastrocnemius

Attachments

- *Above:* Medial head arises from an area behind adductor tubercle and above medial condyle of femur.
  Lateral head arise from area above lateral condyle.
- *Below:* Unites with tendon of soleus to form tendo calcaneus.

Soleus

Attachments

- *Above:* Posterior surface of fibula, soleal line and medial border of tibia, soleal arch
- *Below:* Unites with gastrocnemius to form tendo calcaneus.

Nerve Supply

Tibial nerve S1, S2.

Action

Plantar flexion. Plantaris muscle may sometimes be present with triceps surae to form tendo calcaneus.

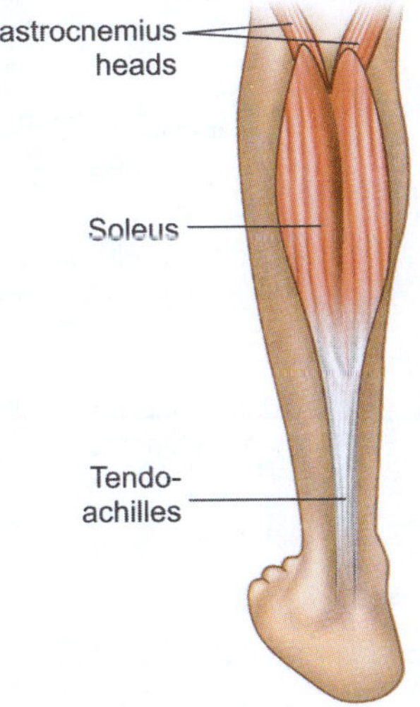

Q. ADDUCTOR HALLUCIS

Adductor hallucis has oblique and transverse heads.

Attachments

- Oblique head arises from 2nd, 3rd, 4th metatarsal base and sheath of peroneus longus tendon
- Oblique head has medial and lateral part:
  - Medial part joins flexor hallucis brevis and attached to lateral hallucial bone
  - Lateral part joins transverse head and attached to lateral hallucial bone and base of first hallucial phalanx.
- Transverse head arises from plantar metatarso phalangeal ligaments of 3rd, 4th, 5th toes and deep transverse metatarsal ligament.

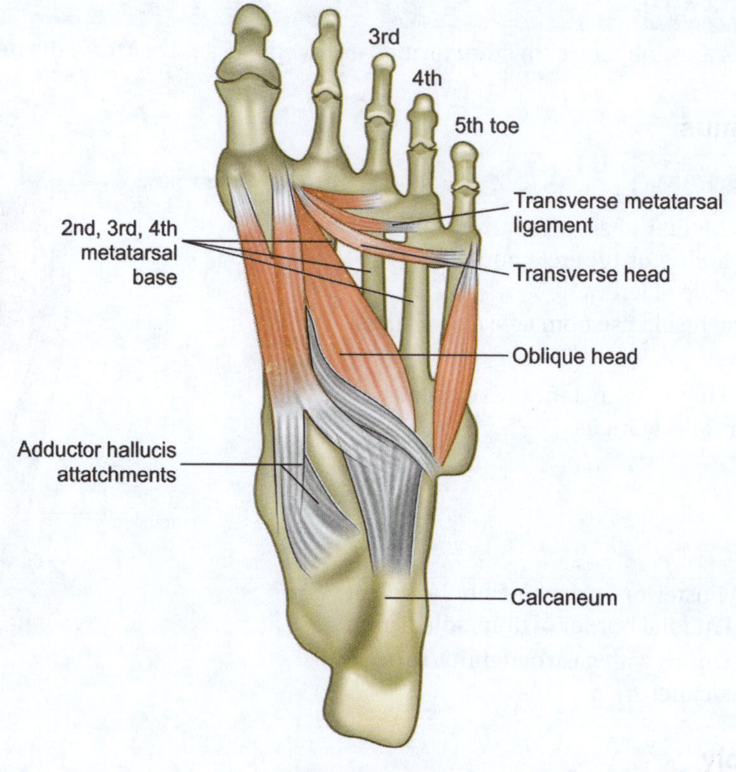

Adductor hallucis

Nerve Supply

Deep branch of lateral plantar nerve.

Action

- Adduction of greater toe
- Maintains transverse arch of foot.

Q. MUSCLE LAYERS OF THE FOOT

First Layer

- Abductor hallucis
- Abductor digiti minimi
- Flexor digitorum brevis (maintains concavity of the sole).

Second Layer

- Flexor digitorum accessorius

- Lumbricals
- Two tendons namely, flexor digitorum longus and flexor hallucis longus.

Third Layer

- Flexor hallucis brevis
- Adductor hallucis
- Flexor digiti minimi brevis.

Fourth Layer

- Dorsal interossei
- Plantar interossei
- Two tendons are tibialis posterior and peroneus longus.

▶ NERVES

Q. LUMBAR PLEXUS

The first three lumbar ventral rami and most of the fourth lumbar ventral rami form the lumbar plexus (L1, L2, L3, L4 ventral rami).

Location

Posterior to psoas major muscle and anterior to transverse process of lumbar vertebra.

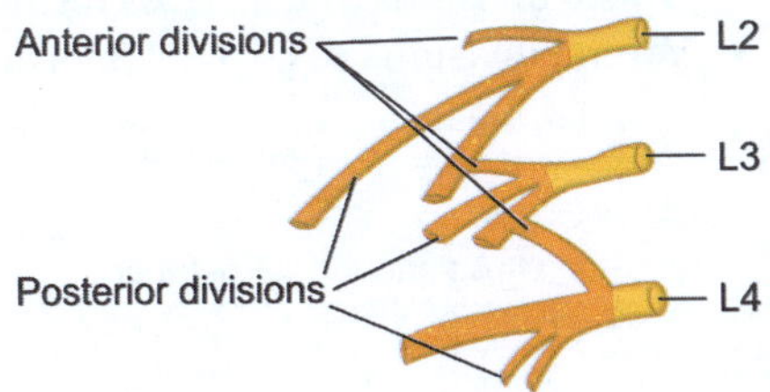

Formation

Ventral rami of L1, L2, L3, L4.

- L1:
  - Divides into upper and lower divisions
  - Upper division redivides into iliohypogastric and ilioinguinal nerves
  - Lower division joins small anterior division of L2 to form genitofemoral nerve.
    Note: L2, L3, L4 each divide into anterior and posterior divisions.
- L2:
  - Anterior and posterior divisions redivide into small and large branches
  - Small anterior division joins with a branch of L1 to form genitofemoral nerve

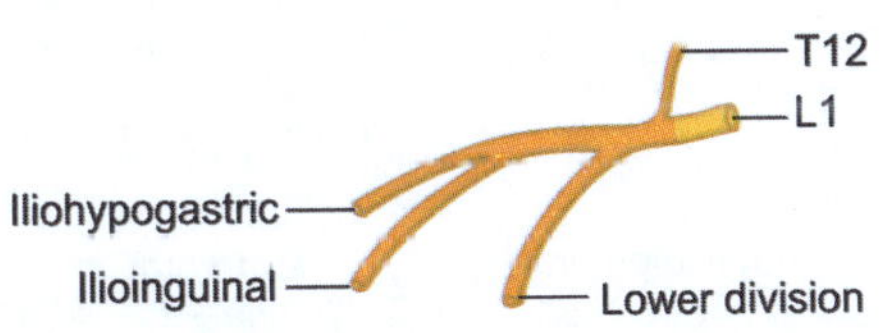

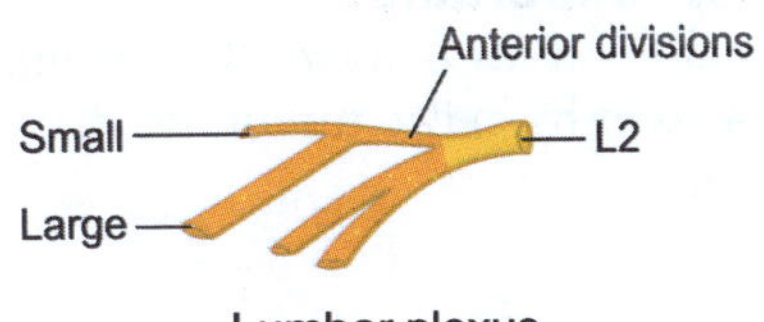

Lumbar plexus

- Large anterior division joins L3 and L4 anterior division to form obturator nerve
- Small posterior division of L2 joins the small posterior division of L3 to form lateral cutaneous nerve of thigh
- Large posterior division of L2 joins large posterior divisions of L3 and L4 to form femoral nerve.
- **L3:**
  - Anterior division of L2 joins anterior divisions of L3 and L4 to form obturator nerve
  - Large posterior division of L2 joins large posterior divisions of L3 and L4 to form femoral nerve.
- **L4:**
  - Anterior division contributes to form obturator nerve
  - Posterior division contributes to form femoral nerve.
- Genitofemoral nerve is formed by union of small anterior divisions of L1, L2 nerve
- Dorsal divisions of L1, L2, L3 form femoral nerve
- Ventral divisions of L1, L2, L3 form obturator nerve.

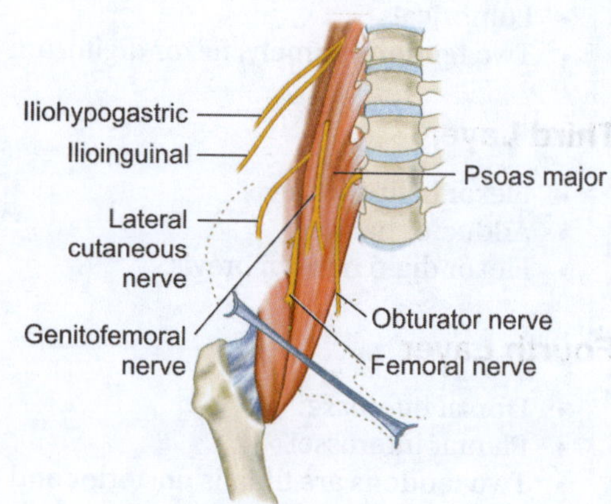

Branches of lumbar plexus

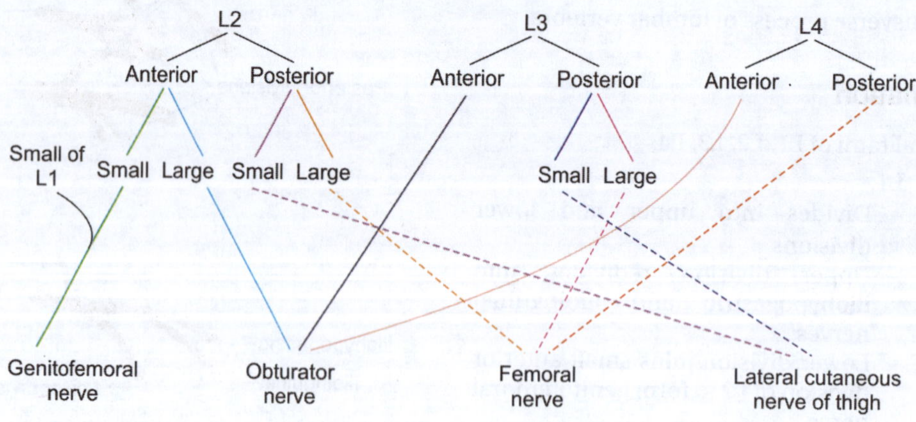

Flow chart of lumbar plexus

Clinical Importance

The major nerves of lower limb begin from lumbar plexus. The lumbosacral trunk may get compressed by pelvic tumors or during pregnancy by fetal head causing severe pain in the lower limb.

Q. FEMORAL NERVE

Femoral nerve is one of the major nerves of lower limb.

Formation

Dorsal branches of ventral rami of L2, L3, L4.

Course and Relations

- The nerve enters the thigh by passing behind the inguinal ligament
- The nerve emerges from lateral border of psoas major in its lower part
- The nerve descends between psoas major and iliacus muscle
- The nerve lies lateral to femoral artery in femoral triangle
- The nerve ends by dividing into anterior and posterior divisions.

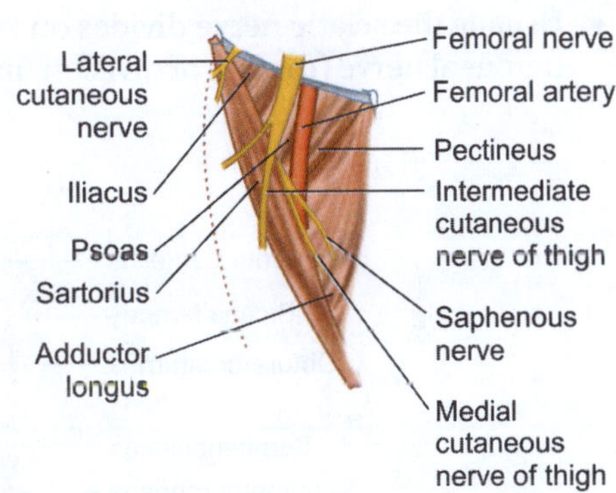

Femoral nerve course and relations in thigh

Branches

Chief branches can be conveniently divided into cutaneous, muscular, vascular and articular.

Anterior division gives fibers to intermediate and medial cutaneous nerve of thigh and a branch to sartorius. Posterior division gives fibers to saphenous nerve and branches to quadriceps femoris and knee joint.

Clinical Importance

The femoral nerve may sometimes get compressed behind the inguinal ligament leading to paralysis of quadriceps femoris and sensory loss on most of the front of the thigh.

Q. SCIATIC NERVE

Sciatic nerve is thickest nerve in the body around 2 cm broad.

Formation

- Ventral rami of L4 (partly), L5 (lumbosacral trunk)
- Ventral rami of S1, S2, S3.

Course and Relations

In pelvis: It lies below levator ani:

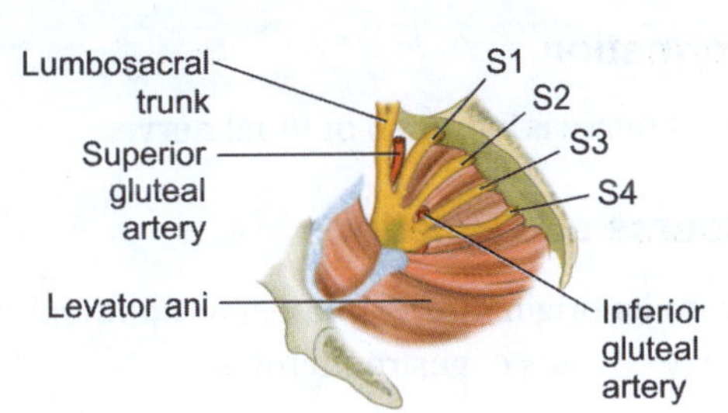

- The nerve leaves the pelvis through greater sciatic foramen and is detected below piriformis on back of thigh
- It runs on the back of thigh between hamstrings and obturator internus with gemelli, quadratus femoris with adductor magnus
- It is medially related to posterior femoral cutaneous nerve and inferior gluteal artery
- Usually the sciatic nerve divides on lower part of back of thigh into tibial and common peroneal nerve (the site of division may be variable).

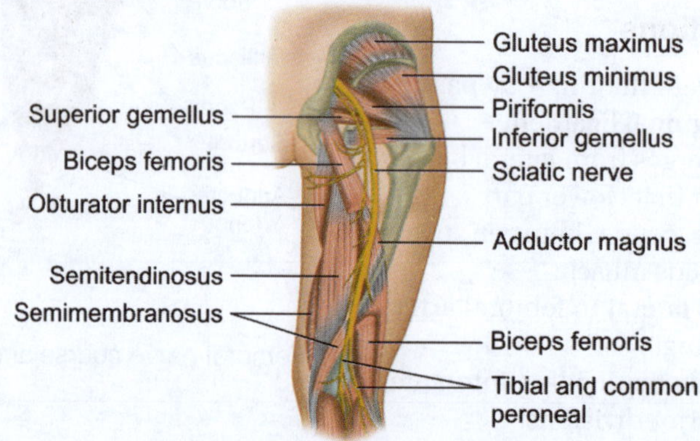

Sciatic nerve on back of thigh

Branches

- Terminal branches are tibial and common peroneal nerve
- Muscular branches to hamstrings (biceps femoris, semitendinosus, semimembranosus) and ischial part of adductor magnus
- Articular branches to hip joint.

Clinical Importance

The nerve may get injured in posterior dislocations or fracture of hip joint in which case, muscles distal to the knee and cutaneous sensation is lost (except the area around saphenous nerve).

Q. SURAL NERVE

Formation

Sural nerve is a branch of tibial nerve.

Course and Relations

From its origin approximately in popliteal fossa the nerve runs down on back of leg between the two heads of gastrocnemius.

It pierces the deep fascia in the upper part of leg to become superficial and then join sural communicating branch of common peroneal nerve.

It runs down to lie lateral to tendocalcaneus and then between lateral malleolus and calcaneum. The nerve during this course is closely related to small saphenous vein.

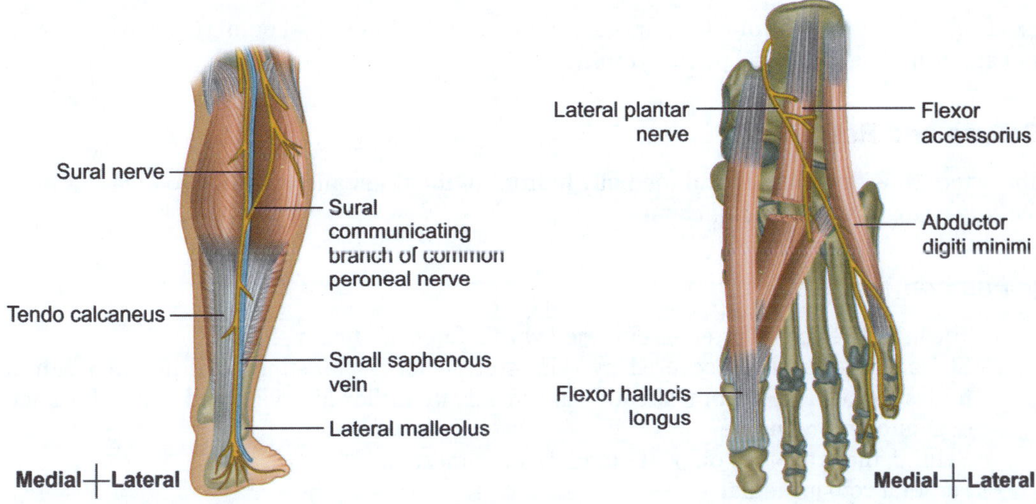

Connections

Sural nerve joins superficial peroneal nerve on dorsum of foot and in the leg it joins the posterior femoral cutaneous nerve.

Branches

Cutaneous branches supply posterior and lateral part of distal leg, lateral border of the foot and little toe.

Clinical Importance

Damage to the nerve may occasionally occur during venesection leading to loss of sensation on lower part of back of leg and lateral part of sole causing pressure sores.

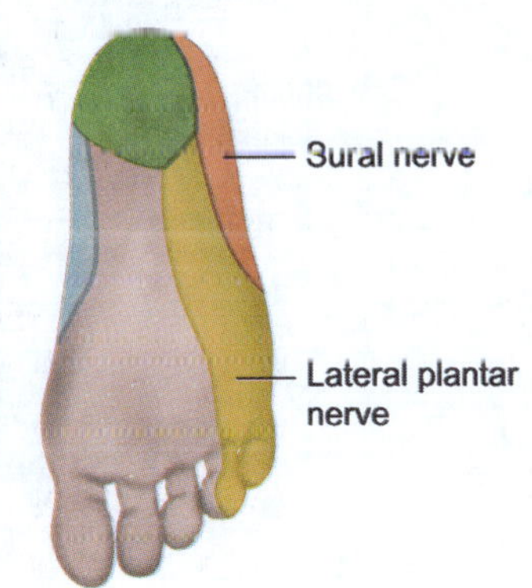

Q. FEMORAL ARTERY

Origin

External iliac artery continues as femoral artery behind midinguinal point (i.e. between anterior superior iliac spine and pubic symphysis).

Course and Relations

The artery runs downwards and medially in front of the thigh and crosses two areas namely, femoral triangle and adductor canal.

In Femoral Triangle

- The initial 3–4 cm of artery is enclosed within femoral sheath
- In front, the artery is covered by skin, superficial fascia, superficial inguinal lymph nodes, fascia lata, femoral sheath, superficial circumflex iliac vein and femoral branch of genitofemoral nerve
- Behind, the artery lies on psoas tendon, femoral sheath
- Femoral vein is medial
- Femoral nerve is lateral.

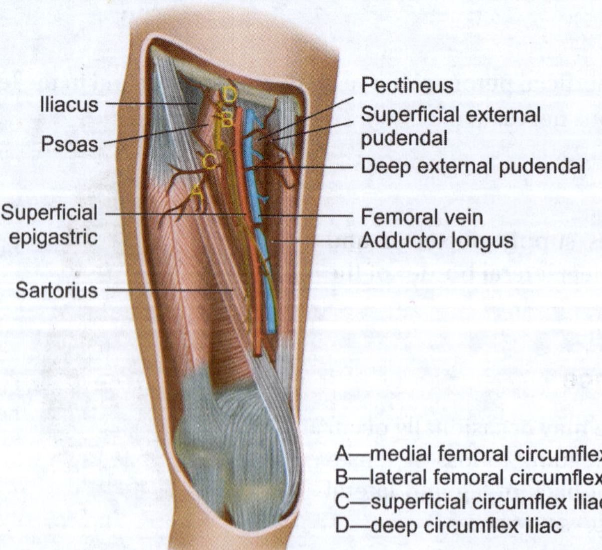

In Adductor Canal

The artery lies under the cover of skin, fascia and sartorius muscle. The saphenous nerve crosses the artery from lateral to medial side. The artery lies on adductor longus magnus.

Branches

Branches of femoral artery can be classified into superficial and deep.

Superficial branches

- Superficial epigastric
- Superficial circumflex iliac
- Superficial external pudendal

Deep branches

- Deep external pudendal
- Muscular
- Arteria profunda femoris

Clinical Importance

In comatosed patient arterial blood is withdrawn from femoral artery for blood gas analysis.

Q. ARTERIA PROFUNDA FEMORIS

Origin

Arteria profunda femoris is a deep branch of femoral artery.

Course and Relations

- It arises from the lateral side of femoral artery and then winds posteriorly to lie between femoral artery and vein medially
- It descends down between pectineus and adductor muscles
- It ends by piercing the adductor magnus and anastomoses with muscular branches of popliteal artery.

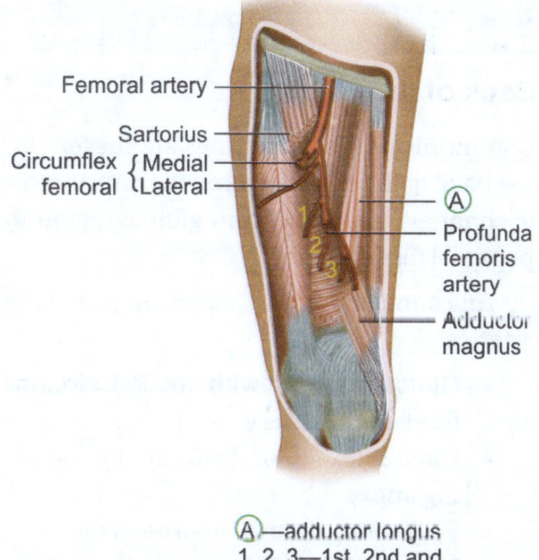

Branches

- Lateral circumflex femoral
- Medial circumflex femoral
- Perforating arteries
- Muscular branches.

Clinical Importance

If femoral artery is ligated proximal to origin of profunda femoris a collateral circulation develops between the branches of internal iliac artery and profunda femoris artery.

Q. POPLITEAL ARTERY

Origin

The artery is the continuation of femoral artery in popliteal fossa.

Course and Relations

Above from opening in adductor magnus the artery runs downwards and laterally toward inter condylar fossa. The artery tilts laterally on back of knee and divides at the lower border of popliteus muscle into anterior and posterior tibial arteries.

Branches

- Cutaneous
- Muscular
- Genicular.

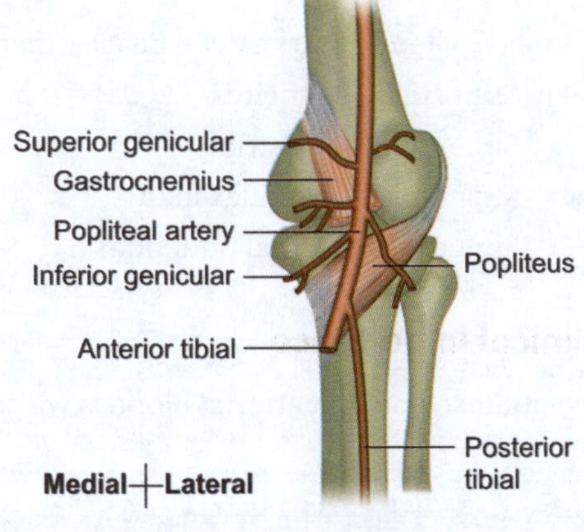

Branches of popliteal artery

Clinical Importance

By virtue of the anastomoses between the branches of the artery a collateral circulation develops in case of blockage in the popliteal artery due to thrombosis.

Q. ANASTOMOSIS

Back of the Thigh

Communicating arterial rings are present on the back of the thigh forming the anastomotic channels extending from gluteal region to popliteal fossa.

Anastomoses exists between following arteries:

- Gluteal arteries with medial circumflex femoral artery
- Circumflex femoral with first perforating artery
- Perforating arteries with each other
- Fourth perforating artery with muscular branches of popliteal artery.

Genicular

This anastomoses exists around the condyles of tibia and femur, and around patella.

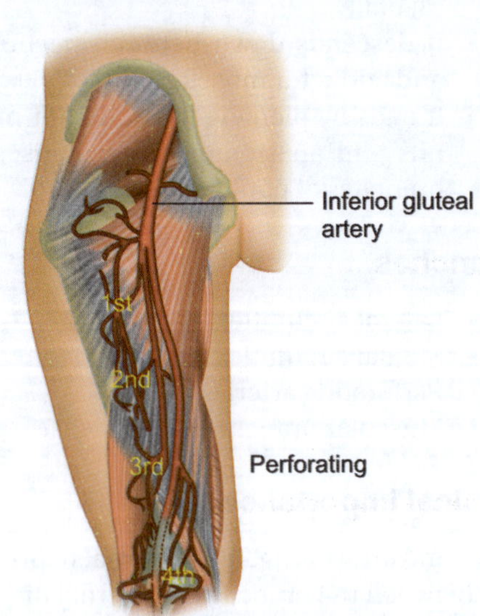

Anastomosis on back of thigh

Superficial anastomosis exists around the skin and superficial fascia in the region of patella and within the fat, deep to ligamentum patellae.

Deep anastomoses exists around the articular surfaces of tibia and femur.

The arteries involved are as follows:

- Medial, lateral, descending genicular
- Lateral circumflex femoral
- Anterior and posterior tibial recurrent.

Clinical Importance

Block in any of the major artery is overcome by the collateral circulation, which develops in the anastomoses.

▶ VEINS

Q. FEMORAL VEIN

Extent

Popliteal vein continues as femoral vein at the level of opening in adductor magnus and ends behind the inguinal ligament to continue as external iliac vein.

Relations

- In the beginning of adductor canal vein lies posterolateral to femoral artery
- Little above and in lower part of femoral triangle the vein lies posterior to femoral artery
- While toward the base of femoral triangle the vein lies medial to femoral artery.

Tributaries

- Several muscular veins
- Vena profunda femoris
- Great saphenous vein
- Circumflex femoral veins.

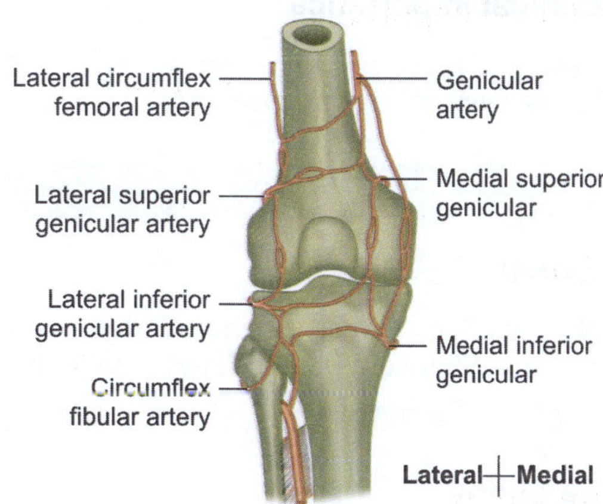

Genicular anastomosis

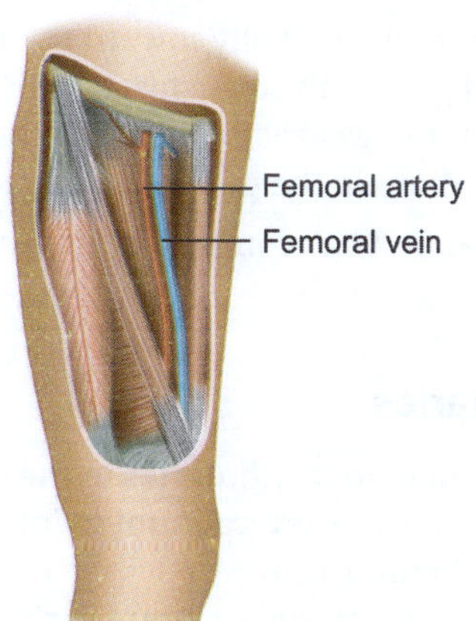

Femoral triangle

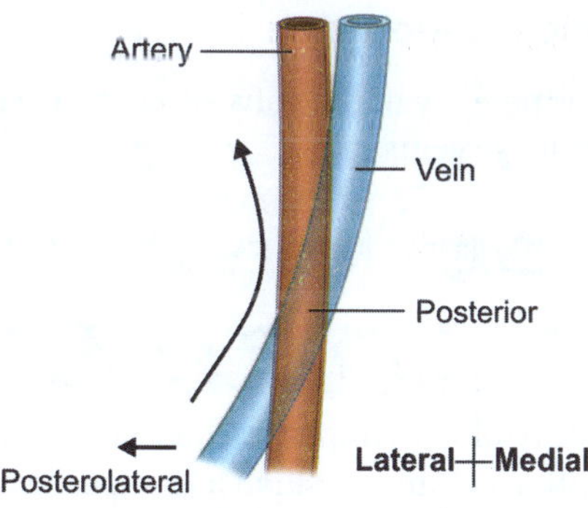

Femoral vein and artery relation

Clinical Importance

In case of incompetence of valves within the femoral vein there may be backflow of venous blood giving rise to varicose veins.

Q. SHORT SAPHENOUS VEIN

Extent

Short saphenous vein is a continuation of lateral marginal vein behind lateral malleolus and ends in popliteal vein.

Relations

In the lower part of the leg the vein lies lateral to tendo calcaneus just below the skin and superficial fascia.

It ascends medially toward the middle of calf and pierces the deep fascia to lie between two heads of gastrocnemius muscle, where it ends to drain in the popliteal vein.

Sural nerve accompanies the vein on the back of leg.

Tributaries

- Cutaneous tributaries in the leg
- Gives out several rami to join great saphenous vein
- Communicating branch to accessory saphenous vein.

There may be 7–13 valves in the vein and one at its termination.

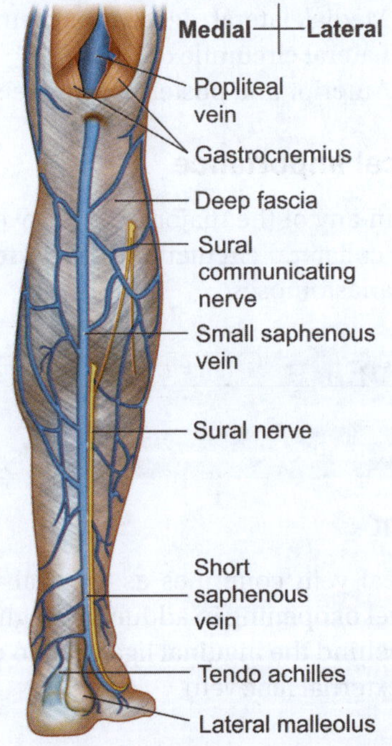

Course of short saphenous vein

Clinical Importance

Incompetency of the valves may cause reversal of flow of venous blood leading to formation of varicose veins.

▶ LYMPH NODES

Q. INGUINAL NODES

Majority of the lymphatic fluid of the lower limb drains into the inguinal nodes. The inguinal lymph nodes are classified into superficial and deep with relation to the deep fascia of the thigh.

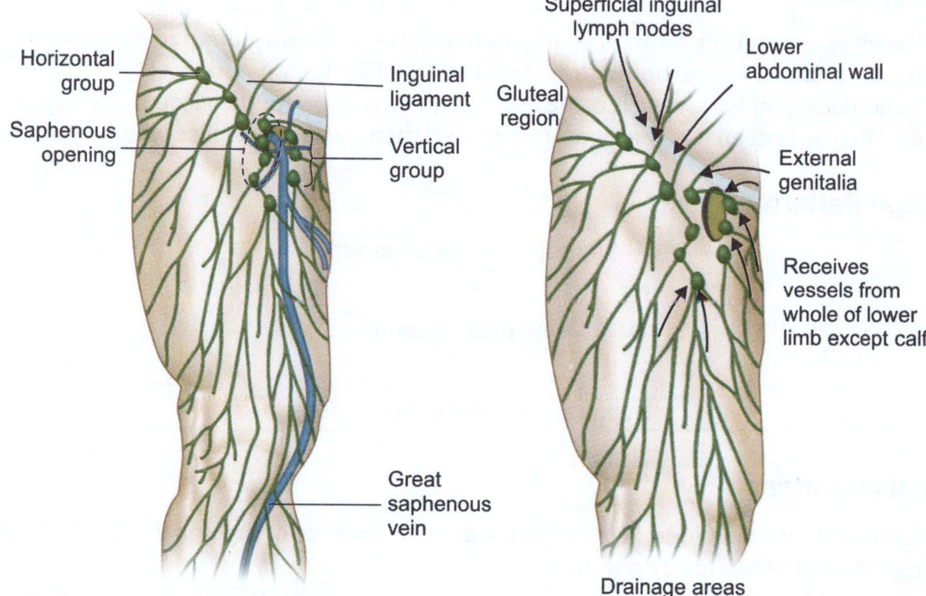

Superficial Inguinal Lymph Nodes

- These nodes are arranged into proximal horizontal group and distal vertical group
- The horizontal group lies under the inguinal ligament and are around five to six in number
- The vertical group lies along the termination of great saphenous vein and are around four to five in number.

Drainage Area

Proximal group medially receives lymph from external genitalia (except glans penis or clitoris), anal canal and area around it, lower part of anterior abdominal wall and round ligament.

Proximal group laterally receives lymph from gluteal and lower part of anterior abdominal wall. Distal vertical group receives lymph through superficial vessels from whole of the lower limb except calf.

Deep Inguinal Lymph Nodes

Located medial to femoral vein. They are three in number, one is close to saphenofemoral junction, another is in the femoral canal and one is close to the femoral ring.

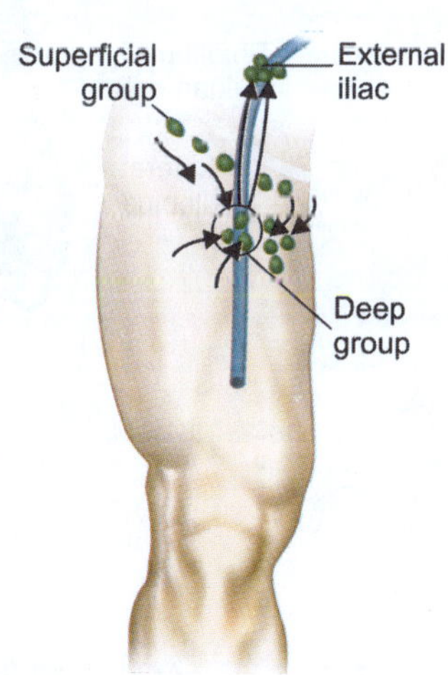

Deep inguinal lymph nodes

Drainage Area

- Receives lymph from superficial inguinal lymph nodes and glans penis or clitoris
- All the inguinal lymph nodes drain into external iliac lymph nodes
- Superficial lymphatic vessels of the lower limb drain into superficial inguinal lymph nodes and then into deep inguinal lymph nodes and then into external iliac lymph nodes.

Drainage Pattern

Superficial inguinal group

↓

Deep inguinal group

↓

Deep external iliac lymph nodes

Clinical Importance

Any lesion like pus collection or cancer in the area of drainage of inguinal lymph nodes leads to enlargement of respective lymph nodes.

▶ JOINTS

Q. ANKLE JOINT

Type: Hinge joint, uniaxial joint, synovial joint.

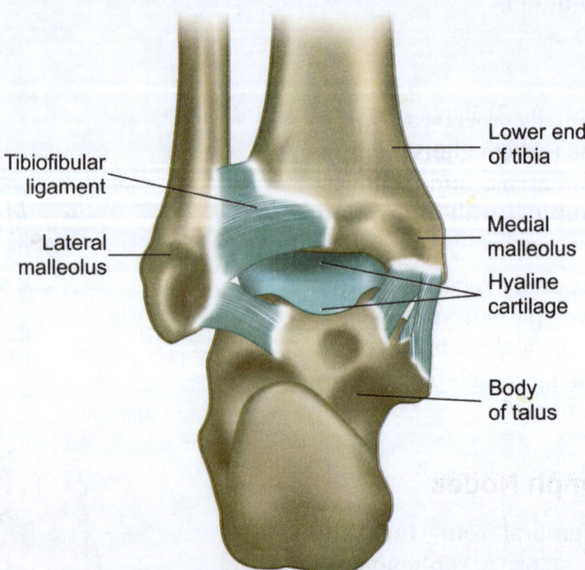

Ankle joint (articular surfaces and ligaments)

Articular Surfaces

Above

- Lower end of tibia, medial malleolus, lateral malleolus of fibula, transverse tibiofibular ligament (all these structures form a socket above).

Below

Body of talus.

Note: Articular surfaces are covered by hyaline cartilage.

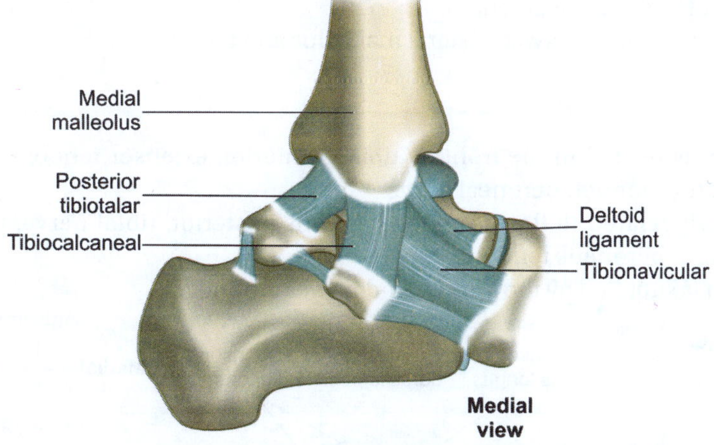

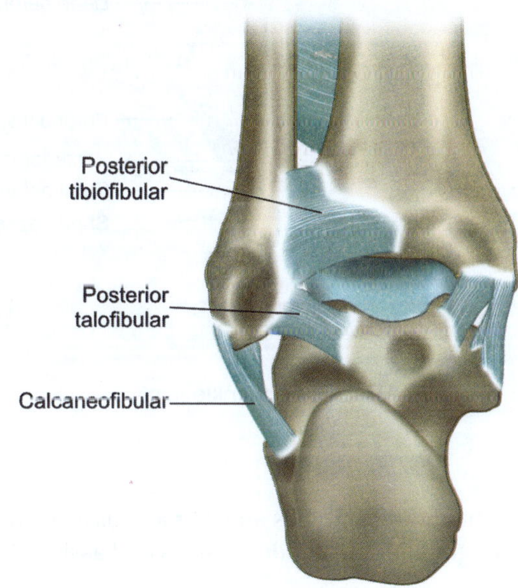

Ankle joint ligaments

Ligaments

Connects the articular surfaces:

- Fibrous capsule:
  - It is thin capsule connecting the articular surfaces
  - The ligaments strengthen the capsule.
- Medial ligament: Deltoid ligament (discussed later):
  - It is a tough triangular band of ligament extending between medial malleolus and calcaneum and talus.
- Anterior talofibular ligament:
  - Extends anteromedially from malleolus of fibula to talus.
- Posterior talofibular ligament:
  - Run horizontally between lateral malleolus and talus.

Relations

- The joint is related in the front by tibialis anterior, extensor tendons, anterior tibial vessels and common peroneal nerve
- Posteriorly related to flexor tendons, tibialis posterior, tibial nerve, posterior tibial vessels and peroneus tendons
- The joint is supplied by the arteries and nerves around it.

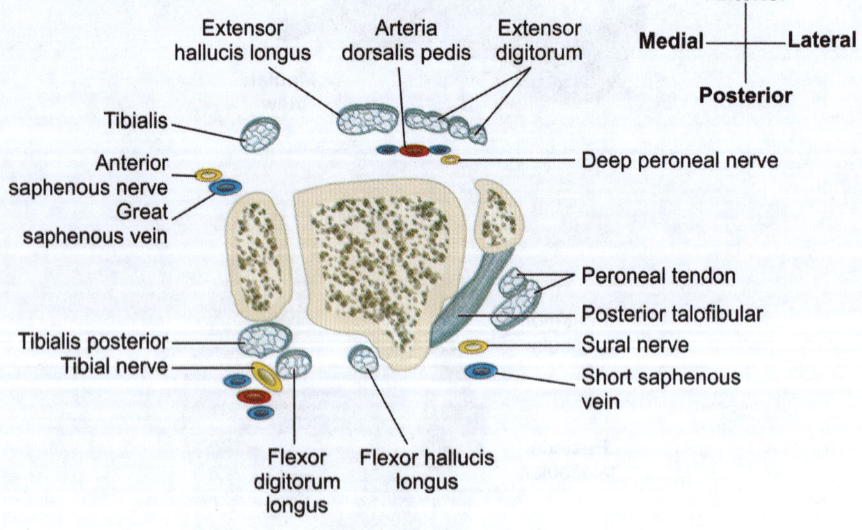

Relations of ankle joint

Movements

- Dorsiflexion is brought about by tibialis anterior and assisted by extensors of the leg
- Plantar flexion is brought about by tendo Achilles and assisted by flexors of the leg.

Clinical Importance

The joint is rarely dislocated because of the structure of articular surfaces. Few fibers of medial ligament may get torn due to sudden movements of foot leading to sprain.

Q. SUBTALAR JOINTS

Definition

The anterior and posterior talocalcaneal joints are termed as subtalar joints.

Type

Synovial, multiaxial joint.

Articular Surface

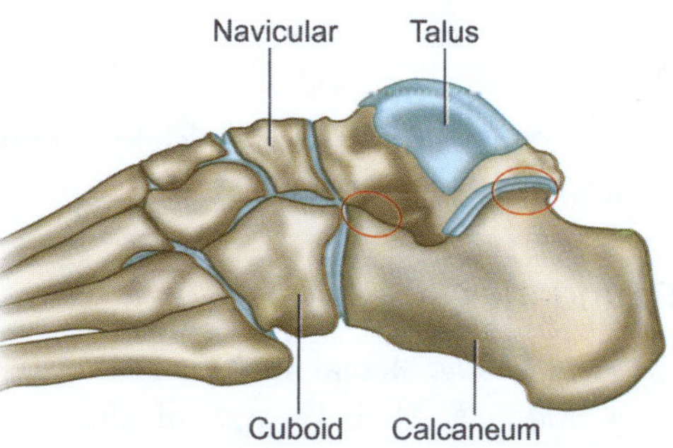

- *Above:* Concave inferior surface of talus
- *Below:* Convex superior surface of calcaneum.

Ligaments

Connects the articular surface:

- Fibrous capsule
- Lateral, medial and interosseous talocalcaneal ligaments connect the respective sides of articular surfaces
- Cervical ligament connects the area next to sinus tarsi to superior calcaneal surface.

Movements

- Inversion is brought about by tibialis anterior and posterior
- Eversion is brought about by peroneus longus and brevis.

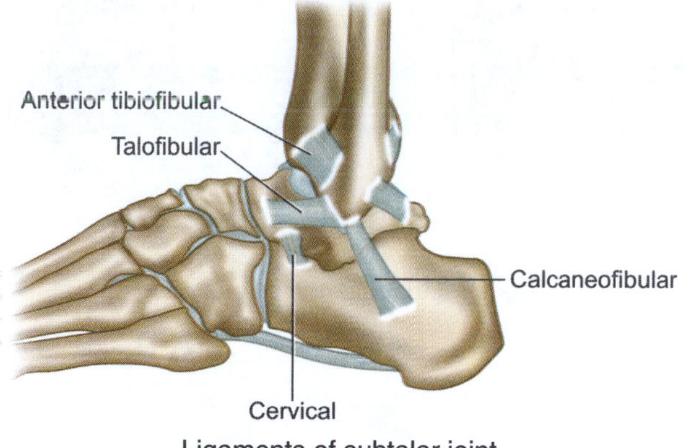

Ligaments of subtalar joint

Clinical Importance

While walking on uneven surface a sudden movement can lead to injury to ligament causing sprain.

▶ MISCELLANEOUS

Q. FEMORAL TRIANGLE

Femoral triangle is also known as Scarpa's triangle. It is marked by a hollow under the inguinal fold.

Roof

Skin, superficial fascia, superficial inguinal lymph nodes, cutaneous nerves and superficial vessels.

Boundaries

- *Laterally:* Medial margin of sartorius
- *Medially:* Medial margin of adductor longus
- *Base:* Inguinal ligament.

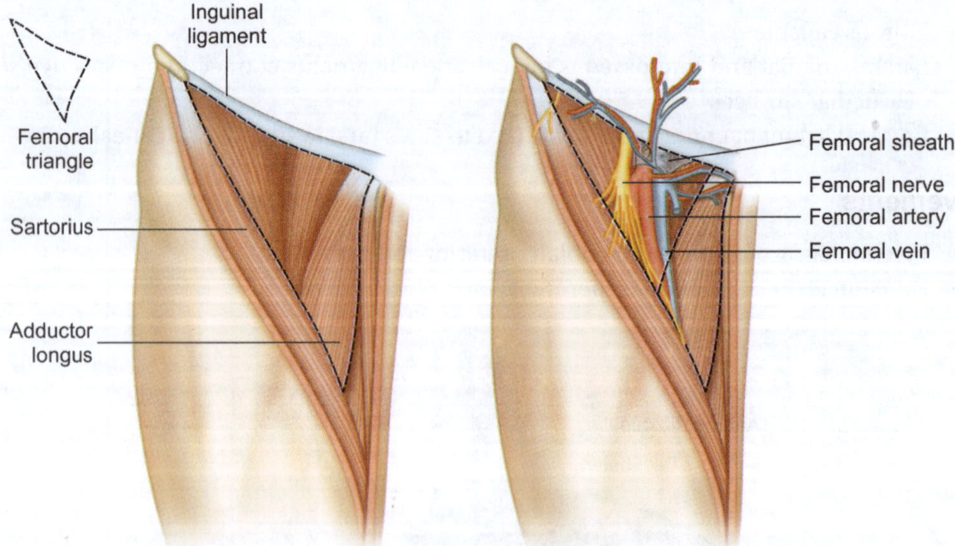

Femoral triangle and its contents

Floor

Following muscles from lateral to medial side form the floor:

- Iliacus
- Psoas major
- Pectineus
- Adductor longus.

Contents

Femoral artery, femoral vein, femoral nerve, inguinal lymph nodes and fat.

Q. FEMORAL SHEATH

Like the half-sleeves of apron the proximal part of femoral vessels is covered by connective tissue known as femoral sheath (like carotid sheath):

- Anteriorly it is the extension of transversalis fascia
- Posteriorly it is the extension of fascia iliaca.

Contents

There are three compartments namely lateral for femoral artery, middle compartment for femoral vein and medial compartment for deep inguinal lymph nodes.

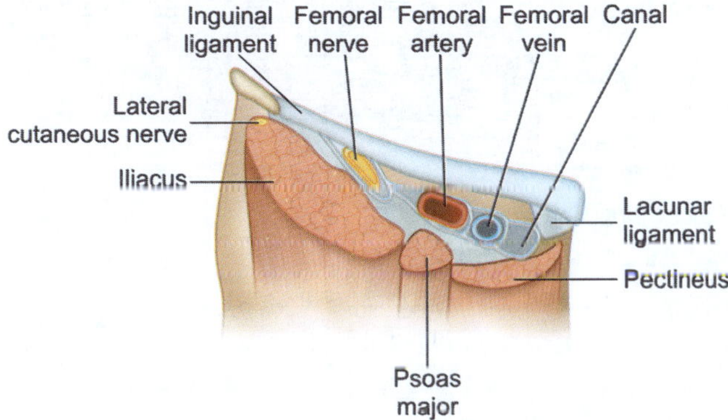

Contents of femoral sheath

The medial compartment known as femoral canal. The proximal end of the canal is thickened to form femoral ring. The femoral ring is bounded anteriorly by inguinal ligament, posteriorly by pectineus, medially by lacunar ligament and laterally by femoral vein.

Q. ADDUCTOR CANAL

Adductor canal is also known as subsartorial canal and proper name is Hunter's canal. It occupies medial side of the thigh in its middle third and is an aponeurotic tunnel.

Extent

Adductor canal extends from apex of the femoral triangle to the opening in the adductor magnus.

Boundaries

Canal is triangular in section:

- Anterolaterally:
  - Vastus medialis.
- Posteriorly:
  - Adductor longus proximally
  - Adductor magnus distally.

- Anteromedially:
  - Sartorius, aponeurosis extending between adductors and vastus medialis.
- Anteriorly sartorius.

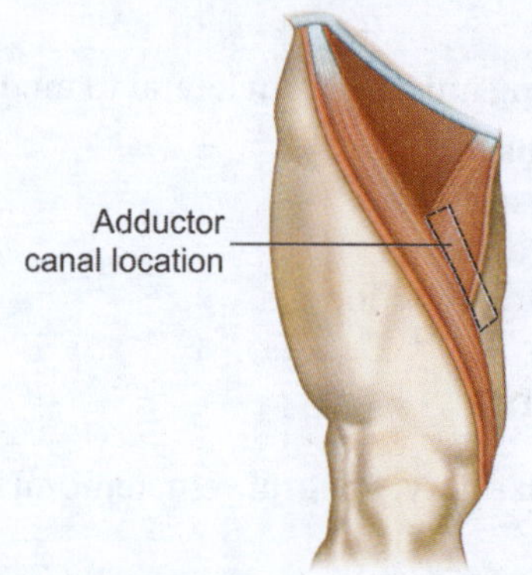

Adductor canal location

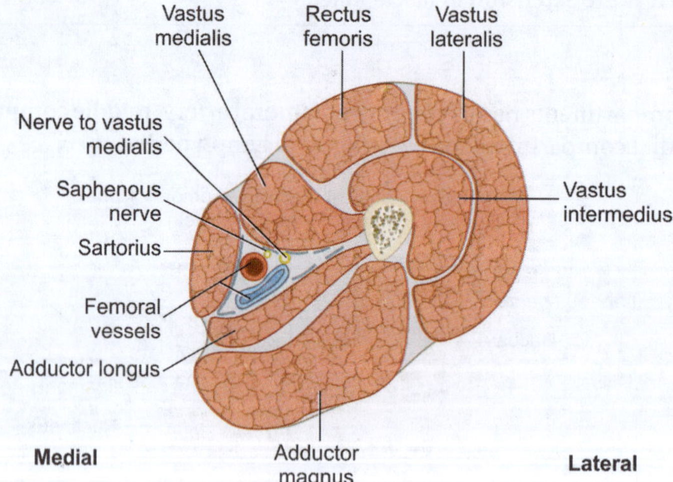

Contents

- Femoral artery
- Femoral vein
- Saphenous nerve
- Nerve to vastus medialis.

Clinical Importance

Femoral artery can be approached in adductor canal for ligation in cases of any aneurysm, thrombosis.

Q. FOOT DROP

The common peroneal nerve is very susceptible to injury due to its superficial location around neck of fibula.

Mode of Injury

Fracture of fibula or pressure on the nerve.

Consequence of Injury

Injury to the nerve leads to paralysis of dorsiflexors and evertors, i.e. tibialis anterior, extensors of leg and peroneal muscles leading to loss of dorsiflexion. Loss of sensation on dorsum of foot and on outer surface of front of leg.

Attitude of Limb

The ankle is plantar flexed, adducted and inverted. However second and third phalanx may be extended by interossei, which is supplied by tibial nerve.

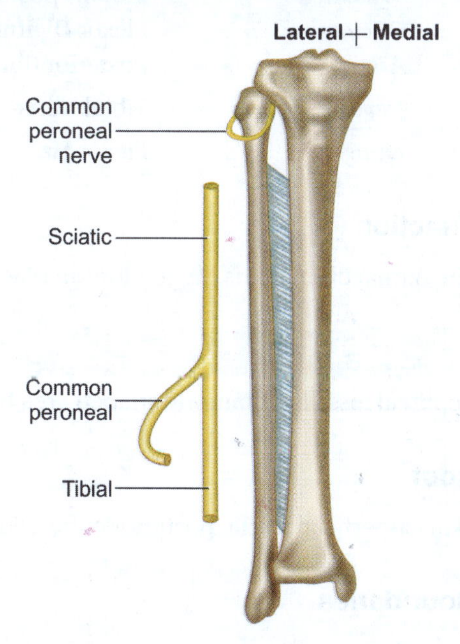

Q. FLEXOR RETINACULUM

Attachments

- Anteriorly—tip of medial malleolus
- Posteriorly—medial calcaneal process
- Structures under the cover of flexor retinaculum from medial to lateral.

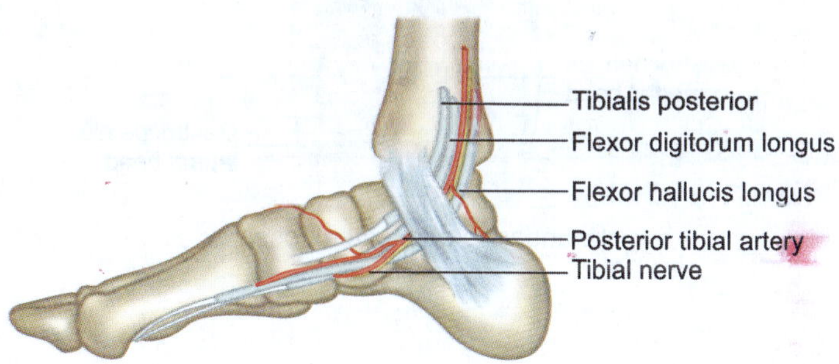

Structures deep to flexor retinaculum

Mnemonic	Structures
"Talented	Tibialis posterior
Doctors	Flexor **D**igitorum longus
ARe	Posterior tibial **AR**tery and vein
Never	Tibial **N**erve
Hungry"	Flexor **H**allucis longus

Function

The retinaculum holds the tendons in place (like logs of wood tied together).

Q. POPLITEAL FOSSA

Popliteal fossa is a diamond shaped area behind the knee joint.

Roof

Skin, superficial fascia, posterior cutaneous nerve of thigh, short saphenous vein.

Boundaries

- *Lateral and above:* Biceps femoris
- *Lateral and below:* Lateral head of gastrocnemius, plantaris
- *Medial and above:* Semitendinosus, semimembranosus
- *Medial and below:* Medial head of gastrocnemius.

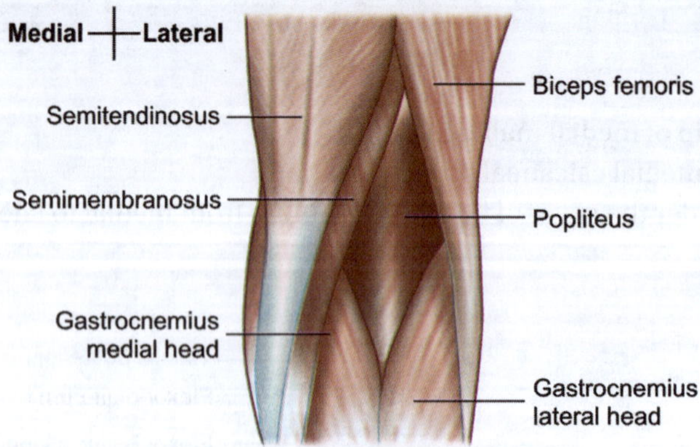

Boundaries of popliteal fossa

Floor

- Femoral popliteal surface
- Oblique popliteal ligament
- Popliteus muscle with its fascia.

Contents

Superficial

Fat, lymph nodes, posterior cutaneous nerve of thigh, articular branch of obturator nerve.

Deep

- Popliteal artery and vein
- Tibial nerve and common peroneal nerve.

Note: The tibial nerve is most superficial, vein is just below it and popliteal artery is the deepest.

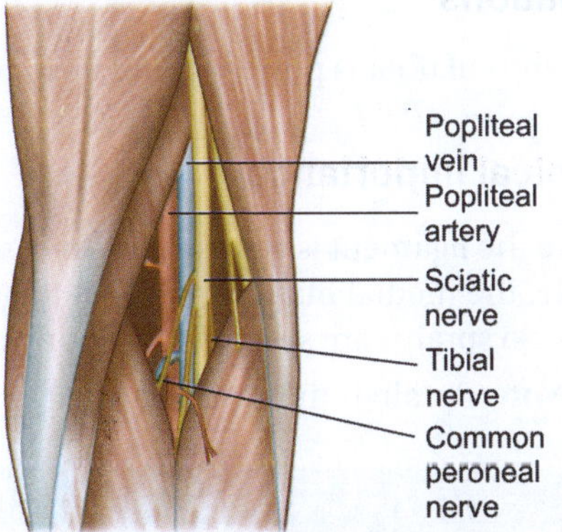

Contents of popliteal fossa

Q. DELTOID LIGAMENT

- Deltoid ligament is a medial collateral ligament of ankle joint
- It consists of superficial and deep fibers and is very tough.

Attachments

Deltoid ligament is attached to apex and anterior, and posterior borders of medial malleolus.

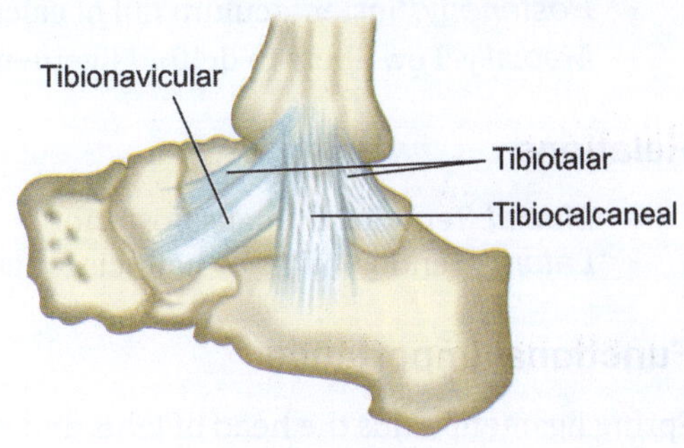

Deltoid ligament

Superficial Fibers

- Anterior tibionavicular fibers
- Intermediate vertical tibiocalcaneal fibers, which reach sustentaculum tali
- Posterior tibiotalar.

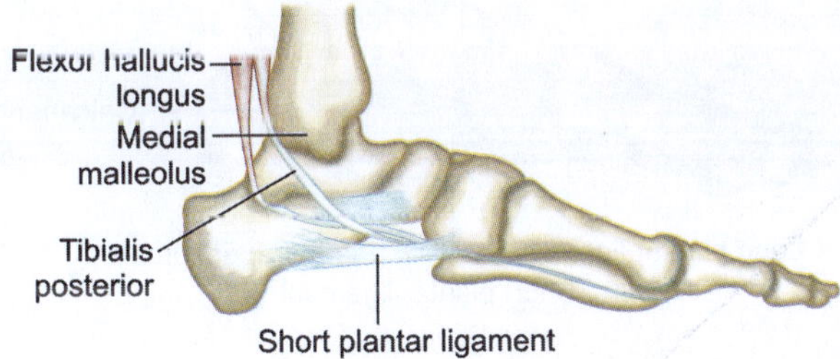

Deep Fibers

- Anterior tibiotalar.

Relations

Tendons of tibialis posterior and flexor digitorum longus cross the ligament.

Clinical Importance

Since the ligament is very strong, in case of sudden movement or injury on the medial side of ankle, the medial malleolus is first to get affected (avulsion) and then only ligament tear occurs. So sprains are secondary to bony injury.

Note: Sprain is injury to ligament.

Q. SPRING LIGAMENT

Spring ligament is plantar calcaneonavicular ligament and is a very strong ligament.

Attachments

- *Anteriorly:* Navicular bone
- *Posteriorly:* Sustentaculum tali of calcaneum
- *Medially:* Few fibers to deltoid ligament.

Relations

- *Medial:* Tendon of tibialis posterior
- *Lateral:* Tendon of flexor hallucis longus and flexor digitorum longus.

Functional Importance

Spring ligament holds the head of talus and maintains the medial longitudinal arch.

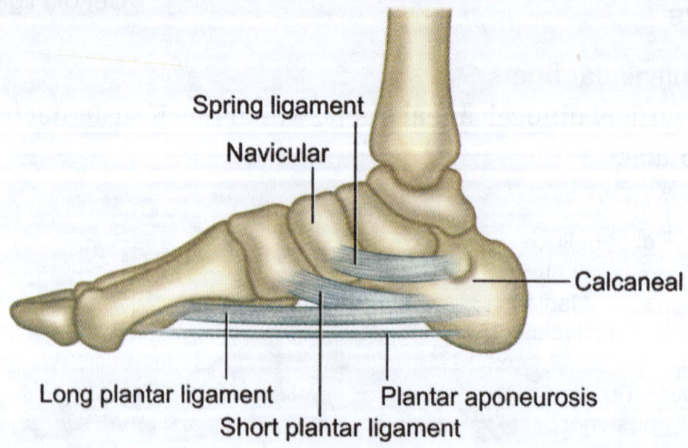

Q. CUTANEOUS INNERVATIONS (DIAGRAM ONLY)

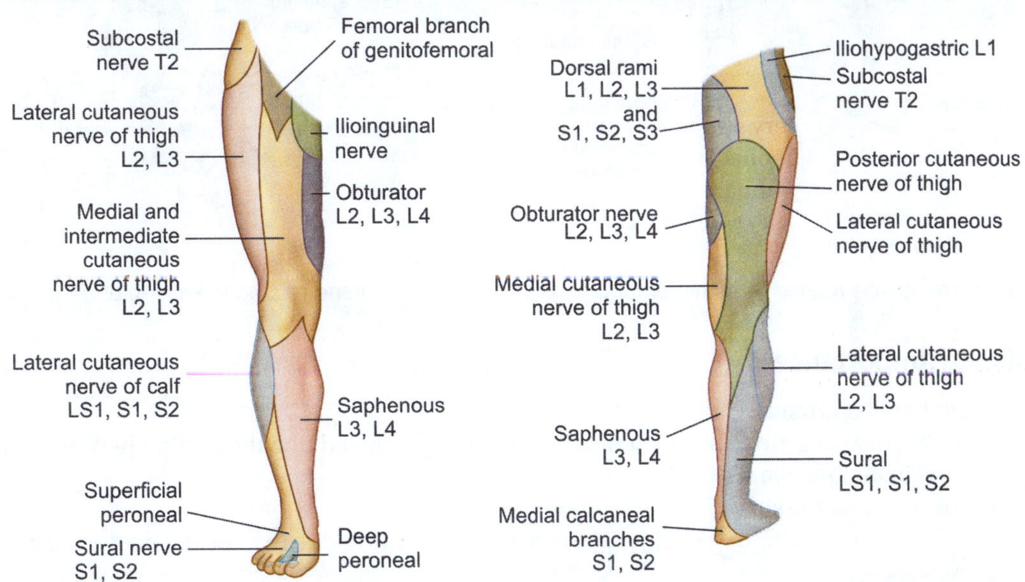

Q. BURSAE AROUND THE KNEE JOINT

Bursae are fluid filled sac, which reduces the friction between articular surfaces and tendon, and bone. There are many bursae in relation to the knee joint, which facilitate smooth movements at the knee joint.

- Suprapatellar:
  - Present between femur bone and tendon of quadriceps
  - It communicates with joint cavity.
- Popliteal:
  - Present between popliteus tendon and lateral condyle of tibia.
- Anserine:
  - Present between tendons of sartorius and gracilis
  - Semitendinosus, tibia bone and tibial collateral ligament.
- Medial bursa of gastrocnemius:
  - It lies deep to medial head of gastrocnemius.
- Semimembranosus bursa:
  - Present between medial head of gastrocnemius and semimembranosus.
- Prepatellar:
  - Lies below the skin and anterior surface of patella.
- Superficial infrapatellar:
  - Lies between skin and tibial tuberosity.
- Deep infrapatellar:
  - Lies between patellar ligament and anterior surface of tibia.

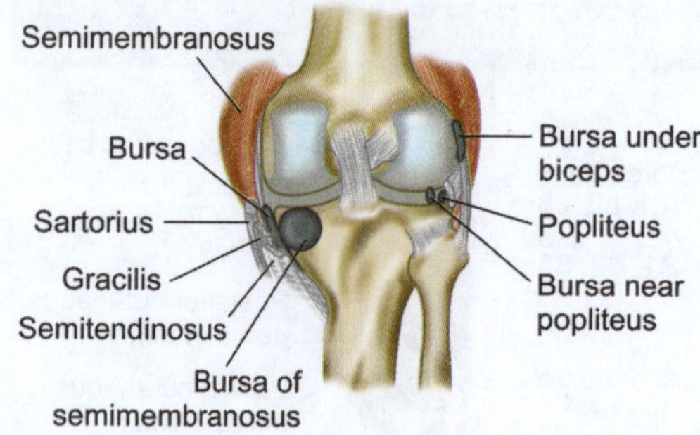

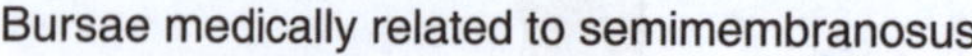

Bursae medically related to semimembranosus

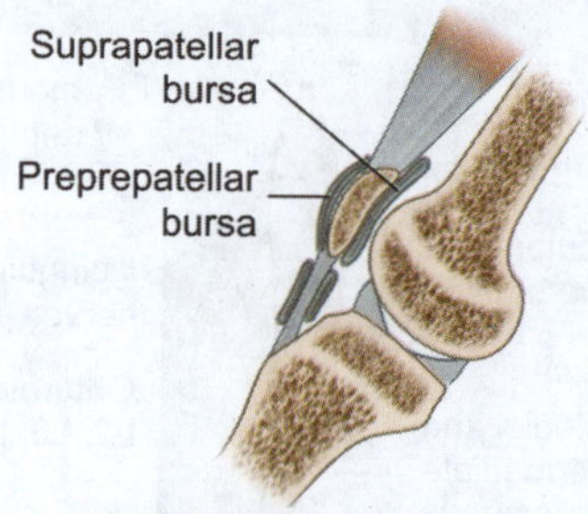

Bursae related to knee joint

Clinical Importance

- Prepatellar bursitis:
  - It is also described as housemaid's knee. It is produced due the friction between the skin and patella.
- Infrapatellar bursitis:
    It is also described as clergyman's knee. It is produced due to kneeling on the knee.
- Baker's cyst:
  - It is herniation of synovial cavity of knee with formation of fluid filled sac, which forms a swelling behind the knee and also extends little below the knee.

Long Questions

Key long questions

- Venous drainage
- Hip joint
- Knee joint
- Arches of foot

Q. DESCRIBE THE VENOUS DRAINAGE OF LOWER LIMB IN DETAIL AND ADD A NOTE ON ITS APPLIED ANATOMY.

Venous drainage of lower limb assumes great significance due to the erect posture of human beings. The venous blood has to flow against gravity upwards, which needs a huge mechanical energy like a motor.

This energy is provided by various factors like negative intrathoracic pressure, the valves within the vein, the musculature and thick condensed superficial fascia of lower limb.

Classification

- Superficial venous system
- Deep venous system
- Perforators.

Superficial Venous System

The major channels included in this system are great (long) saphenous vein and short

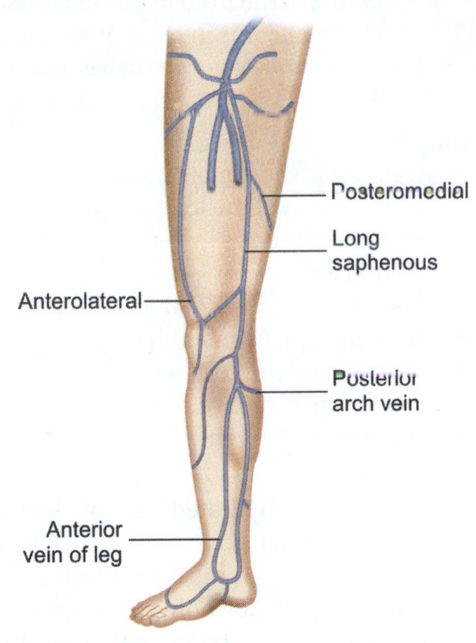

Great saphenous vein with its tributaries

(small) saphenous vein. These veins run in superficial plane in the form of tunnels of superficial fascia.

Great saphenous vein

Great saphenous vein is the longest vein in the body.

Course

1. *In leg:* It begins from the medial end of dorsal venous arch of foot ascends upwards in front of medial malleolus (2–3 cm).

2. The vein further runs straight upwards for short distance in front of leg and then inclines backwards to reach posteromedial side of the knee.

3. *In thigh:* From the backside of the knee the vein again comes in front of the thigh to run obliquely upwards and medially to end in the saphenous opening where it terminates into femoral vein.

Relations

The saphenous nerve is closely related to the vein. The nerve is in the front of the vein at the level of medial malleolus in most of the cases and the nerve lies posterior to the vein at the level of knee.

Tributaries

- Posterior arch vein of the leg
- Anterior vein of the leg
- Short saphenous vein through its tributaries
- Posteromedial vein of thigh
- Anteromedial vein of thigh
- External pudendal vein
- Inferior epigastric vein
- Circumflex iliac vein.

Clinical importance

1. In severely dehydrated patients like in cases of burns great saphenous vein can be chosen for pushing intravenous fluids. So while doing venous cut down one has to be careful about the saphenous nerve.

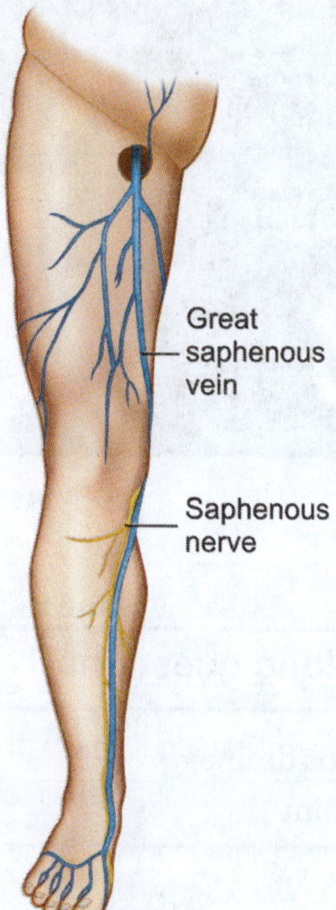

Great saphenous vein

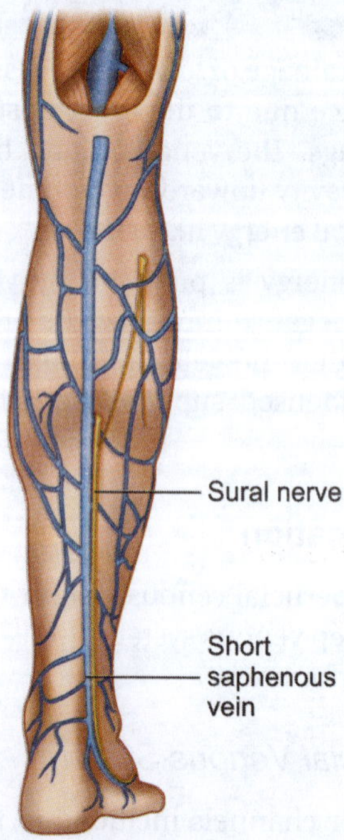

Short saphenous vein

2. Varicosity (tortuous and dilated veins) of great saphenous vein is rarely observed, this is due to the support offered by the condensed fascia around it which helps in venous return. Varicosity is observed in the tributaries of the great saphenous vein.

Short saphenous vein

Course

It begins from the lateral end of dorsal venous arch of foot and runs behind and below lateral malleolus and ascends upwards in back of the leg, pierces the deep fascia to end in popliteal vein in popliteal fossa in most of the cases.

Relations

Initially the vein is lateral to tendo calcaneus and then it lies between the two heads of gastrocnemius. Sural nerve is closely related to the vein on back of the leg.

Tributaries

- Cutaneous veins of the leg
- Accessory saphenous vein.

Clinical importance

While tackling varicosities if the surgeon ligates the vein subcutaneously there may be recurrence of varicose veins because the vein pierces the fascia of the leg and has a sub-fascial course. So the surgeon should ligate (tie) the vein subfascially to avoid recurrence of varicose veins.

Deep Venous System

The deep venous system comprises of:

- Tibial vein
- Peroneal vein
- Popliteal vein
- Femoral vein.

The veins are supported by the musculature of the lower limb and they accompany arteries of the same name. The interior of the veins has valves except the venous sinuses in soleus muscle.

Clinical importance

When a patient is bedridden following a major surgery there is a sluggish movement of blood in the veins leading to high chance of thrombus formation, which may eventually lead to pulmonary embolism.

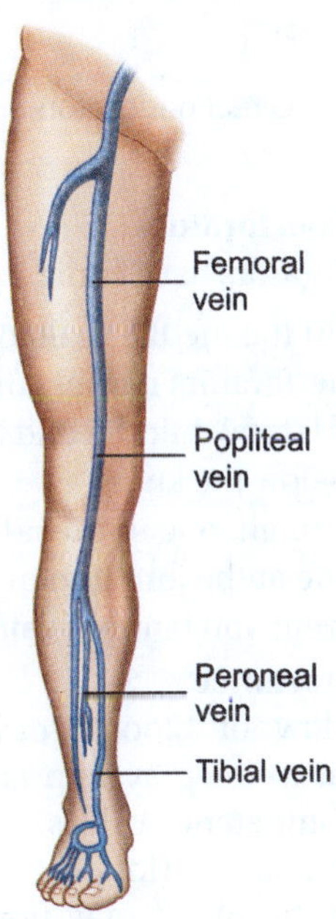

Deep veins

Perforators

Perforators are connecting venous channels between superficial veins and deep veins. They are mostly present within the intermuscular septa and have valves.

Types

- Direct
- Indirect.

Direct: The superficial veins are directly connected through perforator to deep veins by piercing the deep fascia only (without intervening muscle).

Indirect: The superficial veins are first connected to the veins in the muscle and then to the deep veins through the perforators.

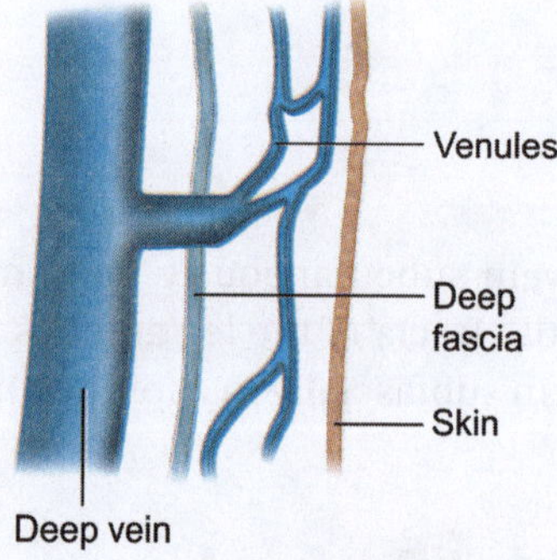

Direct perforators

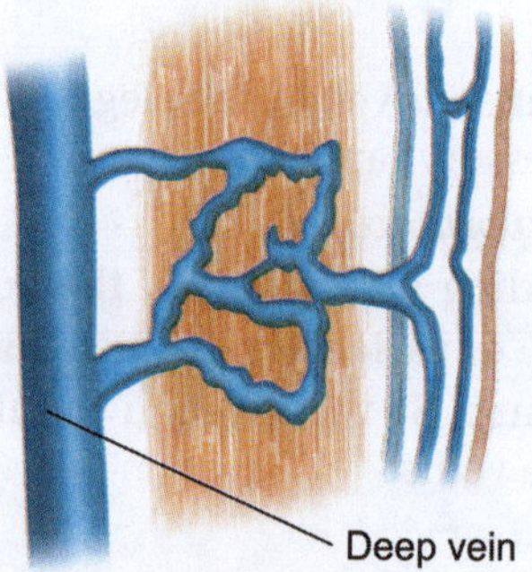

Indirect perforators

Location of perforators

Certain perforators have constant location:

- Around the medial malleolus there are four perforators namely upper medial, upper lateral, middle and low
- One below the knee
- In the thigh, one in the adductor canal and one at the junction of great saphenous vein and femoral vein.

Clinical importance

1. The flow of blood from superficial system to deep system is maintained by competent valves. In case of incompetency (loss of function) of valves the blood may flow in reverse direction leading to varicose veins.
2. The surgical treatment of varicose veins includes removal of incompetent segment.

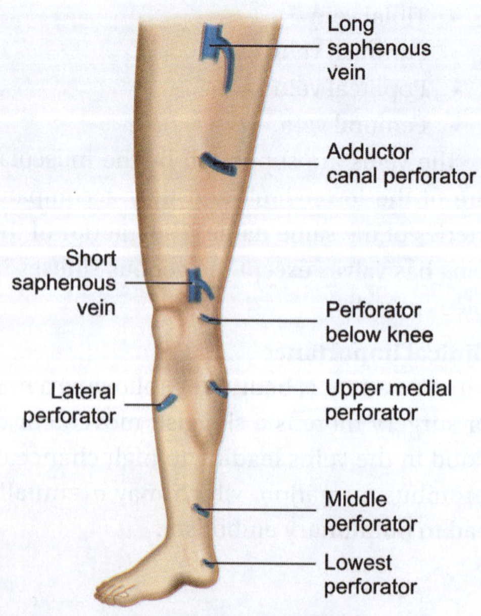

Location of perforators

Q. DISCUSS HIP JOINT IN DETAIL AND ADD A NOTE ON ITS APPLIED ANATOMY.

Hip joint is one of the ideal ball and socket joint with exceptional strength, stability and also mobility.

Type

Synovial joint, ball and socket variety.

Articular Surfaces

- *Above:* Acetabulum of hip bone
- *Below:* Head of the femur.

Peculiarities

The depth of the acetabulum is increased by fringe like covering around the acetabulum.

By virtue of the neck-shaft angle of femur, the range of movement at the hip joint increases. However, this also makes it weak by increasing the vulnerability to fracture.

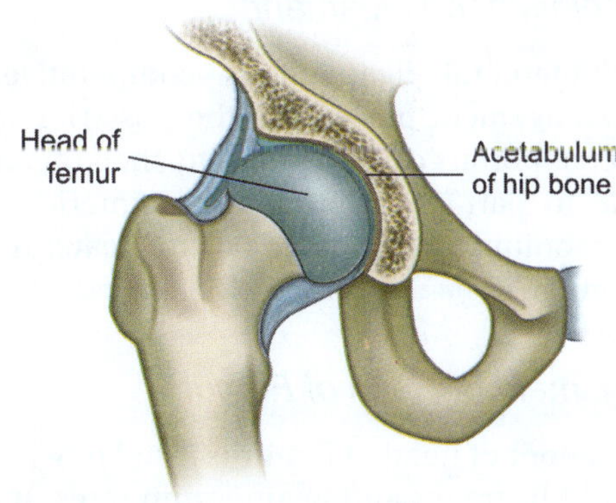

Articulating surfaces of hip bone

Ligaments

Fibrous Capsule

The capsule is very strong and surrounds the joint from all sides. It is attached to the margins of acetabulum and its transverse ligament on one side and to the intertrochanteric line on the femur anteriorly. Posteriorly the capsule is one fingerbreadth in front of the intertrochanteric crest.

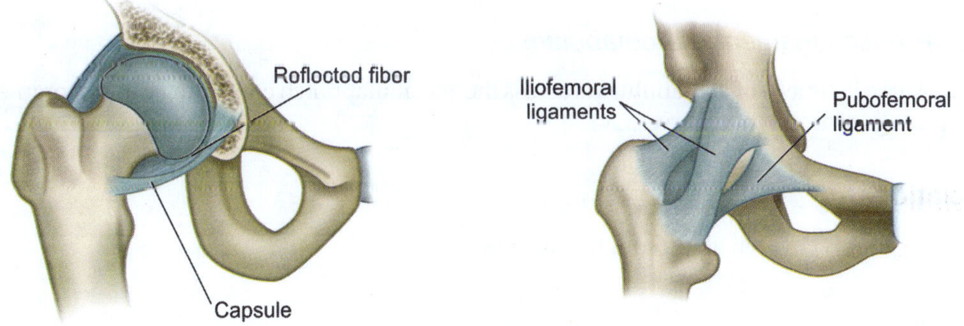

Fibrous capsule

Iliofemoral Ligament

Iliofemoral ligament is the strongest ligament in the body and is attached above to anterior inferior Iliac spine and below it fans out to get attached on intertrochanteric line of femur.

Pubofemoral Ligament

Pubofemoral ligament strengthens the lower and anterior part of fibrous capsule and is attached above to iliopubic eminence and below it blends with iliofemoral ligament.

Ischiofemoral Ligament

Ischiofemoral ligament is comparatively weak ligament present on the posterior aspect of fibrous capsule. It is attached on one side to part of ischium posteroinferior to acetabulum and on other side to greater trochanter.

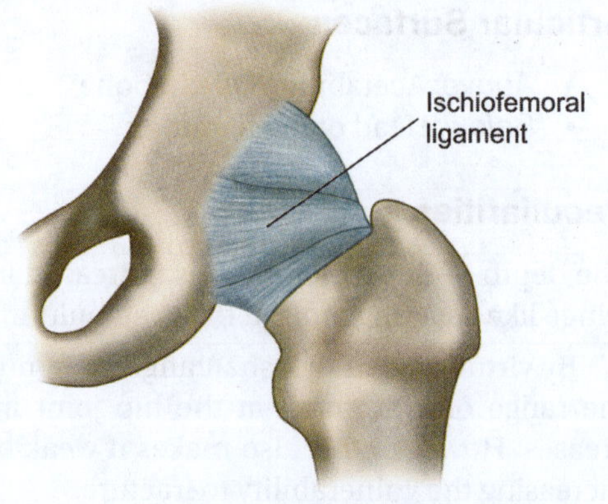

Posterior aspect

Ligament of Head of Femur

Ligament of head of femur is also known as round ligament and ligamentum teres. It is attached to the fovea on head of the femur on one side and transverse ligament and margins of acetabular notch on other side. It is very weak ligament and hardly supports the joint, but helps to spread the synovial fluid during movement of hip joint.

Acetabular Labrum

Acetabular labrum is a fibrocartilaginous ring-like structure attached to the margins of acetabulum. It deepens the cavity of acetabulum.

Transverse Ligament of Acetabulum

Transverse ligament of acetabulum is across the acetabular notch converting it into a foramen for the passage of vessels and nerves.

Relations

The hip joint is covered all around by muscles.

Anterior

- Muscles of the floor of femoral triangle (pectineus, psoas major, iliacus)
- Straight head of rectus femoris more laterally.

Posterior

- Tendon of obturator externus
- Tendon of obturator internus and gemelli.

Superior

- Rectus femoris (reflected head)
- Gluteus minimus.

Inferior

- Pectineus (lateral fibers)
- Obturator externus (few fibers).

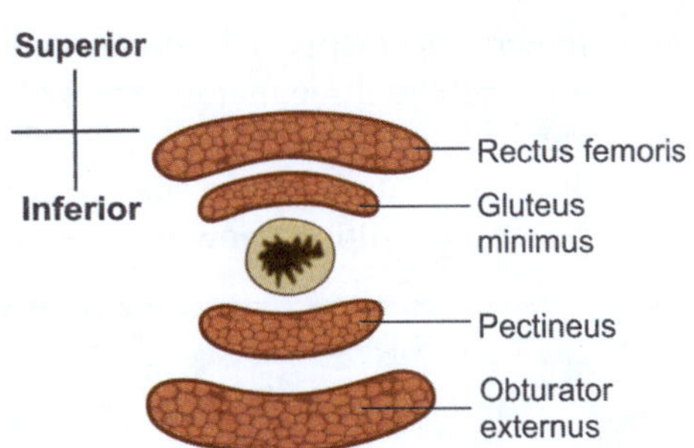

Relations of hip joint

Movements

- Flexion and extension around transverse axis
- Adduction and abduction around anteroposterior axis
- Medial and lateral rotation around vertical axis
- Circumduction is combination of above movements.

Movement	Flexion	Extension	Adduction	Abduction	Medial rotation	Lateral rotation
Muscles	Psoas major, iliacus	Gluteus maximus, hamstrings	Adductors of thigh	Glutei medius, minimus	Tensor lata, few fibers of glutei medius, minimus	Quadratus femoris Obturators with gemelli
Mnemonic	P	G	Adds	Glamor	To	Female Gender

Arterial Supply

Hip joint receives blood from anastomosis around the neck of femur (circumflex femoral arteries and gluteal arteries).

Nerve Supply

All the major nerves of the lower limb supply the hip joint:

- Femoral
- Obturator
- Sciatic.

Clinical Importance

- In cases of joint effusion aspiration of the fluid in the joint can be done by inserting a needle 2 cm lateral to femoral artery and directed posteriorly
- Hip joint can be approached anteriorly, anterolaterally, laterally and posteriorly

- Joint replacement can be done totally by replacing both acetabulum and head of the femur
- Since all the three major nerves of lower limb supply the hip joint, pain in the hip joint can be felt in lower back, knee, calf and around ankle
- The acetabulum can be shallow from birth leading to recurrent dislocations and giving rise to a condition known as acetabular dysplasia.

Q. DESCRIBE KNEE JOINT IN DETAIL (ARTICULAR SURFACES, LIGAMENTS, RELATIONS, MOVEMENTS, BLOOD SUPPLY AND APPLIED ANATOMY).

Knee joint is one of the largest joint in the body susceptible to injuries and pathological conditions.

Type

Synovial joint of modified hinge variety, compound joint (since more than two bones are involved).

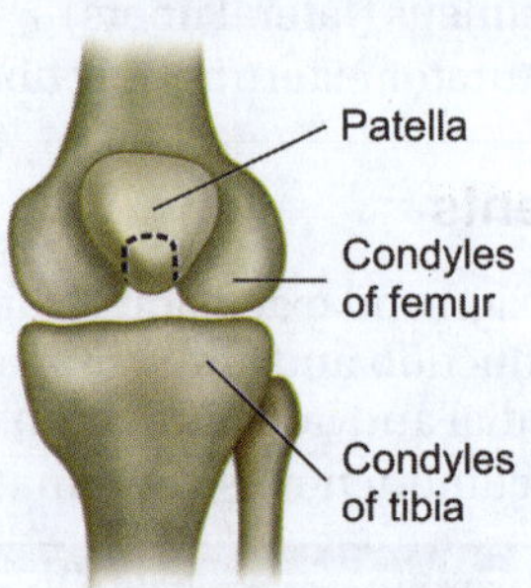

Articular surfaces

Articular Surfaces

- *Above:* Condyles of femur
- *Below:* Condyles of tibia
- Saddle joint between patella and femur.

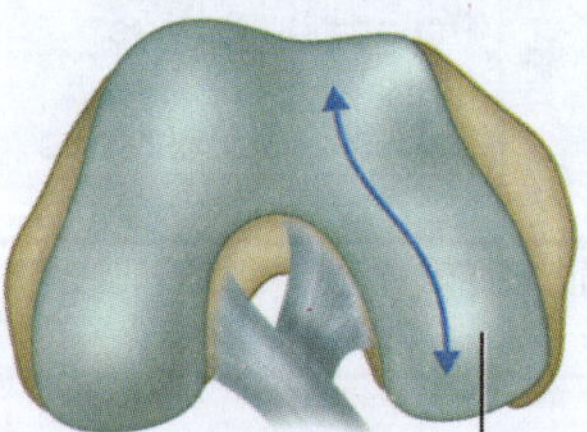

Ligaments

Fibrous Capsule

Attachments on femur

- *Posteriorly:* Margins of femoral condyles and intercondylar fossa
- *Medially:* Articular margin of femur
- *Laterally:* Proximal to the groove of popliteus tendon
- *Anteriorly:* Blends with patellar retinacula, patellar ligament and patella.

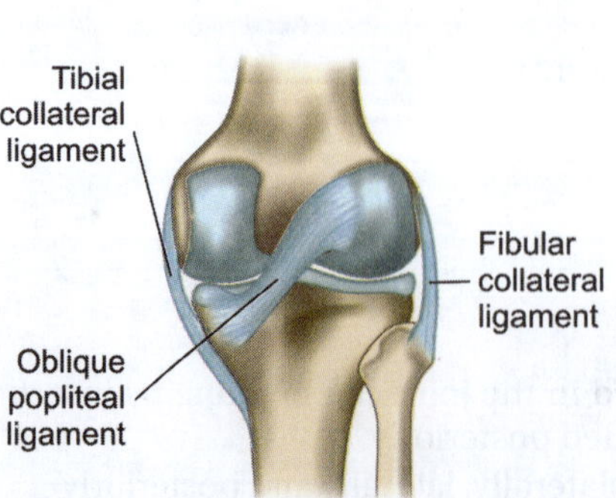

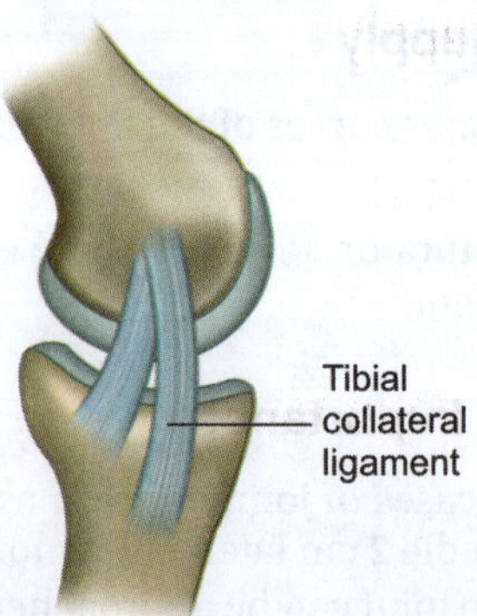

Attachments on tibia
- *Posteriorly:* Margins of tibial condyles and intercondylar area
- *Laterally:* Margins of tibial condyles (laterally—head of fibula also).

Features
- Capsule is deficient above the level of patella for the passage of suprapatellar bursa
- On the lateral condyle of tibia there is an aperture for the passage of popliteus tendon
- Thickening of the capsule medially is deep part of tibial collateral ligament
- Thin fibers from its deep aspect, i.e. coronary ligaments are attached to both menisci.

Tibial Collateral Ligament

Attachments
- *Above:* Medial femoral epicondyle (just distal to adductor tubercle)
- *Below:* Upper part of medial surface of tibia.

Fibular Collateral Ligament

Attachments
- *Above:* Lateral femoral epicondyle (between the attachment of lateral head of gastrocnemius and tendon of popliteus)
- *Below:* Head of fibula.
Note: It is not attached to the capsule and has no connection to the lateral meniscus.

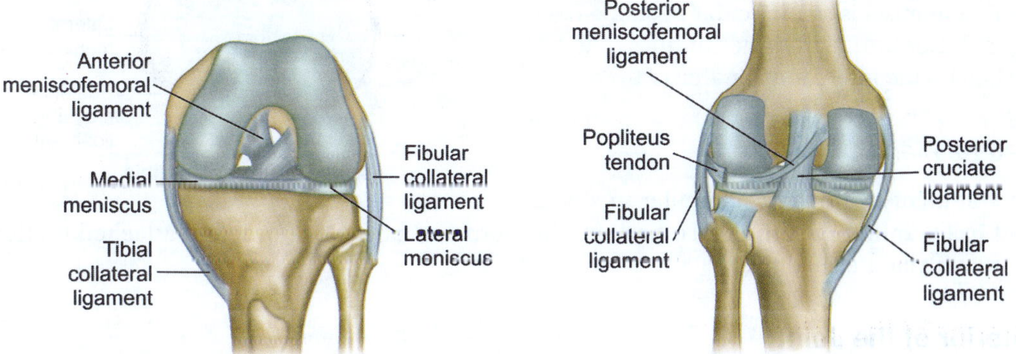

Ligaments of knee joint

Oblique Popliteal Ligament

An expansion of tendon of semimembranosus and it merges with the capsule of knee joint and ascends laterally toward intercondylar fossa and lateral femoral condyle.

Arcuate Popliteal Ligament

A Y-shaped thickening of posterior capsular fiber. At one end it is attached to head of fibula, while the medial limb is attached to the posterior edge of the tibial intercondylar area and the lateral limb is attached to the lateral femoral condyle.

Cruciate Ligaments

Cruciate ligaments are intracapsular ligaments between the tibia and femur. These are two ligaments, which cross each other and hence the name.

Anterior cruciate ligament
This is directed upwards and backwards.

Attachments
- *On tibia:* Anterior part of intercondylar area between the horns of menisci
- *On femur:* Posteromedial area of lateral femoral condyle.

Posterior cruciate ligament
This is directed upwards and forwards.

Attachments
- *On tibia:* Posterior part of intercondylar area between the horns of menisci
- *On femur:* Anteromedial area of medial femoral condyle.

Menisci

Menisci are fibrocartilaginous disks on the tibial condyles. They are mostly avascular structures and receive nutrition from the capillaries in the peripheral rim.

Medial Menisci

Medial menisci is semicircular in shape having anterior horn and posterior horn, and attached on the intercondylar area of tibia.

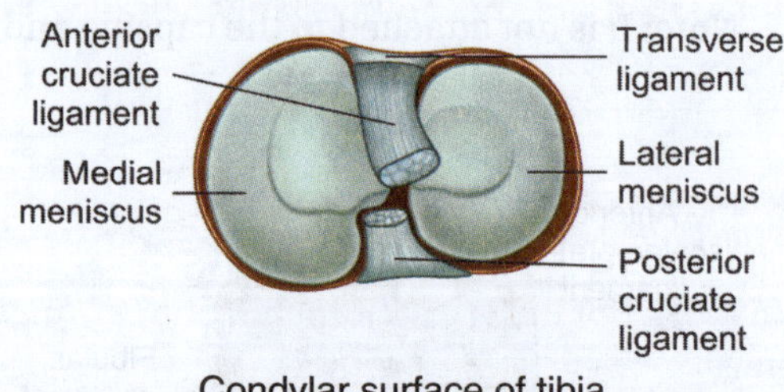

Condylar surface of tibia

Lateral Menisci

Lateral menisci are almost circular in shape and has a uniform width. It also has anterior horn and posterior horn, and attached on the intercondylar area of tibia.

Interior of the Joint

Four cavities coalesce to form the cavity of knee joint. One cavity is between two femoral condyles and another between the tibial condyles. The third is the patellofemoral cavity. And the last is continuous superiorly with the suprapatellar bursa. Synovial membrane lines the cavities except at the articular surfaces, menisci and posterior part of the capsule where it turns forwards to enclose the cruciate ligament.

Relations

Anterior   :   Ligamentum patellae
Posteromedial :   Sartorius, gracilis, semitendinosus, semimembranosus, medial head of gastrocnemius

Posterolateral	:	Biceps, common peroneal nerve, lateral head of gastrocnemius
Posterior	:	Popliteal artery, tibial nerve
Medial	:	Tibial collateral ligament
Lateral	:	Fibular collateral ligament, tendon of popliteus lies between the fibrous capsule and lateral meniscus.

Movements

Movement	Flexion	Extension	Medial rotation	Lateral rotation
Muscles	Hamstrings, gracilis, sartorius, gastrocnemius, popliteus	Quadriceps femoris, tensor fasciae latae	Semimembranosus, semitendinosus	Biceps femoris

Locking of the Knee

In fully extended position, i.e. standing position the knee joint is in a locked state and is in a stable position and a person can stand for a long time without quadriceps fatigue. In this position the tibial tubercles snugly fit into the intercondylar notch, menisci are tightly sandwiched between the tibial and femoral condyles and also the collateral ligaments are taut. This tight situation of the knee joint is known as locking of the knee (medial rotation of femur on tibia in final stages of extension of leg), wherein stability of the knee is maximum, but since there is no movement possible it is vulnerable to injury.

Unlocking of the knee

Unlocking of the knee is brought about by popliteus muscle and is lateral rotation of femur on tibia.

Arterial Supply

Receives blood from the anastomosis around it through branches of popliteal artery, femoral artery and anterior and posterior tibial arteries.

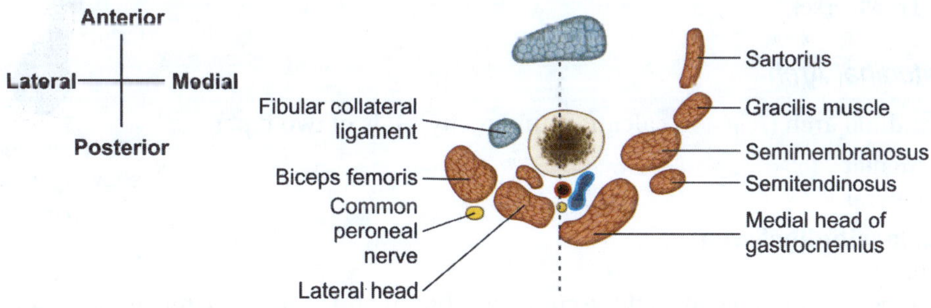

Relation of knee joint

Nerve Supply

All the major nerves of the lower limb supply the knee joint.

- Femoral
- Obturator
- Sciatic.

Clinical Importance

- Knee joint can be surgically approached through anterior vertical midline incision
- The surgeon has to be aware of infrapatellar branch of saphenous nerve, which may get included in the incision
- Posterior approach to knee joint is by giving a 'S' shaped incision
- Direct examination of the knee joint cavity is known as arthroscopy, an anterolateral approach is adopted by surgeons
- Aspiration of the knee joint is carried out by inserting the needle from the side at the upper lateral margin of the patella
- For injecting any medication in the knee joint directly the joint cavity is approached from the lower border of patella from either side of patellar ligament
- Knee joint is prone for athritis almost of every kind.

Q.   DESCRIBE THE ARCHES OF THE FOOT IN DETAIL.

The entire body weight in erect position is supported by foot. Activities like jumping from a height demand extra strength and resilience to sustain the body weight with extra velocity. This is provided by small individual blocks of bone, which are held in position by ligaments, tendons and muscles.

Impression of wet foot on the ground depicts the pressure points of the foot, i.e. the heel, lateral margin of foot, ball of the foot and pads of distal phalanges. The medial margin of the foot does not produce the impression because it arches upwards.

Classification

- Longitudinal
- Transverse.

Longitudinal Arch

Longitudinal arch (rests on calcaneal tuberosity). It is of two types:

- Medial
- Lateral.

Medial longitudinal arch

Formation

It is formed by talus, navicular, three cuneiform bones and inner three metatarsal bones.

Note: Talus is the key bone of this arch.

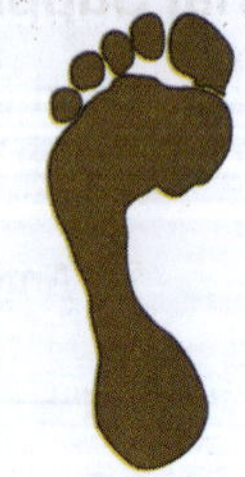

Foot impression showing pressure points

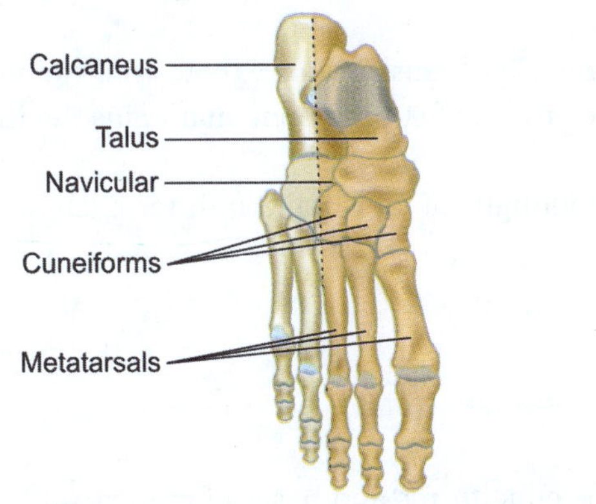

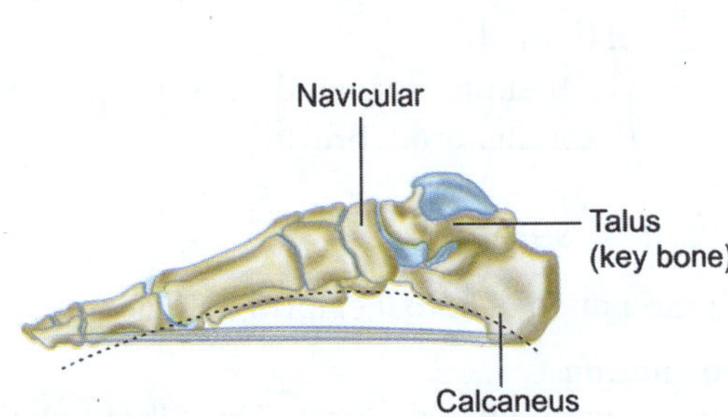

Medial longitudinal arch

Supports
- Head of talus supported on sustentaculum tali
- Plantar aponeurosis stretching from the anterior end of the arch to posterior end
- Spring ligament supports the head of talus
- Tendon of flexor hallucis longus along with flexor digitorum longus act as bow strings
- Accessory support is provided by abductor hallucis and medial half of flexor digitorum brevis
- Tibialis anterior and posterior pull the medial border of the arch and maintain the height of the arch
- While the peroneus longus muscle counters the action of tibialis muscle and evert the foot and lower the height of the arch.

Lateral longitudinal arch

Formation

It is formed by calcaneus, cuboid, lateral two metatarsal.

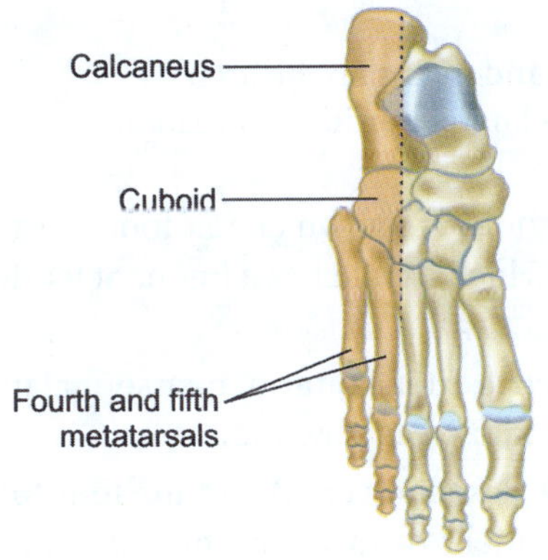

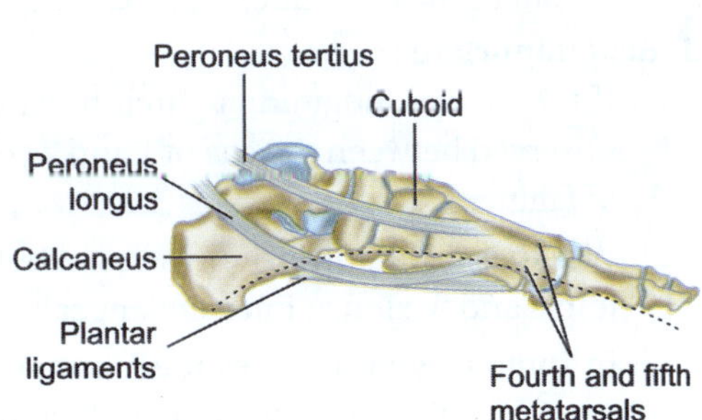

Lateral longitudinal arch

Supports

- Lateral part of plantar aponeurosis and plantar ligaments function as bow strings for the arch
- Peroneus longus tendon as it enters the groove of cuboid bone maintains the integrity of the arch
- Other supports include flexor digitorum longus of fourth and fifth toes, lateral half of flexor digitorum brevis.

Transverse Arch

Combination of both feet form a single transverse arch.

Formation

It is a combined arch, formed by cuboid, three cuneiforms and bases of metatarsal bones of each foot.

> **Note:** Middle cuneiform bone is the key bone of the arch.

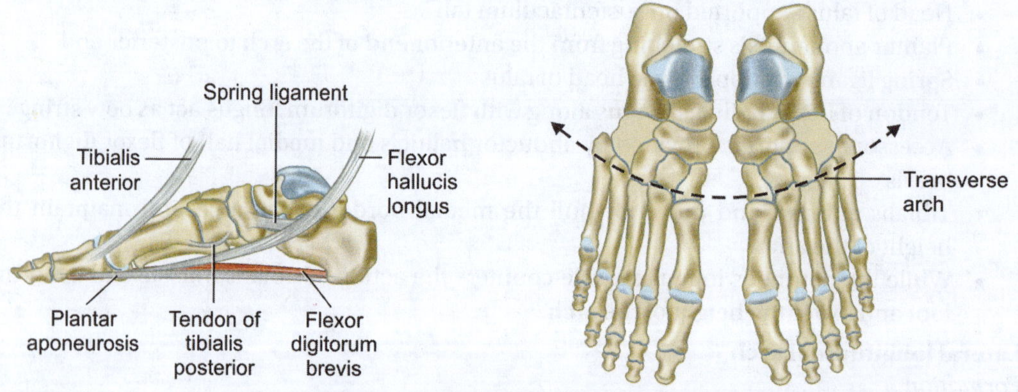

Supports of medial longitudinal arch

Supports

- Interosseus ligaments bind the bones in position and maintain the arch
- Peroneus longus tendon approximate medial and lateral borders of the foot.

Clinical importance

1. If the medial longitudinal arch touches the ground it is known as flat foot. Normally observed between the age of 1 and 2 years due to which a child has a frequent tendency of falling.

2. Weakness in the intrinsic muscles of the foot may lead to extension at metatarsophalangeal joints and flexion at interphalangeal joints. This is known as claw-foot.

3. In some newborn babies the foot may be plantar flexed, inverted and the four foot in varus position. This is known as club-foot. Treatment of this condition should start immediately after birth and each component of the deformity should be corrected.

Key Diagrams with MCQ Tips

Diagrams for

- Ischial tuberosity
- Greater trochanter attachments
- Psoas major muscle
- Gluteus maximus
- Femoral triangle
- Femoral sheath
- Popliteal fossa contents
- Inguinal lymph nodes
- Veins
- Deltoid ligament
- Spring ligament
- Subtalar joints
- Flexor retinaculum
- Popliteus muscle
- Ligaments of knee joint
- Arches of foot
- Dermatomes of lower limb

Q. Ischial tuberosity

Ans.

- Superolateral side of upper area is for semimembranosus muscle
- Inferomedial side of upper area is for biceps femoris and semitendinosus
- Medial side of lower area is covered by fat and this area bears the body weight while sitting
- Margin of ischial tuberosity medially provides attachment to sacrotuberous ligament
- Professions, which demand sitting in one place for long time like tailors are

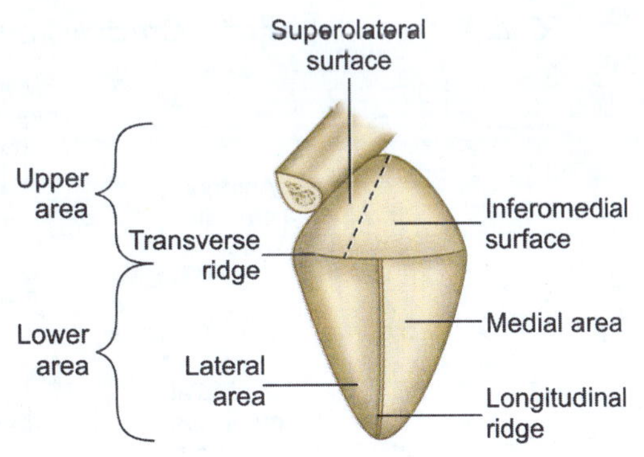

vulnerable to bursitis of ischial tuberosity. This is known as tailor's seat (a bursa is present between ischial tuberosity and gluteus maximus).

Q. Attachments on greater trochanter.

Ans. Very commonly asked in viva, study the diagram carefully.

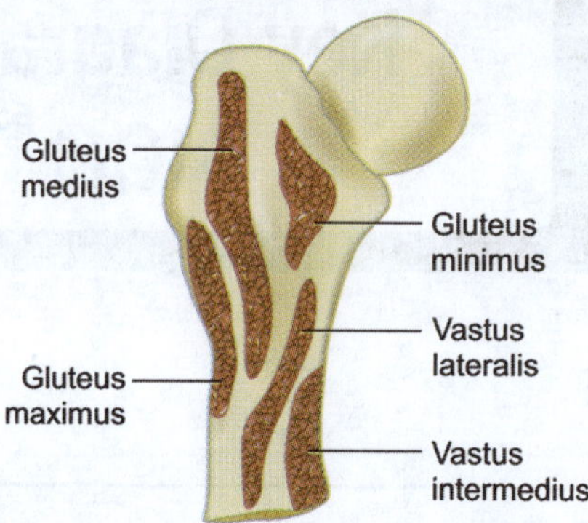

Q. Obturator externus tendon is attached on trochanteric fossa.

Q. Quadratus femoris is attached on quadrate tubercle.

Q. Gluteal tuberosity when prominent is known is third trochanter.

Q. Lesser trochanter anteromedially receives psoas major and iliacus tendon.

Q. Proximal articular surface of tibia.

Ans. Study the diagram carefully.

Mnemonic	Structures
"Medical	Medial meniscus anterior horn
College	Anterior Cruciate ligament
Lucknow	Anterior horn Lateral meniscus
Lucknow	Posterior horn Lateral meniscus
Medical	Posterior horn Medial meniscus
College"	Posterior Cruciate ligament

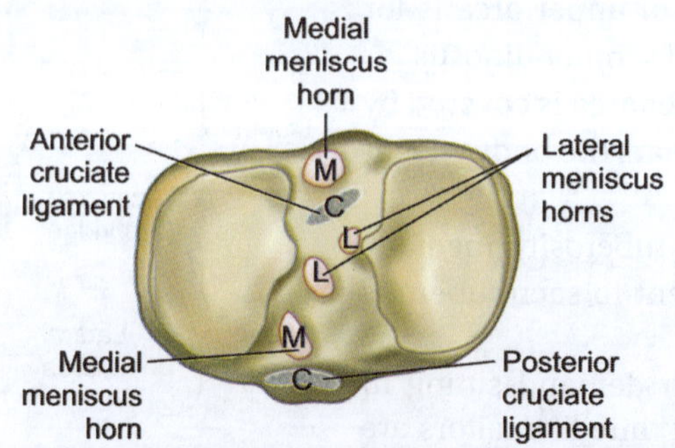

Q. Nerves related to psoas major muscle.

Ans.

- Lateral border from above downwards is related to iliohypogastric nerve, ilio-inguinal nerve, lateral femoral cutane-ous nerve and femoral nerve
- Anterolateral surface is related to geni-tofemoral nerve
- Medial border related to obturator nerve, upper root of lumbosacral trunk.

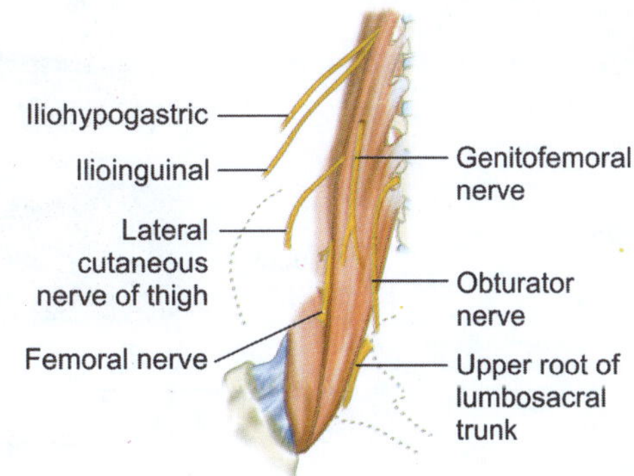

Q. Gluteus maximus supplied by inferior gluteal nerve and extends the flexed thigh.

Q. Gluteus medius and minimus supplied by superior gluteal nerve, and abducts the thigh and also brings about medial rotation of thigh.

Q. Femoral triangle boundaries, floor and contents.

Ans.

- Femoral artery is lateral to femoral vein and lies behind the midinguinal point
- Femoral nerve is lateral to femoral artery.

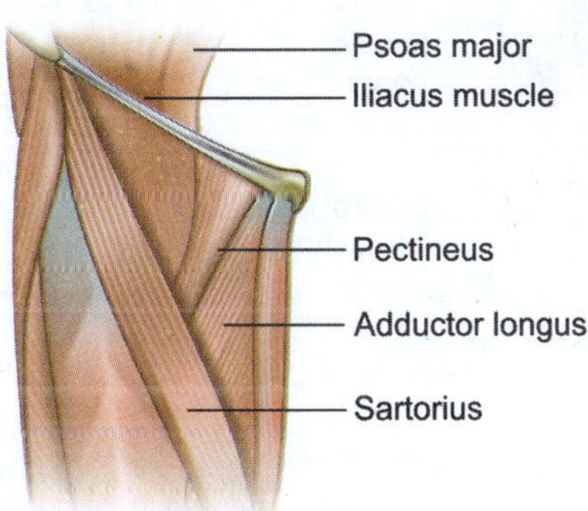

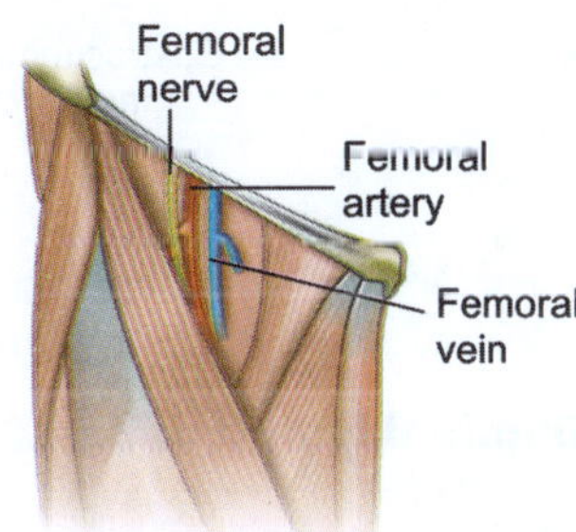

Q. Femoral sheath

Ans.

- Three compartments—lateral for femoral artery, middle for femoral vein and medial for deep inguinal lymph nodes
- Deep inguinal lymph nodes are also known as gland of Cloquet, which drain glans penis in males and clitoris in females
- Anteriorly it is the extension of transversalis fascia
- Posteriorly it is the extension of fascia iliaca.

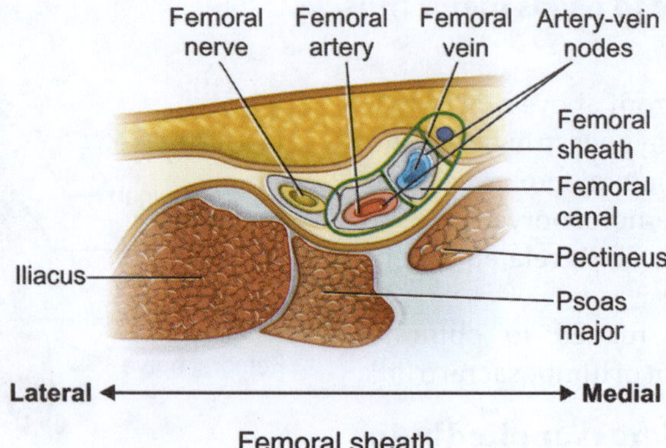

Femoral sheath

Q. Popliteal fossa contents

Ans.

- The tibial nerve is most superficial, vein is just below it and popliteal artery is the deepest
- Sciatic nerve may sometimes divide in popliteal fossa into common peroneal nerve and tibial nerve.

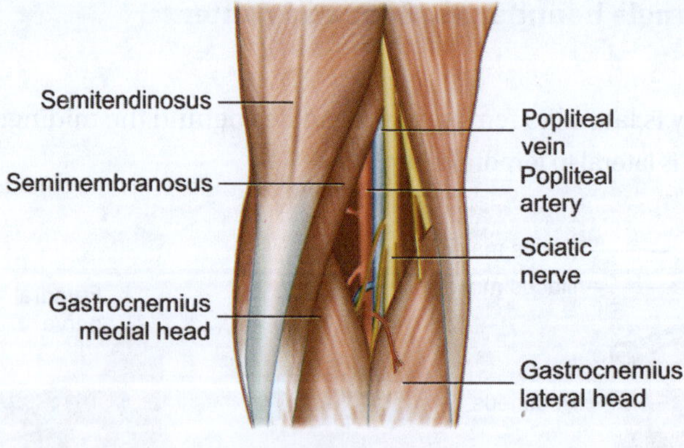

Popliteal fossa

Q. Inguinal lymph nodes

Ans.

- Classified into superficial and deep inguinal lymph nodes
- Deep inguinal lymph nodes are known as glands of Cloquet
- Deep inguinal lymph nodes drain glans penis or clitoris.

Superficial group
Horizontal group
Lateral group
Medial group
Vertical group

Deep group
Femoral vein

Q. Veins

Ans.

Short saphenous vein
Sural nerve

Saphenous opening
Great saphenous vein
Saphenous nerve

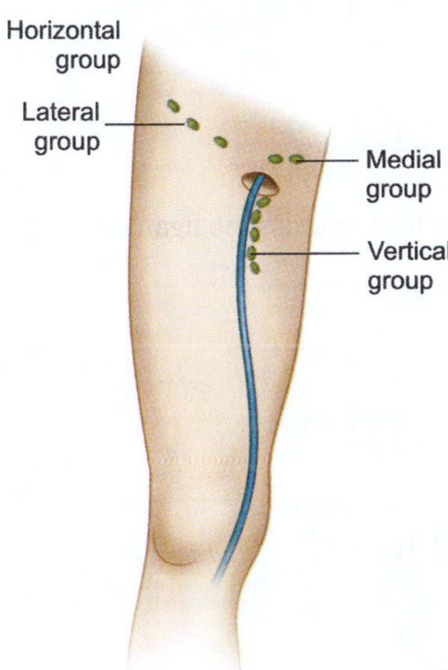

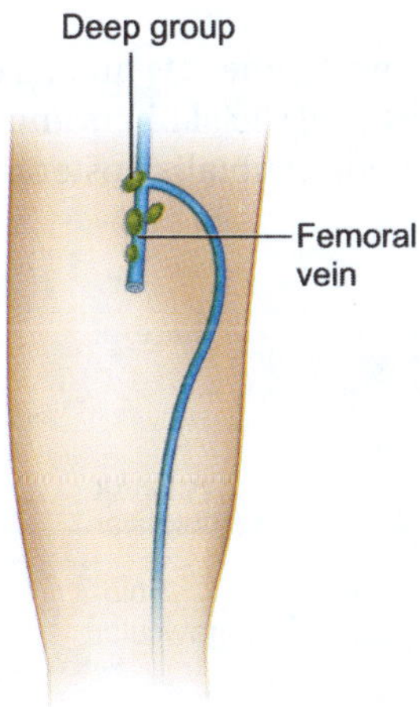

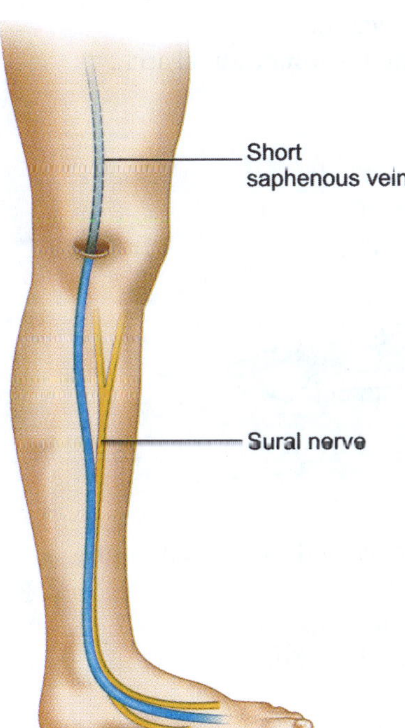

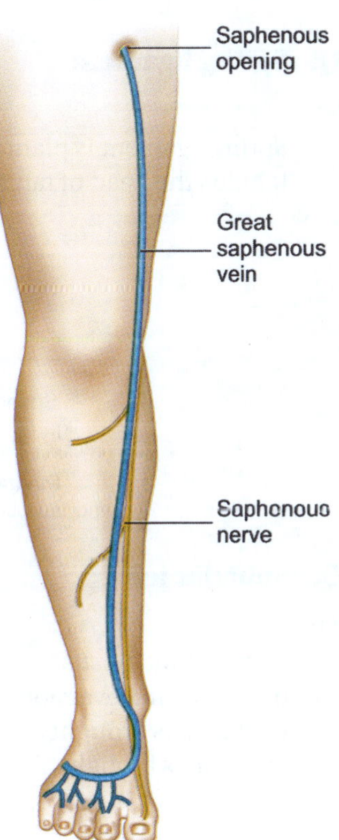

- Great saphenous vein is accompanied by saphenous nerve
- Short saphenous vein is accompanied by sural nerve.

Q. Deltoid ligament

Ans.

- Deltoid ligament is medial collateral ligament of ankle joint
- It has superficial fibers and deep fibers
- Tendons of tibialis posterior and flexor digitorum longus cross the ligament.

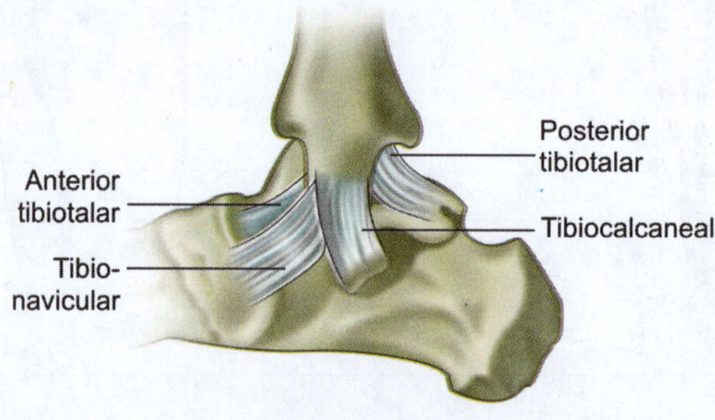

Deltoid ligament

Q. Spring ligament

Ans.

- Spring ligament is plantar calcaneonavicular ligament
- It holds the head of talus and maintains the medial longitudinal arch.

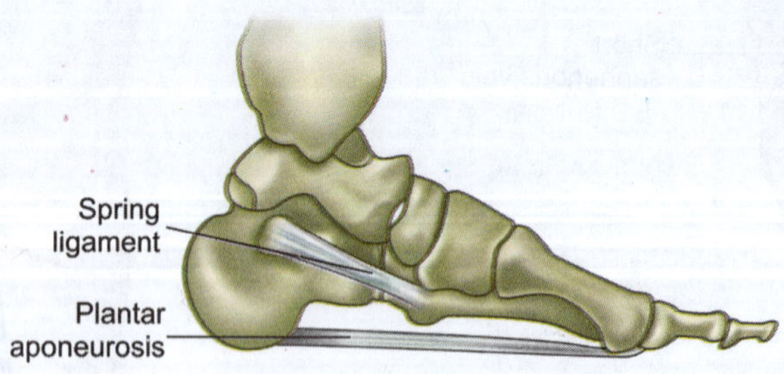

Q. Subtalar joint

Ans.

- Anterior and posterior talocalcaneal joints are termed as subtalar joints
- Inversion and eversion occurs at subtalar joint
- Inversion is brought about by tibialis anterior and posterior
- Eversion is brought about by peroneus longus and brevis.

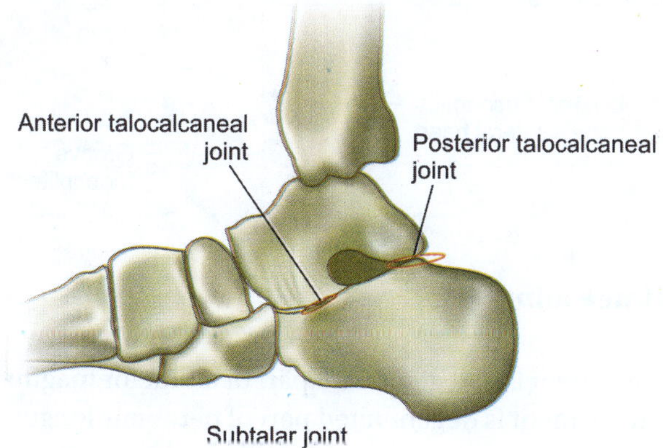

Q. Flexor retinaculum

Ans.

Mnemonic	Structures
"Talented	**T**ibialis posterior
Doctors	Flexor **D**igitorum longus
Are	Posterior tibial **A**rtery and vein
Never	Tibial **N**erve
Hungry"	Flexor **H**allucis longus

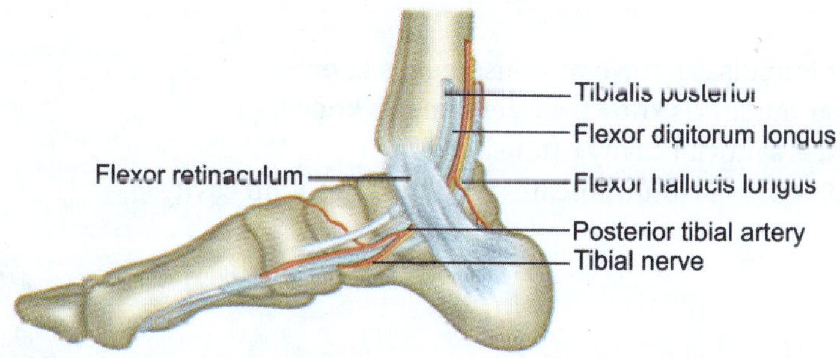

Q. Popliteus muscle

Ans.

- Popliteus muscle tendon is within the cavity of knee joint
- Popliteus muscle unlocks the knee.

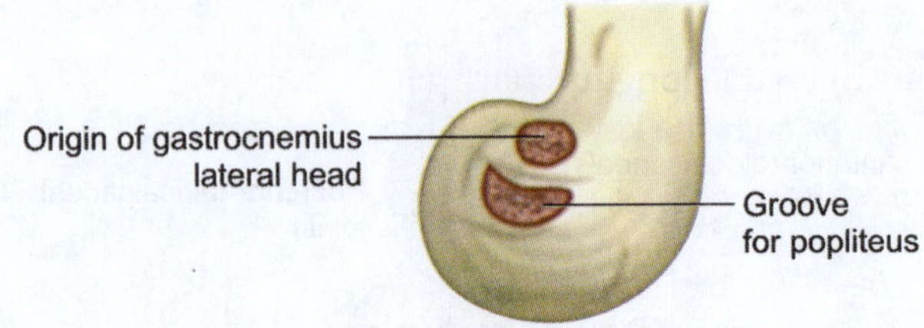

Q. Ligaments of knee joint.

Ans.

- Tibial collateral ligament is a degenerated part of adductor magnus tendon
- Fibular collateral ligament is degenerated part of peroneus longus
- Oblique popliteal ligament is expansion of semimembranosus tendon.

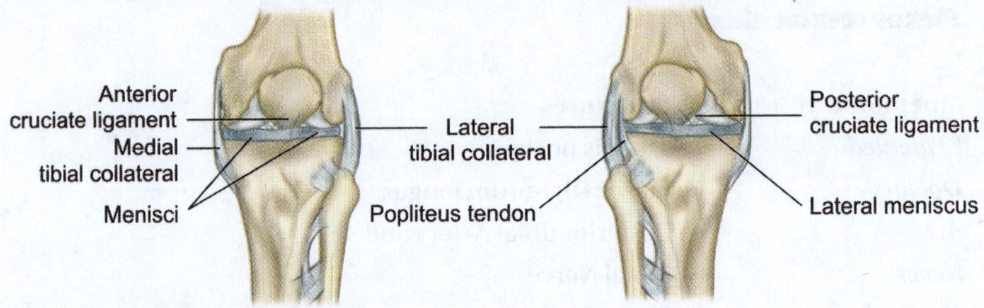

Q. Bursae around the knee joint.

Ans.

- Prepatellar bursitis is known as housemaid's knee
- Infrapatellar bursitis is known as clergyman's knee
- Baker's cyst is synovial cavity extension
- Suprapatellar bursa communicates with the knee joint cavity.

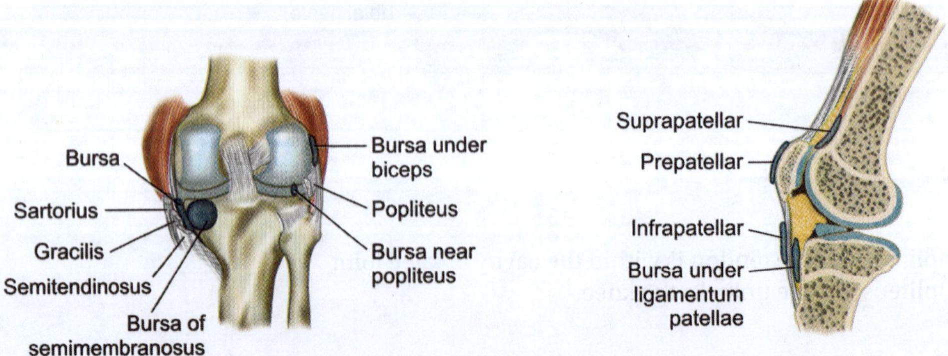

Q. Arches of foot

Ans.

- Talus is key bone of medial longitudinal arch
- Middle cuneiform bone is the key bone of transverse arch.

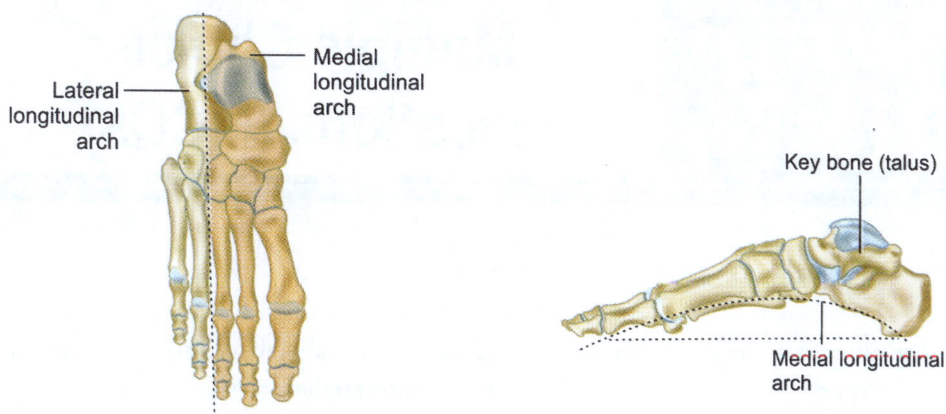

Q. Dermatomes of lower limb (diagram only).

Ans.

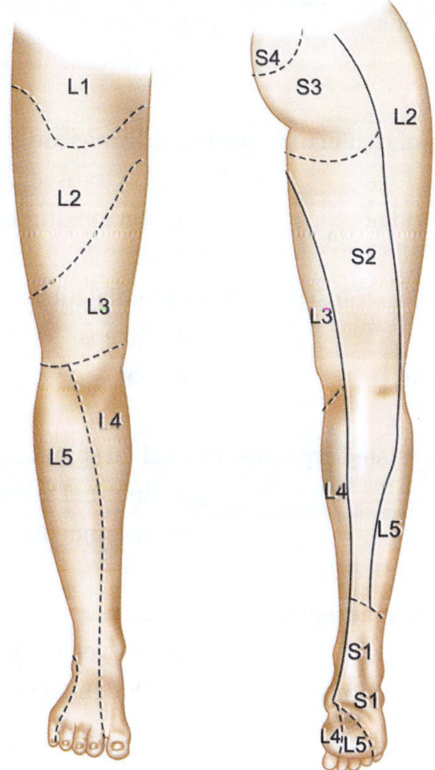

Multiple Choice Questions (MCQs)

1. The tubercle of the iliac crest is on the _____________ lip of iliac bone.
   a. Outer lip
   b. Inner lip
   c. Intermediate area
   d. None

   Answer: a

2. Pubic symphysis is _____________ type of joint.
   a. Primary cartilaginous
   b. Fibrous
   c. Synovial
   d. Fibrocartilaginous

   Answer: d

3. On the following area of ischial tuberosity hamstrings are attached:
   a. Above transverse ridge
   b. Below transverse ridge
   c. On transverse ridge
   d. On longitudinal ridge

   Answer: a

4. On the medial area below transverse ridge of ischial tuberosity what is attached?
   a. Semitendinosus
   b. Semimembranosus
   c. Biceps
   d. Fat

   Answer: d

5. Following structure is related posteriorly to ischial spine _____________
   a. External iliac
   b. External pudendal
   c. Internal pudendal
   d. Internal iliac

   Answer: c

6. The nerve posterior to ischial spine is _____________
   a. Femoral nerve
   b. Nerve to obturator internus
   c. Nerve to obturator externus
   d. Pudendal nerve

   Answer: b

7. The neck shaft angle of femur is _______________
    a. 110
    b. 115

    c. 100
    d. 125

    Answer: d

8. Following muscle is attached to trochanteric fossa _______________
    a. Psoas major
    b. Obturator internus

    c. Obturator externus
    d. Iliacus

    Answer: c

9. All the following muscles are attached on the lesser trochanter except _______________
    a. Psoas major
    b. Psoas minor

    c. Adductor magnus
    d. Iliacus

    Answer: b

10. Neck shaft angle is _______________ at birth.
    a. Widest
    b. Absent

    c. Narrowest
    d. None

    Answer: a

11. Following muscle is attached to quadrate tubercle _______________
    a. Gluteus minimus
    b. Gluteus maximus

    c. Gluteus medius
    d. Quadratus femoris

    Answer: d

12. Third trochanter of femur is _______________
    a. Greater trochanter
    b. Lesser trochanter

    c. Gluteal tuberosity
    d. Quadrate tubercle

    Answer: c

13. Following are the major nerves of the lower limb, except _______________
    a. Femoral
    b. Sciatic

    c. Obturator
    d. Tibial

    Answer: d

14. Which muscle is attached to adductor tubercle?
    a. Adductor longus
    b. Adductor brevis

    c. Adductor magnus
    d. Gluteus maximus

    Answer: c

15. A 25-year-old male, while playing cricket gets a direct hit on the side of leg by bat he develops severe tingling and numbness over the foot, but still could stand on the foot. On taking X-ray, there was fracture of fibula.
    i. The anatomical basis of the patient could stand on foot is _______________
        a. Tibia not fractured
        b. Metatarsals intact

        c. Fibula does not transmit the weight
        d. All of the above

        Answer: c

ii.   Anatomical basis for the tingling and numbness is due to impact on ____________ nerve.

   a. Tibial
   c. Sciatic
   b. Sural
   d. Common peroneal nerve

Answer: d

16. Following muscle is attached to talus bone ____________

   a. Peroneus tertius
   c. Tibialis anterior
   b. Peroneus longus
   d. None

Answer: d

17. Sustentaculum tali is present on ____________ surface of calcaneum.

   a. Lateral
   c. Medial
   b. Dorsal
   d. Ventral

Answer: c

18. Following tendon grooves the inferior aspect of sustentaculum tali ____________

   a. Peroneus longus
   c. Peroneus tertius
   b. Flexor hallucis longus
   d. Flexor digitorum

Answer: b

19. Following muscle fibers are attached to navicular tuberosity ____________

   a. Peroneus longus
   c. Tibialis posterior
   b. Peroneus brevis
   d. Tibialis anterior

Answer: c

20. Fabella is a sesamoid bone in the tendon of ____________ muscle.

   a. Gastrocnemius
   c. Quadriceps femoris
   b. Soleus
   d. Peroneus longus

Answer: a

21. The following nerve is present on the anterolateral surface of psoas major ____________

   a. Obturator nerve
   c. Femoral
   b. Genitofemoral
   d. Ilioinguinal

Answer: b

22. The largest muscle of the quadriceps femoris group is ____________

   a. Vastus medialis
   c. Vastus lateralis
   b. Vastus intermedius
   d. Rectus femoris

Answer: c

23. Literal meaning of patella is ____________

   a. Cup
   c. Plate
   b. Saucer
   d. Flute

Answer: c

24. All of the following form, the group of hamstrings except ____________

   a. Biceps femoris
   c. Semitendinosus
   b. Quadriceps femoris
   d. Semimembranosus

Answer: b

25. All the muscles of hamstrings are supplied by tibial part of sciatic nerve except __________
    a. Semitendinosus
    b. Semimembranosus
    c. Long head of biceps
    d. Short head of biceps

    Answer: d

26. Triceps surae muscles are all except __________
    a. Lateral head of gastrocnemius
    b. Medial head of gastrocnemius
    c. Soleus
    d. Tibialis posterior

    Answer: d

27. A 75-year-old male slipped and fell down. His leg was rotated externally. On X-ray, there was fracture neck of femur. The external rotation of leg was due to action of __________
    a. Gluteus maximus
    b. Psoas major
    c. Psoas minor
    d. Quadratus femoris

    Answer: b

28. Nervus furcalis is ventral rami of __________ nerve.
    a. L2
    b. L3
    c. L4
    d. L5

    Answer: c

29. Dorsal divisions of ventral rami of L2, L3, L4 form __________ nerve.
    a. Obturator
    b. Femoral
    c. Lateral cutaneous
    d. Genitofemoral

    Answer: b

30. Ventral divisions of ventral rami of L2, L3, L4 form __________ nerve.
    a. Femoral
    b. Lateral cutaneous nerve
    c. Obturator nerve
    d. Genitofemoral

    Answer: c

31. The femoral nerve is __________ to femoral artery.
    a. Medial
    b. Anterior
    c. Posterior
    d. Lateral

    Answer: d

32. The terminal divisions of sciatic nerve are __________
    a. Sural nerve and common peroneal nerve
    b. Common peroneal nerve and tibial nerve
    c. Tibial nerve and sciatic nerve
    d. Tibial nerve and peroneal nerve

    Answer: b

33. The sciatic nerve emerges below the lower border of __________ muscle in the upper part of back of thigh.
    a. Gluteus minimus
    b. Gluteus maximus
    c. Piriformis
    d. Obturator internus

    Answer: c

34. A 45-year-old man suffered a direct injury on back of leg close to short saphenous vein. Patient complains of tingling and numbness over lateral part of the leg.
    i. What nerve has got injured?
        a. Saphenous nerve
        b. Sural nerve
        c. Lateral femoral cutaneous nerve
        d. Tibial nerve

        Answer: b

35. The nerve, which crosses the femoral artery from lateral to medial side is _____________
    a. Sural nerve
    b. Saphenous nerve
    c. Femoral nerve
    d. Lateral femoral cutaneous nerve

    Answer: b

36. Femoral artery is a continuation of _____________ artery.
    a. External iliac
    b. Internal iliac
    c. Popliteal
    d. External pudendal

    Answer: a

37. Following are the branches of profunda femoris except _____________
    a. Lateral circumflex femoral
    b. Medial circumflex femoral
    c. Perforating
    d. Medial circumflex iliac

    Answer: d

38. The popliteal artery divides at the lower borders of _____________
    a. Adductor magnus
    b. Tibialis posterior
    c. Soleus
    d. Popliteus

    Answer: d

39. During the ligation of short saphenous vein the surgeon has to be careful of the following nerve:
    a. Saphenous nerve
    b. Sural nerve
    c. Lateral femoral
    d. Ilioinguinal

    Answer: b

40. Following is the drainage area of superficial inguinal lymph nodes, except _____________
    a. Gluteal region
    b. Lower abdominal wall
    c. Glans penis
    d. Anal canal

    Answer: c

41. Deltoid ligament is _____________
    a. Lateral ligament of ankle
    b. Medial ligament of ankle
    c. Transverse tibiofibular
    d. Calcaneonavicular

    Answer: b

42. Subtalar joint is _____________
    a. Talocalcaneal
    b. Talonavicular
    c. Calcaneonavicular
    d. Tibiofibular

    Answer: a

43. Inversion and eversion movements occur at _____________ joint.
    a. Ankle joint
    b. Inferior tibiofibular
    c. Subtalar
    d. All of the above

    Answer: c

44. Following are the boundaries of femoral triangle expect _____________
    a. Adductor longus
    b. Sartorius
    c. Psoas major
    d. Inguinal ligament

    Answer: c

45. Mention the correct statements.
    Regarding femoral ring boundaries __________ mention __________ Yes/No.
    a. Lacunar ligament laterally   Y/ N   **Answer: N**
    b. Lacunar ligament medially   Y/ N   **Answer: Y**
    c. Inguinal ligament superiorly   Y/ N   **Answer: Y**
    d. Inguinal ligament anteriorly   Y/ N   **Answer: Y**
    e. Inguinal ligament posteriorly   Y/ N   **Answer: N**

46. Femoral artery is _____________ to femoral vein.
    a. Medial
    b. Lateral
    c. Anterior
    d. Posterior

    Answer: b

47. A 80-year-old male complains of swelling, in the inguinal region and an ulcer, which bleeds on touch on glans penis. Anatomical basis for the swelling in inguinal region is _____________
    a. Superficial inguinal lymph nodes enlargement
    b. Deep inguinal lymph nodes enlargement
    c. Tumor in inguinal region
    d. All of the above

    Answer: b

48. A 35-year-old diabetic developed a swelling in upper part of the thigh following an injury to big toe, leading to abscess. The reason for the swelling is _____________
    a. Enlargement of inguinal lymph nodes
    b. Collection of blood
    c. Tumor in upper thigh
    d. None of above

    Answer: a

49. Following are the parts of deltoid ligament except _____________
    a. Calcaneonavicular
    b. Tibionavicular
    c. Tibiocalcaneal
    d. Tibiotalar

    Answer: a

50. Cervical ligament forms a support to ____________ joint.
    a. Inferior tibiofibular joint
    b. Ankle joint
    c. Subtalar joint
    d. Knee joint

Answer: c

51. Spring ligament is ____________
    a. Calcaneonavicular
    b. Tibionavicular
    c. Talocalcaneal
    d. Tibiotalar

Answer: a

52. The popliteal fascia forms the ____________ of popliteal fossa.
    a. Roof
    b. Floor
    c. Both
    d. None

Answer: b

53. Plantaris forms ____________ boundary of popliteal fossa.
    a. Lateral and above
    b. Lateral and below
    c. Medial and above
    d. Medial and below

Answer: b

54. Deltoid ligament is crossed by following tendon ____________
    a. Tibialis anterior
    b. Flexor hallucis longus
    c. Tibialis posterior
    d. Peroneus longus

Answer: c

55. Great saphenous vein is closely related to ____________ nerve.
    a. Sural nerve
    b. Tibial nerve
    c. Common peroneal nerve
    d. Saphenous nerve

Answer: d

56. Short saphenous vein is related to ____________ nerve.
    a. Sural nerve
    b. Tibial nerve
    c. Common peroneal nerve
    d. Saphenous nerve

Answer: a

57. Strongest ligament of the body is ____________
    a. Pubofemoral
    b. Iliofemoral
    c. Ischiofemoral
    d. All of above

Answer: b

58. Prepatellar bursitis is also known as ____________
    a. Housemaid's knee
    b. Clergyman's knee
    c. Baker's cyst
    d. None

Answer: a

59. Clergyman's knee is ____________ bursitis.
    a. Prepatellar
    b. Infrapatellar
    c. Suprapatellar
    d. Synovial cyst

Answer: b

60. Baker's cyst is _____________
    a. Prepatellar bursitis
    b. Infrapatellar
    c. Synovial cavity extension
    d. Suprapatellar bursitis

    Answer: c

61. Tibial collateral ligament is a degenerated part of _____________ tendon.
    a. Adductor longus
    b. Peroneus longus
    c. Peroneus tertius
    d. Adductor magnus

    Answer: d

62. Fibular collateral ligament is degenerated part of _____________
    a. Adductor longus
    b. Peroneus longus
    c. Peroneus tertius
    d. Adductor magnus

    Answer: b

63. A housemaid was complaining of pain and swelling in front of the knee.
    The most probable reason would be _____________
    a. Infrapatellar bursitis
    b. Prepatellar bursitis
    c. Baker's cyst
    d. Fracture patella

    Answer: b

64. Oblique popliteal ligament is expansion of _____________ tendon.
    a. Semitendinosus
    b. Semimembranosus
    c. Gracilis
    d. Sartorius

    Answer: b

65. Unlocking of the knee is brought about by _____________ muscle.
    a. Semitendinosus
    b. Quadriceps femoris
    c. Popliteus
    d. Biceps femoris

    Answer: c

66. A traffic police can stand for a long time, on the road by the virtue of _____________ of knee joint.
    a. Strength of quadriceps femoris muscle
    b. Strength of the leg bones
    c. Locking of the knee
    d. All of the above

    Answer: c

67. Key bone of medial longitudinal arch _____________
    a. Calcaneus
    b. Cuboid
    c. Talus
    d. Navicular

    Answer: c

68. Single important tendon, which forms key support of lateral longitudinal arch is _____________
    a. Peroneus tertius
    b. Peroneus longus
    c. Abductor digiti minimi
    d. Flexor digitorum brevis

    Answer: b

69. Following bone is the key bone of transverse arch:
    a. Lateral cuneiform
    b. Medial cuneiform
    c. Middle cuneiform
    d. Cuboid

    Answer: c

70. A chain smoker is diagnosed of having lung cancer. A segmental lobectomy can be done by virtue of _______________ structure of lungs.
    a. Arterial supply of lung
    b. Venous drainage of lung
    c. Bronchopulmonary segment
    d. All of the above

    Answer: c

Section - III

ABDOMEN AND PELVIS

Key Questions

> **Key questions**
>
> - Typical lumbar vertebra
> - Atypical lumbar vertebra
> - Sacralization of fifth lumbar vertebra
> - Ala of sacrum
> - Male and female pelves
> - Pelvic brim index
> - Pelves classification
> - Strong ligament in female pelvis
> - Events occurring at L1

Q. What are the features of 'typical' lumbar vertebra?

Ans. Following are the features of 'typical' lumbar vertebra:

- Body of the vertebra is large, strong and stout
- Transverse diameter is greater than anteroposterior diameter
- Vertebral foramen is relatively large and triangular in shape
- Pedicles are short and strong
- Inferior vertebral notch is deeper than superior vertebral notch
- Laminae are short, thick and broad, and directed backwards and medially
- Spine is in the form of quadrilateral plate
- Transverse processes are thin
- Superior articular processes have concave facet facing medially and backwards, and they lie quite apart from each other
- Posterior border of superior articular process has a rough tubercle known as mammillary process
- Inferior articular processes are relatively close to each other.

Q. Which is the 'atypical' lumbar vertebra?

Ans. Fifth lumbar vertebra is the 'atypical' vertebra.

Q. What do you understand by sacralization of fifth lumbar vertebra?

Ans. The fifth lumbar vertebra or its transverse process may be fused with sacrum and this is known as sacralization of fifth lumbar vertebra.

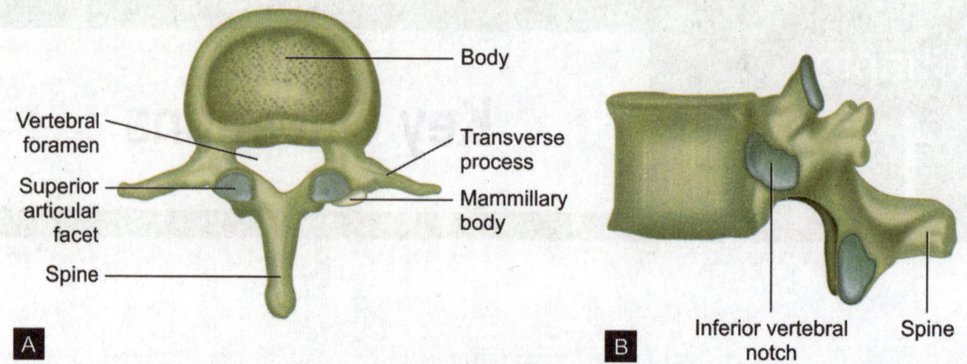

Fifth lumbar vertebra. **A.** Axial view; **B.** Lateral view.

Q. Depict the relations of ala of sacrum.

Ans.

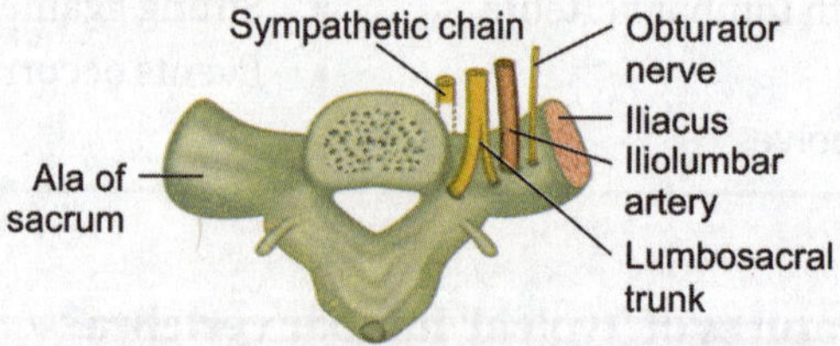

Relations of ala of sacrum

Q. What are the differences between male and female pelves?

Ans.

Criteria	Male	Female
Greater sciatic notch	Narrow	Wider
Acetabulum	Larger	Smaller
Iliac crest	More prominent	Less prominent
Iliac fossa	Shallow	Deeper
Pubic crest	Shorter	Longer
Ischiopubic rami	Everted	Not everted
Preauricular sulcus	Less prominent	More prominent
Ischial spine	Inturned	Straight, pointed
Obturator foramen	Large, oval	Small, triangular

Q. What is pelvic brim index?

Ans.

$$\text{Pelvic brim index} = \frac{\text{Anteroposterior diameter}}{\text{Transverse diameter}} \times 100$$

Q. How are the pelves classified depending on pelvic brim index?

Ans. The pelves are classified as follows:

- Platypellic: Transversely flat
- Mesatipellic: Intermediate
- Dolicopellic: Anteroposteriorly flat.

Q. Which ligament is considered strong in female pelvis?

Ans. Interosseous sacroiliac ligament is the strongest ligament in female pelvis.

Q. What are the events occurring at L1?

Ans. Following are the events:

- Transpyloric plane passes through L1
- Superior mesenteric artery arises at L1
- Body of pancreas lies at L1
- Pylorus of stomach lies at L1
- First part of duodenum lies at L1
- Superior duodenal flexure lies at L1
- Celiac plexus lies at L1
- Upper part of the hilus of right kidney lies at L1
- Lower part of the hilus of left kidney lies at L1
- Cisterna chyli lies against L1 and L2.

Short Notes

Key short notes

MUSCLE

- External oblique
- Internal oblique
- Transversus abdominis
- Rectus sheath
- Perineal body
- Supports of uterus
- Pelvic diaphragm
- Anal sphincters

PERITONEUM

- Greater omentum
- Lesser omentum
- Epiploic foramen
- Vertical disposition of peritoneum
- Horizontal section of supracolic compartment of colon
- Hepatorenal pouch
- Peritoneal reflections and bare areas on liver
- Mesentery
- Rectouterine pouch
- Duodenal fossae

TRIANGLES IN ABDOMEN

- Lumbar triangle
- Hesselbach's triangle
- Calot's triangle

ARTERIES

- Celiac trunk
- Superior mesenteric artery
- Differences between the vascular arcades of jejunum and ileum
- Inferior mesenteric artery
- Marginal artery
- Branches of internal iliac artery

Contd...

Contd...

LYMPHATICS

- Cisterna chyli
- Lymphatic drainage of stomach
- Lymphatic drainage of rectum

NERVES

- Urinary bladder innervation

MISCELLANEOUS

- Regions of abdomen
- Inguinal ligament
- Coverings of testis
- TS of body of penis
- Inguinal canal
- Spermatic cord
- Differences between small and large intestine
- Meckel's diverticulum
- Pudendal canal
- Perineal membrane in male
- Perineal membrane in female
- Stomach bed
- Anterior impressions on right and left kidney
- Urogenital region of male perineum
- Urogenital region of female perineum
- Posterior relations of cecum
- Posterior relations of kidney
- Visceral relations on inferior surface of liver
- Anatomical and surgical importance of pectinate line
- Holden's line

► MUSCLE

Q. EXTERNAL OBLIQUE MUSCLE

External oblique muscle is the most superficial muscle of the anterolateral side of abdominal wall. The fibers of the muscle are directed downwards, forwards and medially (like hands in pocket).

Attachments

- Arises from lower eight ribs (upper fibers mingle with serratus anterior and lower fibers mingle with latissimus dorsi)
- Muscle fibers get inserted into anterior two third of outer lip of iliac crest.

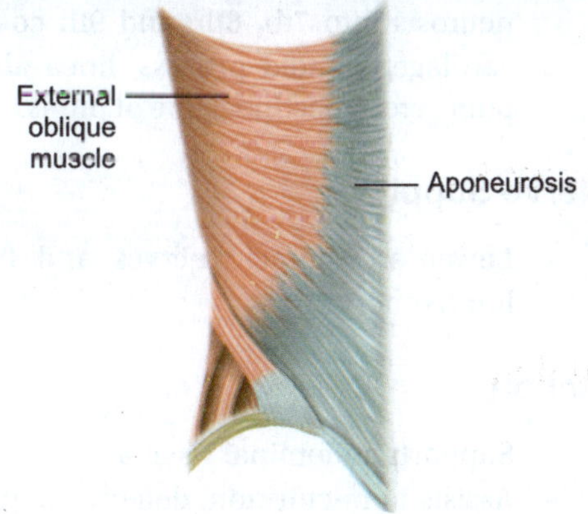

External oblique muscle

Aponeurosis gets inserted into xiphoid process, linea alba, pubic symphysis, pubic crest and pectineal line of pubis.

Nerve Supply

- Lower six thoracic nerves.

Action

- Supports abdominal viscera
- Assists in micturition, defecation, parturition, coughing, sneezing, etc.
- Lateral flexion and rotation of trunk.

Peculiarities

- Gets inserted in the form of flattened aponeurosis
- Lower edge of the aponeurosis gets folded on itself to form inguinal ligament
- Opening in the aponeurosis is known as superficial inguinal ring.

Q. INTERNAL OBLIQUE MUSCLE

The muscle lies on the anterolateral side of abdominal wall and below external oblique muscle. The fibers of the muscle are directed upwards, forwards and medially (muscle fibers are at right angle to external oblique muscle fibers).

Attachments

- Arises from lateral two third of inguinal ligament, anterior two third of inter-mediate area of iliac crest and thoraco-lumbar fascia
- Gets inserted in the form of broad apo-neurosis into 7th, 8th, and 9th costal cartilage, xiphoid process, linea alba, pubic crest, pectineal line of pubis.

Nerve Supply

- Lower six thoracic nerves and first lumbar nerve.

Action

- Supports abdominal viscera
- Assists in micturition, defecation, par-turition, coughing, sneezing, etc.
- Lateral flexion and rotation of trunk.

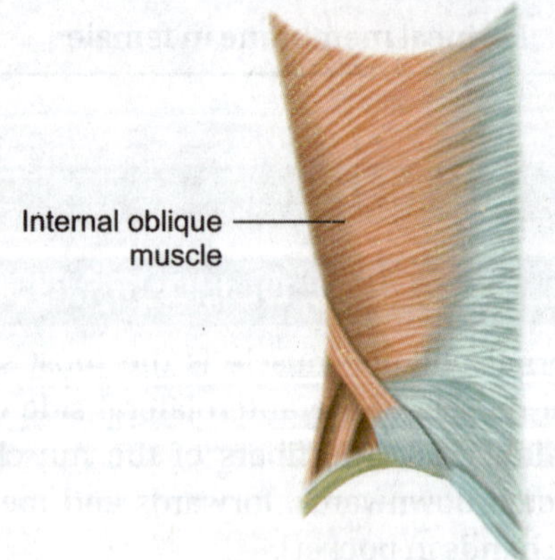

Internal oblique muscle

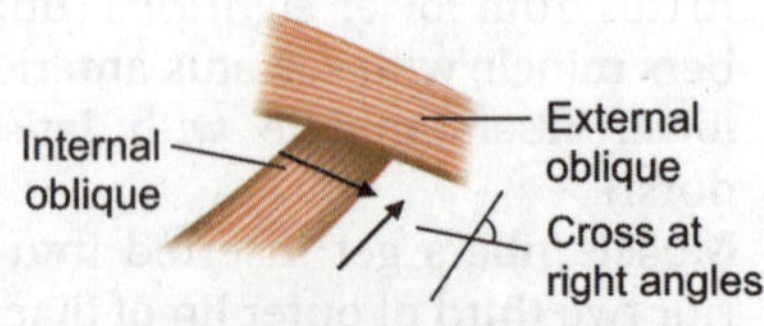

Disposition of oblique fibers

Q. TRANSVERSUS ABDOMINIS

Transversus abdominis is a deeper muscle on the anterolateral side of the abdominal wall. The fibers run transversely and hence the name.

Attachments

- Arises from lateral one third of inguinal ligament, anterior two third of inner lip of iliac crest, thoracolumbar fascia, inner surface of lower six costal cartilages
- Gets inserted in the form of broad aponeurosis into xiphoid process, linea alba, pubic crest, pectineal line of pubis.

Nerve Supply

- Lower six thoracic nerves and first lumbar nerve.

Action

- Supports abdominal viscera
- Assists in micturition, defecation, parturition, coughing, sneezing, etc.
- Lateral flexion and rotation of trunk.

Peculiarities

- Lower fibers of the muscle fuse with fibers of internal oblique to form conjoint tendon
- Fascia transversalis lines the inner surface of the muscle
- An oval opening is present in the fascia transversalis, around half inch above midinguinal point and is known as deep inguinal ring.

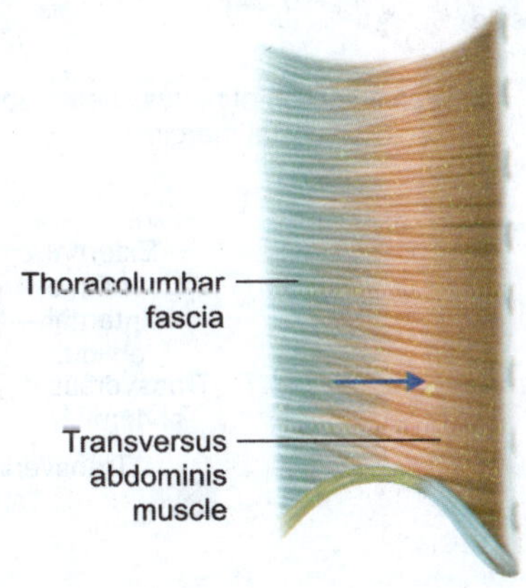

Transversus abdominis

Q. RECTUS SHEATH

Rectus sheath is an aponeurosis of internal oblique muscle, which splits into anterior and posterior layer to enclose rectus abdominis muscle.

Peculiarities

- External oblique aponeurosis fuses with anterior layer
- Transversus aponeurosis fuses with posterior layer
- Below the umbilicus all the three aponeuroses lie in front of rectus muscle

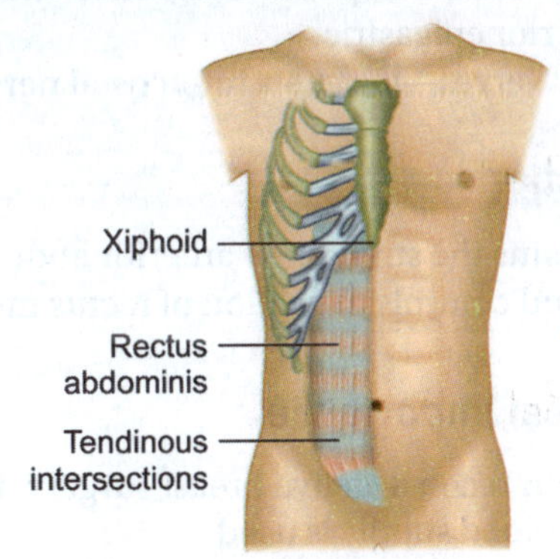

Rectus abdominis muscle

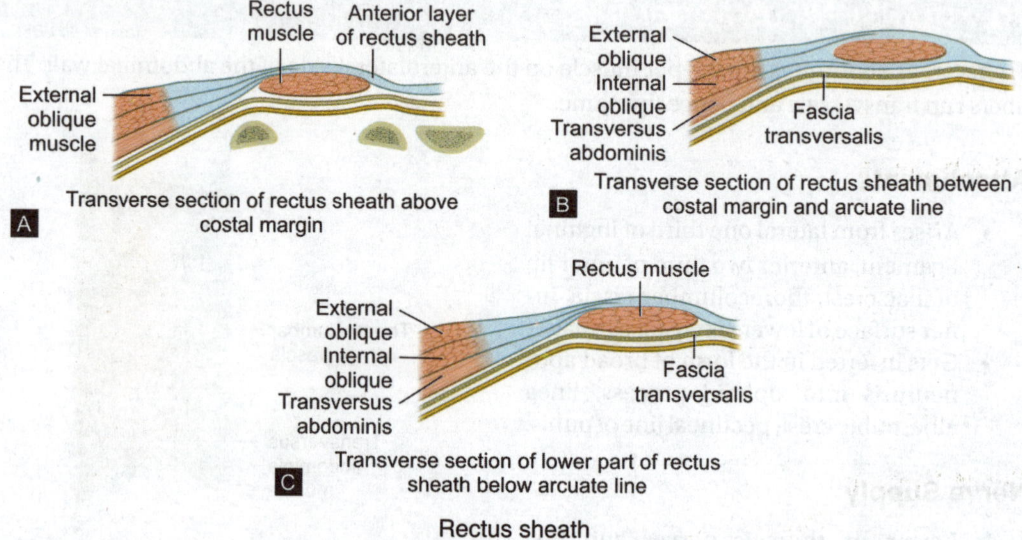

Rectus sheath

- Posterior layer of the sheath has a free concave margin known as arcuate line
- Aponeuroses of all the three muscles intersect in the midline to form linea alba
- Linea alba is wide above the umbilicus and narrow below the umbilicus.

Formation

- Above costal margin only external oblique and its aponeurosis is present
- Between umbilicus and costal margin the rectus muscle is completely enclosed in split internal oblique aponeurosis
- All the three aponeuroses are in front of the rectus muscle below the arcuate line.

Contents

- Muscles—rectus abdominis and pyramidalis
- Vessels—superior epigastric and inferior epigastric
- Nerves—lower six intercostal nerves.

Contents of rectus sheath

Functions

Maintains the strength of anterior abdominal wall and controls the action of rectus muscle.

Clinical Importance

- In reconstructive breast surgery, in cases of breast cancer, flap of rectus muscle with its blood supply is used

- After multiple pregnancies, the linea alba may weaken giving rise to a condition known as divarication of recti
- Supraumbilical median incisions provide bloodless operative field and are safe, but postoperative healing may cause weakness of abdominal wall
- Infraumbilical incisions hardly cause weakness of abdominal wall since natural gap between recti is very less.

Q. PERINEAL BODY

Perineal body is also known as the central tendon of perineum. It provides stability and support to pelvic structures.

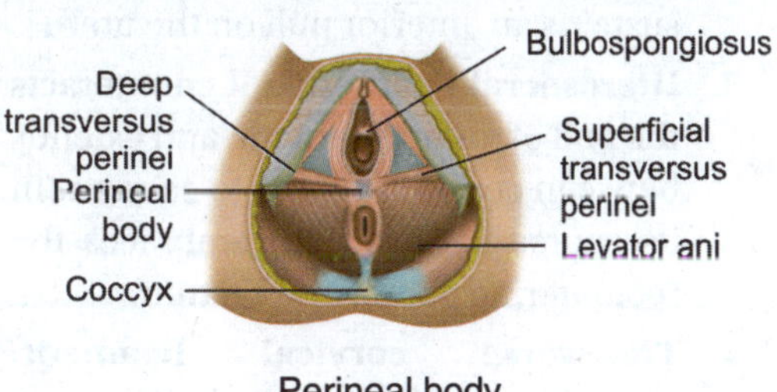

Perineal body

Locations

- Lies at posterior border of perineal membrane
- Located between anal canal and vagina or bulb of penis.

Formation

Following muscles gain attachment to this midline muscular mass:

- External anal sphincter
- Pubovaginalis (puboprostaticus)
- Levator ani partly
- Bulbospongiosus
- Superficial transversus perinei
- Deep transversus perinei.

Functions

Perineal body provides stability and support to pelvic structures.

Clinical Importance

Perineal body may weaken during childbirth giving rise to prolapse (herniation of organs to the exterior due to gravity) of pelvic organs.

Q. SUPPORTS OF UTERUS

Supports of the uterus can be classified into true supports and false supports.

True Supports

1. **Uterine position:** Angulation of body and fundus of uterus to cervix (angle of anteflexion) and angulation of cervix to vagina (angle of anteversion) itself provides positional support to uterus.

2. **Round ligament of uterus:** It maintains the uterine angulation by virtue of its attachment. It extends from upper part of uterus at the level of attachment of ligament of ovary to deep inguinal ring. It passes through the inguinal canal and gets attached to the fibrofatty tissue of labium majus. It sustains an anterior pull on the uterus.

3. **Uterosacral ligaments:** It counteracts the pull of round ligament, and extends between cervix of uterus to sacrum. In its course backwards it embraces the rectouterine pouch and rectum.

4. **Transverse cervical ligament:** Also known as cardinal ligament, Mackenrodt's ligament. It is the condensation of connective tissue between cervix and vaginal fornix to lateral wall of pelvis. It gives lateral support to the uterus and is considered as an cardinal support of uterus.

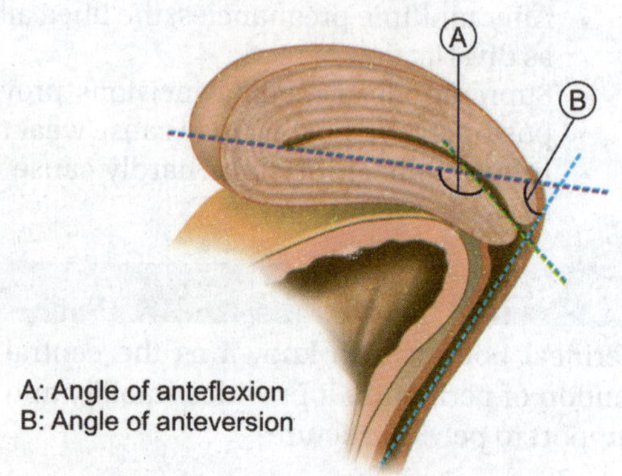

Positional support to uterus

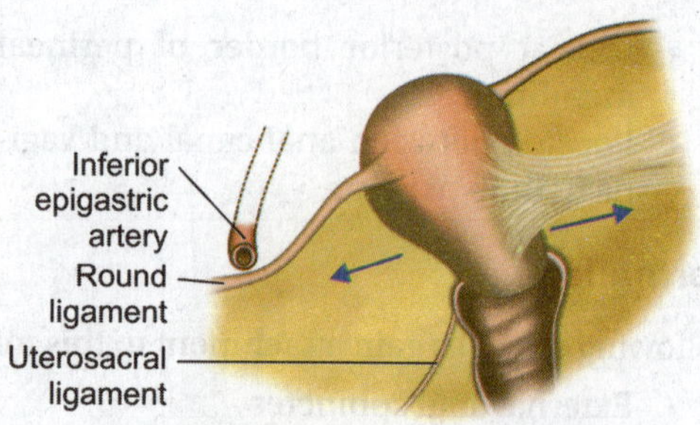

Counteraction of forward and backward pull

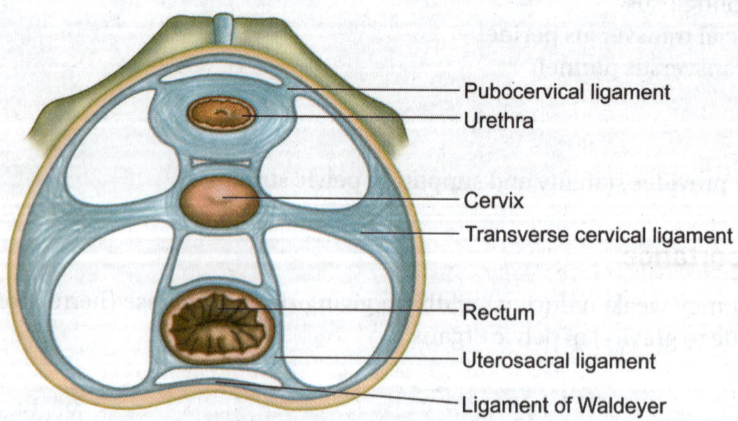

Condensations of pelvic fascia

5. **Pubovaginalis:** This part of levator ani and perineal body with its muscular attachment primarily support the vagina thus indirectly maintain the position of cervix.

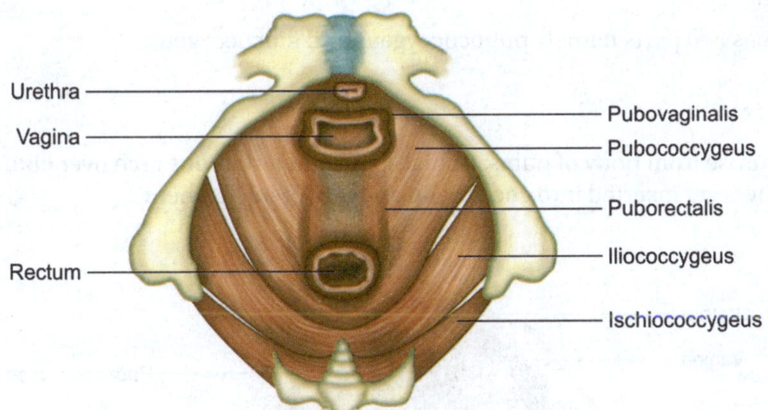

Pelvic diaphragm

False Supports

1. **Broad ligament:** It is not a true ligament, but a double-layered fold of peritoneum extending between lateral wall of uterus and pelvic wall. The upper free border contains the uterine tube and forms the mesosalpinx. The ureter adheres posteriorly while the line of lateral attachment crosses the obturator nerves and vessels.

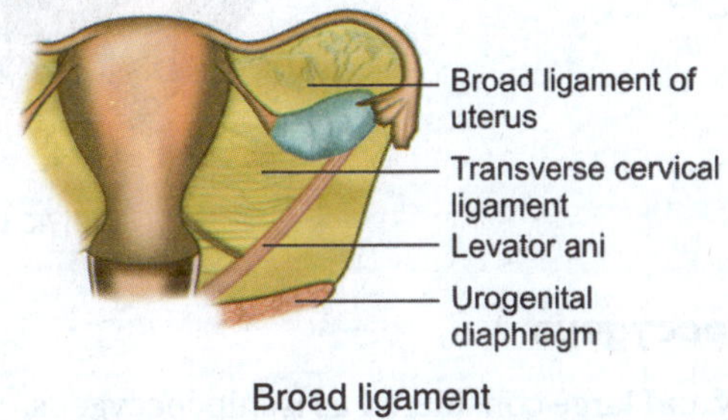

Broad ligament

2. **Anterior ligament:** It is the peritoneal fold reflected on to the bladder from the uterus. Hence known as uterovesical fold.
3. **Posterior ligament:** It is the peritoneal fold reflected from vaginal fornix to the anterior wall of rectum. Hence known as rectovaginal fold.

Clinical Importance

- Posterior inclination of uterus is known as Retroversion wherein the cervix faces forwards
- Sometimes the uterus may have a posterior curvature of the body and this is known as retroflexion
- Due to the weakness of pelvic floor muscles secondary to childbirth the uterus may protrude out of vagina this is known as prolapse of uterus.

Q. PELVIC DIAPHRAGM

The pelvic floor muscles form the pelvic diaphragm. These muscles suspend the pelvic structures like a hammock. It comprises of levator ani group of muscles and coccygeus.

Levator Ani

The muscle has two parts namely pubococcygeus and iliococcygeus.

Attachments

- Fibers arise from body of pubis, ischial spine and tendinous arch over obturator fascia
- The fibers get inserted into coccyx and anococcygeal ligament.

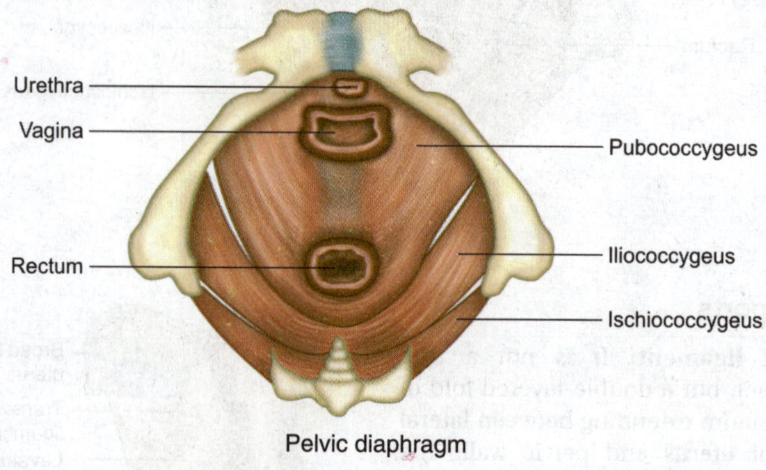

Pelvic diaphragm

Coccygeus

By and large considered as ischiococcygeus.

Attachments

- Arises from ischial spine
- Gets inserted into side of coccyx and lower part of sacrum.

Nerve Supply

Chiefly supplied by branches of sacral plexus through S3 and S4.

Actions

- Supports the pelvic viscera
- Contraction of pelvic floor counteracts the raised intra-abdominal pressure during sneezing, coughing or lifting heavy weights
- Assists during childbirth to expel the head of fetus
- Few fibers assist the urethral sphincter at the end of micturition.

Q. ANAL SPHINCTERS

The continence of anus and the sphincter mechanism of anus comprise of external and internal anal sphincters:

1. Internal anal sphincter is a downward extension of circular muscle layer of rectum.
2. External anal sphincter surrounds the internal muscle and conventionally thought to have deep superficial and subcutaneous portions. However it is considered to be a single sheet of muscle variably divided by fibers from longitudinal muscle layer of rectum.

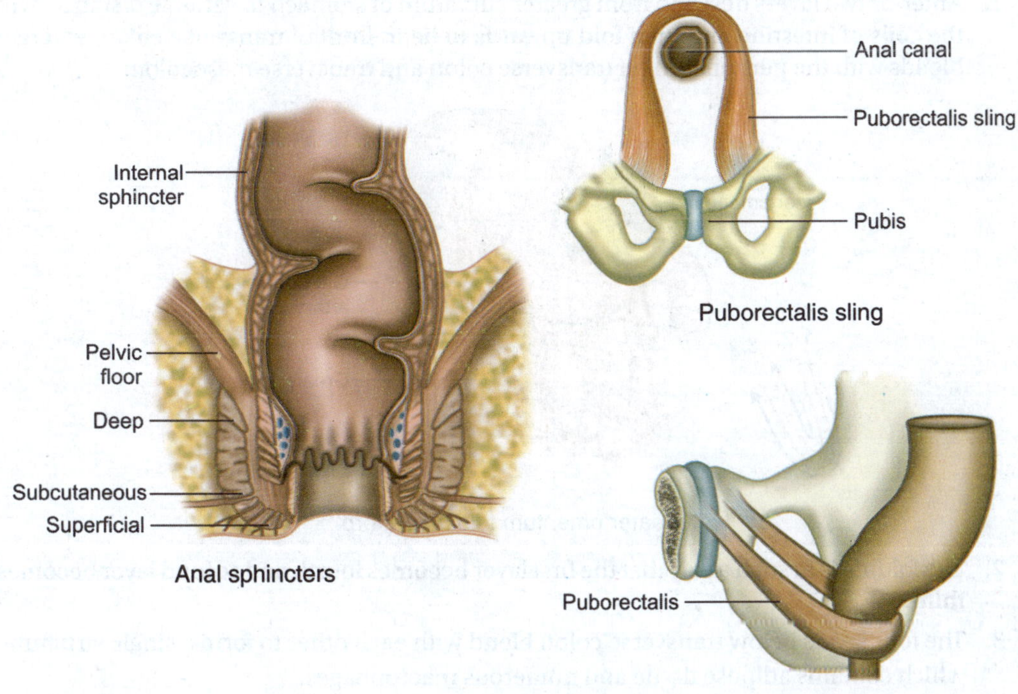

Peculiarities

- Internal anal sphincter is involuntary
- External anal sphincter is under voluntary control.

Nerve Supply

- Internal anal sphincter receives autonomic innervations
- External anal sphincter supplied by inferior rectal branch of pudendal nerve and perineal branch of S4.

Clinical Importance

- Damage to pudendal nerve during perineal surgeries can cause anal incontinence.

▶ PERITONEUM

Q. GREATER OMENTUM

Greater omentum is a double fold of peritoneum hanging from the greater curvature of stomach. It is made up of four layers folded upon itself.

Architecture

1. Anterior two layers descend from greater curvature of stomach to variable distance over the coils of intestine and then fold upwards to lie in front of transverse colon, where it blends with the peritoneum on transverse colon and transverse mesocolon.

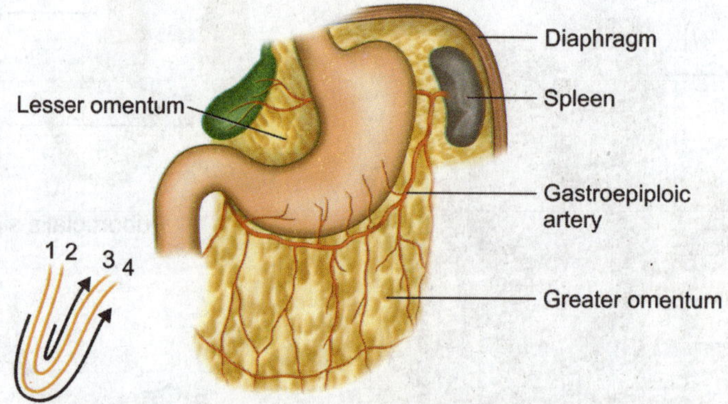

Greater omentum folding pattern

2. The folding is in such a way that the first layer becomes fourth and second layer becomes third.
3. The four layers below transverse colon blend with each other to form a single structure, which contains adipose tissue and numerous macrophages.

Subdivisions

- The part of greater omentum between stomach and transverse colon is named as gastro-colic omentum
- Double-layered fold of peritoneum between greater curvature of stomach and hilum of spleen is known as gastrosplenic ligament
- Double-layered fold of peritoneum between hilum of spleen and anterior surface of left kidney is known as splenorenal (lienorenal) ligament.

Contents

- Right and left gastroepiploic vessels
- Fat.

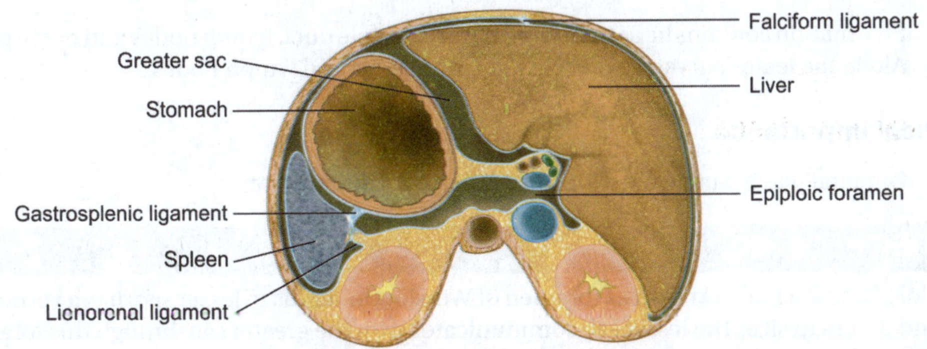

Transverse section of supracolic compartment

Functions

- Storehouse of fat
- Macrophages in the omentum protect against infection
- It limits the spread of infection by engulfing the site of infection.

Clinical Importance

Lesser sac can be approached through gastrocolic omentum.

Q. LESSER OMENTUM

Lesser omentum is a double-layered fold of peritoneum, which can be appreciated in the cadaver by lifting the liver away from stomach.

Attachments

1. Gastric attachment extends from right side of abdominal esophagus, lesser curvature of stomach and first 2 cm of duodenum.
2. Hepatic attachment is in the form of letter inverted 'L' wherein it is attached to fissure for ligamentum venosum and margins of porta hepatis.

Features

- Between the duodenum and the liver is the free margin of lesser omentum where the anterior and posterior layers are continuous
- Free margin forms anterior boundary of epiploic foramen.

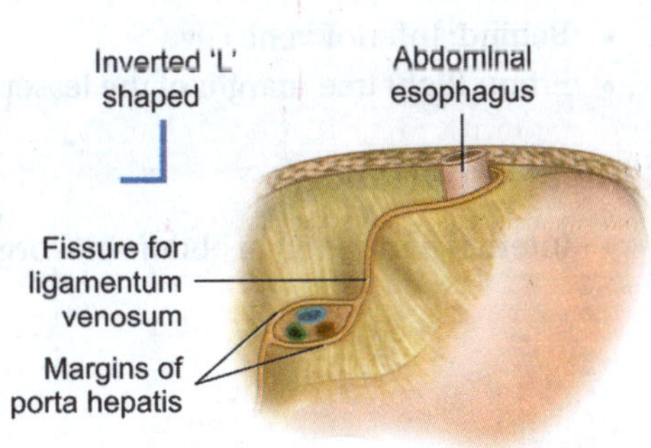

Lesser omentum (attachments and contents)

Contents

- Free margin contains hepatic artery, portal vein, bile duct, lymph nodes and nerve plexus
- Along the lesser curvature there are gastric vessels and lymph nodes.

Clinical Importance

- Omental patch can be used for closure of gastric perforation.

Q. EPIPLOIC FORAMEN

Epiploic foramen is also known as foramen of Winslow or aditus to lesser sac. It is a vertical slit around 2.5 cm in size. The lesser sac communicates with the greater sac through this foramen.

Location

- Epiploic foramen is located at the right border of the lesser sac and at the level of T12 vertebra.

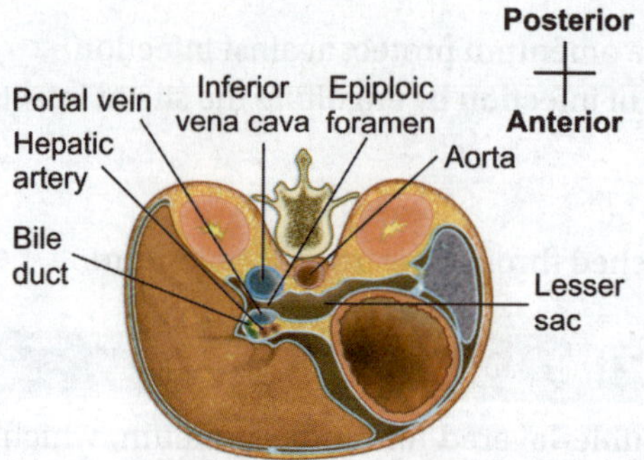

Transverse section at T12 showing epiploic foramen

Boundaries

- Above: Caudate process of liver
- Below: First part of duodenum
- Behind: Inferior vena cava
- Front: Right free margin of the lesser omentun.

Clinical Importance

- Internal herniation of abdominal organs may occur throw this foramen.

Q. VERTICAL DISPOSITION OF PERITONEUM (DIAGRAM ONLY).

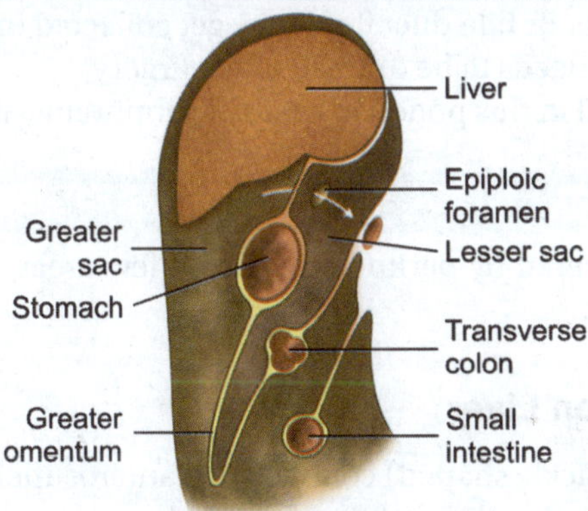

Vertical disposition of peritoneum (sagittal section)

Q. HORIZONTAL SECTION THROUGH SUPRACOLIC COMPARTMENT OF PERITONEUM (DIAGRAM ONLY).

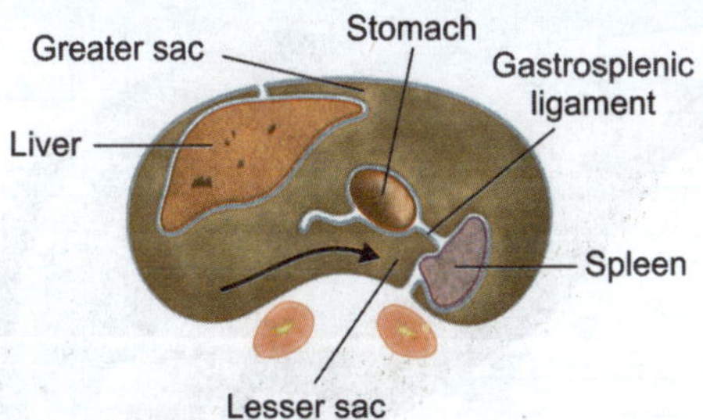

Transverse section of supracolic compartment of peritoneum

Q. HEPATORENAL POUCH (MORISON'S POUCH)

Hepatorenal pouch is the most dependent space of the supracolic peritoneal cavity in horizontal position.

Location

- Hepatorenal pouch is a deep recess located above the upper pole of right kidney lined by peritoneal cavity (right subhepatic space, right posterior space).

Boundaries

- Front: Inferior surface of liver
- Above: Coronary ligament of liver
- Behind: Peritoneum of diaphragm.

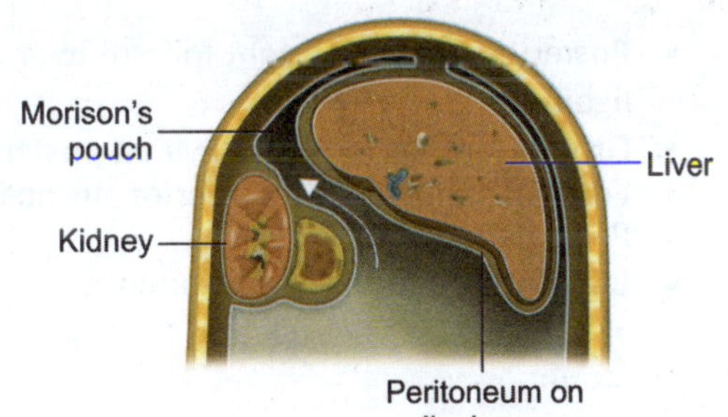

Hepatorenal pouch (Morison's pouch)

Clinical Importance

- After surgeries on liver or bile duct fluid may get collected in this pouch due to its position. Thus the pouch needs to be drained after surgery.
- The pus gets collected in this pouch in cases of subphrenic abscess.

Q. PERITONEAL REFLECTIONS AND BARE AREAS ON LIVER.

Large surface of liver is covered by peritoneum except few areas, which are not covered are known as bare areas of liver.

Peritoneal Ligaments on Liver

- Falciform ligament (sickle shaped) connects the anterosuperior surface of liver to anterior abdominal wall and under surface of diaphragm
- Left triangular ligament—connects superior surface of left lobe of liver to diaphragm
- Right triangular ligament—connects lateral part of posterior surface of right lobe of liver to the diaphragm
- Coronary ligaments—encloses the bare area on posterior surface of right lobe of liver.

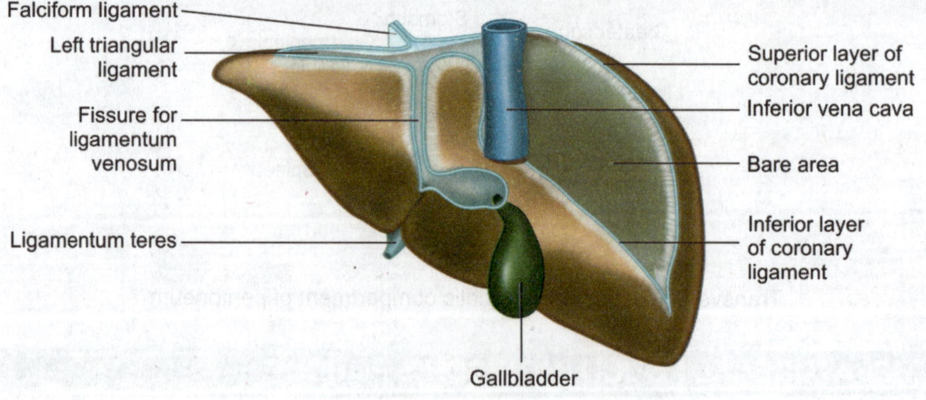

Peritoneal ligaments on liver

Bare Areas on Liver

- Posterior surface of right lobe of liver between coronary ligament and right triangular ligament
- Groove for inferior vena cava on posterior surface of right lobe of liver
- Fossa of gallbladder on inferior surface of right lobe of liver
- Porta hepatis
- Lines of reflections of peritoneum.

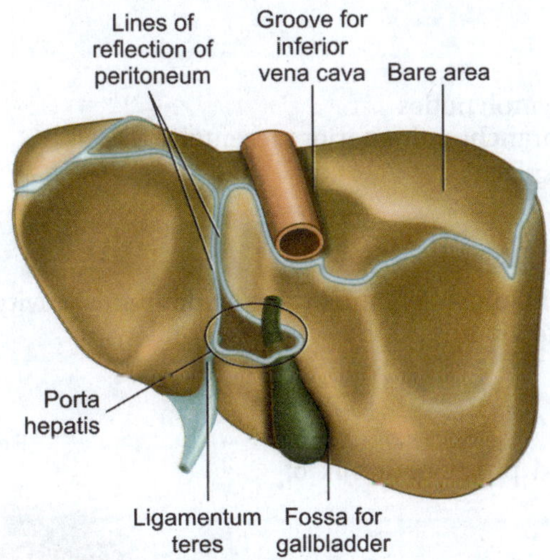

Bare areas of liver (inferior view of liver)

Q. MESENTERY

The coils of jejunum and ileum suspend from the posterior abdominal wall with the help of mesentery.

Attachment and Disposition

- Root of the mesentery is the fixed portion, disposed obliquely across duodenojejunal flexure to upper part of right sacroiliac joint
- Free border of the mesentery is thrown in folds in the form of fan held in hand.

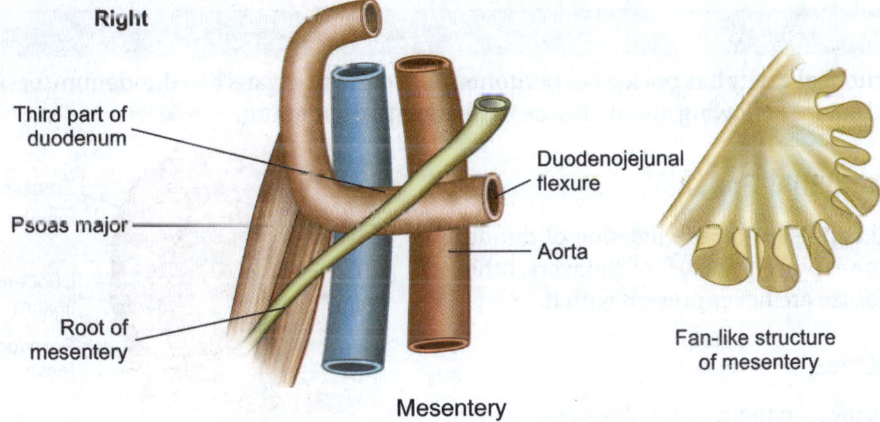

Mesentery

Relations

- Mesentery crosses third part of duodenum, abdominal aorta, inferior vena cava, right ureter and right psoas major.

Contents

- Fat
- Lymphatics and lymph nodes
- Jejunal and ileal branches of superior mesenteric vessels
- Autonomic nerve plexus.

Q. RECTOUTERINE POUCH (POUCH OF DOUGLAS)

Rectouterine pouch is the most dependent part of peritoneal cavity in standing position. So the fluid gets accumulated in this pouch by virtue of gravity.

Boundaries

- Front: Uterus and posterior fornix of vagina
- Behind: Rectum
- Above: Connected to peritoneal cavity
- Below: Rectovaginal fold of peritoneum.

Clinical Importance

- In cases of abscess formation in pelvis the pus may get collected in the pouch
- The pouch can be approached through posterior fornix or rectum
- In per-rectal or per-vaginal examination, the pouch can be felt 5.5 cm above anus.

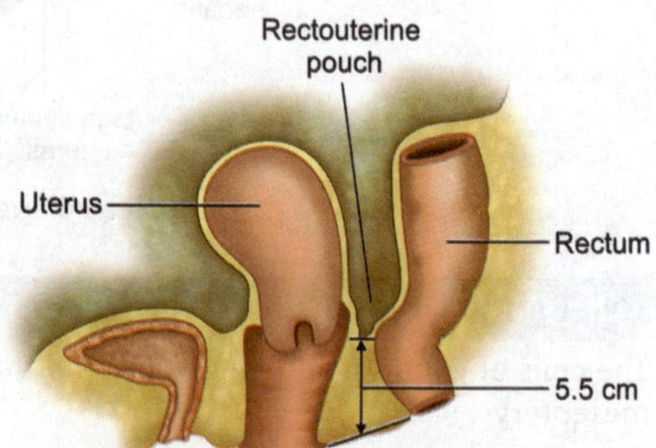

Female pelvis showing rectouterine pouch (sagittal section)

Q. DUODENAL FOSSAE

The peritoneal cavity has pockets of peritoneal fold close to organs like duodenum, cecum and sigmoid colon. Following are the fossae in relation to duodenum.

Paraduodenal Fossa

- It is present on the left side of duodenum, present in 20% of cadavers, other fossae are never present with it.

Boundaries

- Above—pancreas, renal vessels
- Front—inferior mesenteric vein
- Right—aorta
- Left—kidney.

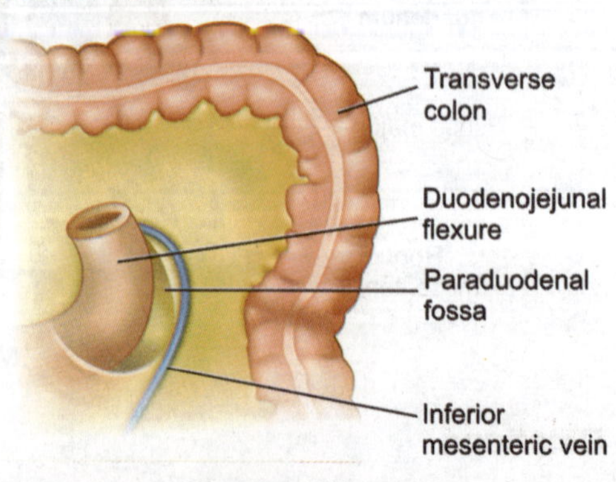

Duodenal fossae

Clinical Importance

- In case of internal herniation, while opening the fossa, surgeon has to be careful of the inferior mesenteric vein in front.

Superior and Inferior Duodenojejunal Fossa

- These fossae are often present
- They are to the left of duodenum
- Superior fossa looks downwards, is 2–3 cm in depth and is in front of L2 vertebra
- Inferior fossa looks upwards and lies in front of L3.

Inferior Duodenal Fossa

- Inferior duodenal fossa is present below the third part of duodenum.

Mesentericoparietal Fossa of Waldeyer

- Mesentericoparietal fossa of Waldeyer lies behind the superior mesenteric artery close to beginning of jejunum
- The fossa looks to the left
- Superior mesenteric artery lies in front.

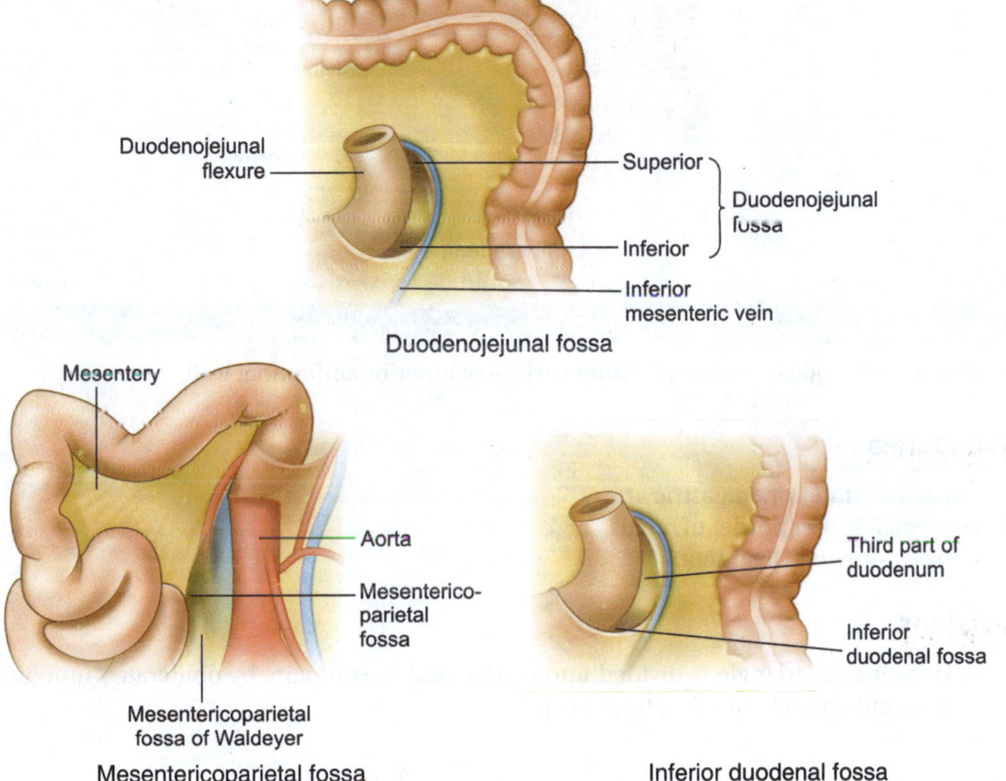

Duodenojejunal fossa

Mesentericoparietal fossa

Inferior duodenal fossa

Clinical Importance

- Surgeon has to be vigilant of superior mesenteric artery, while approaching the fossa.

▶ TRIANGLES IN ABDOMEN

Q. LUMBAR TRIANGLE

Lumbar triangle is also known as Petit's triangle.

Boundaries

- Laterally—posterior border of external oblique
- Medially—lateral and lower margin of latissimus dorsi
- Base—Iliac crest.

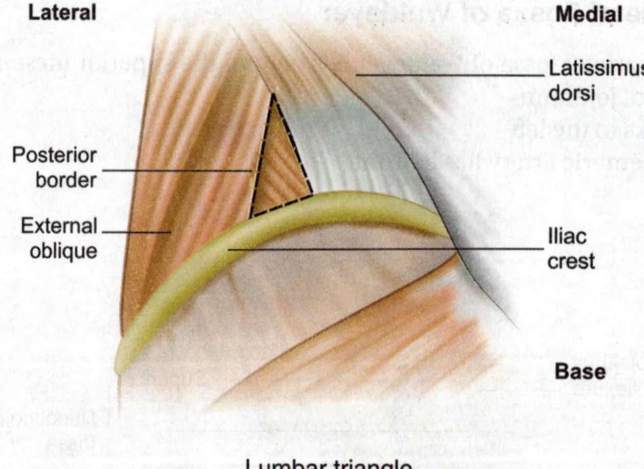

Lumbar triangle

Q. HESSELBACH'S TRIANGLE

Hesselbach's triangle is seen at the inner surface of anterior abdominal wall.

Boundaries

- Lateral—inferior epigastric artery
- Medial—outer border of rectus
- Base—inguinal ligament.

Divisions

- Hesselbach's triangle is divided into medial and lateral parts by obliterated umbilical ligament (lateral umbilical ligament).

Clinical Importance

- Direct inguinal hernia leaves the abdominal cavity through this triangle.

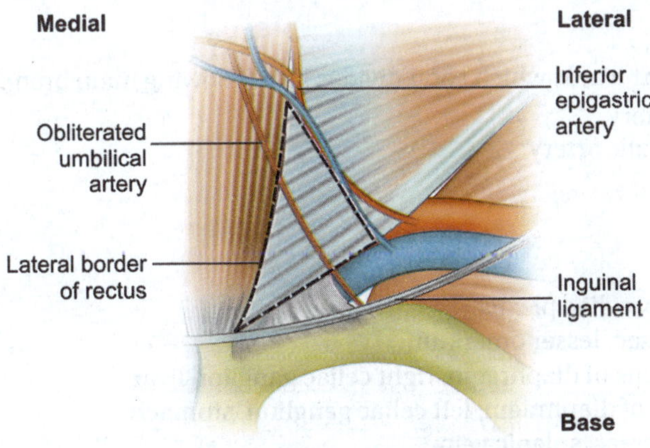

Hesselbach's triangle

Q. CALOT'S TRIANGLE

A triangle can be identified, while doing cholecystectomy (removal of gallbladder), following are the boundaries of Calot's triangle.

Boundaries

- Left—common hepatic duct
- Right—cystic duct
- Above—liver.

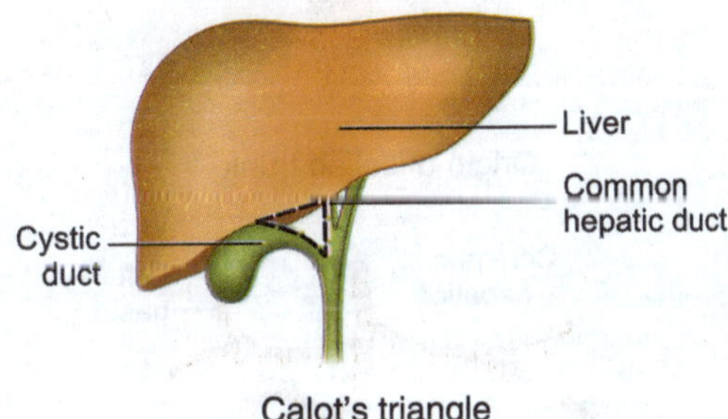

Calot's triangle

Contents

- Cystic artery
- Right hepatic artery.

Clinical Importance

- While doing cholecystectomy surgeon has to be aware of the variations of the vessels in Calot's triangle
- While performing cholecystectomy dissection can begin from Calot's triangle.

▶ ARTERIES

Q. CELIAC TRUNK

Celiac trunk is the artery of foregut supplying lower part of esophagus, stomach, upper part of duodenum, liver, spleen and pancreas.

Origin

- Arises from front of aorta at the level between T12 and L1 vertebra.

Main Branches

Celiac trunk is a short trunk, which soon divides into following main branches:
- Left gastric artery
- Common hepatic artery
- Splenic artery.

Relations

- Surrounded by celiac plexus
- Front—lesser sac, lesser omentum
- Right—right crus of diaphragm, right celiac ganglion liver
- Left—left crus of diaphragm, left celiac ganglion, stomach
- Inferior—pancreas, splenic vein.

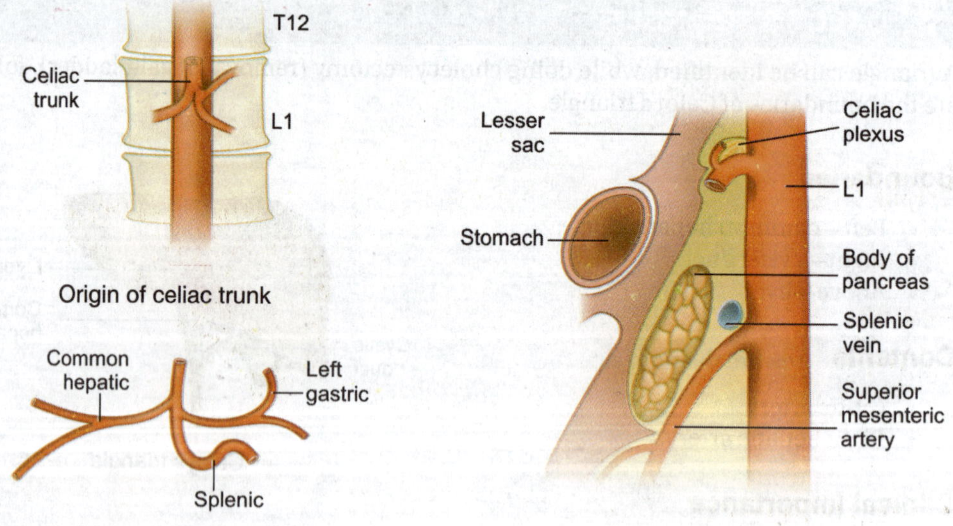

Subdivisions of Main Branches

- Left gastric artery—esophageal branches
- Common hepatic artery—right gastric, gastroduodenal, hepatic artery proper
- Splenic artery—left epiploic, short gastric, arteria pancreatica magna.

Clinical Importance

Sometimes the origin of celiac trunk may get compressed by median arcuate ligament, giving rise to median arcuate ligament syndrome. Commonly seen in women, wherein blood supply to abdominal viscera may get compromised causing severe epigastric pain following food intake.

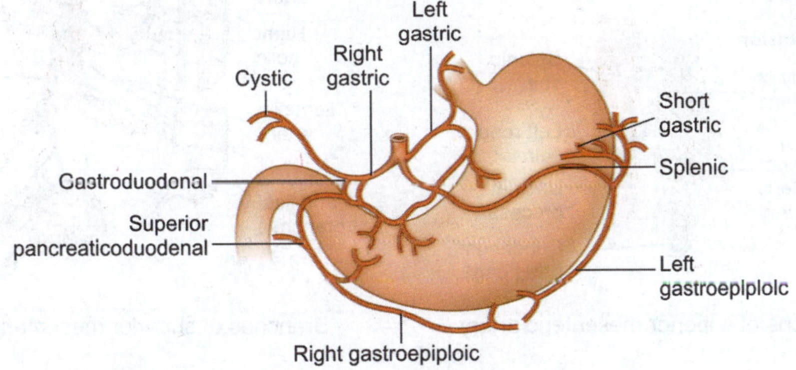

Celiac trunk and its branches

Q. SUPERIOR MESENTERIC ARTERY

Superior mesenteric artery is the artery of midgut. The artery supplies the portion of the gut from the entrance of bile duct to a level just proximal to splenic flexure of colon.

Origin

- Front of aorta, at the level of L1 vertebra.

Course

- Curved toward the right side (like a sword).

Clinical Importance

- Pressure of the artery on the renal vein can give rise to left sided varicocele
- Pressure on the duodenum will give rise to symptoms of intestinal obstruction.

Relations

- Front—splenic vein, body of pancreas
- Behind—left renal vein, uncinate process of pancreas, third part of the duodenum

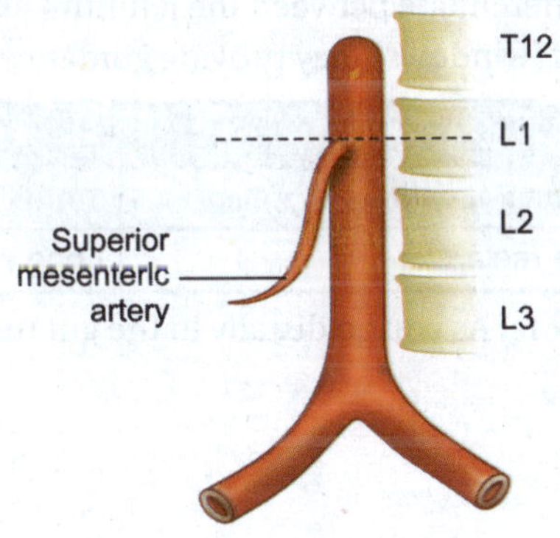

Superior mesenteric artery

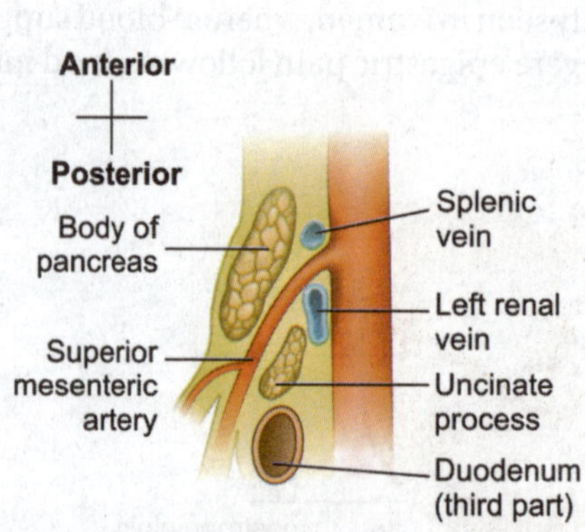

Relations of superior mesenteric artery

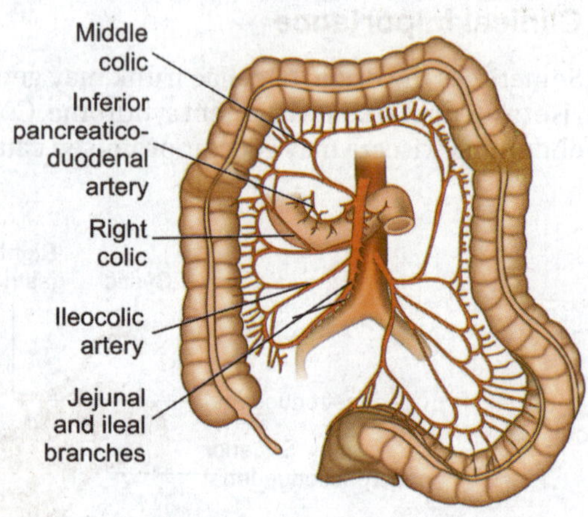

Branches of superior mesenteric artery

- Right—superior mesenteric vein
- Left—root of mesentery.

Branches

- Inferior pancreaticoduodenal
- Jejunal and ileal branches
- Ileocolic
- Right colic
- Middle colic.

Q. DIFFERENCES BETWEEN THE VASCULAR ARCADES OF JEJUNUM AND ILEUM.

To differentiate between the jejunum and ileum, the arrangement and number of vascular arcades (windows) may provide guidance during surgery.

Parts	Jejunum	Ileum
Vascular arcades	1 or 2	3–5
Vasa recta	Long and few	Short and many

Note: As you go distally in the gut the number and density of arterial arcades increases.

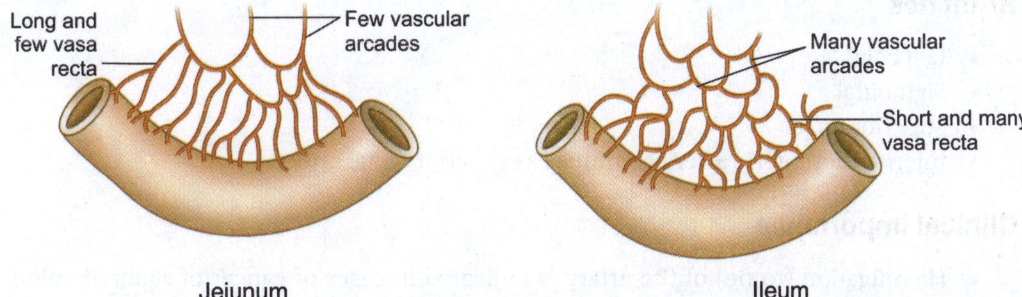

Jejunum   Ileum

Q. INFERIOR MESENTERIC ARTERY

Inferior mesenteric artery is the artery of hindgut. It supplies the left one third of transverse colon, descending colon, sigmoid colon and proximal part of anal canal above the pectinate line.

Origin

- Front of aorta at the level of L3
- Proximal to bifurcation of aorta by 3.8 cm.

Course

- Inferior mesenteric artery runs downwards to the left retroperitoneally.

Relations

- Behind—left common iliac artery
- Lateral—ureter, inferior mesenteric vein.

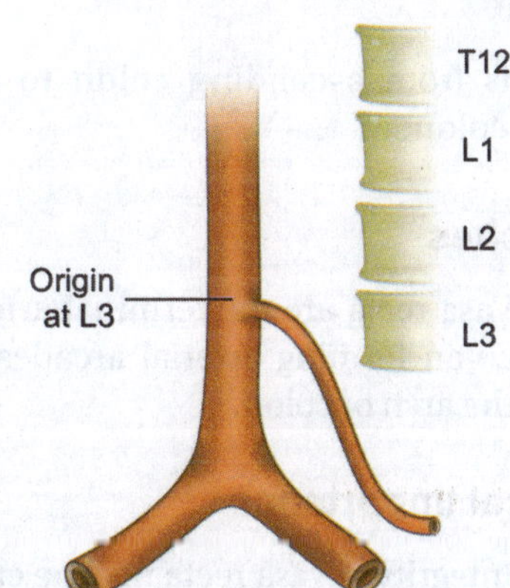

Inferior mesenteric artery

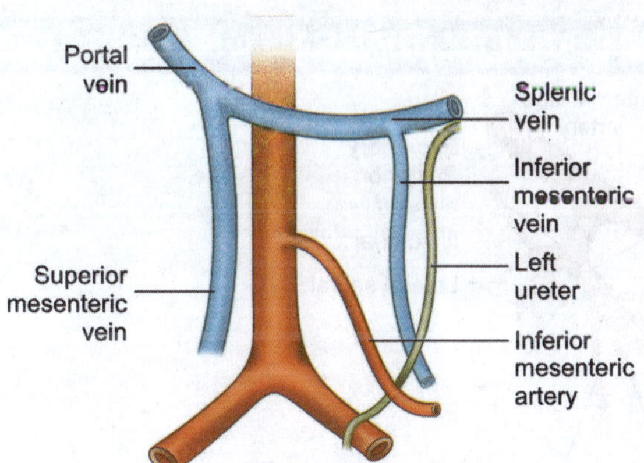

Relations of inferior mesenteric artery

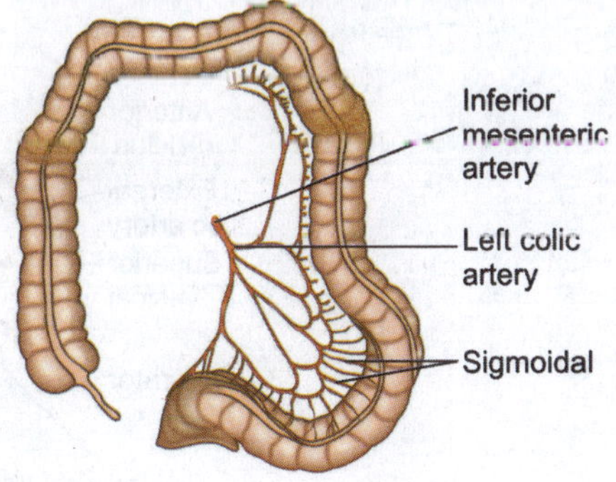

Branches of inferior mesenteric artery

Branches

- Left colic
- Sigmoidal
- Superior rectal
- Inferior mesenteric artery continues as superior rectal artery.

Clinical Importance

- High ligation (to tie) of the artery is indicated in cases of cancer of sigmoid colon or rectum.

Q. MARGINAL ARTERY

Marginal artery is a paracolic vessel under the arch of colon, formed by the anastomosis between the branches of colic arteries.

Extent

Extends from ascending colon to end of pelvic colon.

Branches

- Vasa recta are the terminal arteries to colon forming arterial arcades below the arch of colon.

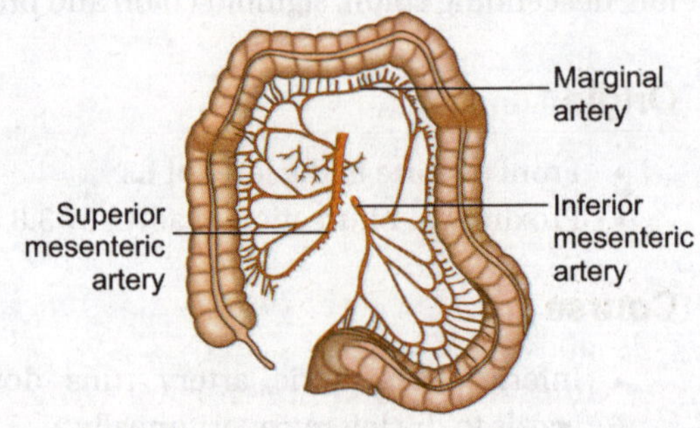

Marginal artery

Clinical Importance

- Integrity of vasa recta may be crucial to maintain blood supply of bowel when the mesenteric arteries are ligated.

Q. BRANCHES OF INTERNAL ILIAC ARTERY (DIAGRAM ONLY).

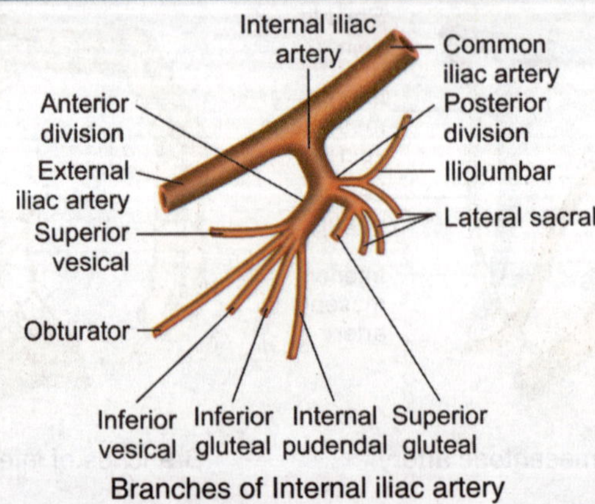

Branches of Internal iliac artery

▶ LYMPHATICS

Q. CISTERNA CHYLI

Cisterna chyli is a lymph sac from which the thoracic duct begins.

Location

- Lies in front of L1 and L2.

Relations

- Lies between aorta, right crus of diaphragm and inferior vena cava.

Tributaries

- Right lumbar trunk
- Left lumbar trunk
- Intestinal trunk.

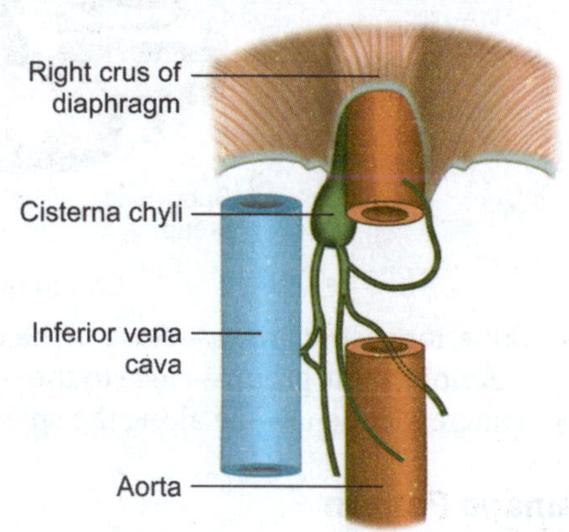

Drainage Areas

- Lumbar trunks drain the lymph from lower limbs, pelvic viscera, kidney, adrenals and abdominal walls
- Intestinal lymph drains lymph from stomach, pancreas, spleen, most of liver and intestines.

Q. LYMPHATIC DRAINAGE OF STOMACH.

The knowledge of lymphatic drainage of stomach is very important in managing gastric cancer. Stomach is divided into three lymphatic territories similar to the vascular territories of celiac artery.

Divisions of Lymphatic Areas

There are three territories identified on the stomach:
- Right two third upper area along the lesser curvature of stomach
- Left lower one third area along greater curvature of stomach
- Left upper area close to the spleen
- The efferents of all the lymph of stomach goes to celiac group of lymph nodes.

Lymph Groups of Stomach

- Hepatic group—lies in lesser omentum, receives lymph from liver and gallbladder
- Subpyloric group—lie in the angle between first and second part of duodenum, close to the bifurcation of gastroduodenal artery, receives lymph through inferior gastric nodes draining right two third of lesser curvature of stomach

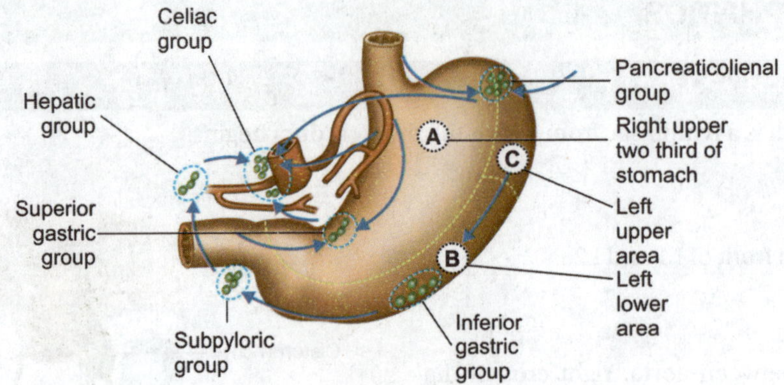

Lymph groups of stomach

- Superior gastric group—close to the cardiac end of stomach
- Inferior gastric group—close to the pylorus within the layers of greater omentum
- Pancreaticolienal—lie along the splenic artery.

Drainage Pattern

- Lesser curvature of stomach is drained by superior gastric nodes and finally celiac nodes
- Region close to pylorus drains into inferior gastric nodes, thence to subpyloric and then to celiac nodes
- Upper gastric area close to the spleen is drained by pancreaticolienal nodes and finally into celiac nodes.

Clinical Importance

- While operating cases of cancer stomach, surgeon has to be aware of the drainage pattern of lymph nodes to clear all those lymphatic areas likely to get involved.

Q. LYMPHATIC DRAINAGE OF RECTUM.

The lymph from the rectum is drained by various lymphatic groups thus cancer can spread in various directions.

Lymph Groups Involved

- Inguinal group
- Internal iliac group
- Sacral group
- Left common iliac group.

Efferent Lymph Vessels of Rectum

- Downwards to involve perianal skin, ischiorectal fossa, external anal sphincter
- Laterally involves levator ani muscles, urinary bladder, seminal vesicles (in females involves vagina, cervix and base of broad ligament)

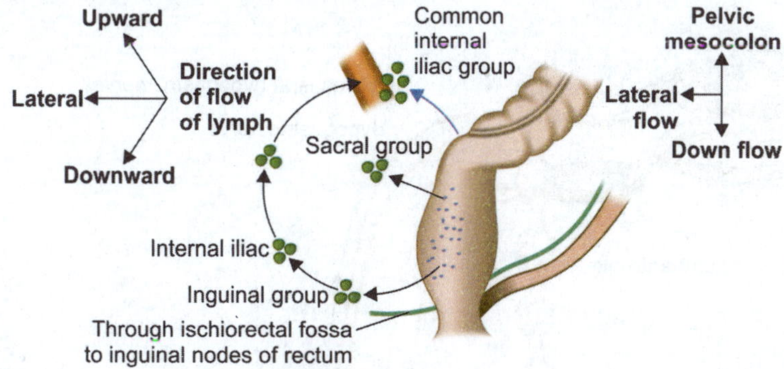

Lymphatic drainage of rectum

- Upwards involves pelvic peritoneum, pelvic mesocolon and nodes close to inferior mesenteric artery.

Clinical Importance

- Cancer of rectum can spread along these lymphatic channels and secondary involvement can be seen in these areas
- The surgeries in cancer rectum, may mandate removal of pelvic colon with mesocolon, rectum, anus perianal skin, ischiorectal fossa (fat filled) and levator ani with the fascia.

▶ NERVES

Autonomic nervous system is concerned with innervations of viscera, glands, blood vessels and smooth muscles.

Q. URINARY BLADDER INNERVATION

General Features

- The nerves supplying the bladder comprises of sympathetic and parasympathetic components
- These nerves form the vesical plexus
- Both efferent and afferent components are present in sympathetic and parasympathetic fibers.

Bladder Innervation

- Parasympathetic nerve fibers arise from S2, S3, S4 segments of the spinal cord (nervi erigentes)
- Sympathetic fibers arise from T11, T12, L1 and L2 segments of spinal cord
- Parasympathetic fibers are excitatory to detrusor muscle and inhibitory to sphincter urethrae
- Sympathetic nerves have vice versa function, i.e. inhibitory to detrusor and excitatory to sphincter urethrae
- The pudendal nerve supplies the skeletal muscle, sphincter urethrae.

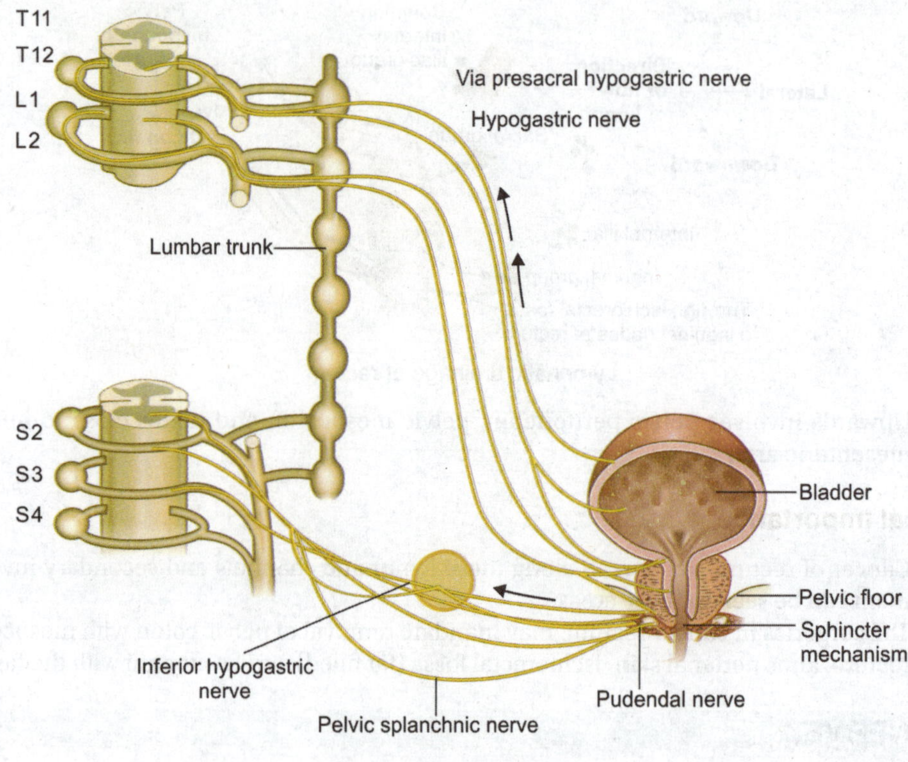

Bladder innervation

Functional Aspects

1. Normal emptying of the bladder occurs by contraction of detrusor muscle and simultaneous relaxation of urethral sphincter and pelvic floor.
2. Accumulation of urine initially adjusts the tone and then stimulates the stretch receptors, which carry the afferent sensation along pelvic splanchnic nerve to the sacral segments (S2, S3, S4).
3. Parasympathetic cell bodies are stimulated and efferent impulses flow down through pelvic splanchnic nerve to postganglionic cells within the bladder and cause bladder contraction.
4. This is autonomic stretch reflex.
5. With training, higher centers in brain, i.e. inferior frontal gyrus takes control over the spinal stretch reflex. This center has a inhibitory activity.

Clinical Importance

- In spinal cord section above S2, the cortical control is lost and sacral reflex is intact and bladder automatically empties on distension
- If the sacral segments itself are not functional the detrusor muscle is paralyzed and the bladder distends, but emptying is not possible leading to urinary incontinence.

▶ MISCELLANEOUS

Q. REGIONS OF ABDOMEN (DIAGRAM ONLY).

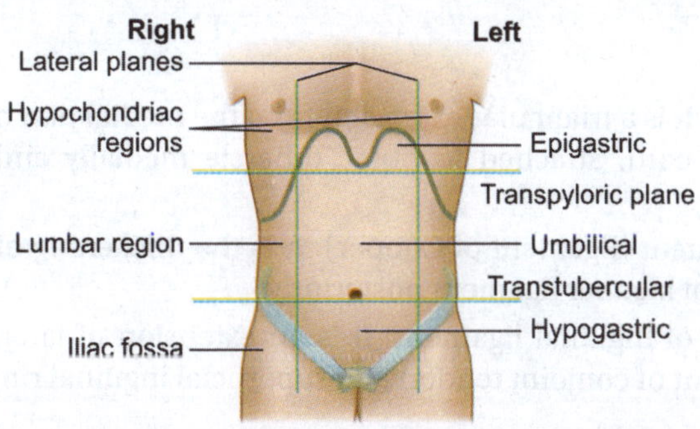

Regions of abdomen

Q. INGUINAL LIGAMENT

The lower border of external oblique aponeurosis folds upon itself to form the inguinal ligament.

Location

- Lies beneath the fold of groin.

Extent

- Anterior superior iliac spine to pubic tubercle.

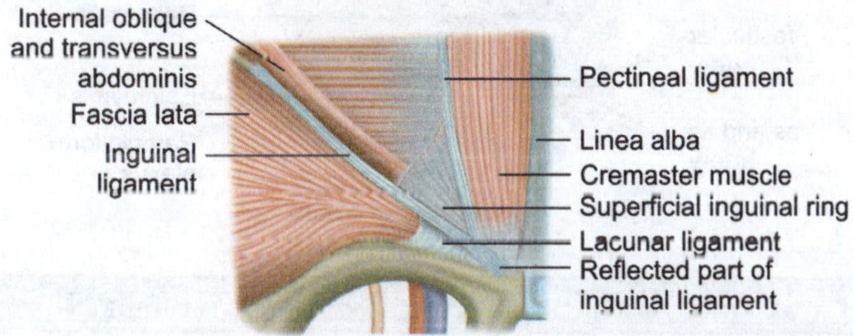

Extensions of inguinal ligament

Structures Attached to the Ligament

- Fascia lata is attached to outer lower border, thus is convex downwards
- Internal oblique and transversus oblique take origin from its upper surface lateral part
- Cremaster muscle is attached to its middle part.

Relations

- Medial half forms the floor of inguinal canal
- Spermatic cord in males and round ligament in females is lodged on the superior surface of ligament.

Extensions

1. Pectineal part: It is a triangular extension from the medial part of the ligament, supports the spermatic cord, attached to pubic tubercle medially and laterally supports the inguinal ring.
2. Pectineal ligament (ligament of Cooper): It is the thickening of pectineal fascia and is the extension of lacunar ligament posteriorly.
3. Reflected part of inguinal ligament: It is an extension of lateral crus of inguinal ring medially in front of conjoint tendon and superficial inguinal ring.

Q. COVERINGS OF TESTIS (DIAGRAM ONLY).

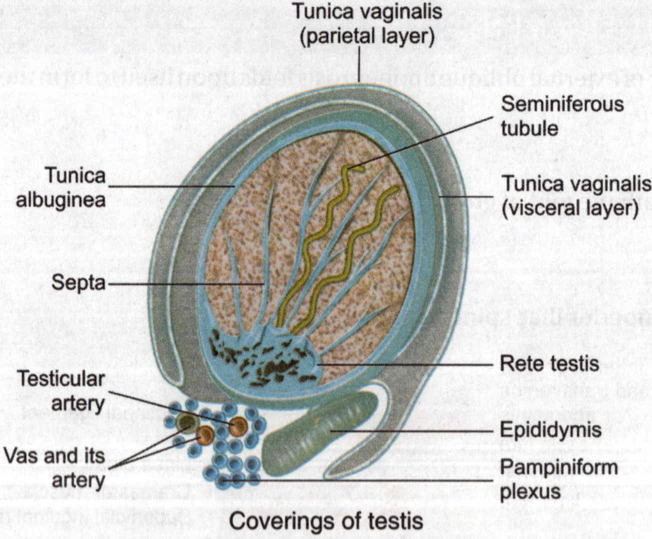

Coverings of testis

Q. INGUINAL CANAL

Inguinal canal is an oblique intermuscular slit above the medial half of inguinal ligament, placed horizontally:

- Length: 4 cm
- Extent: Lies between the deep inguinal ring and superficial inguinal ring.

Boundaries

- Anterior wall—external oblique aponeurosis and assisted laterally by internal oblique muscle

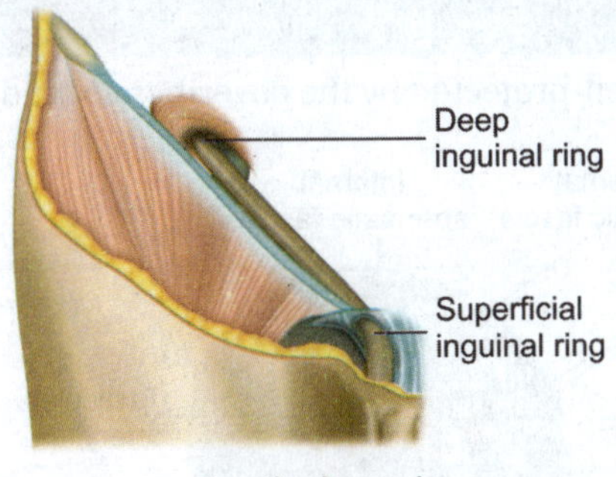

Inguinal canal

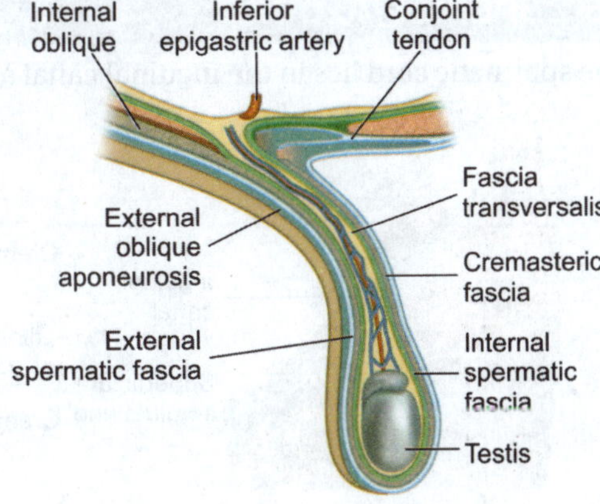

Boundaries of inguinal canal

- Posterior wall—transversalis fascia, reinforced medially by conjoint tendon
- Floor—inrolled lower edge of inguinal ligament, strengthened medially by lacunar ligament
- Roof—arched fibers of internal oblique and transversus abdominis muscle.

Contents

- In males—spermatic cord, ilioinguinal nerve
- In females—round ligament, ilioinguinal nerve.

Clinical Importance

- Indirect inguinal hernia occurs through deep inguinal ring lateral to inferior epigastric artery
- Direct inguinal hernia occurs medial to inferior epigastric artery
- Incomplete hernia does not cross superficial inguinal ring.

Q. TRANSVERSE SECTION OF PENIS (DIAGRAM ONLY).

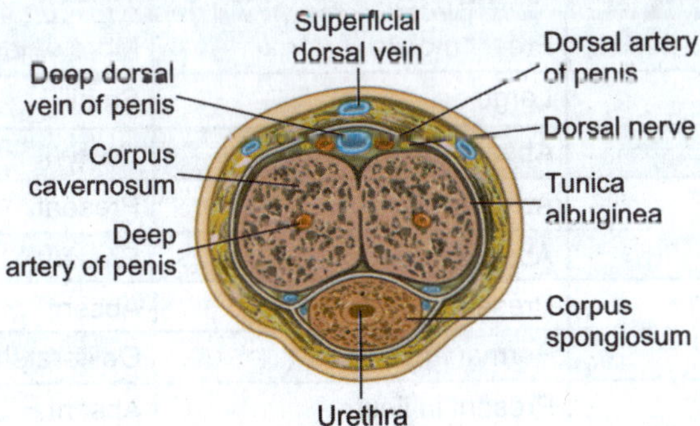

Transverse section of penis

Q. SPERMATIC CORD

The spermatic cord lies in the inguinal canal and is well-protected by the coverings around it.

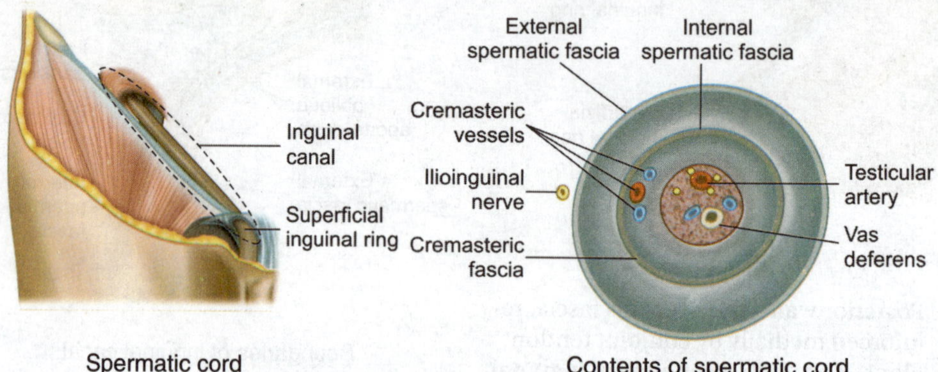

Spermatic cord   Contents of spermatic cord

Following are the coverings and their derivatives:

- Internal spermatic fascia derived from transversalis fascia
- Cremasteric fascia derived from cremaster muscle
- External spermatic fascia is derived from external oblique aponeurosis.

Contents

- Vas deferens
- Testicular artery, cremasteric artery, artery to vas
- Pampiniform plexus
- Testicular lymphatics
- Genital branch of genitofemoral nerve
- Processus vaginalis.

Q. DIFFERENCES BETWEEN SMALL AND LARGE INTESTINE.

Features	Small intestine	Large intestine
Mobility	Freely mobile	More or less fixed
Caliber	Large	Small
Appendices epiploicae	Absent	Present
Teniae coli	Absent	Present
Sacculations	Absent	Present
Villi	Present	Absent
Transverse mucosal fold	Permanent	Obliterated
Peyer's patches	Present in ileum	Absent

Q. MECKEL'S DIVERTICULUM

Normally the vitellointestinal duct disappears around 6th week of intrauterine life, but if it persists it is known as Meckel's diverticulum.

Features

- Present in 2% cases
- 2 inches in length
- 2 feet proximal to ileocecal junction
- Present on the antimesenteric border
- Caliber of the diverticulum is equal to ileum
- In 2% cases, accessory pancreatic tissue may be found.

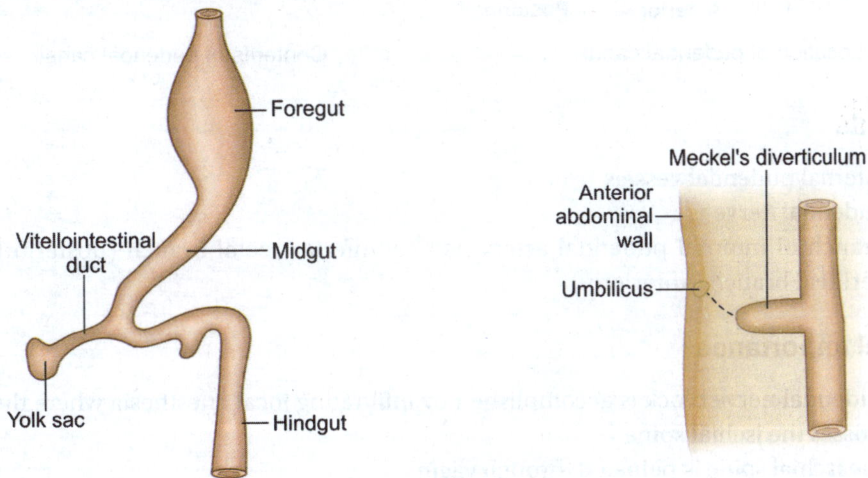

Meckel's diverticulum

Clinical Importance

- It may cause intestinal obstruction
- Could be site of peptic ulcer
- Acute inflammation may resemble appendicitis
- Tumors may occur in Meckel's diverticulum.

Q. PUDENDAL CANAL

Pudendal canal is also known as Alcock's canal. It runs on the lateral wall of ischiorectal fossa forwards anteriorly.

Location and Extent

- Pudendal canal is 3.8 cm in length
- Above lower border of ischial tuberosity
- Extends between lesser sciatic foramen posteriorly to perineal membrane anteriorly.

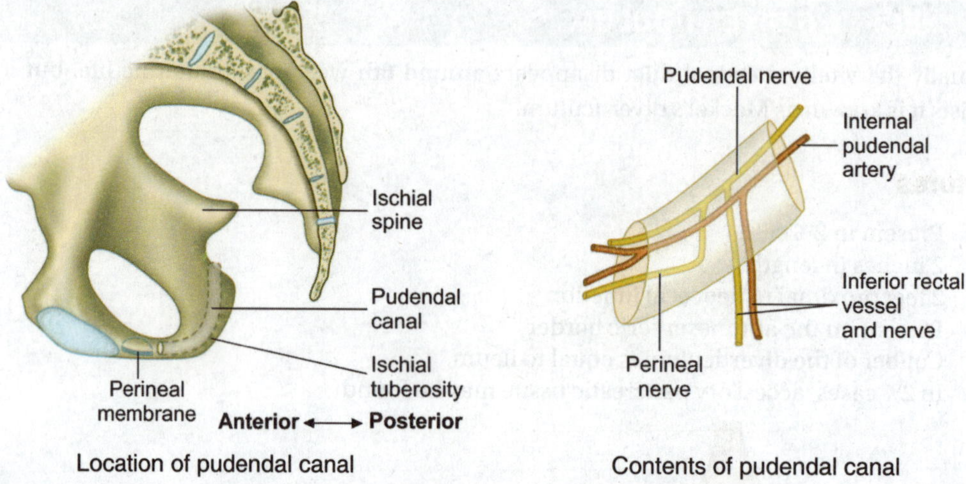

Location of pudendal canal   Contents of pudendal canal

Contents

- Internal pudendal vessels
- Pudendal nerve
- Branch of internal pudendal artery namely inferior rectal branch (posteriorly) and perineal branch (anteriorly).

Clinical Importance

- Pudendal nerve block is accomplished by infiltrating local anesthesia where the nerve crosses the ischial spine
- The ischial spine is palpated through vagina.

Q. PERINEAL MEMBRANE IN MALE (DIAGRAM ONLY).

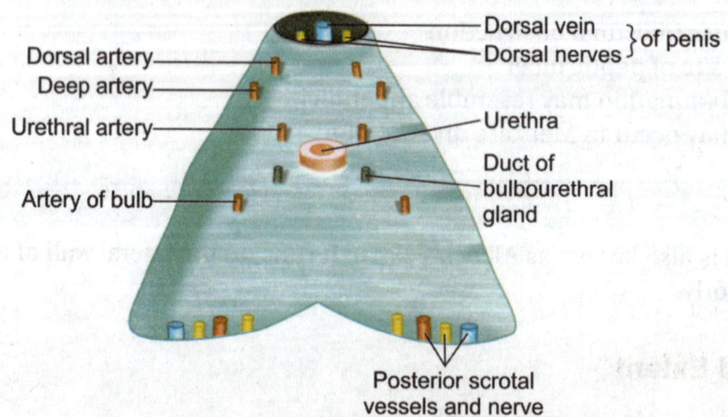

Perineal membrane in male

Q. PERINEAL MEMBRANE IN FEMALE (DIAGRAM ONLY).

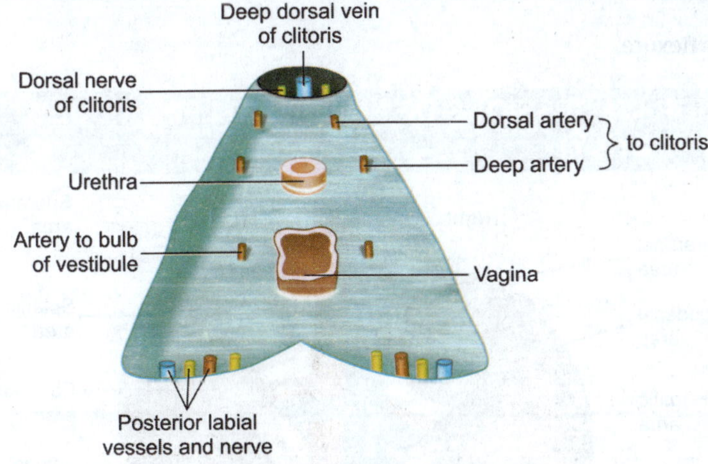

Perineal membrane in female

Q. STOMACH BED

The posterior relations of stomach comprise the stomach bed. Group of structures lying behind the stomach is known as stomach bed.

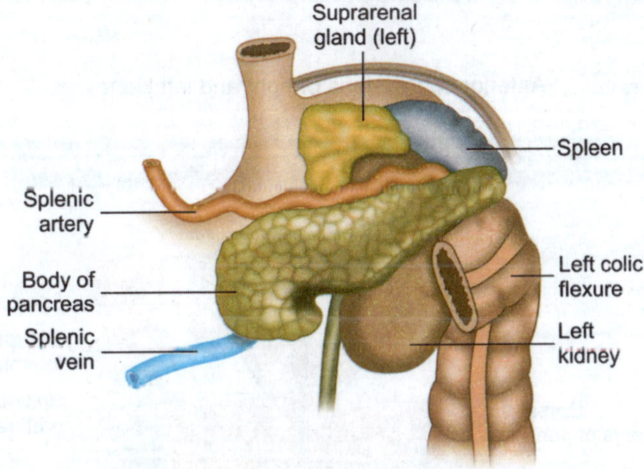

Stomach bed

Following structures form stomach bed:

- Anterior wall of lesser sac covers the posterior wall of stomach
- Bed is covered by the posterior wall of lesser sac
- Left crus and dome of diaphragm
- Splenic artery
- Body of pancreas
- Transverse mesocolon

- Upper part of left kidney
- Left suprarenal gland
- Spleen
- Left colic flexure.

Q. ANTERIOR IMPRESSIONS OF RIGHT AND LEFT KIDNEY (DIAGRAM ONLY).

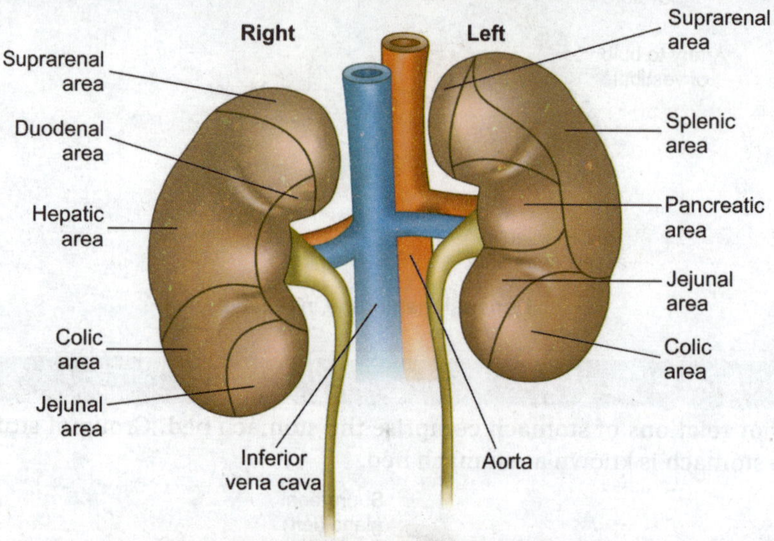

Anterior impressions of right and left kidney

Q. UROGENITAL REGION OF MALE PERINEUM (CORONAL SECTION).

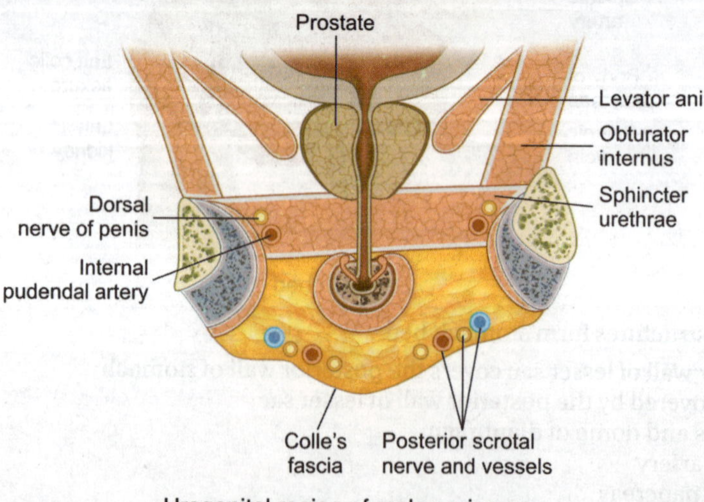

Urogenital region of male perineum

Q. UROGENITAL REGION OF FEMALE PERINEUM (CORONAL SECTION).

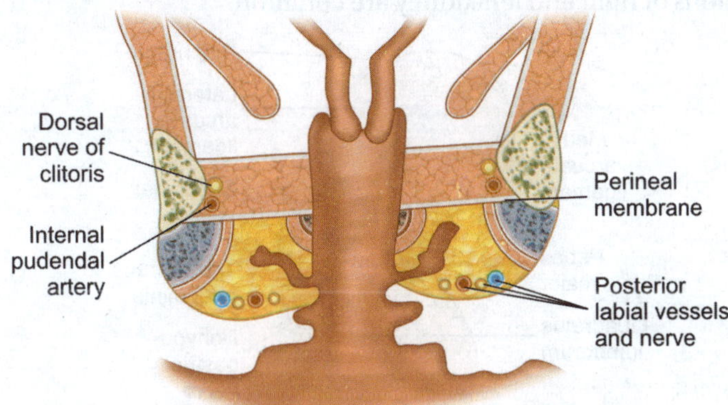

Urogenital region of female perineum

Q. POSTERIOR RELATIONS OF CECUM

Posterior relations of cecum assume importance due to the surgical cases of appendicitis especially when the appendix is retrocecal.

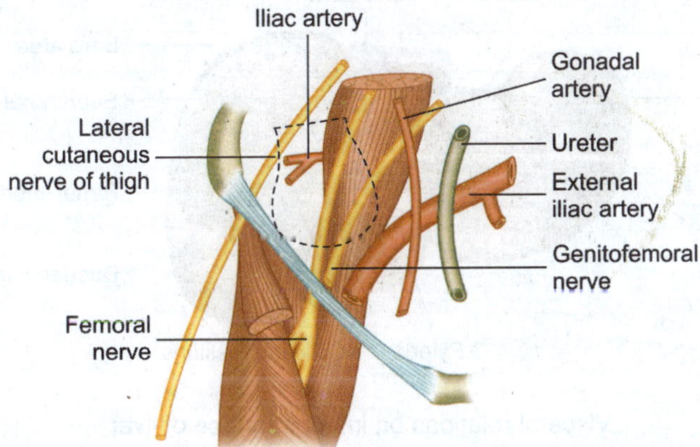

Posterior relations of cecum

- Right psoas and iliacus
- Right genitofemoral nerve
- Right femoral nerve
- Right lateral cutaneous nerve of thigh
- Right gonadal vessels (testicular or ovarian)
- Appendix in retrocecal position.

Q. POSTERIOR RELATIONS OF KIDNEY (DIAGRAM ONLY).

The posterior relations of right and left kidney are common.

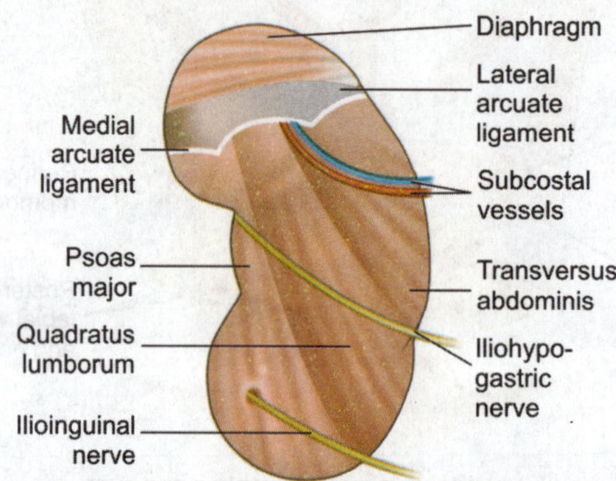

Posterior relations of kidney

Q. VISCERAL RELATIONS ON INFERIOR SURFACE OF LIVER.

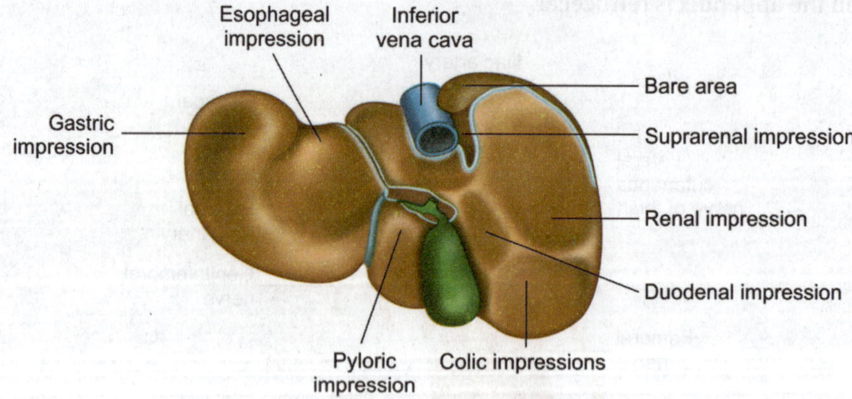

Visceral relations on inferior surface of liver

Q. ANATOMICAL AND SURGICAL IMPORTANCE OF PECTINATE LINE.

The dentate line represents the former site of embryonic anal membrane. At the dentate line transverse folds of mucosa form ring of anal valves above which are the anal sinuses. Anal glands open in the anal sinuses wherein anal abscesses and fistula develop.

Following is the anatomical and surgical importance of pectinate line:

- It is embryological watershed between visceral structures above and somatic structures
- Mucosa above has autonomic nerve supply thus insensitive to pain, while skin below is supplied by inferior rectal branch sensitive to pain and other stimuli

- Venous drainage above is to portal circulation, while below is to systemic venous circulation
- Lymphatic drainage above the pectinate line goes to iliac group of lymph nodes and below to inguinal group
- Internal hemorrhoids develop above the dentate line
- Infection in anal gland may lead to anal abscess formation
- A midline crack or fissure in the wall of anal canal is associated with severe pain during defecation
- Stimulation of nerve endings around the dentate line may lead to voluntary changes in the tone of sphincters.

Q. HOLDEN'S LINE

The superficial fascia of thigh and abdomen are continuous with each other and made up of two layers. The two layers are:

- Superficial fatty layer
- Deep membranous layer.

The membranous layer is loosely attached over the deep fascia of the thigh except in the region of inguinal ligament.

In the region of inguinal ligament the membranous layer is firmly attached to the deep fascia. This line of firm attachment is known as Holden's line.

Clinical Importance

In bladder injuries, extravasation of urine occurs between membranous layer and deep fascia of abdomen, however the urine cannot go down in the thigh due the Holden's line.

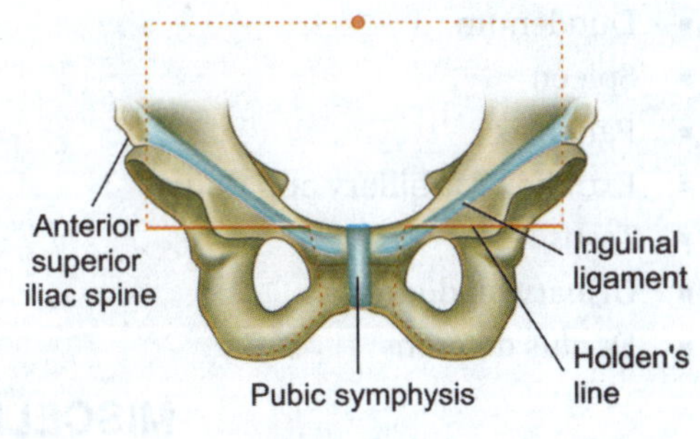

Holden's line

Long Questions

ORGANS

- Stomach
- Duodenum
- Spleen
- Pancreas
- Extrahepatic biliary apparatus
- Testis
- Urinary bladder
- Ductus deferens

- Male urethra
- Prostate
- Ureter
- Uterus
- Uterine tubes
- Ovary
- Rectum
- Anal canal

MISCELLANEOUS

- Ischiorectal fossa

- Portal vein and sites of portosystemic anastomosis

▶ ORGANS

The student should know any organ under following headings location, gross features, relations, blood supply, lymphatic drainage and clinical importance.

Q. STOMACH

Stomach is the most dilated part of the alimentary canal, lying between esophagus and duodenum. The stomach has a variable shape depending upon the volume of fluid or water in stomach. The position of stomach varies depending upon erect or supine position.

Locations

- Occupies mainly left hypochondriac region, epigastric and umbilical region.

Gross Features

- Size: 10 inches, approximately 1.5 liters capacity in adult (30 mL at birth)
- Parts: Cardiac end, fundus, body, pyloric end, lesser curvature, greater curvature
- Mucosa of empty stomach has folds known as rugae.

Salient Features of Each Part of Stomach

- The gastroesophageal junction is the cardia:
    - Most fixed part of the organ
    - Lies 2.5 cm to the left of midline
    - At T10 vertebra
    - Behind seventh left costal cartilage
    - 40 cm from incisor tooth.
- The gastroduodenal junction is the pylorus
- Fundus is the part of stomach above the cardia of stomach
- Body is the largest part of stomach lying between fundus and notch along lesser curvature known as angular incisure
- Greater curvature, lesser curvature
- Pylorus extends from angular notch to gastroduodenal junction. It can be subdivided into two parts proximal pyloric antrum and distal pyloric canal. Distal palpable circular muscle on the pyloric canal is known as pyloric sphincter.

Relations

Can be divided into peritoneal and visceral relations.

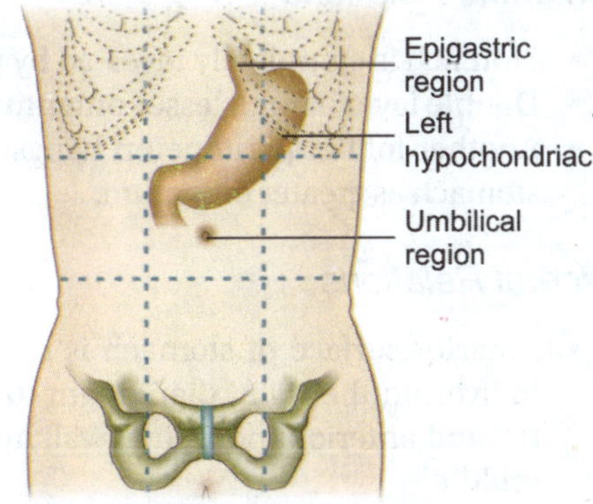

Location of stomach

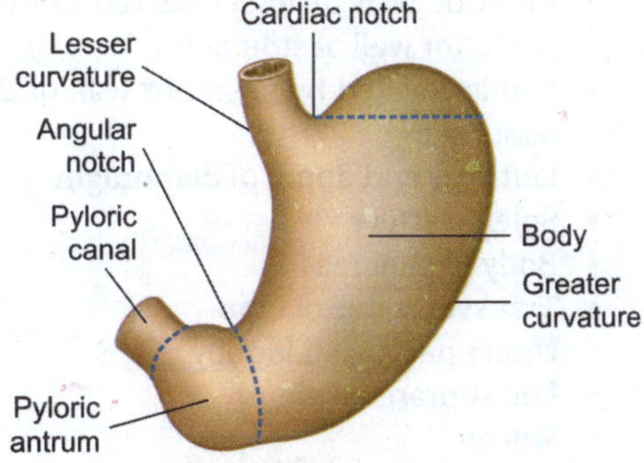

Parts of stomach

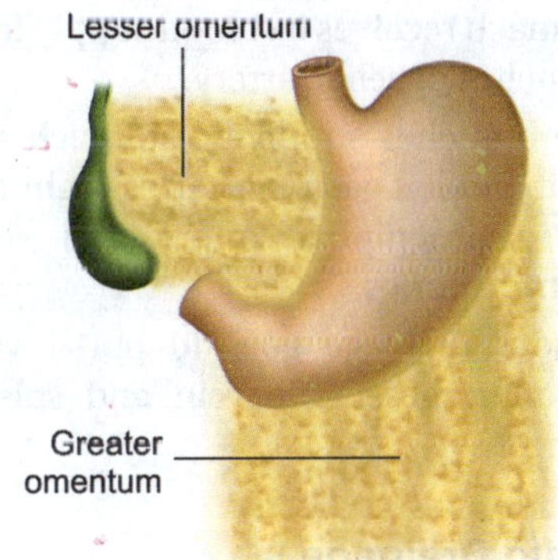

Peritoneal Relations

- Stomach is completely invested by peritoneum
- Double layer of fold, lesser omentum extends between lesser curvature and liver
- Another fold of peritoneum hangs down from the fundus and the greater curvature of stomach as greater omentum.

Visceral Relations

- Anterior surface of stomach is related to liver on the right, diaphragm to the left and anterior abdominal wall in the middle
- Posterior surface is related to the structures, which form the stomach bed.

Following structures form stomach bed:

- Anterior wall of lesser sac covers the posterior wall of stomach
- Bed is covered by posterior wall of the lesser sac
- Left crus and dome of diaphragm
- Splenic artery
- Body of pancreas
- Transverse mesocolon
- Upper part of left kidney
- Left suprarenal gland
- Spleen
- Left colic flexure.

Blood Supply

1. Stomach receives its blood supply from branches of celiac artery.
2. The branches supplying stomach are- right and left gastric arteries, right and left gastroepiploic artery and short gastric arteries.
3. Venous drainage goes to portal vein, superior mesenteric vein and splenic vein.

Lymphatic Drainage

Stomach is divided into three lymphatic territories similar to the vascular territories of celiac artery.

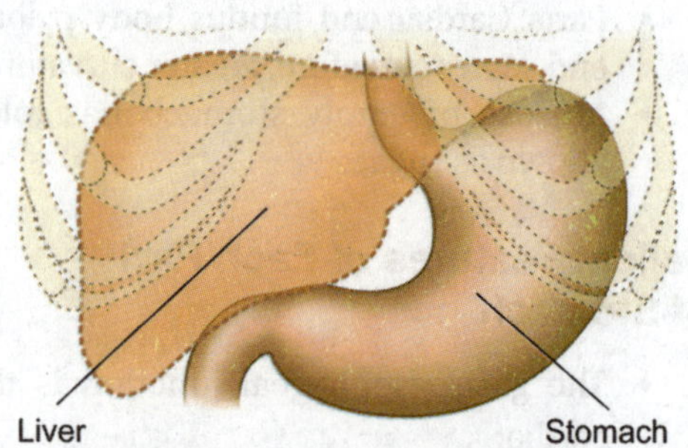

Anterior relations of stomach

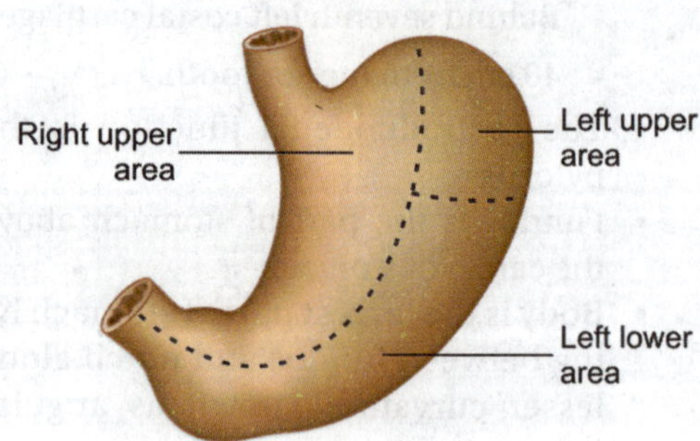

Lymphatic drainage areas

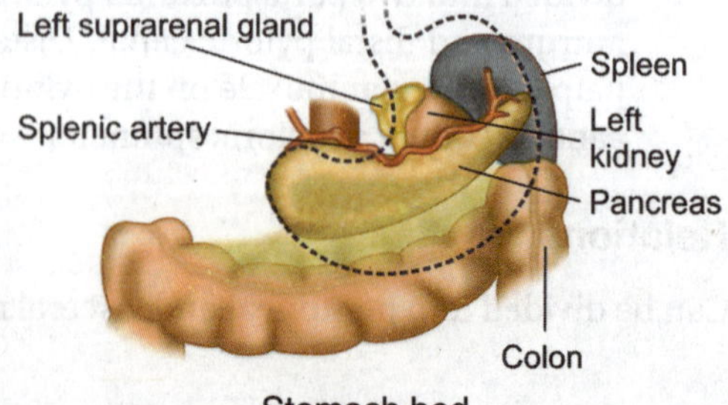

Stomach bed

Divisions of Lymphatic Areas

There are three territories identified on the stomach:

- Right two third upper area along the lesser curvature of stomach
- Left lower one third area along greater curvature of stomach
- Left upper area close to the spleen
- The efferents of all the lymph of stomach goes to celiac group of lymph nodes.

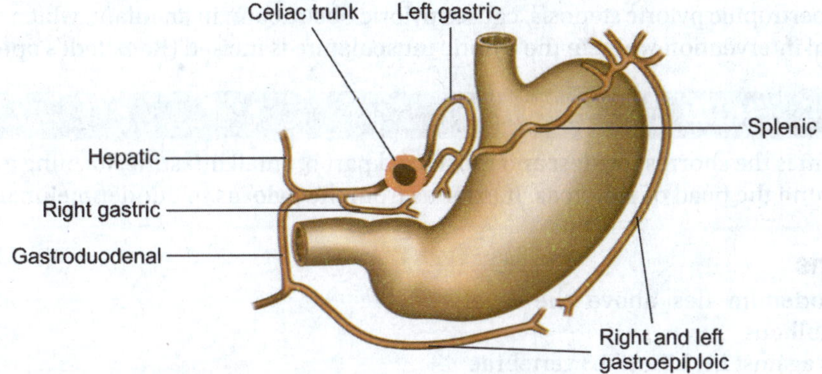

Arterial supply of stomach

Lymph Groups of Stomach

- **Hepatic group:** Lies in lesser omentum, receives lymph from liver and gallbladder
- **Subpyloric group:** Lies in the angle between first and second part of duodenum, close to the bifurcation of gastroduodenal artery, receives lymph through inferior gastric nodes draining right two third of lesser curvature of stomach
- **Superior gastric group:** Close to the cardiac end of stomach
- **Inferior gastric group:** Close to the pylorus within the layers of greater omentum
- **Pancreaticolienal:** Lies along the splenic artery.

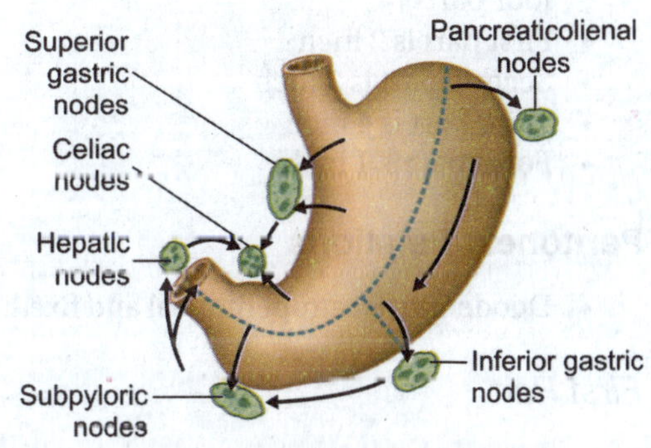

Lymph groups of stomach

Drainage Pattern

- Lesser curvature of stomach is drained by superior gastric nodes and finally celiac nodes
- Region close to pylorus drains into inferior gastric nodes, thence to subpyloric and then to celiac nodes
- Upper gastric area close to the spleen is drained by pancreaticolienal nodes and finally into celiac nodes.

Clinical Importance

- Gastric disturbance gives rise to symptoms like anorexia, nausea, vomiting known as dyspepsia
- Peptic ulcer occurs typically along lesser curvature of stomach
- Gastric carcinoma occurs along greater curvature of stomach
- While operating cases of cancer stomach, surgeon has to be aware of the drainage pattern of lymph nodes to clear all those lymphatic areas likely to get involved
- Hypertrophic pyloric stenosis, causes pyloric obstruction in an infant, which needs surgical intervention wherein the pyloric musculature is incised (Ramstedt's operation).

Q. DUODENUM

Duodenum is the shortest, widest and most fixed part of small intestine, forming a C-shaped curve around the head of pancreas. It extends from the pylorus to duodenojejunal flexure.

Locations

- Duodenum lies above the level of umbilicus
- It is against L1, L2 and L3 vertebrae
- Present on either side of midline.

Gross Features

- Duodenum is 10 inches long and has four parts
- First part is 2 inch
- Second part is 3 inch
- Third part is 4 inch
- Forth part is 1 inch.

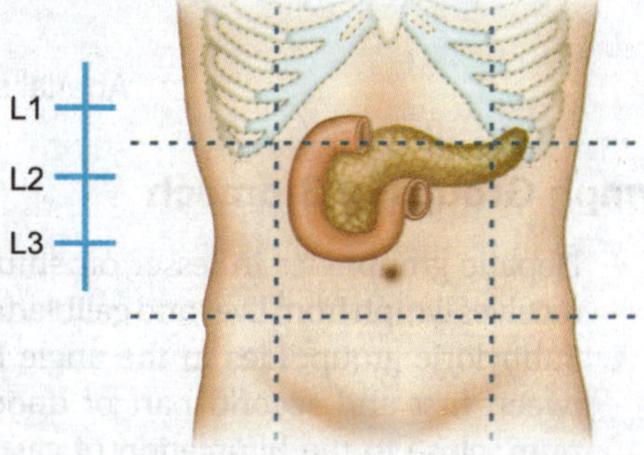

Locations of duodenum

Peritoneal Relations

- Duodenum is retroperitoneal and fixed.

First Part

- Extends between pylorus and superior duodenal flexure
- Directed backwards, upwards and to the right
- Proximal part has lesser omentum attachment.

Visceral relations

- In front: Quadrate lobe of liver and gallbladder
- Behind: Gastroduodenal artery, portal vein and bile duct

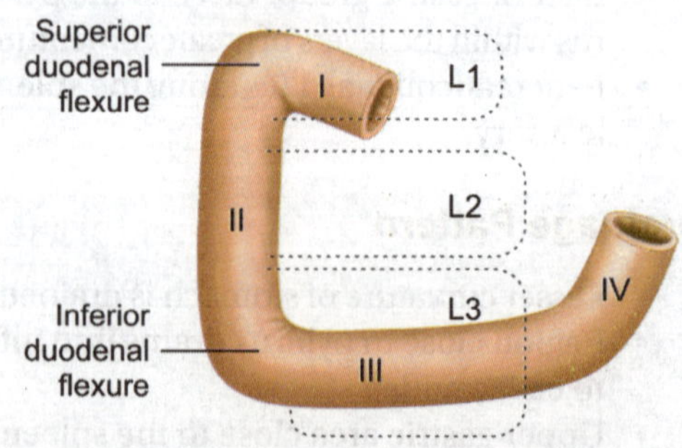

Parts of duodenum

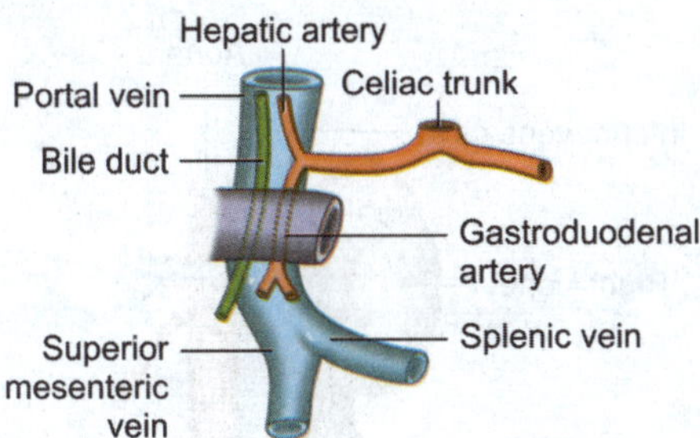

Posterior relations of first part

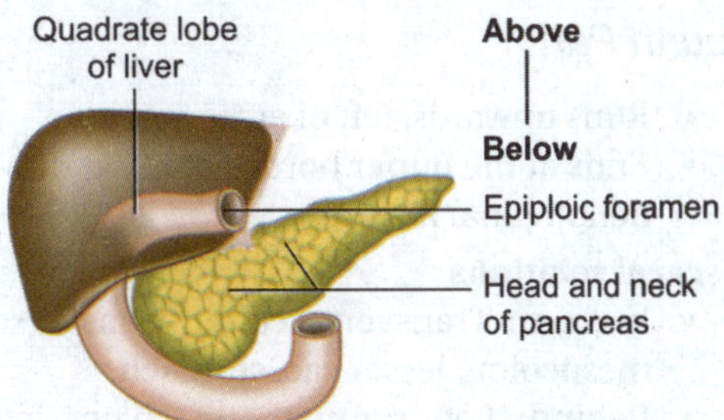

Visceral relations of first part

- Superior: Epiploic foramen
- Inferior: Head and neck of pancreas.

Second Part

- Extends between superior duodenal flexure to inferior duodenal flexure
- Major and minor duodenal papillae are present on the inner side.

Visceral relations
- In front: Right lobe of liver, transverse colon, coils of intestine
- Behind: Right kidney, right renal vessels, right edge of inferior vena cava, right psoas major
- Medially: Head of pancreas, bile duct
- Laterally: Hepatic flexure of colon.

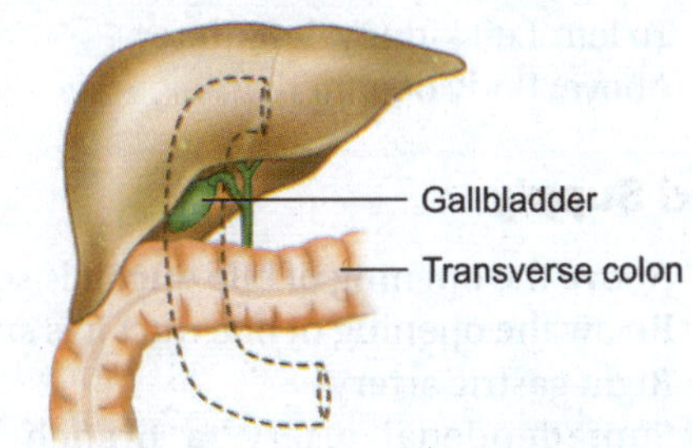

Third Part

- Lies across L3 horizontally
- Extends from inferior duodenal flexure
- Ends in front of aorta.

Visceral relations
- In front: Superior mesenteric vessels, root of mesentery
- Behind: Right ureter, right psoas major, right gonadal vessel, inferior vena cava, abdominal aorta with the origin of inferior mesenteric artery
- Superior: Head of pancreas with uncinate process
- Inferior: Coils of intestine.

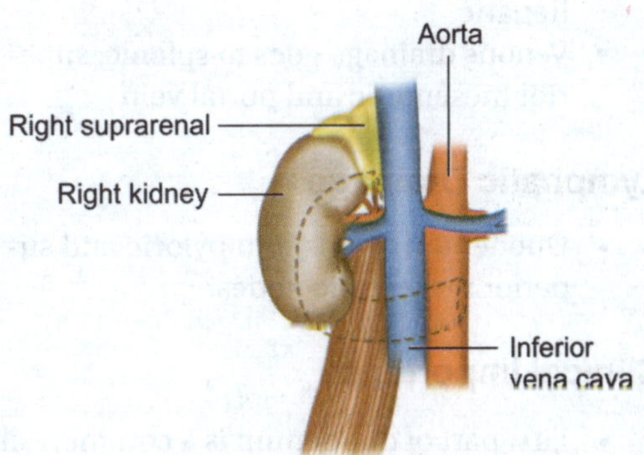

Visceral relations of second part

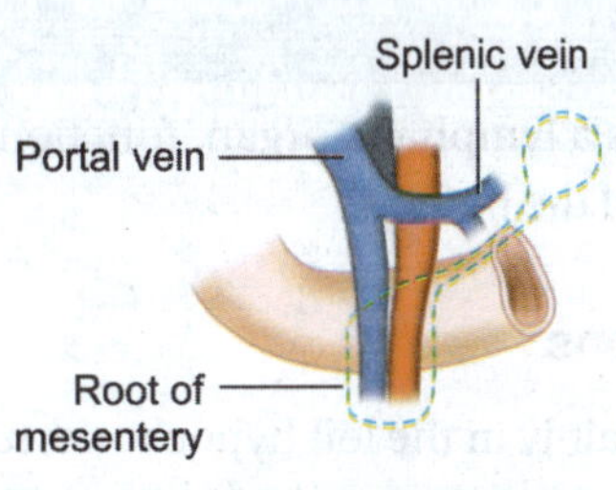

Visceral relations of third part

Fourth Part

- Runs upwards, left of aorta
- Ends at the upper border of L2, at duodenojejunal flexure.

Visceral relations

- In front: Transverse colon, transverse mesocolon, lesser sac, stomach
- Behind: Left sympathetic chain, left psoas major, left renal vessels, left gonadal vessels, inferior mesenteric vein
- To right: Root of mesentery
- To left: Left kidney, left ureter
- Above: Body of pancreas.

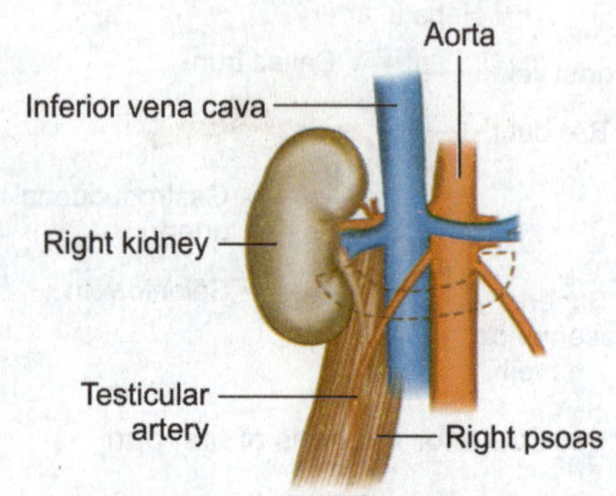

Posterior relations of third and fourth part

Blood Supply

- Above the opening of bile duct it is supplied by superior pancreaticoduodenal artery
- Below the opening of bile duct it is supplied by inferior pancreaticoduodenal artery
- Right gastric artery
- Supraduodenal artery, a branch of hepatic
- Venous drainage goes to splenic, superior mesenteric and portal vein.

Lymphatic Drainage

- Duodenum drains into pyloric and superior mesenteric nodes.

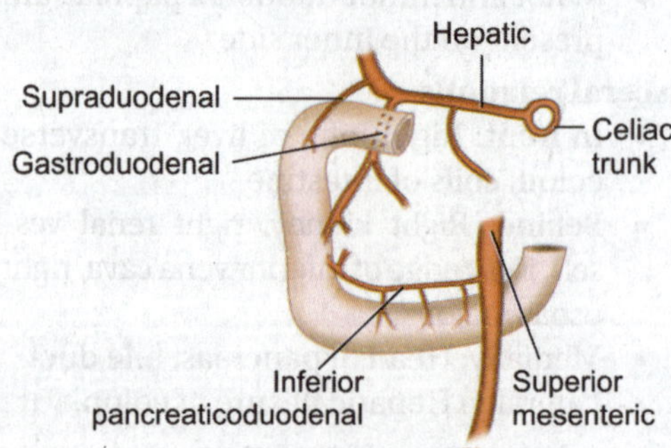

Arterial supply of duodenum

Clinical Importance

- First part of duodenum is a common site of peptic ulcer
- Second part of duodenum is commonly involved in congenital stenosis
- Widening of duodenal loop is seen in carcinoma of head of pancreas.

Q.   SPLEEN

Spleen is a lymphatic organ, functions as a filter of blood and plays vital role in the immune system of the body.

Locations

- Mainly in the left hypochondrium
- Posterior end extends into epigastrium
- Placed between left dome of diaphragm and fundus of stomach
- Related to left 9–11 ribs.

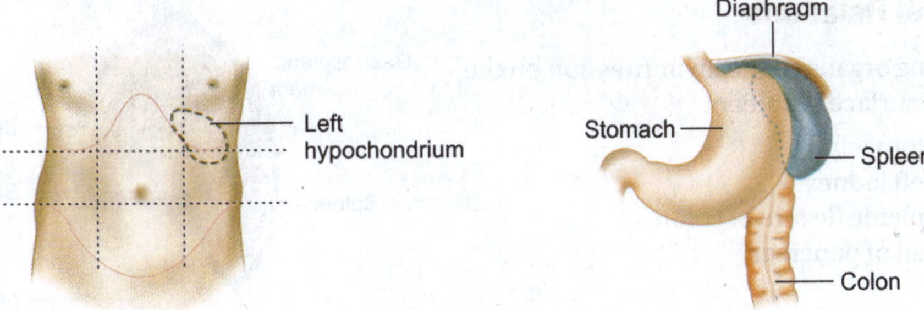

Gross Features

- Shape varies depending upon colic impression
- 5 x 3 inches in dimension, 7 ounces in weight
- Directed downwards, forwards and laterally
- Makes angle of 45° with the horizontal

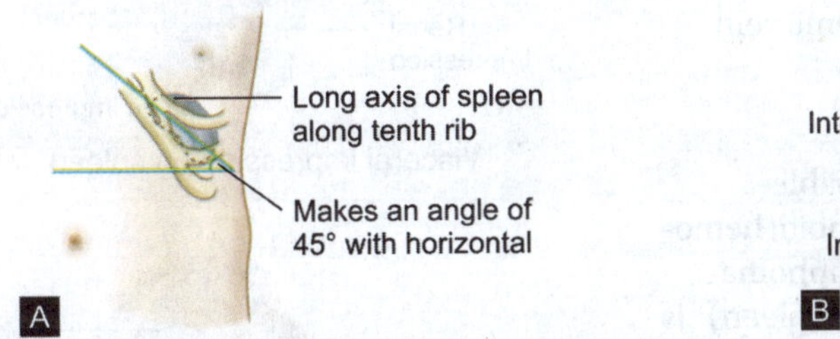

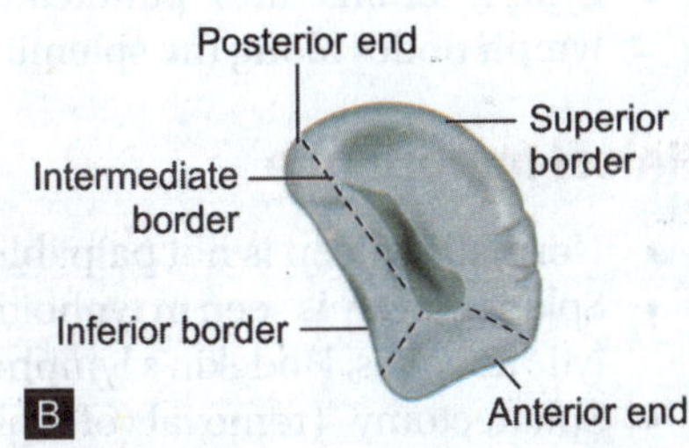

Spleen. **A.** Disposition of spleen; **B.** Gross features.

- Has two ends anterior end (like a border) and posterior end
- Three borders superior border (has a notch), inferior border, intermediate border
- Two surfaces diaphragmatic and visceral.

Peritoneal Relations

Spleen is surrounded by peritoneum and has following ligaments:

- Gastrosplenic ligament between hilum of spleen and greater curvature of stomach
- Lienorenal ligament between hilum of spleen and anterior surface of kidney
- Phrenicocolic ligament supports the anterior end of spleen the ligament extends from splenic flexure of colon and diaphragm.

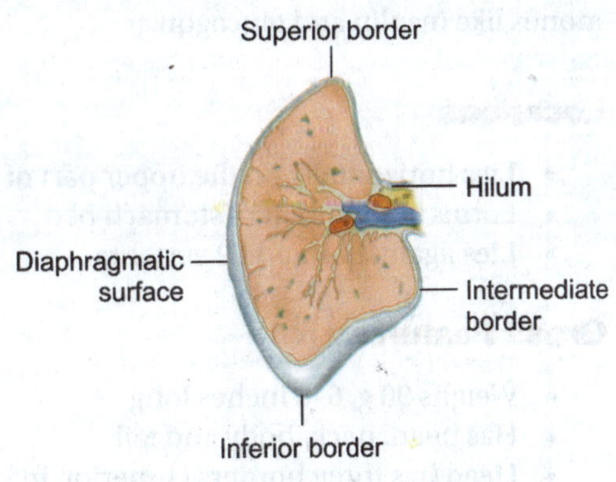

Visceral Relations

Following organs create an impression on the visceral surface of spleen:

- Stomach
- Left kidney
- Splenic flexure of colon
- Tail of pancreas.

Blood Supply

- Splenic artery, a branch of celiac artery, enters the spleen through the lienorenal ligament
- Splenic vein, drains the spleen.

Lymphatic Drainage

- Lymph drains into pancreaticolienal lymph nodes along the splenic vein.

Clinical Importance

- Normally spleen is not palpable
- Splenomegaly is seen in typhoid, hemolytic anemias, Hodgkin's lymphoma
- Splenectomy (removal of spleen) is done in splenic rupture.

Q. PANCREAS

Pancreas is a partly exocrine and endocrine gland, secreting digestive enzymes and hormones like insulin and glucagon.

Locations

- Lies horizontally on the upper part of the posterior abdominal wall
- Forms component of stomach bed
- Lies against L1 and L2 vertebra.

Gross Features

- Weighs 90 g, 6–8 inches long
- Has head, neck, body and tail
- Head has three borders (superior, inferior, right lateral), two surfaces (anterior, posterior) and a uncinate process

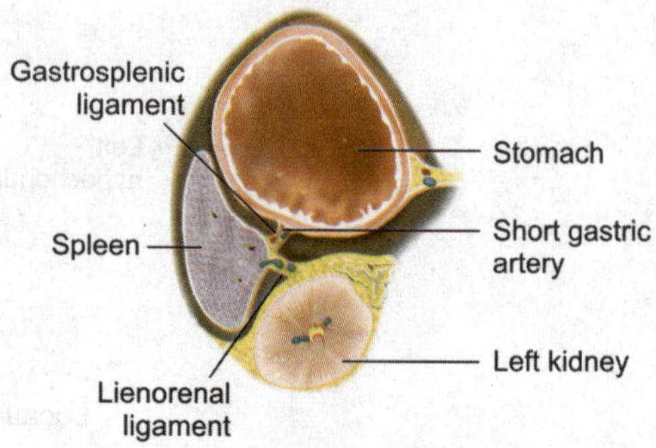

Peritoneal ligaments

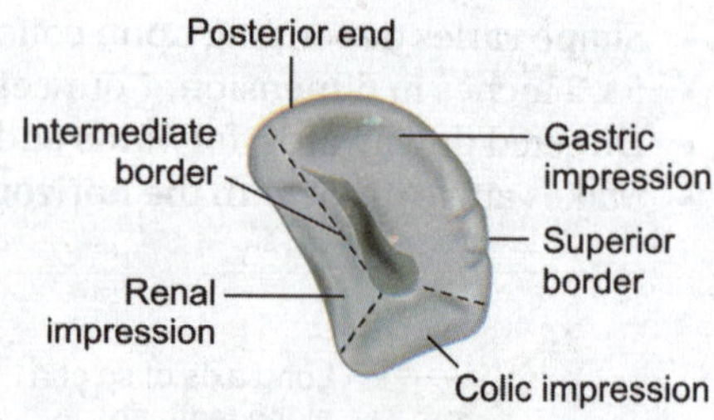

Visceral impression on spleen

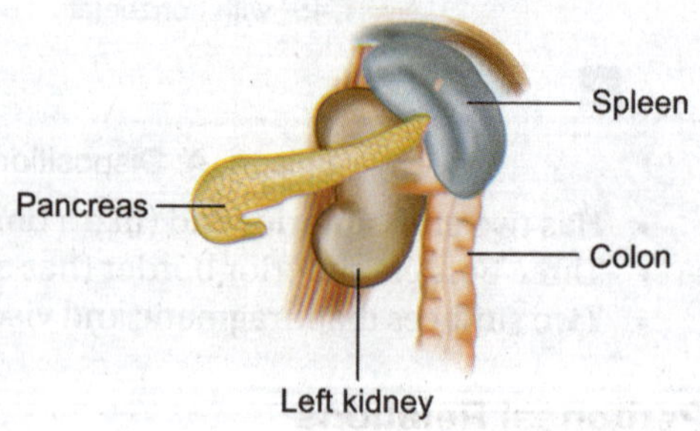

Stomach bed

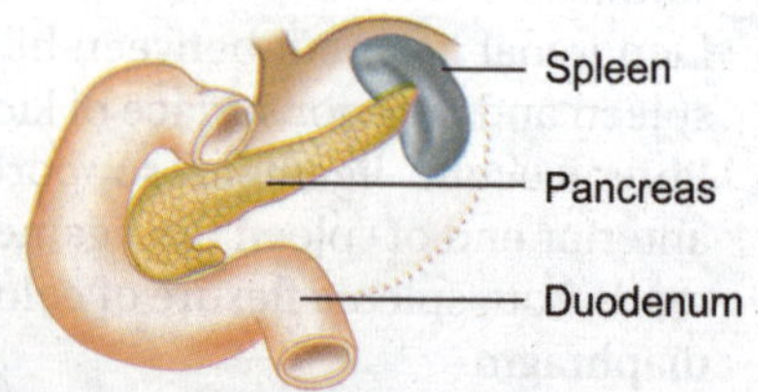

Location of pancreas

- Neck has two surfaces (anterior and posterior)
- Body has three borders (anterior, superior and inferior), three surfaces (anterior, posterior and inferior)
- Pancreatic duct is placed superficially on the posterior surface of the gland
- Accessory pancreatic duct is frequently present.

Peritoneal Relation

- Pancreas is a retroperitoneal organ.

Visceral Relations

Head

- Lies within the curve of duodenum
- Anteriorly related to gastroduodenal artery, transverse colon and jejunum
- Posteriorly related to inferior vena cava, renal veins, right crus of diaphragm and bile duct
- Uncinate process is related anteriorly to superior mesenteric vessels and posteriorly to aorta.

Neck

- Anteriorly is related to pylorus
- Posteriorly related to superior mesenteric vein and portal vein.

Body

- Anterior border gives attachment to root of transverse mesocolon
- Superior border is related to splenic artery
- Anteriorly related to stomach
- Posteriorly related to aorta, left kidney, left suprarenal gland, left crus of diaphragm, left renal vessels
- Inferiorly related to duodenojejunal flexure, left colic flexure.

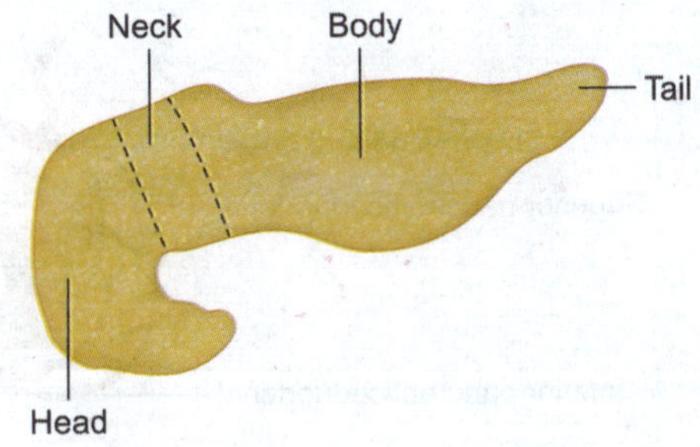

Visceral relations of pancreas

Tail

- Lies in the lienorenal ligament.

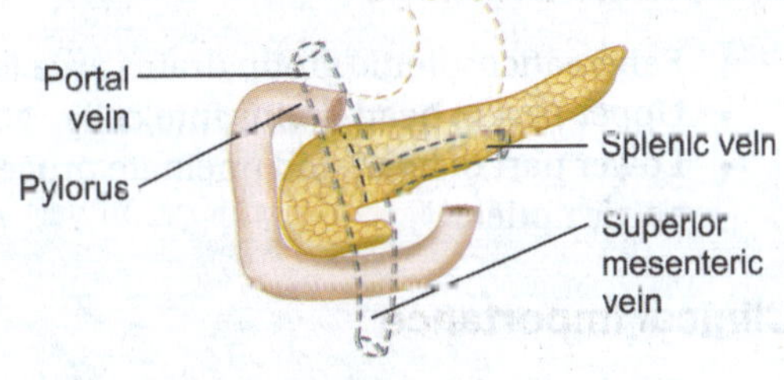

Parts of pancreas

Blood Supply

- Pancreatic branches of splenic artery
- Superior pancreaticoduodenal artery, branch of celiac artery
- Inferior pancreaticoduodenal, a branch from superior mesenteric artery
- Arteria pancreatica magna, a large branch

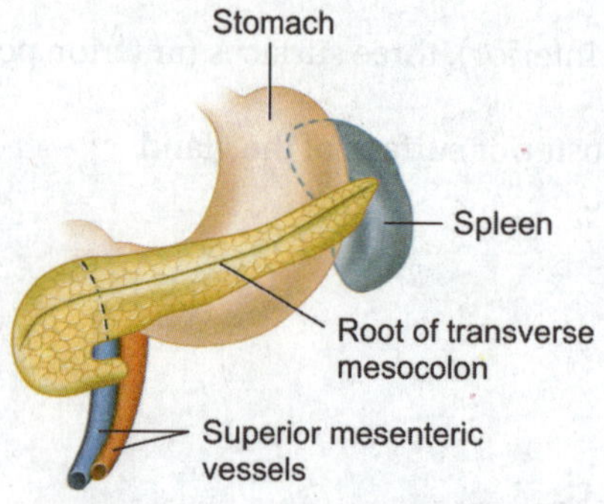

Anterior relations of body of pancreas

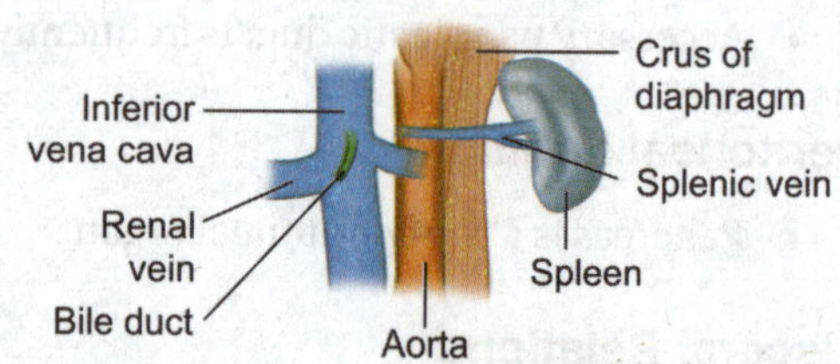

Posterior relations of body of pancreas

- By small veins into splenic vein
- By superior pancreaticoduodenal vein into portal vein
- By inferior pancreaticoduodenal vein into superior mesenteric vein.

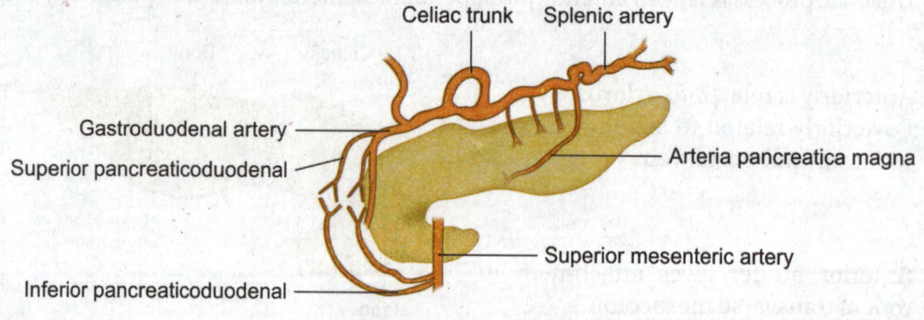

Arterial supply of pancreas

Lymphatic Drainage

- Pancreaticosplenic group drains area left to neck of pancreas
- Upper part of head drains into celiac group
- Lower part of head and uncinate process drains into superior mesenteric group of pre-aortic nodes.

Clinical Importance

- The head of pancreas and duodenum can be mobilized by incising peritoneum along the right edge of second part of duodenum and turning duodenum medially known as Kocher's manoeuvre
- Deficiency of insulin causes diabetes mellitus
- Inflammation of pancreas is known as pancreatitis
- Carcinoma of head of pancreas can cause obstructive jaundice
- Pseudocysts of pancreas can follow pancreatitis and can be drained by incising the anterior wall of stomach and opening made through posterior wall of stomach into pseudocyst.

Q. EXTRAHEPATIC BILIARY APPARATUS

The extrahepatic biliary apparatus is concerned with the collection, storage and transportation of bile. The components of extrahepatic biliary apparatus are:

- Right and left hepatic ducts
- Common hepatic duct
- Gallbladder
- Cystic duct
- Bile duct.

Hepatic Ducts

1. The bile canaliculi within the substance of liver form bile ductules, which in turn form interlobular ducts, these unite to form hepatic ducts.
2. The hepatic ducts emerge from porta hepatis and join each other to form common hepatic duct.
3. At porta hepatis the portal vein lies behind, in between is hepatic artery and in front is hepatic duct.

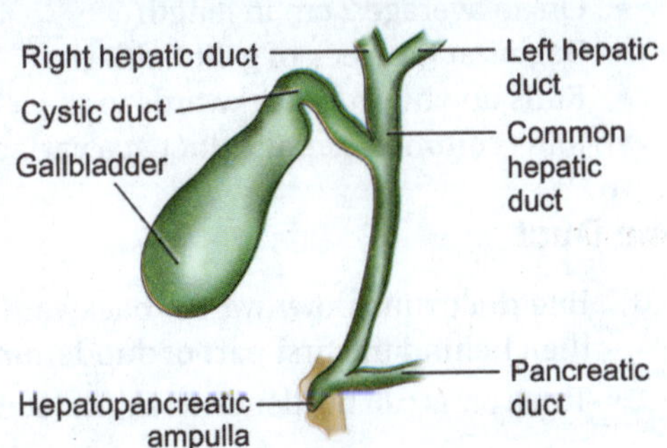

Components of extrahepatic biliary apparatus

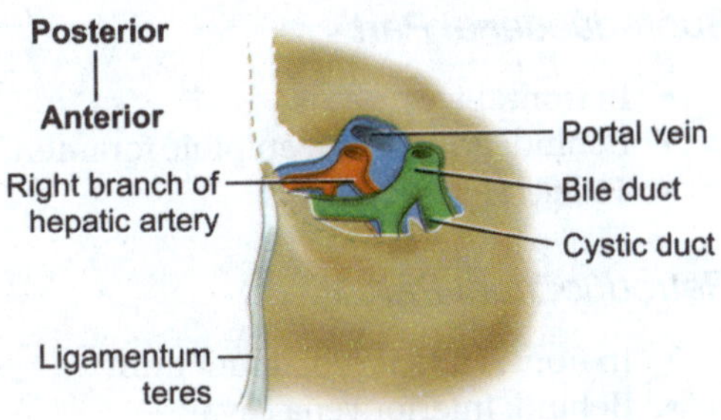

Porta hepatis structures

Gallbladder

- Gallbladder is a piriform-shaped storage chamber of bile, in a shallow fossa on the right edge of quadrate lobe of liver
- Has three parts fundus, body and neck
- Fundus protrudes from the inferior margin of liver and touches the anterior abdominal wall
- Fundus and body lie on the first and second part of duodenum
- Posteromedial wall of the neck is dilated to form Hartmann's pouch.

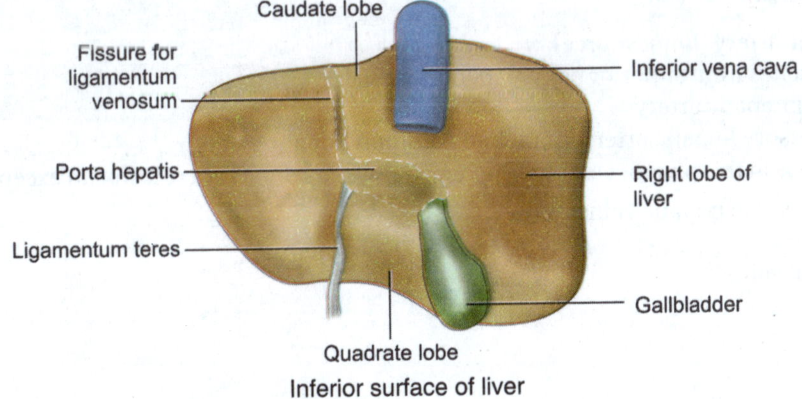

Inferior surface of liver

Cystic Duct

- On an average 2 cm in length
- Begins at the neck of gallbladder
- Runs downwards, backwards to the left
- Joins common hepatic duct at a variable point to form bile duct.

Bile Duct

1. Bile duct runs downwards, backwards initially in the free margin of lesser omentum, then behind the first part of duodenum and then behind head of pancreas.
2. Three parts can be identified supraduodenal, retroduodenal and infraduodenal.

Visceral Relations

Supraduodenal Part

- In front: Liver
- Behind: Portal vein, epiploic foramen
- To left: Hepatic artery.

Retroduodenal Part

- In front: First part of duodenum
- Behind: Inferior vena cava
- To left: Gastroduodenal artery.

Infraduodenal Part

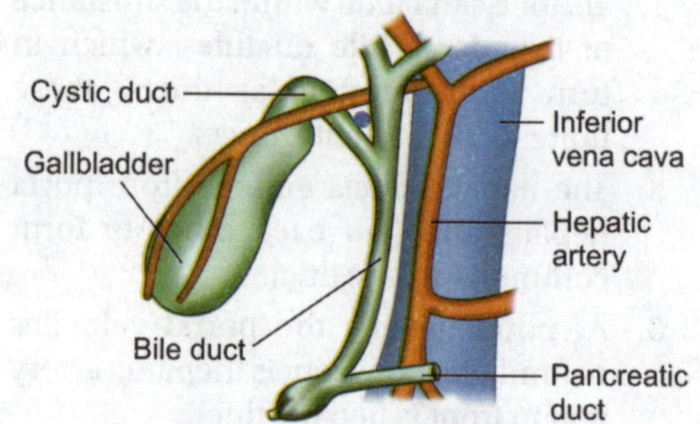

Relations of biliary apparatus

- In front: Groove on posterior surface of pancreas
- Behind: Inferior vena cava
- The union of common bile duct and pancreatic duct forms ampulla of Vater. There is circular muscle around it known as sphincter of Oddi, which is present at a point where it opens in the second part of duodenum.

Blood Supply

- Cystic artery (main source)
- Branches from superior pancreaticoduodenal
- Right hepatic artery
- Accessory hepatic artery, branch of common hepatic artery.

Variations in this region, i.e. course of hepatic, cystic arteries is a rule not an exception.

- Drains into hepatic veins
- Cystic vein
- Portal vein.

Lymphatic Drainage

- Cystic nodes
- Hepatic nodes
- Pancreaticosplenic nodes.

Clinical Importance

- Acute cholecystitis occurs in adult women, presents with sharp agonizing pain in right hypochondrium referring to the scapula behind
- Chronic cholecystitis occurs in fat, females above 40 years age
- Variations are very common in the anatomy of biliary apparatus, a surgeon should be aware of the variations, while operating in this region
- A triangle can be identified, while doing cholecystectomy that is known as Calot's triangle; it is bounded by common hepatic duct on left, cystic duct on right and liver above
- Biliary system can be visualized by injecting a radiopaque dye in biliary system a procedure known as cholangiography.

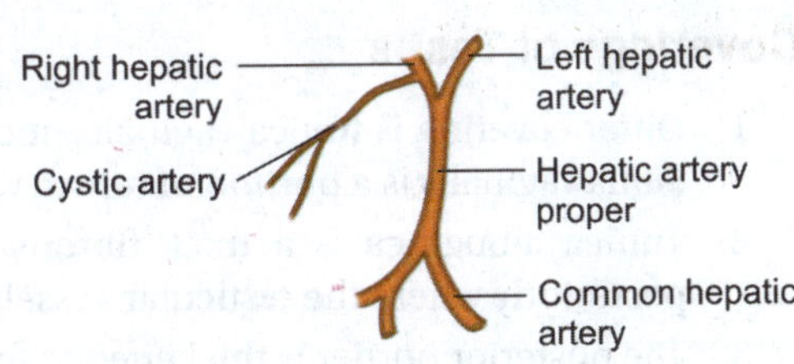

Arterial tree supplying biliary apparatus

Q. TESTIS

Testis is the male reproductive organ, suspended by spermatic cord into the scrotum.

Locations

- Suspended in scrotum
- Lies obliquely in a way that upper pole is tilted forwards and laterally and lower pole backwards and medially.
- Left testis is lower to right.

Gross Features

- Testis is oval in shape and is 10–15 g
- Has two poles—upper and lower, two borders anterior and posterior, two surfaces medial and lateral, appendix
- Spermatic cord attached to upper pole, both the poles are convex and smooth
- Anterior border convex and smooth, posterior border is straight
- Epididymis is attached to posterolateral surface
- Medial and lateral surfaces are convex and smooth
- Appendix is remnant of paramesonephric duct.

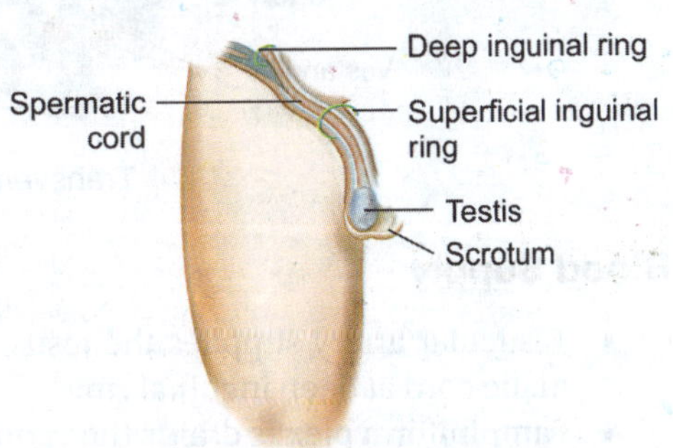

Location of testis in scrotum

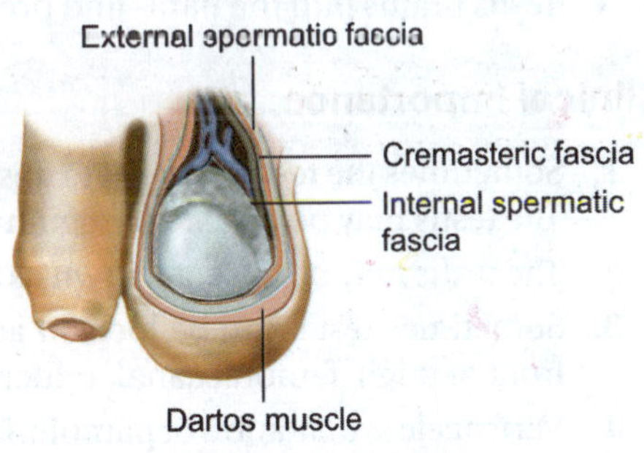

Coverings of testis

Coverings of Testis

1. Outer covering is tunica vaginalis, it covers whole of the testis except posterior border. Sinus vaginalis is a portion of tunica vaginalis between testis and epididymis.
2. Tunica albuginea is a thick fibrous layer surrounding the testis all around except posteriorly where the testicular vessels and nerves enter the testis.
3. The posterior border is thickened to form a septum, known as mediastinum.
4. Tunica vasculosa is the innermost covering lining the lobules of testis.

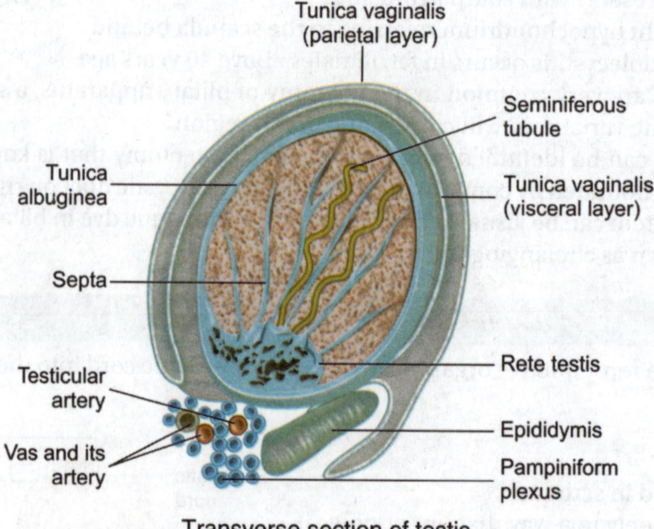

Transverse section of testis

Blood Supply

- Testicular artery supplies the testis, it is a branch of aorta at L2 level, enters the spermatic cord at deep inguinal ring
- Pampiniform plexus drains the venous blood of testis.

Lymphatic Drainage

- Testis drains into the para- and pre-aortic group.

Clinical Importance

1. Sometimes the testis may fail to descend in the scrotum this is known as cryptorchidism. The testis may be located in inguinal, lumbar or upper scrotal region.
2. The testis may be absent known as anarchism.
3. Sometimes testis can be located at abnormal sites like, under skin of lower abdomen, front of thigh, femoral canal, under skin of penis or in perineum.
4. Varicocele is dilatation of pampiniform plexus, it commonly occurs on the left side since left testicular vein is longer and drains at a right angle to renal vein. Also crossed by loaded colon giving rise to varicocele formation.

5. Hydrocele is a condition where the fluid accumulates in the processus vaginalis.
6. Acute orchitis may occur following mumps.

Q. URINARY BLADDER

Urinary bladder is a reservoir of urine and is a muscular organ.

Locations

- An empty bladder is present entirely within the pelvis
- Posterior to the pubic bones separated from it by a retropubic space
- When full it extends into the abdominal cavity up to the umbilicus.

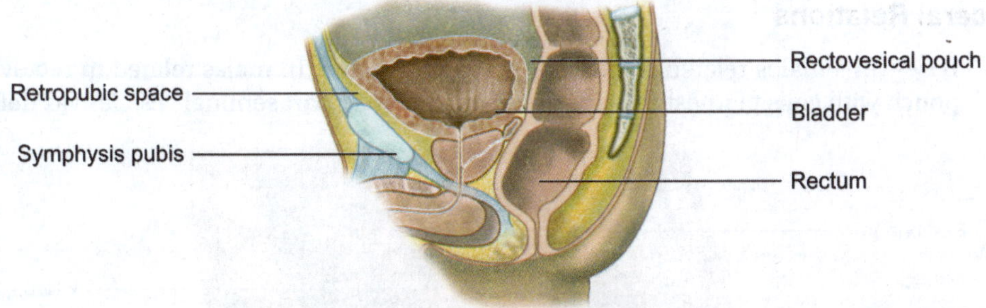

Location of urinary bladder in pelvis

Gross Features

Empty Bladder

- Tetrahedral in shape
- Apex directed forwards
- Base directed backwards
- Neck most fixed and lowest part of bladder
- Three surfaces—superior, two inferolateral surfaces
- Four borders—two lateral, one anterior, one posterior.

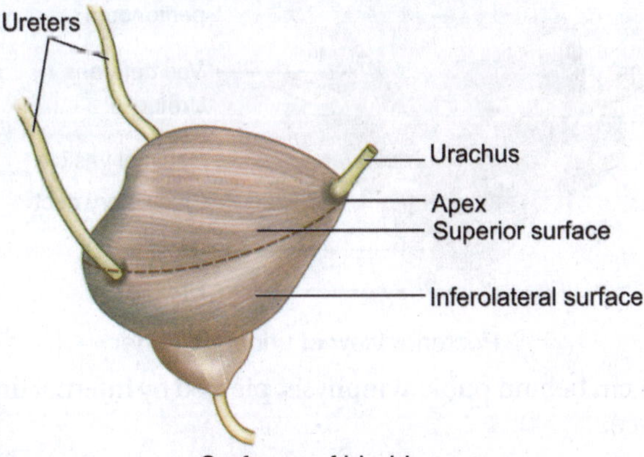

Surfaces of bladder

Full Bladder

- Ovoid in shape
- Apex directed upwards, towards umbilicus.

Peritoneal Relations

- Apex has remains of urachus, which forms the median umbilical ligament
- Uppermost part of the base between the two vas deferens is covered by peritoneum
- Separated from rectum by rectovesical pouch in males
- Peritoneum is reflected from superior surface of bladder onto the anterior wall of uterus
- Superior surface is covered by peritoneum.

Visceral Relations

- Base—in females related to uterine cervix and vagina. In males related to rectovesical pouch with coils of intestine within, rectum, in lower part seminal vesicles vas deferens

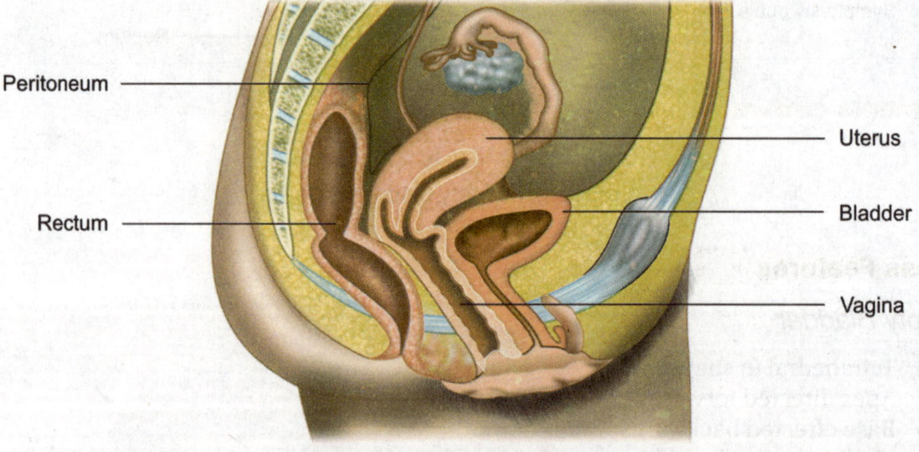

Sagittal section of female pelvis

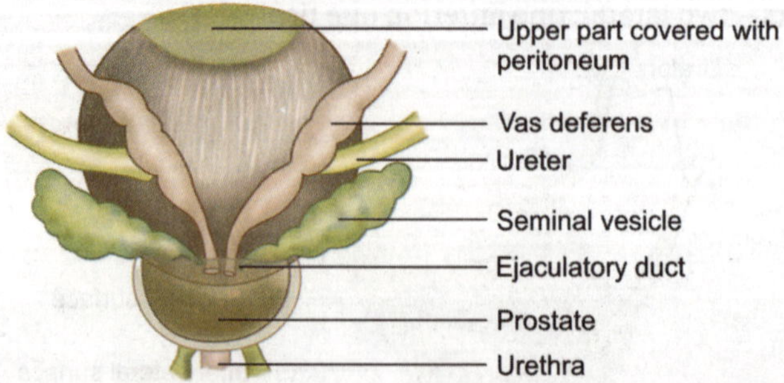

Posterior view of urinary bladder

- Neck—lies 3–4 cm behind pubic symphysis, pierced by internal urethral orifice
- Superior surface:

- In males—lies in contact with sigmoid colon, coils of ileum
- In females—small area near posterior border related to supra-vaginal part of cervix.

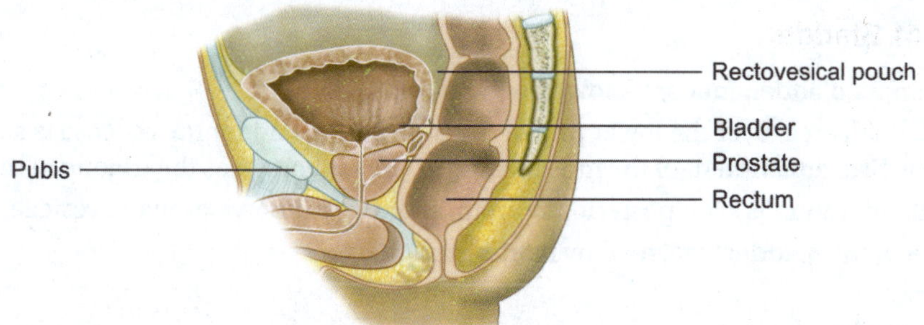

Sagittal section of male pelvis

- Inferolateral surface:
  - In males—puboprostatic ligament, retropubic fat, levator
  - Ani, obturator internus
  - In females—pubovesical ligament, retropubic fat, levator ani, obturator internus.

Ligaments of Bladder

- Lateral true ligament extends from side of bladder to tendinous pelvic arch

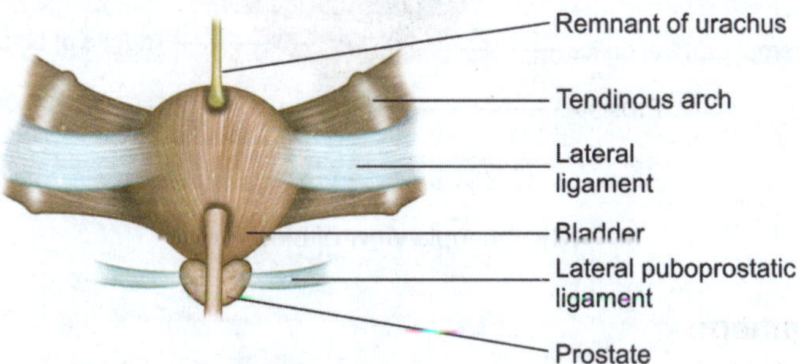

Ligaments of bladder anterior view

- Lateral puboprostatic ligament extends from anterior end of tendinous arch to prostatic sheath, is directed medially and backwards
- Medial puboprostatic ligament extends from pubic bone to prostatic sheath
- Median umbilical ligament is a remnant of urachus
- Posterior ligament of bladder is directed backwards and upwards

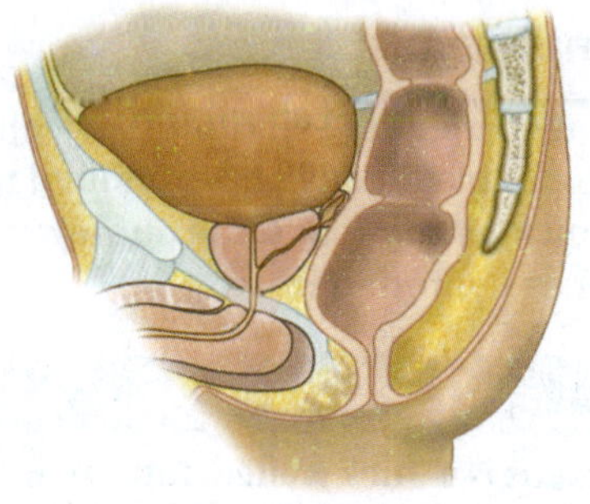

Side view of male pelvis

- False ligaments include peritoneal folds namely median umbilical fold, medial umbilical fold, lateral and posterior false ligament.

Interior of Bladder

1. In empty bladder, mucosa shows irregular folds.
2. In a small area, over the lower part of the base of the bladder the mucosa is smooth due to the firm attachment of the muscular layer. This is known as the trigone of the bladder.
3. Slight elevation is seen posterior to urethral orifice is known as uvula vesicae.
4. Base of the bladder is formed by interureteric ridge.

Blood Supply

- Superior and inferior vesical arteries branches of internal iliac artery
- Obturator, inferior gluteal arteries (vaginal and uterine arteries in females)
- Vesical venous plexus drains into internal iliac veins.

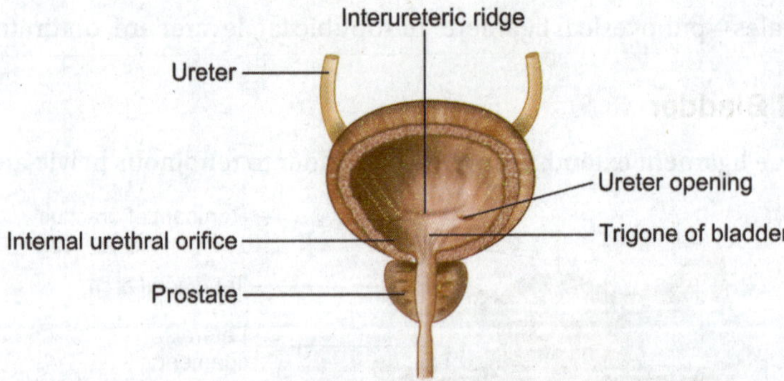

Cystoscopic view of bladder

Lymphatic Drainage

- Mostly to external iliac nodes
- Few to internal iliac nodes via lateral aortic nodes.

Clinical Importance

- Distended bladder can rupture by injuries on anterior abdominal wall
- Interior of bladder can be examined by cystoscopy
- Chronic obstruction to the outflow of urine can cause hypertrophy of bladder, hydro-ureter or hydronephrosis.

Q. DUCTUS DEFERENS

Ductus deferens is a thick walled, muscular tube, which carries the spermatozoa from epididymis to prostatic urethra via ejaculatory duct.

Location and Course

- The duct courses from the posterior border of testis through spermatic cord to the pelvis
- It lies in the posterior part of cord and then traverses the canal
- The duct leaves the spermatic cord at the deep inguinal ring
- It passes medially, backwards to enter the lesser pelvis
- Runs downwards and backwards in lesser pelvis and take a sharp turn medially
- Toward its end it runs downwards, forwards and medially behind base of bladder
- The duct is dilated at the base of bladder known as ampulla of vas.

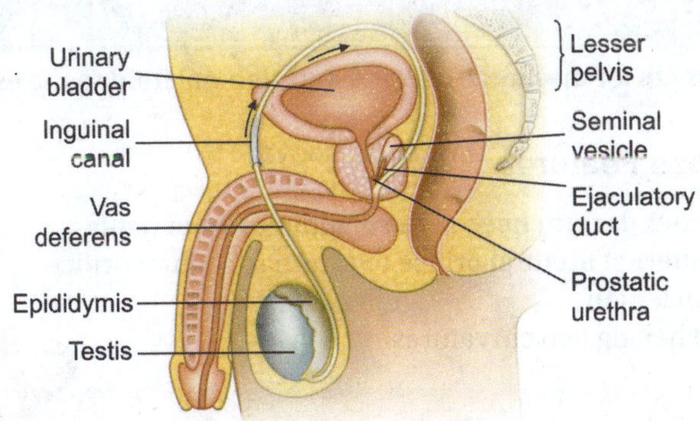

Course of ductus deferens

Relations

- Begins as a continuation of epididymis
- Lies along posterior border of testis
- Lies on the posterior aspect of spermatic cord
- In pelvis lies lateral to inferior epigastric artery and cross the external iliac vessels
- It is retroperitoneal in pelvis, it crosses the obturator nerve, obliterated umbilical artery and obturator vessels and vesical vessels
- Crosses the ureter runs in the sacrogenital fold of peritoneum
- Lies behind the base of bladder and medial to seminal vesicle
- Ductus deferens joins the duct of seminal vesicle to form ejaculatory duct.

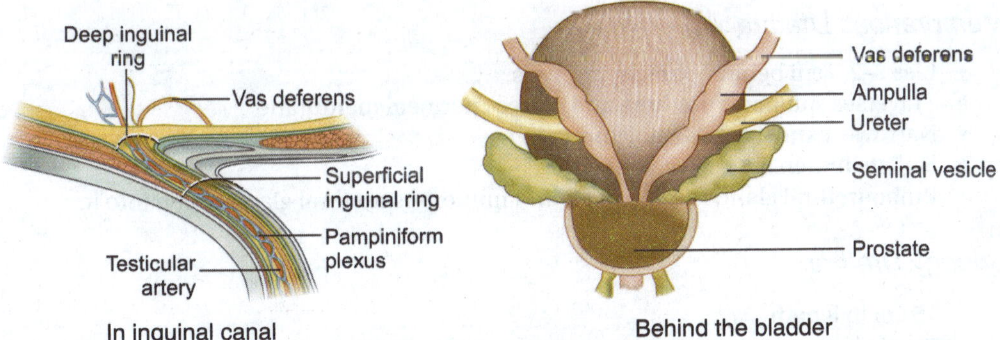

In inguinal canal

Behind the bladder

Relations of vas deferens

Blood Supply

- Artery to vas is a branch of superior or inferior vesical artery
- Vesical venous plexus drains the vas and opens into internal iliac vein.

Clinical Importance

- Vasectomy is a procedure for male sterilization wherein a part of vas is cut and ligated (tied).

Q. MALE URETHRA

Male urethra is a passage for discharge of urine and seminal fluid to the exterior.

Location and Gross Features

- Male urethra extends from neck of the bladder to tip of penis
- Lies between internal urethral orifice to external urethral orifice
- It is 18–20 cm in length
- 'S'-shaped and having two curvatures.

Parts

- Prostatic urethra as it traverses prostate
- Membranous urethra as it lies surrounded by sphincter urethrae
- Spongy part as it lies within the corpus spongiosum of penis.

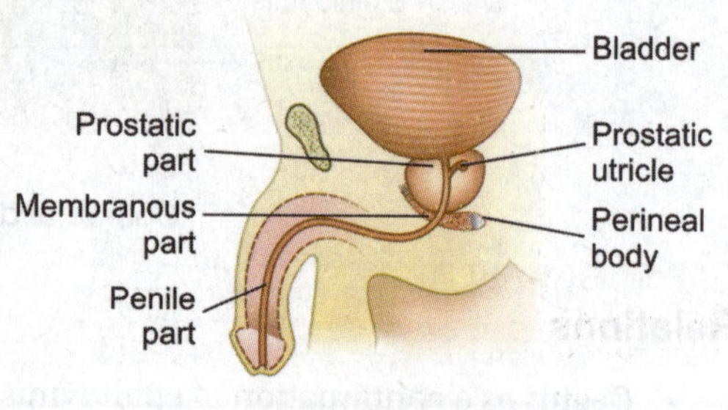

Male urethra

Prostatic Urethra

- Widest and dilatable part—3 cm
- Posterior wall has a crest known as urethral crest (verumontanum)
- Middle part of the crest also has another elevation known as colliculus seminalis, which lodges the orifice of prostatic utricle
- On the either side of the utricle are the openings of ejaculatory ducts.

Membranous Urethra

- Lies 2–2.5 cm behind pubic symphysis
- Traverses sphincter urethrae and pierces perineal membrane
- Narrowest and least dilatable part
- Stellate lumen in transverse section
- Bulbourethral glands lie around it and numerous urethral glands open into it.

Spongy Urethra

- 15 cm in length
- Fixed part runs forwards and upwards in the bulb of penis

- It bends forwards and downwards as the free part
- It is dilated at the commencement as the intrabulbar fossa and at its end as the navicular fossa
- Lumen is oblong horizontally in transverse section
- Ducts of bulbourethral gland open in the proximal part of urethra
- Urethral glands open into it.

Sphincters of Urethra

1. Internal urethral sphincter is involuntary in nature lies at the neck of the bladder.
2. External urethral sphincter is voluntary in nature, made up of striated muscles supplied by perineal branch of pudendal nerve. Voluntary holding of the urine is possible by this sphincter.

Blood Supply

- Receives branches from inferior vesicle, middle rectal and internal pudendal arteries
- Venous drainage is through internal pudendal vein into the internal iliac vein and vesical veins.

Clinical Importance

- In retention of urine the urethra is catheterized with rubber tube
- Rupture of urethra is common following pelvic fractures
- External urethral meatotomy can be done to widen the external orifice in cases of obstruction
- Urethritis can occur in infections leading to stricture urethra.

Anterior view of urethra
(schematic representation)

Q. PROSTATE

Prostate is a glandular tissue with fibromuscular stroma and is an accessory organ of male reproductive system, which adds to the bulk of seminal fluid.

Locations

- Surrounds the first 3 cm of urethra
- Lies within the lesser pelvis, below the neck of the bladder

- In front of ampulla of rectum
- Behind lower part of pubic symphysis.

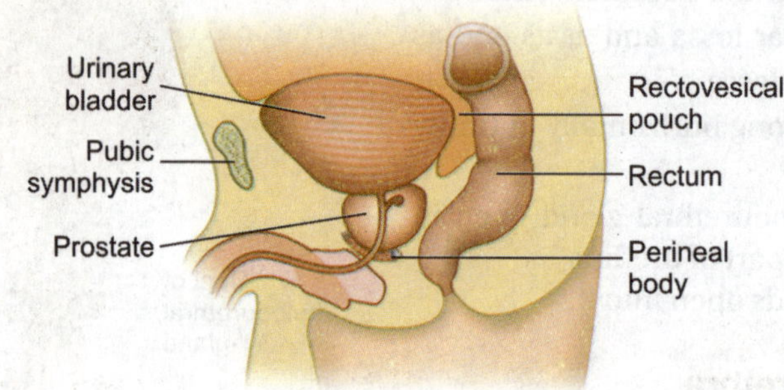

Location of prostate

Gross Features

- Inverted cone shaped
- Has apex, base, four surfaces—anterior, posterior and two inferolateral; five lobes—anterior, posterior, median and two lateral
- Anterior lobe—lies in front of urethra and has little glandular tissue
- Posterior lobe—lies behind median lobe
- Median lobe—lies at the neck of the bladder, in between the urethra and ejaculatory ducts, produces an elevation in the lower part of the trigone known as uvula vesicae
- Lateral lobes—lie on either side of urethra, has enough glandular tissue.

Surfaces

- Base: Continuous with neck of bladder
- Apex: Rests on upper surface of urogenital diaphragm
- Posterior: Rests on rectum
- Inferolateral: Lies on levator ani
- Anterior: Lies behind symphysis pubis.

Capsules

- True: Formed by condensation of prostatic tissue, deep to false capsules
- False: Formed by visceral layer of pelvic fascia.

The prostatic venous plexus lies between the two capsules.

Structures Within the Prostate

- Prostatic urethra
- Prostatic utricle
- Ejaculatory ducts.

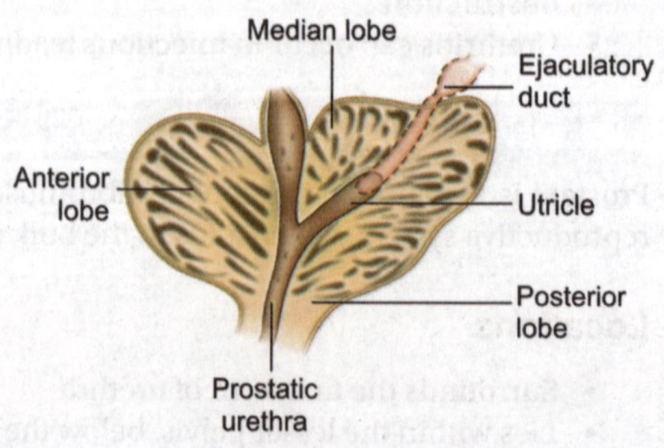

Sagittal section of prostate

Blood Supply

1. Branches of inferior vesical, middle rectal and internal pudendal arteries supply the gland.
2. Veins form a rich plexus around the gland; it communicates with vesical plexus and internal pudendal vein and then drains into vesical and internal iliac vein.

Lymphatic Drainage

- Mainly drains into internal iliac and sacral nodes
- Partly into external iliac.

Age Changes in Prostate

- At birth it is small in size with only a simple glandular system
- At puberty under the influence of hormones the gland grows in size and stroma condenses
- 20–30 years—marked proliferation of glandular tissue occurs
- 30–40 years—involution begins
- 40–45years—prostate enlarges causing prostatic hypertrophy or reduces in size causing senile atrophy.

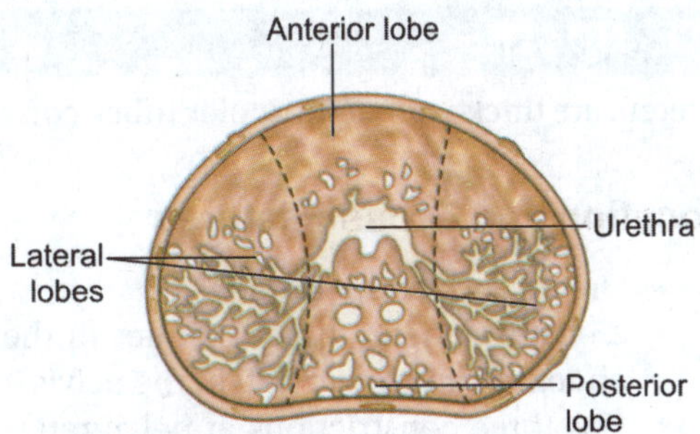

Lobes of prostate in transverse section

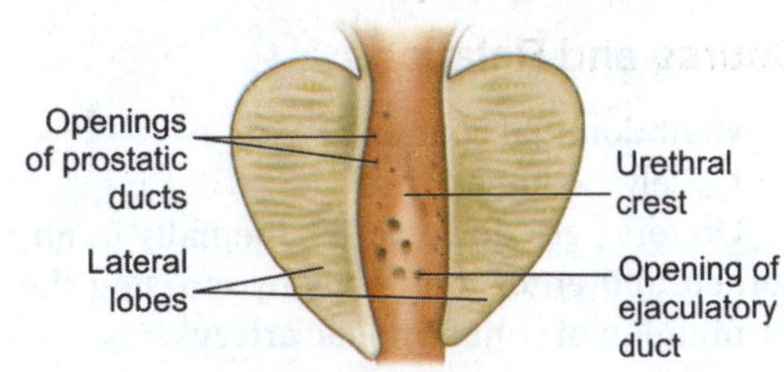

Coronal section of prostate

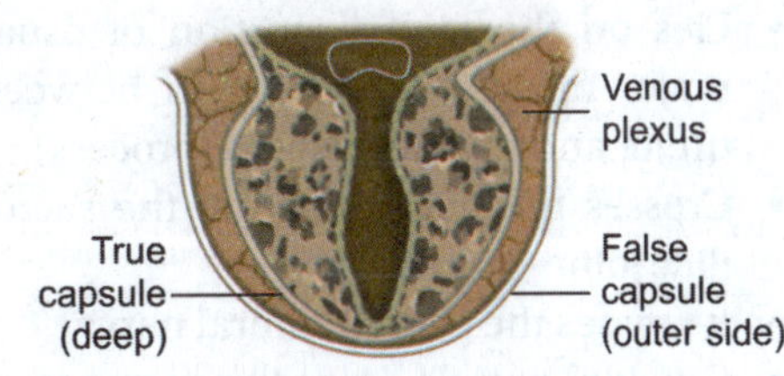

Capsules of prostate

Clinical Importance

1. Prostatic enlargement can cause urinary retention.
2. Per-rectal examination is clinically useful to detect prostatic enlargement.
3. Prostatectomy can be done by various approaches through bladder, i.e. transvesical through prostatic capsule, i.e. retropubic or through perineum by incising fascia of Denonvillier's, i.e. perineal approach. Both capsules are left behind to avoid damage to venous or benign plexus in prostatectomy.
4. Inflammation of prostate is known as prostatitis, it causes frequency of micturition, pain in perineum and tenderness in prostate.
5. Posterior lobe is the site of beginning of primary carcinoma of prostate.
6. Median lobe is a common site of adenoma or benign hypertrophy.
7. Valveless communication exists between prostatic and vertebral venous plexus leading to the spread of prostatic cancer.

Q. URETER

Ureters are thick-walled muscular tubes conveying urine from the kidneys to the bladder.

Location and Gross Features

- Ureters are retroperitoneal
- 25 cm in length, upper half lies in the abdomen and lower half in the pelvis
- Has three constrictions at pelviureteric junction, at brim of pelvis and as it passes through the bladder wall.

Course and Relations

- Abdominal course
- Pelvic course.

Ureters pass downwards, medially in abdomen and enter the pelvis by crossing the termination of common iliac artery.

Abdominal Course

- Lies on the medial portion of psoas major muscle (muscle is in between ureter and tip of transverse process)
- Crosses the pelvic brim at the sacroiliac joint
- It crosses the genitofemoral nerve
- Gonadal vessels cross the ureter from front
- Right ureter is covered by second part of duodenum and crossed by right colic and ileocolic vessels
- Left ureter crossed by left colic vessels
- Left ureter lies behind the pelvic mesocolon and its mesentery.

Pelvic Course

- Lies in front of internal iliac artery and its anterior division
- At the ischial spine it leaves the pelvic wall by turning medially
- Uterine artery crosses the ureter 2 cm lateral to cervix

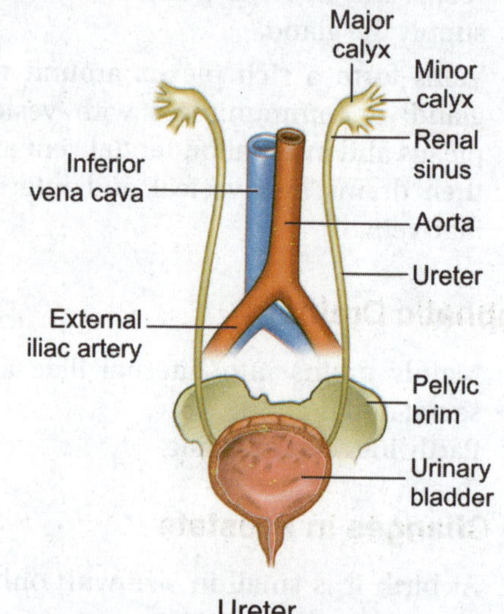

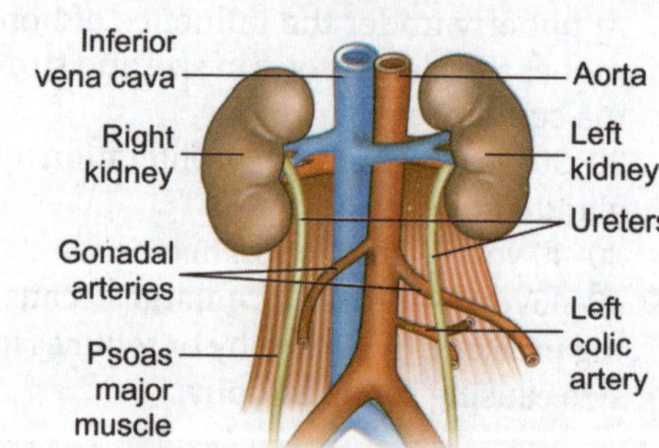

Abdominal course of ureter

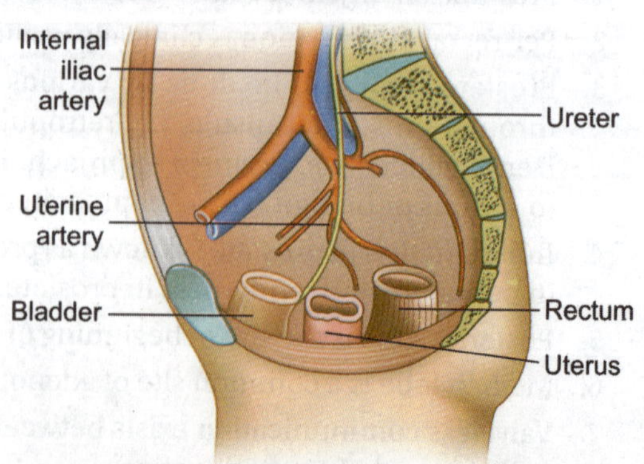

Pelvic course of ureter in females

- Ureter passes above the lateral fornix of vagina and lies close to the anterior wall of vagina
- Ureter lies behind and below infundibulopelvic ligament of ovary.

Blood Supply

- Upper part is supplied by the branches of renal, gonadal or adrenal arteries
- In pelvis it gets blood from internal iliac artery and its branches
- Arteries from the posterior abdominal wall form a plexus on the ureter
- Arteries enter the ureter from lateral side in the pelvic portion and from the medial side in the abdominal portion
- Similarly, renal, gonadal, adrenal and internal iliac veins drain the ureters.

Clinical Importance

- While ligating colic vessels during hemicolectomy the ureter may get injured
- During excision of rectum, inferior mesenteric artery ligation is needed ureter may get accidentally injured since it lies close to it
- Ureter lies behind and below infundibulopelvic ligament of ovary, it may get cut, while during ovariectomy
- While ligating uterine artery surgeon needs to remember that ureters are 2.0 cm lateral to the cervix
- Ligation of lateral ligament of rectum can damage ureters
- Application of clamps on the vagina can damage the ureter
- Ureteric colic due to kidney stone as it passes through the ureter may cause severe pain
- Sometimes the ureter may be duplicated.

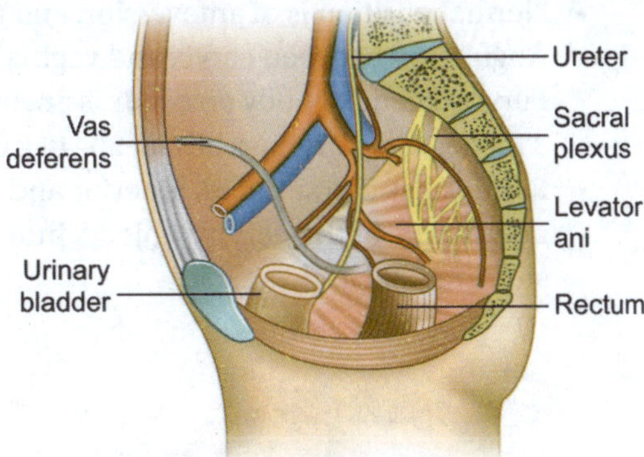

Pelvic course of ureter in males

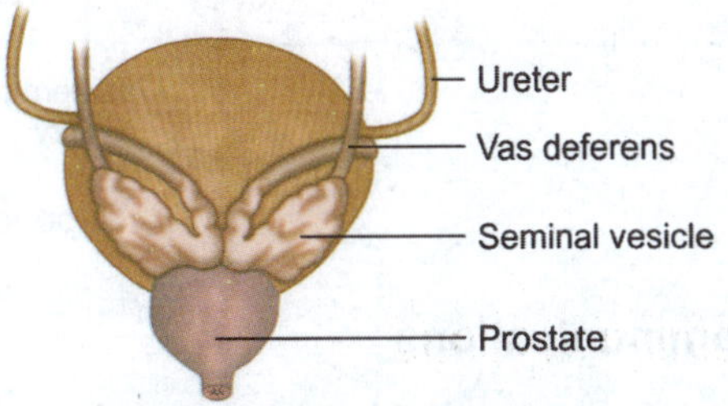

Posterior view of bladder

Q. UTERUS

Uterus is a muscular organ, which retains the developing embryo.

Locations and Gross Features

- Uterus is located in lesser pelvis between bladder and rectum
- Parts—fundus, body and cervix
- Constriction between body and cervix is isthmus

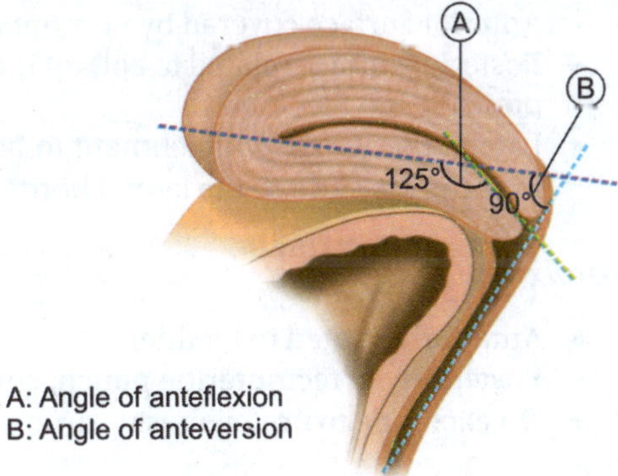

- Normal position is of anteversion and anteflexion
- Angulation between cervix and vagina is angle of anteversion
- Forward bend of body on cervix is angle of anteflexion
- 3 inches long, 2 inches broad, 30–40 g weight
- Fundus has two surfaces, anterior and posterior, two lateral borders
- Lower part of the cervix projects into the vagina, dividing the cervix into two parts—supravaginal and vaginal.

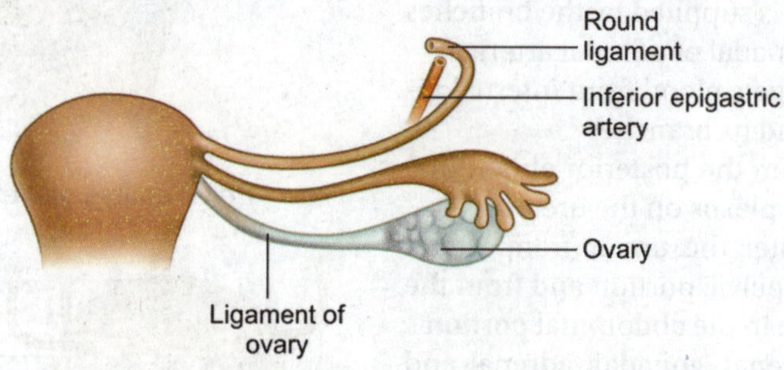

Superior view of uterus

Communications

- One on each side with the uterine tubes
- Below with the vagina.

Cavity

- Slit like in sagittal section
- Triangular in shape in coronal section
- Internal os is at the site between the body and the cervix
- External os is at the site where the cervical canal opens into the vagina.

Relations

Body

- Anterior surface covered by peritoneum and related to bladder
- Posterior surface related to coils of intestine, sigmoid colon, anterior wall of rectouterine pouch
- Lateral border gives attachment to broad ligament, uterus is in its upper part and uterine artery is close to the lateral border between the layers of broad ligament.

Cervix

- Anteriorly related to bladder
- Posteriorly to rectouterine pouch, coils of intestine and rectum
- On each side to ureter, uterine artery.

Supports of Uterus

Supports of the uterus can be classified into true supports and false supports.

True Supports

1. Uterine position: Angulation between body and fundus of uterus to cervix (angle of anteflexion) and angulation of cervix to vagina (angle of anteversion) itself provides positional support to uterus.

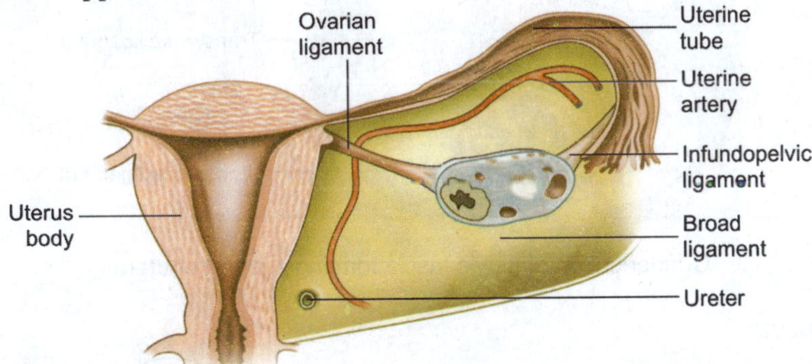

Relations of uterus

2. Round ligament of uterus: It maintains the uterine angulation by virtue of its attachment. It extends from upper part of uterus at the level of attachment of ligament of ovary to deep inguinal ring. It passes through the inguinal canal and gets attached to the fibrofatty tissue of labium majus. It sustains an anterior pull on the uterus.
3. Uterosacral ligaments: It counteracts the pull of round ligament and extends between cervix of uterus to sacrum. In its course backwards it embraces the rectouterine pouch and rectum.
4. Transverse cervical ligament: Also known as cardinal ligament, Mackenrodt's ligament. It is the condensation of connective tissue between cervix and vaginal fornix to lateral wall of pelvis. It gives lateral support to the uterus and is considered as cardinal support of uterus.

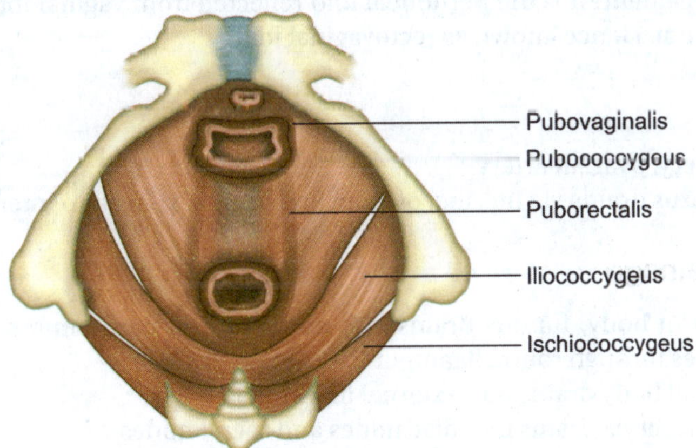

Pelvic diaphragm

5. Pubovaginalis part of levator ani and perineal body with its muscular attachment primarily support the vagina thus indirectly maintain the position of cervix.

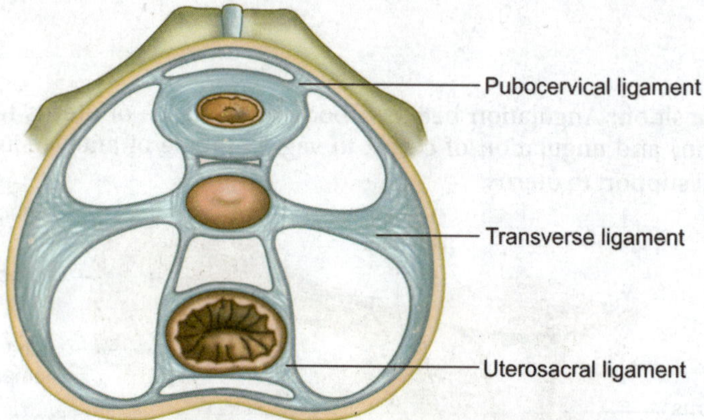

Condensation of pelvic fascia forming support of uterus

False Supports

1. **Broad ligament:** It is not a true ligament, but a double layered fold of peritoneum extending between lateral wall of uterus and pelvic wall. The upper free border contains the uterine tube and forms the mesosalpinx. The ureter adheres posteriorly, while the line of lateral attachment crosses the obturator nerves and vessels.

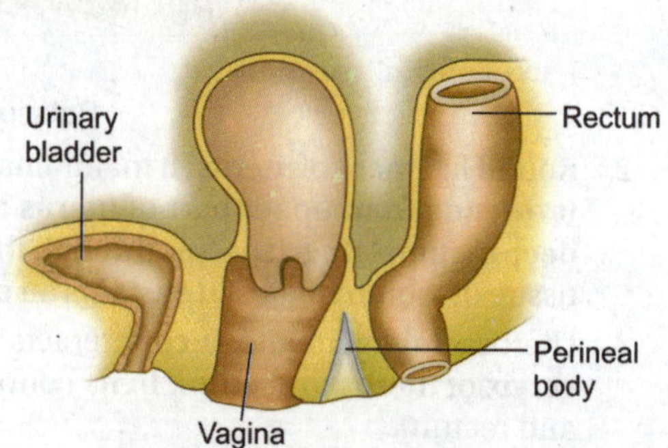

False supports of uterus

2. **Anterior ligament:** It is the peritoneal fold reflected on to the bladder from the uterus. Hence known as uterovesical fold.

3. **Posterior ligament:** It is the peritoneal fold reflected from vaginal fornix to the anterior wall of rectum. Hence known as rectovaginal fold.

Blood Supply

- Uterine artery, ovarian artery
- Uterine plexus drains via uterine, ovarian and vaginal veins into internal iliac veins.

Lymphatic Drainage

- Upper part of body, fundus drains into aortic nodes, partly into superficial inguinal lymph nodes through round ligament
- Lower part of body drains into external iliac nodes
- Lymph from cervix drains into iliac nodes and sacral nodes.

Clinical Importance

- Posterior inclination of the uterus is known as retroversion wherein the cervix faces forwards
- Sometimes the uterus may have a posterior curvature of the body and this is known as retroflexion
- Due to the weakness of pelvic floor muscles secondary to childbirth the uterus may protrude out of vagina this is known as prolapse of uterus
- Cancer cervix is a common cancer in Indian women
- Hysterectomy is removal of uterus.

Q. UTERINE TUBES

Uterine tubes are tortuous ducts, which carry the ovum from ovary to uterus and sperms from uterus to uterine tubes.

Location and Gross Features

- Located in the free upper margin of the broad ligament of uterus
- Each tube is 10 cm long
- Parts—intramural part, isthmus, ampulla and infundibular:
  - Intramural part is 1 cm, lies within the wall of uterus, opens through ostium in the uterine cavity
  - Isthmus narrow part, 2–3 cm
  - Ampulla thin walled, dilated part, 6–7 cm
  - Infundibulum—funnel-shaped end of tube, which opens in peritoneum.

Relations

- Isthmus and ampulla are directed posterolaterally in horizontal plane
- Ampulla arches on the ovary and is related to its posterior and anterior borders
- Infundibulum opens in abdominal cavity beyond free border of broad ligament
- Part of broad ligament between mesovarium and uterine tube is mesosalpinx.

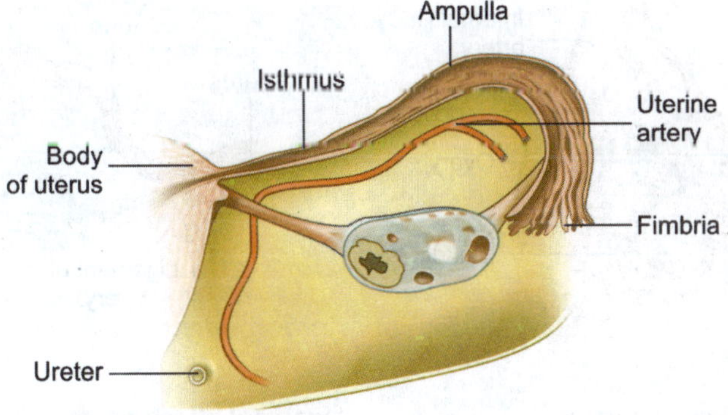

Parts of uterine tube and relations

Blood Supply

- Uterine artery supplies the medial two third of tube, while lateral one third is supplied by ovarian artery
- Tube is drained by pampiniform plexus into uterine veins.

Lymphatic Drainage

- Lymph of tube drains into lateral aortic and preaortic nodes
- Lymph from isthmus drains through round ligament into superficial inguinal ligament.

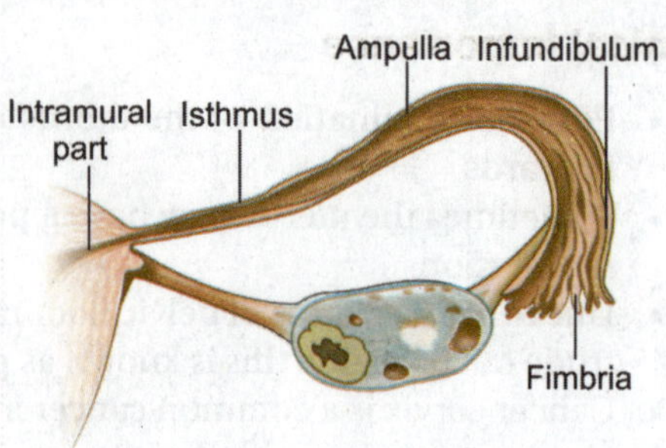

Parts of uterine tube

Clinical Importance

- Inflammation of tube is known as salpingitis; it commonly occurs secondary to tuberculosis leading to fibrosis of the tube causing secondary infertility
- 2–3 cm length of tube is cut and ligated, in tubectomy for sterilization
- Sometimes the embryo may adhere to the tube instead of uterus giving rise to tubal pregnancy.

Q. OVARY

Ovaries are pair of female reproductive organs, which lie in the pelvis.

Locations

- Located in the ovarian fossa on the lateral pelvic wall
- Ovarian fossa is bounded by in front by obliterated umbilical artery, and behind by ureter and internal iliac artery.

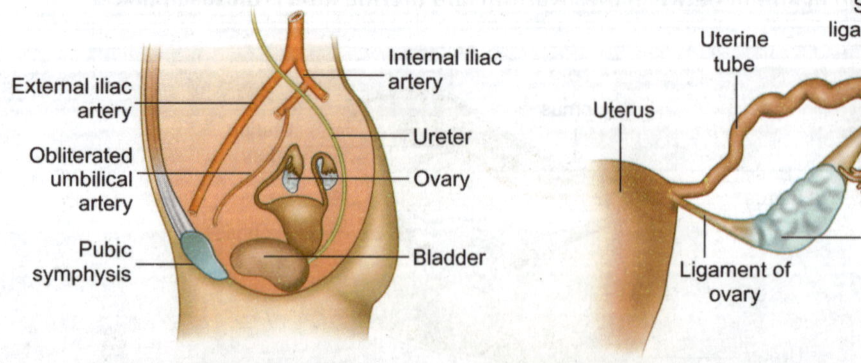

Locations of ovary

Ligament attachments on ovary (in nulliparous), position of ovary is vertical

Gross Features

- Almond shaped, grayish pink in color
- Has anterior and posterior border
- Two surfaces lateral and medial.

Peritoneal Relations

1. Entirely covered by peritoneum except anterior border where the layers of peritoneum are reflected on posterior layer of broad ligament.
2. Ovary is connected to posterior layer of broad ligament by a fold of peritoneum known as mesovarium.
3. Lateral part of broad ligament of uterus extending from infundibulum to the upper pole forms a fold of peritoneum is known as suspensory ligament of ovary.

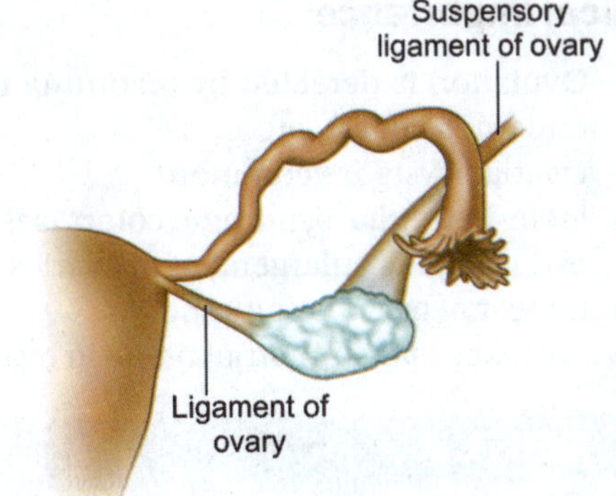

Ligament of ovary (in multiparous), position of ovary is horizontal

Visceral Relations

- Upper pole: Related to uterine tube, external iliac vein, fimbria and suspensory ligament are attached to upper pole
- Lower pole: Related to pelvic floor, it is connected to lateral angle of uterus by ligament of ovary
- Anterior border: Related to uterine tube, obliterated umbilical artery
- Posterior border: Related to uterine tube, ureter
- Lateral surface: Ovarian fossa, obturator vessels and nerves
- Medial surface: Covered by uterine tube, peritoneal recess between mesosalpinx and medial surface is known as ovarian bursa.

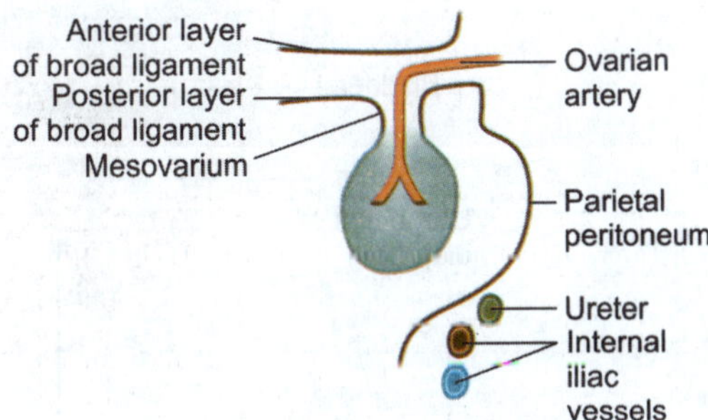

Superior view of ovarian fossa

Blood Supply

- Ovarian artery, supplies through suspensory ligament
- Uterine artery also supplies the ovary
- Pampiniform plexus of ovary drains into ovarian vein.

Lymphatic Drainage

- Lateral aortic and preaortic.

Clinical Importance

- Ovulation is detected by recording the basal body temperature, cervical mucus test, endometrial test, etc.
- Ovarian cysts are common
- Stein-Leventhal syndrome comprises of mild hirsutism, hoarse voice, secondary amenorrhea, cystic enlargement of ovaries
- Cancer of ovary is common
- Presence of endometrial tissue in ovary produces endometrial cysts.

Q. RECTUM

Rectum lies between sigmoid colon above and anal canal below. The rectum is not straight as the name suggests, but curved anteroposteriorly and side to side. However, the features of large intestine, i.e. teniae coli, sacculations and appendices epiploicae are absent.

Locations

- Closely fit into the concavity of sacrum and coccyx
- Lies against S3, S4, S5 and coccyx
- Ends 2–3 cm in front and below coccyx
- Is about 4 cm above the anal verge.

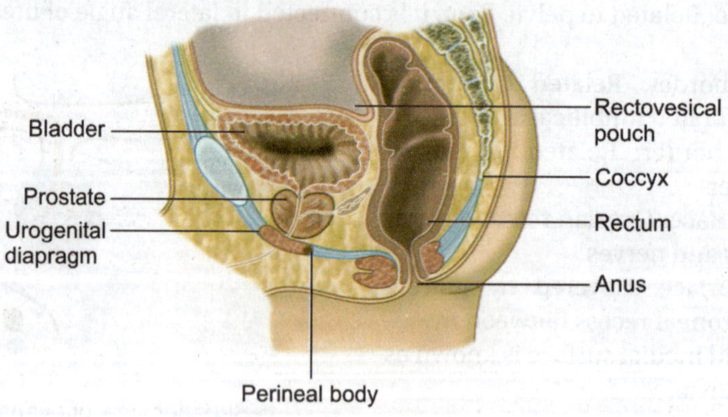

Location of rectum (sagittal section)

Gross Features

- 12 cm long, lower part dilated to form ampulla
- Runs forwards and downwards, then backwards and downwards
- Two anteroposterior curvatures sacral flexure follows sacral curve, perineal flexure is backward bend
- Three lateral curvatures convex to right, convex to left and lower curve again convex to right.

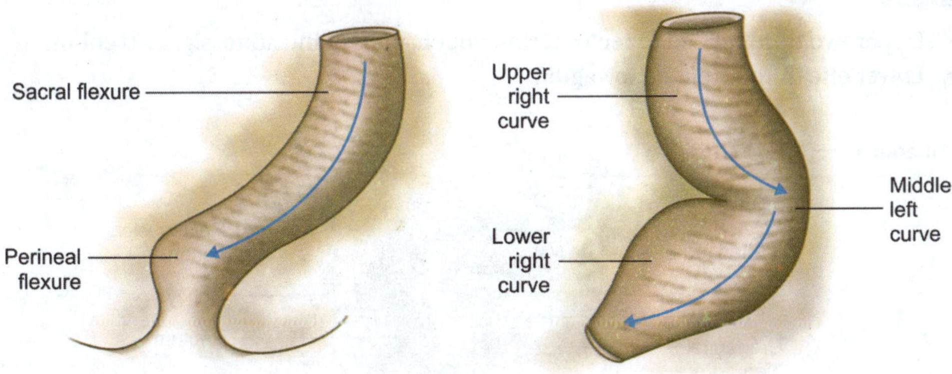

Curvatures of rectum

Peritoneal Relations

- Upper one third of rectum is covered in front and sides
- Middle one third of rectum is covered only in front
- Lower one third is not covered by peritoneum
- Posteriorly fascia of Waldeyer suspends rectum from the sacrum
- Pelvic fascia condenses laterally to support rectum to form lateral ligaments
- Rectovesical fascia lies between rectum behind and seminal vesicles, prostate and bladder in front.

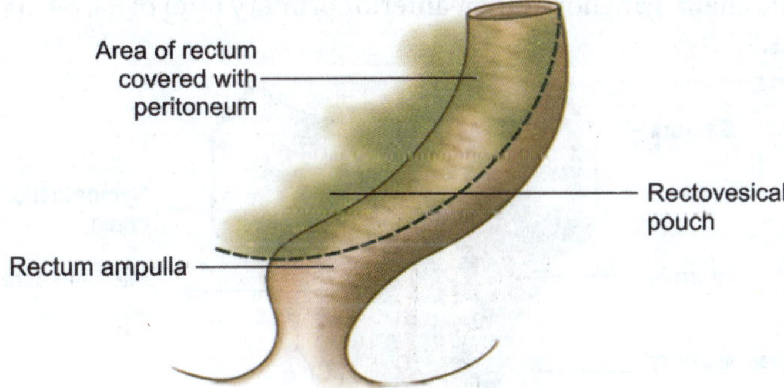

Peritoneal relations of rectum

Visceral Relations

Anteriorly

In males:

- Upper two third related to rectovesical pouch, coils of intestine, sigmoid colon
- Lower one third related to base of urinary bladder, ureters, seminal vesicles, vas deferens, prostate.

In females:

- Upper two third related to rectouterine pouch, coils of intestine, sigmoid colon
- Lower one third is related to vagina.

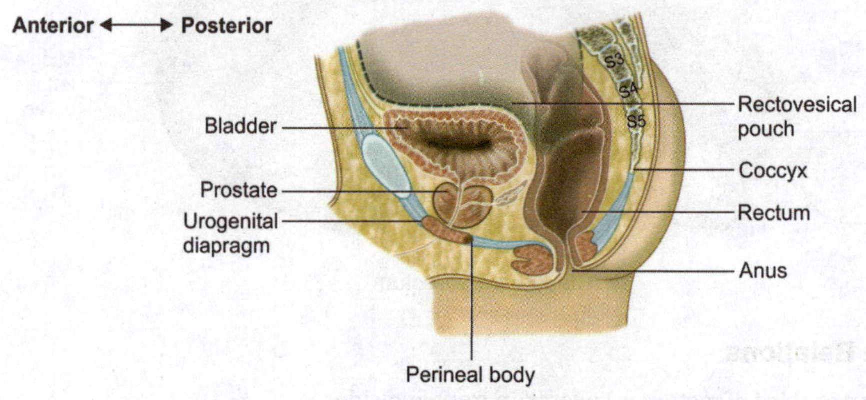

Relations of rectum

Posteriorly

- Sacrum, coccyx, anococcygeal ligament
- Piriformis, coccygeus and levator ani
- Median sacral, superior rectal, lower lateral sacral vessels
- Sympathetic chain, ganglion impar, anterior primary rami of S3, S4, S5
- Lymphatics.

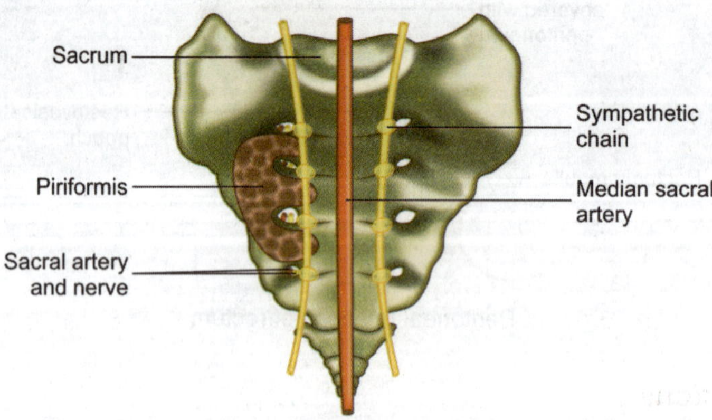

Posterior relations of rectum

Mucous Membrane

- Temporary longitudinal folds are present in empty rectum
- Permanent horizontal folds—upper, middle and lower.

Blood Supply

- Superior rectal artery, is continuation of inferior mesenteric artery is the main supply to rectum, also receives blood from middle rectal and median sacral artery
- Internal rectal venous plexus forms superior rectal vein, which drains into inferior mesenteric vein. Rectum is also drained by middle rectal vein, which opens into internal iliac vein.

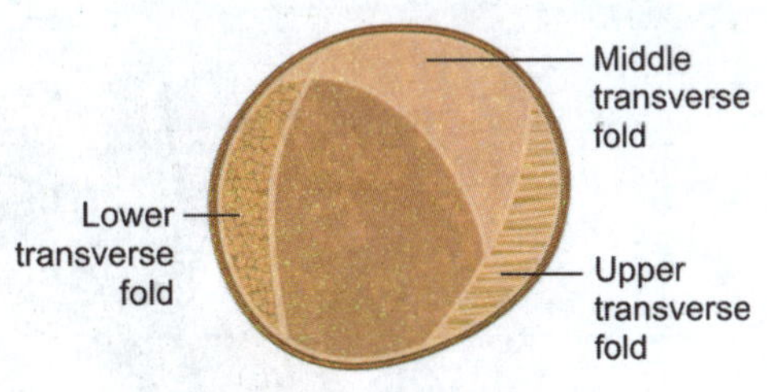

Horizontal mucosal folds

Lymphatic Drainage

- Upper rectum drains via pararectal and sigmoid nodes to inferior mesenteric nodes
- Lower rectum drains along middle rectal vessels to internal iliac nodes.

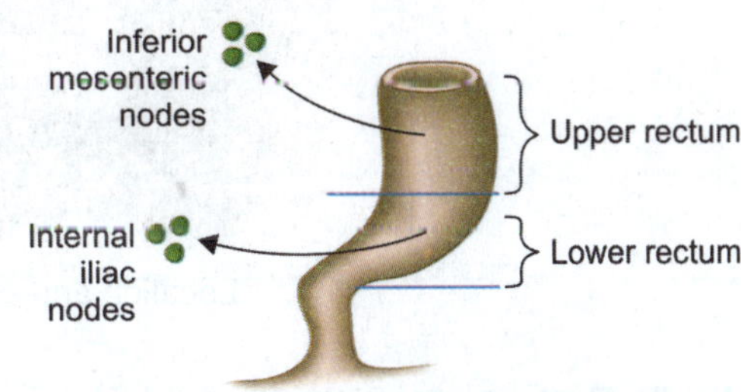

Lymphatic drainage of rectum

Clinical Importance

- In digital examination of rectum (per rectal) following structures are felt prostate, seminal vesicles, vas deferens, anorectal ring, sacrum, coccyx (in females perineal body, cervix can be palpated)
- Direct visualization of interior of rectum and anal canal is possible by sigmoidoscope and proctoscope
- Violent straining may cause prolapse of rectum.

Q. ANAL CANAL

Anal canal is a muscular canal, which has a significant sphincter mechanism, present at the distal end of gastrointestinal tract.

Location and Gross Features

- Length is 4 cm
- Extends from anorectal junction to anus
- Separated posteriorly from tip of coccyx by fibrofatty tissue and anococcygeal ligament
- Ischiorectal fossa on either side of rectum.

Interior of Anal Canal

Upper Part

Upper part is 15 mm, lined by columnar epithelium, vertical mucosal folds known as anal columns, with rectal anal valves toward the base of the columns, anal sinuses are pockets above the valves, pectinate line along the attachment of anal valves can be appreciated.

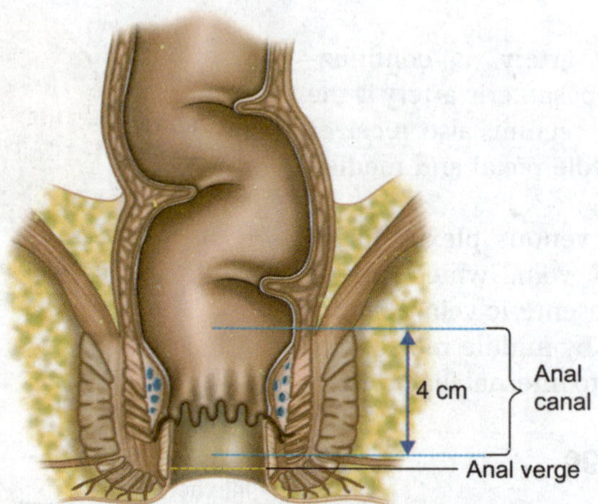

Location and extent of anal canal

Middle Part

Middle part is 15 mm, lies between pectinate above and Hilton's line below (lies between the subcutaneous part of external sphincter and lower border of internal sphincter).

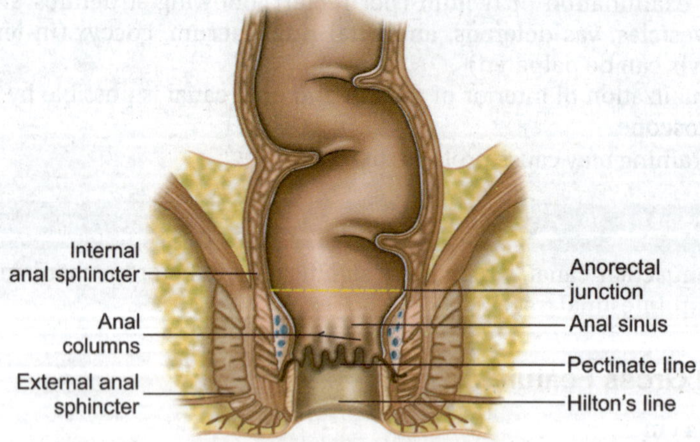

Interior of anal canal

Lower Part

Lower part is 8 mm, lined by skin (has stratified squamous epithelium, sweat and sebaceous glands).

Anal Sphincters

External Anal Sphincter

- Has three parts—subcutaneous, superficial and deep
- Is striated muscle, under voluntary control
- Supplied by inferior rectal, perineal branch of S4
- Surrounds the whole length of anal canal
- At the level of anorectal junction it forms a sling of puborectalis muscle.

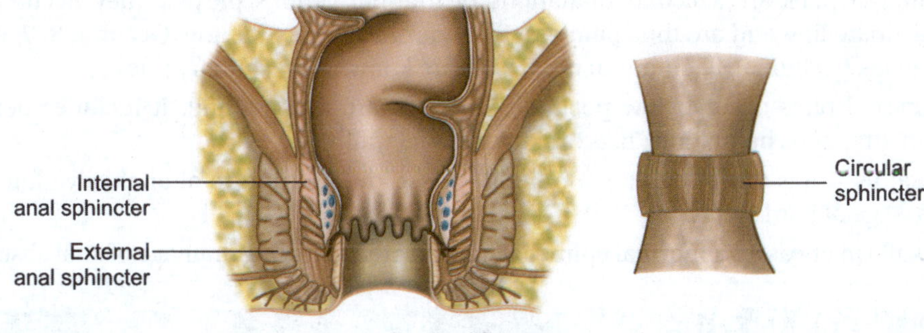

Anal sphincters

Internal Anal Sphincter

- Internal anal sphincter is the downward extension of circular muscle layer of rectum
- It is partly muscular and partly fibrous
- The fibers run down the perianal fat and lower part of external sphincter and get attached to the skin.

Blood Supply

- Above the pectinate line, it is supplied by superior rectal artery and below the pectinate line is supplied by inferior rectal artery
- Internal rectal venous plexus in the submucosa of anal canal drains into superior rectal vein
- External rectal venous plexus lies outside the muscular layer of anal canal, communicates with internal plexus and drains into internal pudendal vein, internal iliac vein and inferior mesenteric vein.

Lymphatic Drainage

- Above the pectinate line drains into internal iliac nodes
- Below pectinate line drains into superficial inguinal lymph nodes.

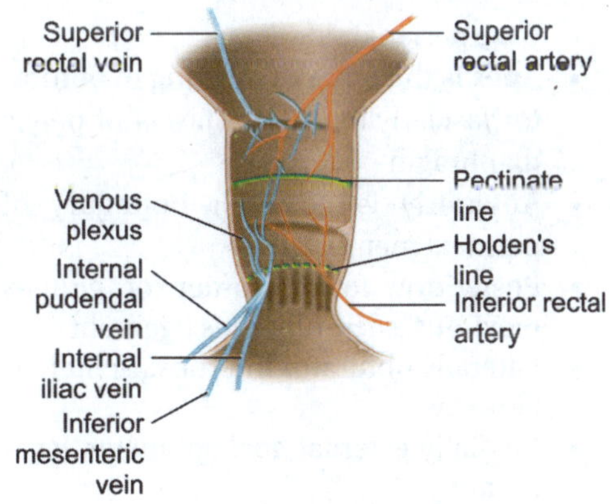

Blood supply of anal canal

Nerve Supply

- Above the pectinate line it is supplied by autonomic nerves
- Below pectinate line it is supplied by somatic nerves
- Internal sphincter is supplied by autonomic nerves
- External sphincter is supplied by somatic nerve.

Clinical Importance

1. Internal piles are saccular dilatations of internal venous plexus. They occur above pectinate line and are thus painless. Bleed profusely by straining. Occur at 3, 7 and 11 O'clock position. Dilatations at other sites are known as secondary piles.

2. External piles occur below pectinate line and are thus painful. It includes perianal subcutaneous hematoma, tags of skin and anal wall.

3. Anal fissure is a very painful condition caused due to rupture of anal valve following passage of hard stools.

4. Fistula in ano is an abnormal epithelial tract created following drainage of anal abscess.

▶ MISCELLANEOUS

Q. ISCHIORECTAL FOSSA

Ischiorectal fossa is a conical space around the anal canal with the apex upwards and base downwards. The presence of the space on either side of anal canal allows the dilatation of anus during defecation.

Locations

- On each side of anal canal
- Below the pelvic diaphragm.

Boundaries

- Base perianal skin
- Apex is the point of meeting of obturator fascia with inferior fascia of pelvic diaphragm
- Anteriorly is posterior boundary of perineal membrane
- Posteriorly lower border of gluteus maximus, sacrotuberous ligament
- Laterally obturator internus, ischial tuberosity
- Medially external anal sphincter, levator ani.

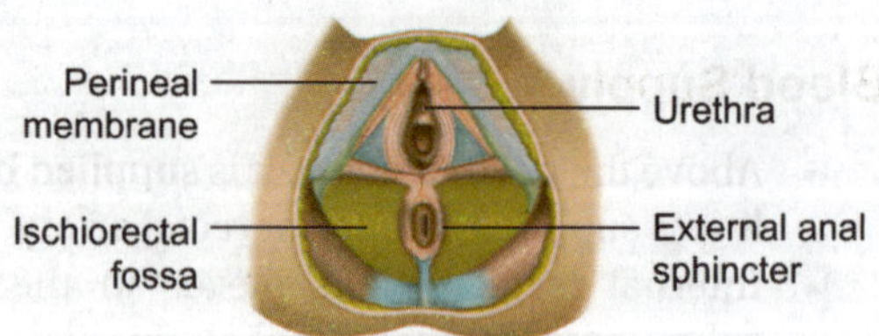

Contents of ischiorectal fossa

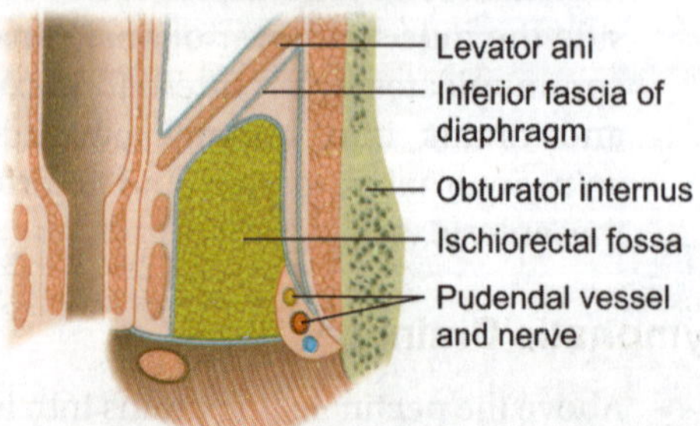

Boundaries of ischiorectal fossa

Recesses

- Anterior recess is an extra space beyond the boundaries, above the urogenital diaphragm
- Posterior recess deep to sacrotuberous ligament
- Horseshoe recess connects the two fossae.

Spaces Around the Fossa

- Perianal space with subcutaneous fat, tightly arranged in the form of loculi
- Ischiorectal space, fat is loosely arranged
- Pudendal canal is in the lateral wall of fossa.

Contents

- Fat
- Inferior rectal vessels and nerve
- Posterior scrotal nerves and vessels
- Perineal branch of S4, S2, S3 cutaneous branches.

Clinical Importance

1. Ischiorectal abscess is common due to the close proximity of anal canal. Abscess anywhere in the body should be incised and drained and in ischiorectal fossa the drainage can be carried out safely due to less vascularity.
2. Fat in the fossa acts as a support to rectum and anal canal and prevents prolapse of rectum.

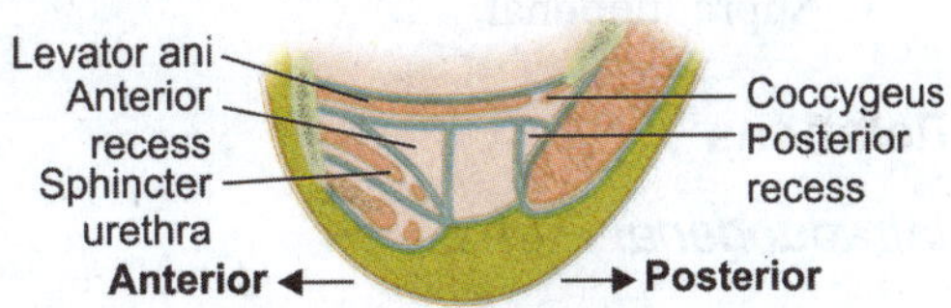

Recesses of ischiorectal fossa (schematic view)

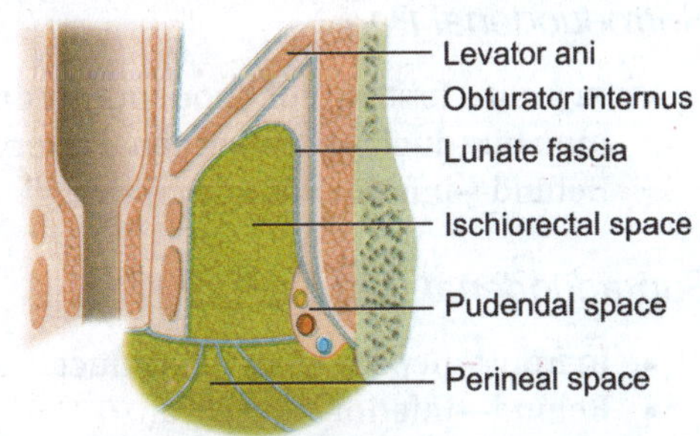

Spaces around ischiorectal fossa

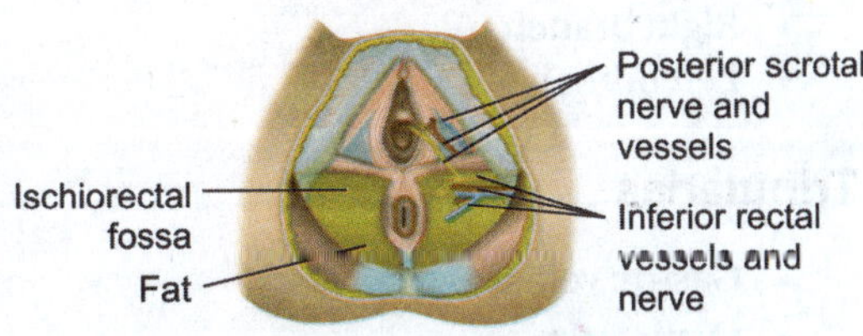

Contents of ischiorectal fossa

Q.   PORTAL VEIN AND SITES OF PORTOSYSTEMIC ANASTOMOSIS.

Portal system of vein begins and ends in capillaries. Portal vein is a major vein which collects blood from abdominal organs and carries it to liver. In the liver the portal vein breaks into sinusoids, which drain into hepatic veins and then into inferior vena cava.

Formation and Course

- Formed by the union of superior mesenteric vein and splenic vein
- Begins behind the neck of pancreas, ascends upwards to the right lying behind first part of duodenum and then in the free margin of lesser omentum
- It ends at the right end of porta hepatis by dividing into right and left branch.

Parts

- Infraduodenal
- Retroduodenal
- Supraduodenal.

Relations

Infraduodenal Part

- In front—neck of pancreas
- Behind—inferior vena cava.

Retroduodenal Part

- In front—first part of duodenum, common bile duct, gastroduodenal artery
- Behind—inferior vena cava.

Supraduodenal Part

- In front—hepatic artery, bile duct
- Behind—inferior vena cava.

Branches

- Right branch
- Left branch.

Tributaries

- Gastric veins
- Cystic vein
- Paraumbilical vein
- Superior pancreaticoduodenal vein.

Portosystemic Anastomosis Sites

- At the lower end of esophagus veins of stomach (portal) communicate with esophageal veins (systemic)
- Around umbilicus—veins of liver (portal) communicate with veins around the umbilicus, i.e. epigastric veins (systemic)
- At lower end of rectum, superior rectal vein (portal) communicates with middle and inferior rectal veins (systemic)

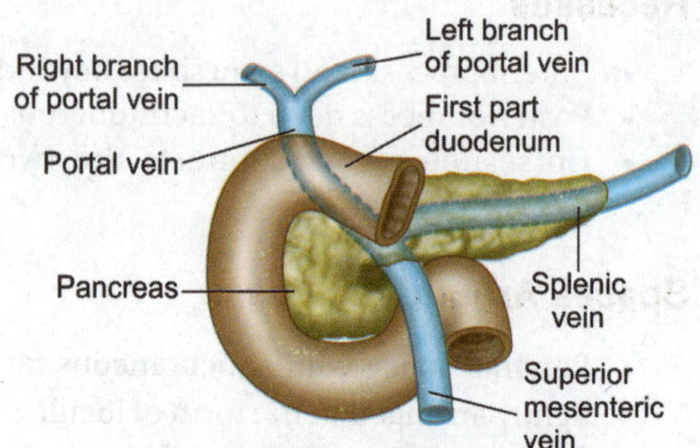

Formation and course of splenic vein

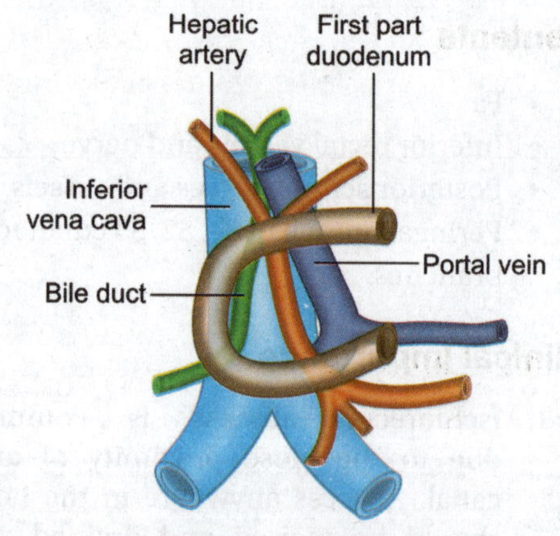

Relations of portal vein

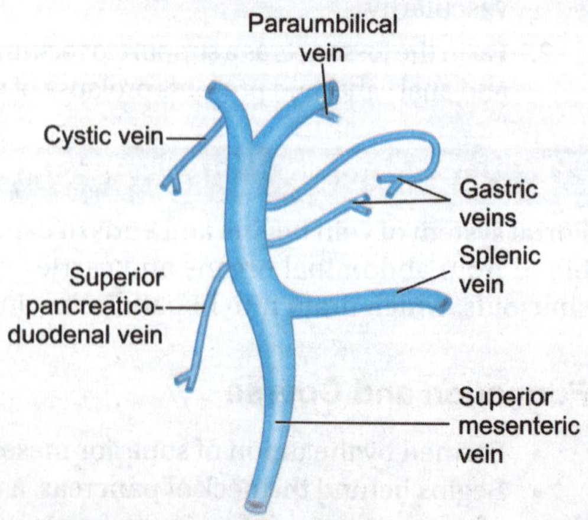

Tributaries of portal vein

- Bare area of liver—hepatic veins (portal) communicate with phrenic and intercostal veins (systemic)
- Posterior abdominal wall veins of peritoneum, colon (portal) communicate with vessels of kidney (systemic).

Clinical Importance

1. Normal portal pressure is 7–10 cm of saline and at the junction of hepatic vein and inferior vena cava is 0 cm.

2. In portal hypertension, there is an abnormally high pressure within the portal venous system by and large due to mechanical obstruction. Obstruction can occur in hepatic veins (Budd-Chiari syndrome) or intrahepatic (due to cirrhosis, tumor) or in portal vein (due to thrombosis, tumor).

3. Signs of portal hypertension are ascites (fluid collection in abdomen), enlarged spleen, caput medusa (dilated and tortuous veins around umbilicus) hematemesis due to esophageal varices (dilated and tortuous veins at the lower end of esophagus), bleeding per rectum.

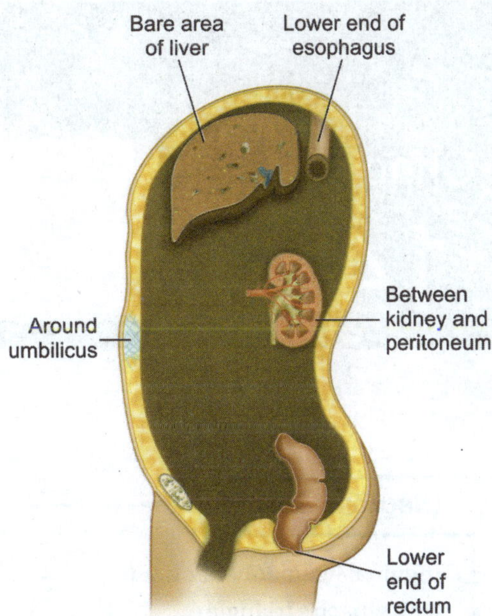

Sites of portosystemic anastomosis (schematic representation)

Key Diagrams with MCQ Tips

Diagrams for

- Inguinal ligament of Poupart
- Hesselbach's triangle
- Transverse section of spermatic cord
- Posterior relations of kidney
- Mesentery
- Epiploic foramen
- Branches of abdominal aorta
- Celiac artery main branches
- Superior mesenteric artery branches
- Inferior mesenteric artery
- Posterior relations of cecum
- Portal vein
- Perineal body
- Per-rectal examination
- Forward angulation between cervix and vagina
- Relation of ureter to uterine artery
- Pectinate line
- Branches of internal iliac artery

Q. Inguinal ligament of Poupart

Ans.

- Folded border of external oblique aponeurosis
- Attached to anterior superior iliac spine and pubic tubercle
- Fascia lata, internal oblique, transversus abdominis, cremaster muscle are attached
- Parts are reflected part, pectineal part, lacunar part.

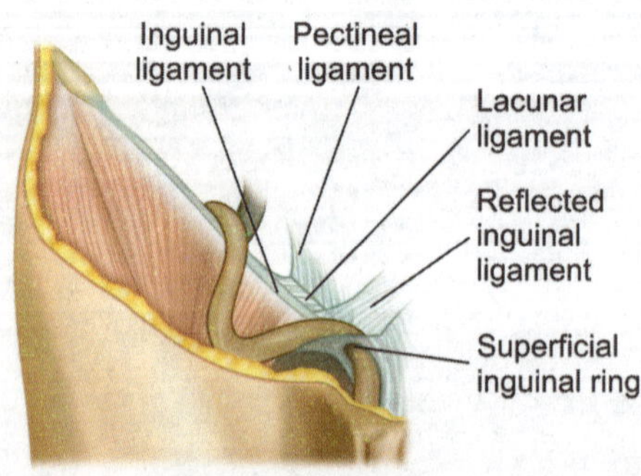

Inguinal ligament

Q. Hesselbach's triangle

Ans.
- Bounded laterally by inferior epigastric artery, medially lateral border of rectus abdominis and base by inguinal ligament
- Divided into two parts by obliterated umbilical artery (lateral umbilical ligament)
- Direct inguinal hernia traverses this triangle.

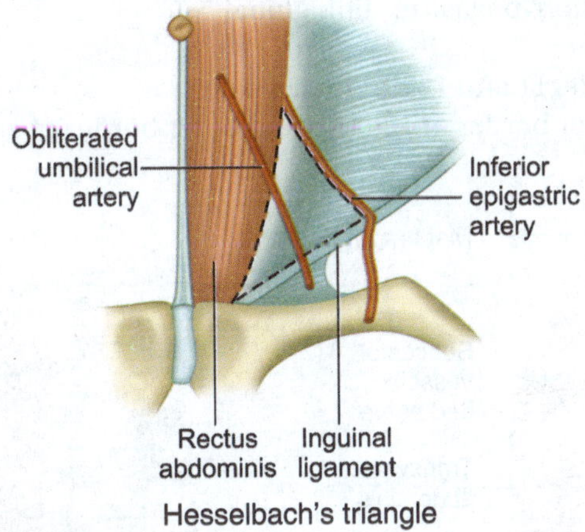

Hesselbach's triangle

Q. Superficial inguinal ring is a triangular gap in the external oblique aponeurosis.

Q. Deep inguinal ring is an oval opening in the fascia transversalis.

Q. Transverse section of spermatic cord.

Ans.
- Internal spermatic fascia is derived from fascia transversalis
- Cremasteric fascia is derived from internal oblique and transversus abdominis muscle
- External spermatic fascia is derived from external oblique aponeurosis.

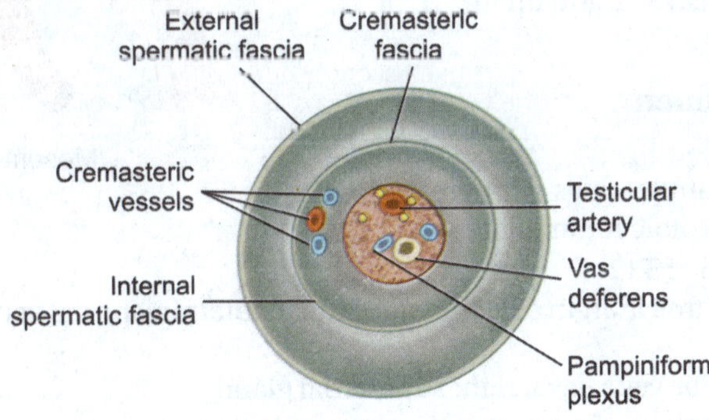

Transverse section of spermatic cord

Q. Rectouterine pouch is pouch of Douglas.

Q. Hepatorenal pouch is Morison's pouch.

Q. Posterior relations of kidney.

Ans.

- Muscles—diaphragm, psoas major, quadratus lumborum, transversus abdominis
- Nerves subcostal, iliohypogastric, ilioinguinal
- Subcostal vessels
- 12th rib on right side, 11 and 12 ribs on left side
- Angle between lower border of 12th rib and outer border of erector spinae is known as renal angle.

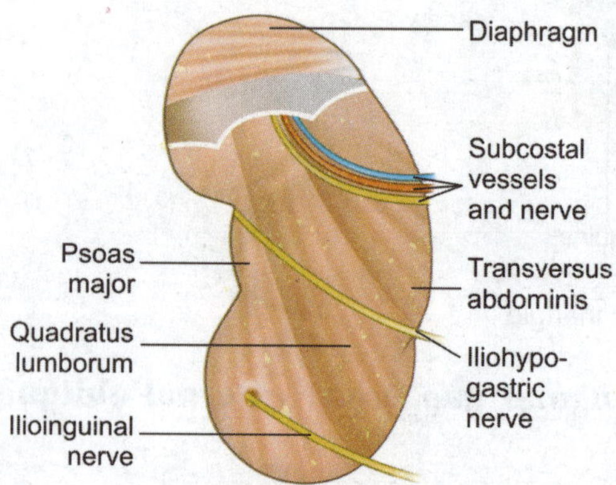

Posterior relations of kidney

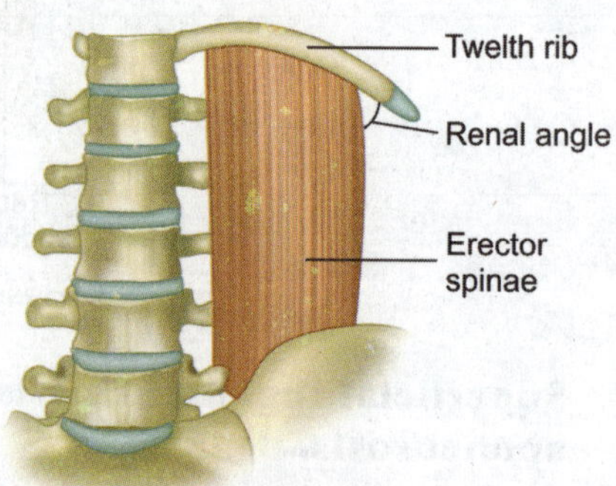

Renal angle

Q. Mesentery

Ans.

- Root of mesentery 6 inches long, directed obliquely to right
- Crosses third part of duodenum, aorta, inferior vena cava, right ureter, right psoas.

Q. Epiploic foramen

Ans.

- Lesser sac communicates with greater sac through epiploic foramen
- Lies at the level of T12
- In front is right free margin of lesser omentum containing portal vein, hepatic artery and bile duct
- Behind is inferior vena cava, right suprarenal gland
- Above—liver; below—first part of duodenum, hepatic artery.

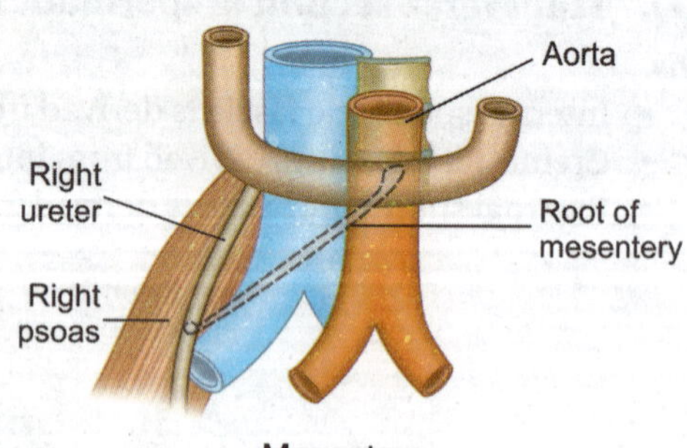

Mesentery

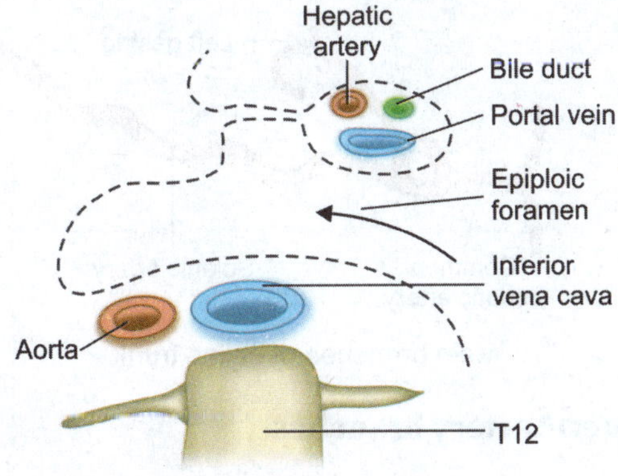

Epiploic foramen

Q. Branches of abdominal aorta

Ans.

- Celiac artery between T12 and L1
- Superior mesenteric artery at L1
- Renal artery between L1 and L2
- Gonadal artery at L2
- Inferior mesenteric artery at L3
- Divides into two common iliacs at L4.

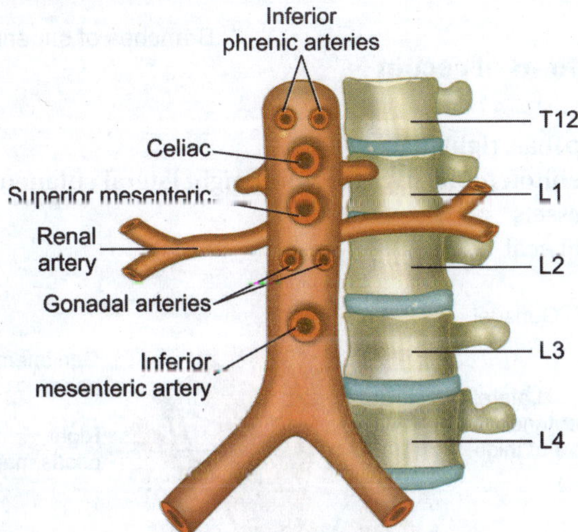

Branches of abdominal artery

Q. Celiac artery main branches

Ans.

- Left gastric artery
- Splenic artery
- Common hepatic artery.

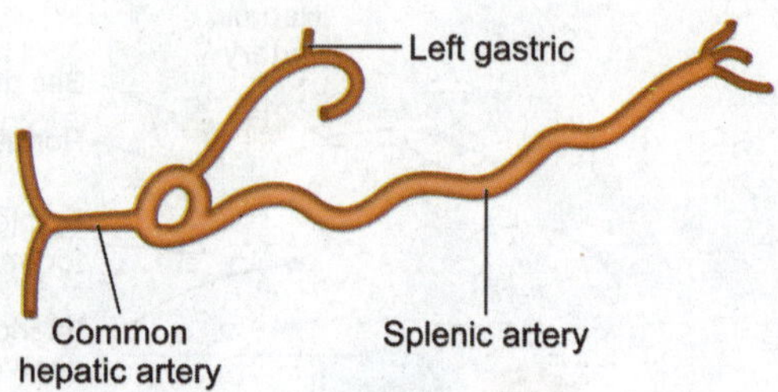

Main branches of celiac trunk

Q. Superior mesenteric artery branches

Ans.

- Inferior pancreaticoduodenal
- Jejunal, ileal
- Ileocolic
- Right colic
- Middle colic.

Q. Inferior mesenteric artery

Ans.

- Left colic
- Sigmoid
- Superior rectal.

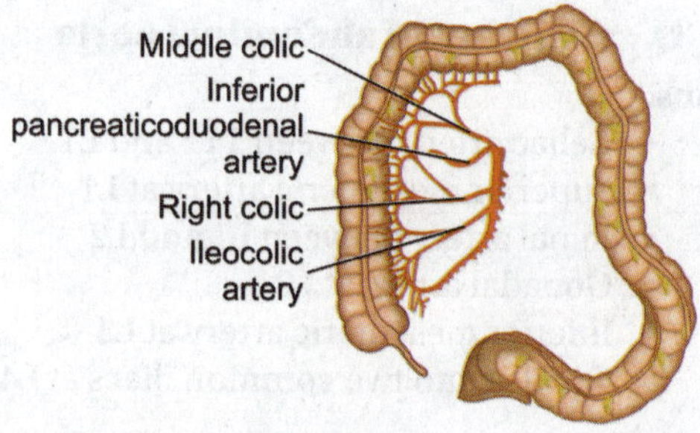

Branches of superior mesenteric artery

Q. Posterior relations of cecum

Ans.

- Muscles—right psoas, right iliacus
- Nerves—right genitofemoral, right femoral, right lateral cutaneous nerve of thigh
- Right gonadal vessels
- Appendix if retrocecal.

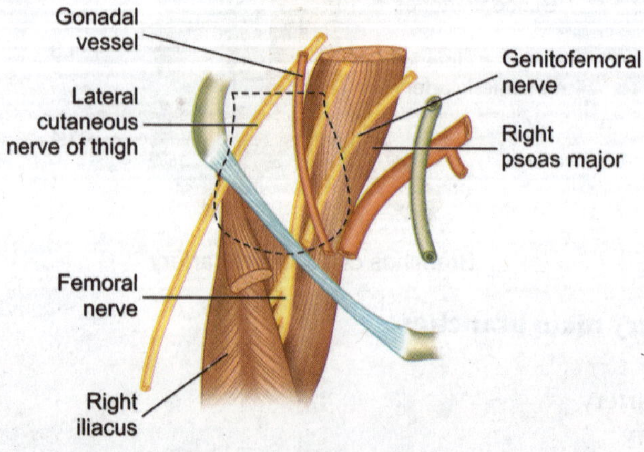

Posterior relations of cecum

Q. Third part of duodenum is anteriorly related to superior mesenteric vessels.

Q. Abdominal tonsil means appendix.

Q. Pudendal canal is in lateral wall of ischiorectal fossa.

Q. Portal vein

Ans.

- Formed by union of superior mesenteric vein with splenic vein
- At L2
- Behind neck of pancreas.

Q. Gonadal vessels lie in front of ureter.

Q. Perineal body

Ans.

- 1.25 cm in front of anal margin
- Three paired muscles—superficial and deep transversus perinei, levator ani
- Three unpaired muscles—external anal sphincter, bulbospongiosus, longitudinal muscle coat of rectal ampulla
- Central tendon of perineum, key support of pelvic organs.

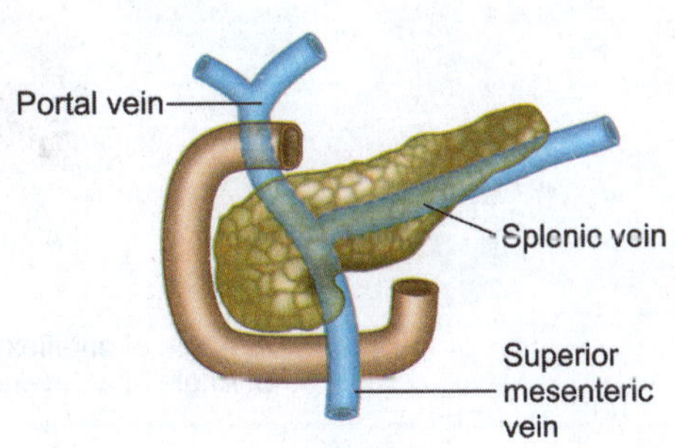

Portal vein

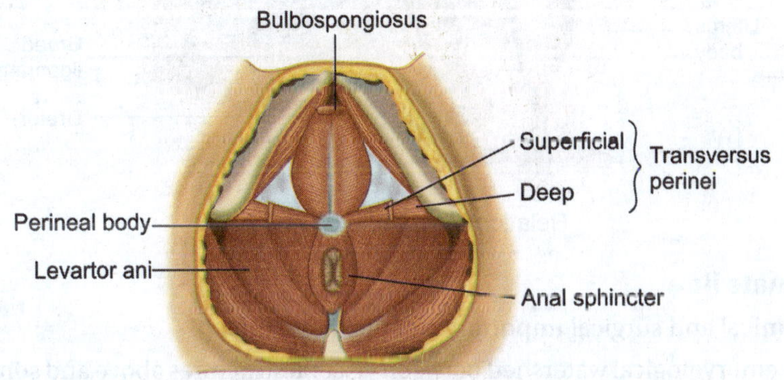

Perineal body

Q. Per-rectal examination

Ans.

- In males—posterior surface of prostate, seminal vesicles, vas deferens
- In females—cervix, perineal body ovaries (sometimes).

Q. Forward angulation between cervix and vagina is angle of anteversion angulation between body and cervix is angle of anteflexion (diagram only).

Ans.

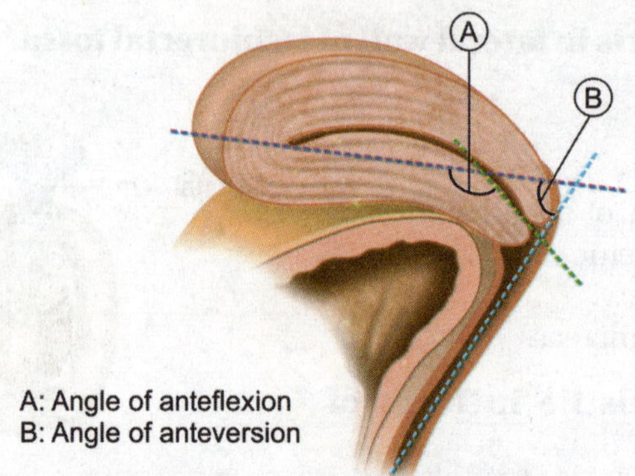

Position of uterus

Q. Uterine artery initially runs medially towards cervix then crosses ureter above lateral fornix of vagina and lies 2 cm lateral to cervix (diagram only).

Ans.

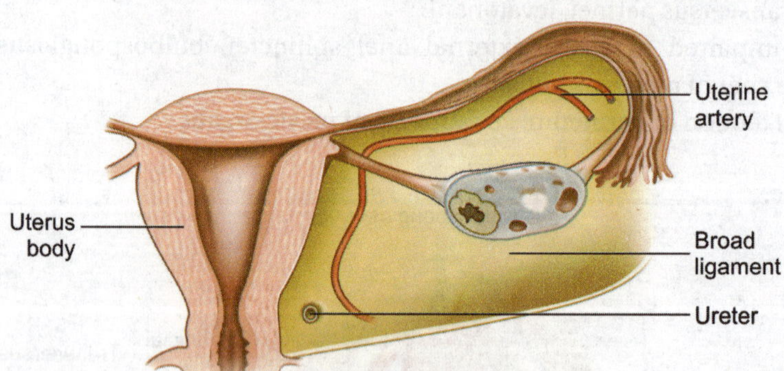

Relation of ureter to uterine artery

Q. Pectinate line

Ans. Anatomical and surgical importance of pectinate line:

- It is an embryological watershed between visceral structures above and somatic structures
- Mucosa above has autonomic nerve supply thus insensitive to pain while skin below is supplied by inferior rectal branch sensitive to pain and other stimuli
- Venous drainage above is to portal circulation, while below is to systemic venous circulation
- Lymphatic drainage above the pectinate line goes to iliac group of lymph nodes and below to inguinal group
- Internal hemorrhoids develop above the dentate line.

Q. Branches of internal iliac artery

Ans.

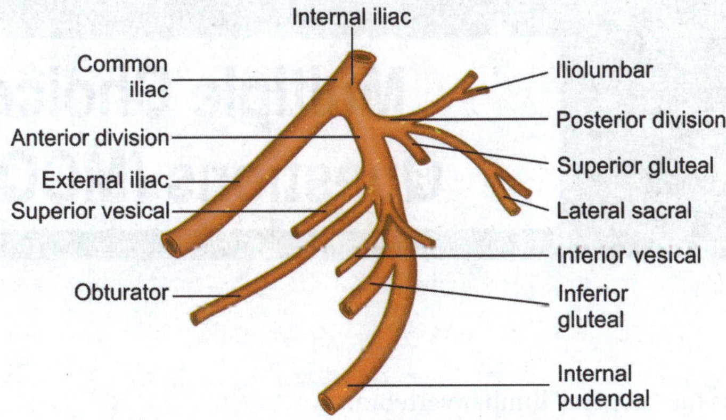

Branches of internal iliac artery

Anterior Division

- Superior vesical
- Obturator
- Middle rectal
- Inferior vesical/vaginal
- Inferior gluteal
- Internal pudendal.

Posterior Division

- Iliolumbar
- Lateral sacral
- Superior gluteal.

Multiple Choice Questions (MCQs)

1. Following is the 'atypical' lumbar vertebra:
   a. L1
   b. L5
   c. L3
   d. L4

   Answer: b

2. Following events occur at L1 except ______________
   a. Superior duodenal flexure
   b. Celiac plexus
   c. Upper part of the hilus of right kidney
   d. Upper part of the hilus of left kidney

   Answer: d

3. Superficial inguinal ring is an opening in ______________ muscle aponeurosis.
   a. External oblique
   b. Internal oblique
   c. Transversus abdominis
   d. All of the above

   Answer: a

4. Deep inguinal ring is an opening in ______________ fascia.
   a. Fascia iliaca
   b. Cremasteric fascia
   c. Fascia transversalis
   d. None of the above

   Answer: c

5. All of the following are posterior abdominal muscles except ______________
   a. Psoas major
   b. Quadratus lumborum
   c. Transversus abdominis
   d. Iliacus

   Answer: c

6. Following muscles get inserted into the perineal body except ______________
   a. Puborectalis
   b. Pubovaginalis
   c. Transversus perinei
   d. Levator ani

   Answer: a

7. Following muscles form the pelvic floor except _____________
   a. Pubococcygeus
   b. Iliococcygeus
   c. Deep transversus perinei
   d. Coccygeus

   Answer: c

8. Urogenital diaphragm consists of following muscles _____________
   a. Sphincter urethrae
   b. Deep transversus perinei
   c. Both a and b
   d. None of above

   Answer: c

9. Perineal membrane is _____________
   a. Superior fascia of urogenital diaphragm
   b. Inferior fascia of urogenital diaphragm
   c. Obturator fascia
   d. Pelvic fascia

   Answer: b

10. The root of mesentery crosses _____________ part of duodenum.
    a. First
    b. Second
    c. Third
    d. Fourth

    Answer: c

11. One of the following is not the boundary of Hesselbach's triangle _____________
    a. Linea alba
    b. Rectus muscle
    c. Inferior epigastric artery
    d. Inguinal ligament

    Answer: a

12. Following structure divides the Hesselbach's triangle:
    a. Obliterated umbilical vein
    b. Obliterated umbilical artery
    c. Ligamentum teres
    d. Inferior epigastric artery

    Answer: b

13. Point out the incorrect statement about the boundaries of Calot's triangle _____________
    a. Right: Cystic duct
    b. Left: Common hepatic duct
    c. Right: Common hepatic duct
    d. Above: Liver

    Answer: c

14. Following structure is present in front of paraduodenal fossa _____________
    a. Inferior mesenteric vein
    b. Inferior mesenteric artery
    c. Superior mesenteric artery
    d. Superior mesenteric vein

    Answer: a

15. The superior mesenteric artery arises at _____________ level.
    a. L1
    b. L2
    c. L3
    d. L4

    Answer: a

16. Following are the main branches of celiac artery except _____________
    a. Left gastric
    b. Common hepatic
    c. Right gastric
    d. Splenic

    Answer: c

17. Following structures form the stomach bed _____________
    a. Right crus of diaphragm
    b. Left crus of diaphragm
    c. Transverse mesocolon
    d. Spleen

    Answer: a

18. The nerves posterior to the cecum are all except _____________
    a. Right genitofemoral
    b. Left genitofemoral
    c. Right femoral
    d. Right lateral cutaneous nerve of thigh

    Answer: b

19. Celiac artery lies at _____________ level.
    a. L1
    b. L2
    c. Between L1 and L2
    d. Between T12 and L1

    Answer: d

20. All of the following are the main branches of celiac trunk except _____________
    a. Common hepatic artery
    b. Right gastric artery
    c. Splenic artery
    d. Left gastric artery

    Answer: b

21. While doing resection of the small intestine, the surgeon can differentiate between jejunal and ileal segment depending on following criteria mainly _____________
    a. Length of intestine
    b. Diameter of intestine
    c. Vascular arcades
    d. All of the above

    Answer: c

22. Following are the branches of inferior mesenteric artery except _____________
    a. Right colic
    b. Left colic
    c. Sigmoidal
    d. Superior rectal

    Answer: a

23. While operating, the surgeon has ligated both the mesenteric arteries what maintains the blood supply to the colon in the operating time _____________
    a. Superior mesenteric vein
    b. Inferior mesenteric vein
    c. Vasa recta
    d. Superior rectal artery

    Answer: c

24. A 60-year-old male, had a lump in epigastrium, it turned out to be carcinoma stomach. Following lymphatic areas need to be scanned except _____________
    a. Hepatic
    b. Gastric
    c. Subpyloric
    d. Diaphragmatic

    Answer: d

25. A surgeon was operating a case of cancer rectum, following areas need to be excised except ___________
    a. Pelvic colon
    b. Anal skin
    c. Ischiorectal fossa
    d. Mesentery

    Answer: d

26. Following structures are attached to the inguinal ligament except ___________
    a. External oblique
    b. Fascia lata
    c. Internal oblique
    d. Cremaster

    Answer: a

27. Direct inguinal hernia is ___________ to inferior mesenteric artery.
    a. Posterior
    b. Lateral
    c. Medial
    d. Anterior

    Answer: c

28. Indirect inguinal hernia is ___________ to inferior mesenteric artery.
    a. Lateral
    b. Medial
    c. Anterior
    d. Posterior

    Answer: a

29. Following statements of spermatic cord are true except ___________
    a. External spermatic fascia is derived from internal oblique
    b. Internal spermatic fascia is derived from transversalis fascia
    c. Cremasteric fascia derived from cremasteric muscle
    d. External spermatic fascia is derived from external oblique

    Answer: a

30. All are features of large intestine except ___________
    a. Appendices epiploicae present
    b. Teniae coli absent
    c. Sacculations present
    d. Peyer's patch absent

    Answer: b

31. The anatomical landmark for pudendal nerve block is ___________
    a. Ischial tuberosity
    b. Pubic tubercle
    c. Ischial spine
    d. Rectum

    Answer: c

32. The structure forming stomach bed ___________
    a. Posterior wall of lesser sac
    b. Liver
    c. Anterior wall of lesser sac
    d. Left suprarenal gland

    Answer: c

33. The surgeon while doing appendicectomy has to be careful of all nerves except ___________
    a. Right genitofemoral nerve
    b. Left genitofemoral nerve
    c. Right femoral nerve
    d. Lateral cutaneous nerve of thigh

    Answer: b

34. Following nerves are posterior to kidney except _______________
    a. Iliohypogastric nerve
    b. Ilioinguinal nerve
    c. Subcostal nerve
    d. Genitofemoral nerve

    Answer: d

35. Mother of a 12-year-old child complained of a lump (swelling) in left hypochondriac region. What organ is likely to be enlarged _______________
    a. Liver
    b. Spleen
    c. Stomach
    d. Kidney

    Answer: b

36. Which vessels lie in front of third part of duodenum?
    a. Inferior mesenteric
    b. Superior mesenteric
    c. Splenic
    d. Celiac

    Answer: b

37. Vas deferens begins from _______________ border of testis.
    a. Anterior
    b. Medial
    c. Lateral
    d. Posterior

    Answer: d

38. The prostate gland surrounds _______________ of urethra.
    a. Initial 1 cm
    b. Distal 3 cm
    c. Initial 3 cm
    d. Distal 3 cm

    Answer: c

39. Following are the sites of portosystemic anastomosis except _______________
    a. Upper end of esophagus
    b. Lower end of esophagus
    c. Lower end of rectum
    d. Bare area of liver

    Answer: a

SECTION - IV

THORAX

Key Questions

Q. How many thoracic vertebrae are there?

Ans. There are 12 thoracic vertebrae.

Q. How many ribs are there?

Ans. There are 12 pairs of ribs (the number may increase or decrease with the development of cervical/lumbar rib).

Q. How are the ribs classified?

Ans. Ribs are classified according to its attachment:

1. True ribs or vertebrosternal ribs—1–7 ribs are true ribs.
2. Vertebrochondral ribs—cartilage of one rib is attached to next higher cartilage 8th, 9th and 10th ribs.
3. Floating ribs—free ends of 11th and 12th cartilage are floating.

Q. Which are the atypical ribs?

Ans. The 1st, 2nd, 10th, 11th, 12th are atypical ribs.

Q. Which of the ribs are typical ribs?

Ans. The 3rd to 9th ribs are the typical ribs.

Q. What are the features of typical ribs?

Ans. The features of typical ribs are:

1. Each typical rib has anterior end, posterior end and shaft.
2. Anterior end is costal end, oval and concave.
3. Posterior end has head, neck and tubercle.
4. Shaft is flattened, convex upwards, inner surface is smooth and marked by a ridge.
5. There is costal groove between the ridge and inferior border.
6. Upper border is thick and has outer and inner lips.

Q. How do you identify first rib?

Ans. First rib is identified by the presence of following features:

- It is short, broad and acutely curved
- Shaft is not twisted
- It is flattened from above downwards.

Q. Draw a diagram to show the superior relations of first rib.

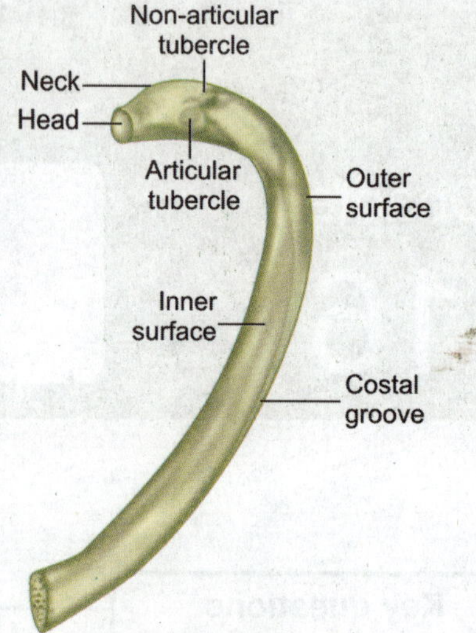

Parts of typical rib

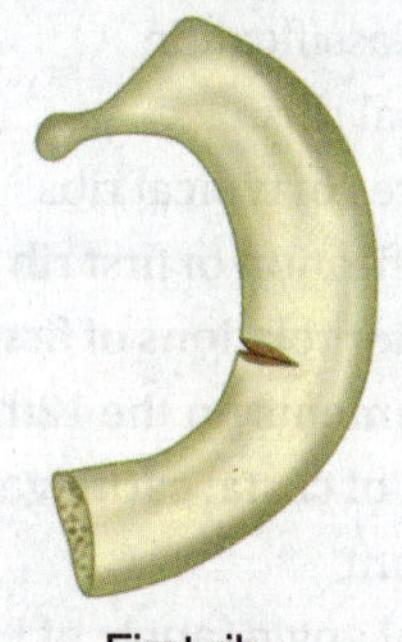

First rib

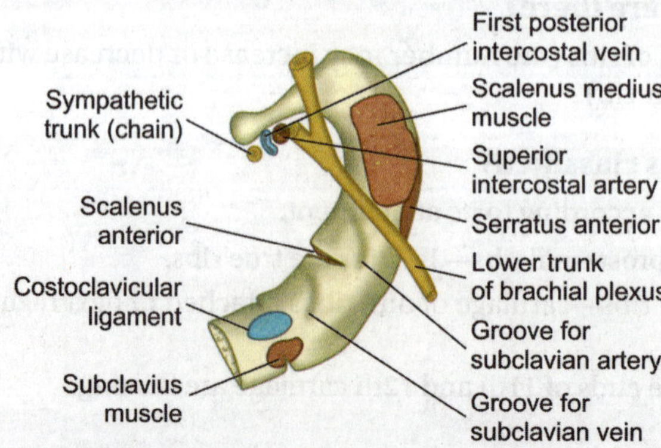

Q. **What are the attachments on the 12th rib (diagram only)?**

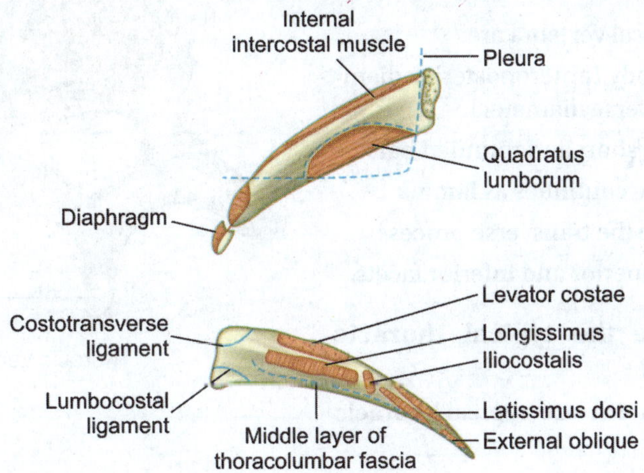

Q. **What is the 'type' of costal cartilage?**

Ans. The 'type' of costal cartilage is hyaline cartilage.

Q. **What is the meaning of sternum?**

Ans. The meaning of sternum is 'chest'.

Q. **What are the events occurring at the sternal angle (angle of Louis)?**

Ans. Following events occur at the sternal angle:

1. Second costal cartilage and rib lies at this level.
2. Superior and inferior mediastinum are demarcated.
3. Ascending aorta ends.
4. Arch of aorta begins.
5. Arch of aorta ends.
6. Descending aorta begins.
7. Trachea divides into two principal bronchi.
8. Azygos vein arches over root of right lung.
9. Pulmonary trunk divides.
10. Thoracic duct crosses from right to left side.
11. Base of heart lies at this level.
12. Cardiac plexus is located at this level.

Q. **What is the meaning of xiphoid?**

Ans. Xiphoid means 'sword like'.

Q. What are the parts of typical vertebra?

Ans. Parts of typical vertebra are:

- Rounded body (anteroposterior diameter = transverse diameter)
- Pedicles are short and rounded bars
- Each pedicle continues as lamina
- Laterally are the transverse process
- There are superior and inferior facets.

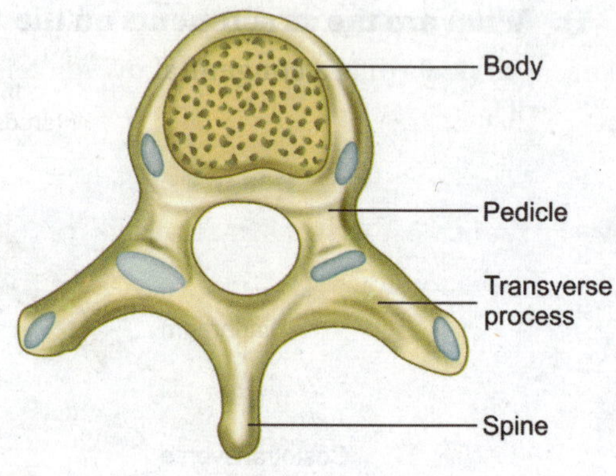

Thoracic vertebra

Q. Which are the typical thoracic vertebrae?

Ans. The 2nd to 8th are typical thoracic vertebrae.

Q. How do you identify thoracic vertebrae?

Ans. Thoracic vertebrae are identified by following features:

- Rounded, heart-shaped body (anteroposterior diameter = transverse diameter)
- Presence of costal facets on lateral aspect of the body.

Q. Morphologically, how is the transverse process of thoracic vertebra formed?

Ans. Morphologically, the transverse process has two elements:

- Costal element
- Transverse element.

Costal element forms the rib in thoracic region.

Q. What type of joint is manubriosternal joint?

Ans. The type of manubriosternal joint is a secondary cartilaginous joint.

Q. What is the structure of intervertebral disk?

Ans. The structure of intervertebral disk is:

- These are fibrocartilaginous in nature
- They have two parts:
  - Central—nucleus pulposus
  - Peripheral—annulus fibrosus.

Q. What is the 'type' of intervertebral joint?

Ans. The 'type' of intervertebral joint is a secondary cartilaginous joint.

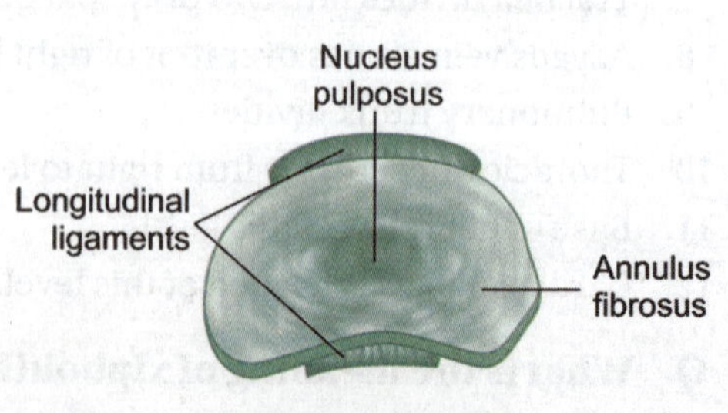

Intervertebral disk

Q. What is cervical rib?

Ans. Cervical rib is a congenital overdevelopment (bony or fibrous) of the costal process of C7.

Q. What are the types of cervical rib?

Ans. There are four types of cervical rib as shown below.

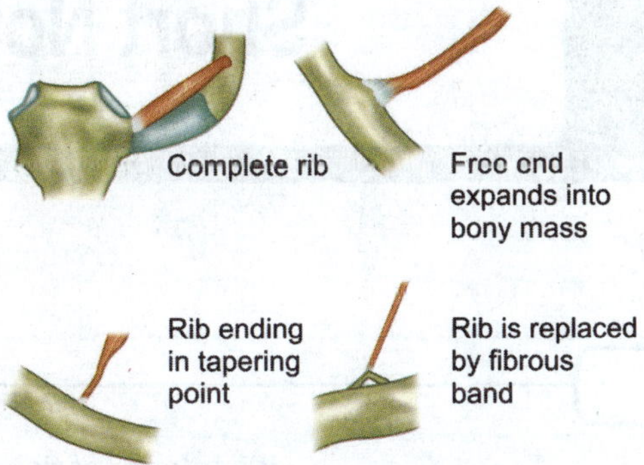

Types of cervical rib

Q. What is Adson's test?

Ans. On turning the head to the side, where cervical rib is present or on deep breathing, the radial pulse disappears.

Q. How do you treat cervical rib?

Ans. In 70% of cases, even if cervical rib is not recognized, symptoms are relieved by dividing scalenus anterior.

Note: One must excise cervical rib along with its periosteum.

Q. How many splanchnic nerves are there?

Ans. There are three splanchnic nerves:
- Greater splanchnic nerve
- Lesser splanchnic nerve
- Least splanchnic nerve.

Q. What are splanchnic nerves?

Ans. Splanchnic nerves are medial branches of thoracic ganglia 7, 8, 9, 10, 11 and 12, relaying into celiac ganglion. They are preganglionic branches of medial branches of thoracic ganglia, as given below:
- Greater—5, 6, 7, 8, 9
- Lesser—10, 11
- Least—12.

Short Notes

Key short notes

- Intercostal space
- Internal thoracic artery
- Pleural recesses
- Mediastinal suture of lungs
- Hilum of right and left lungs
- Pericardium
- Fibrous skeleton of heart
- Cardiac silhouette
- Sinuses of pericardium
- Interior of right atrium
- Surface projection of the heart valves
- Veins of the heart
- Cardiac plexus
- Constrictions of esophagus
- Sibson's fascia
- Triangle of Koch
- Atrioventricular valves
- Semilunar valves

Q. INTERCOSTAL SPACE

The gap between the ribs is the intercostal space. It is filled by intercostal muscles, intercostal nerves, vessels and lymphatics.

Intercostal Muscles

Intercostal muscles are:

- External intercostal muscle
- Internal intercostal muscle
- Transversus thoracis.

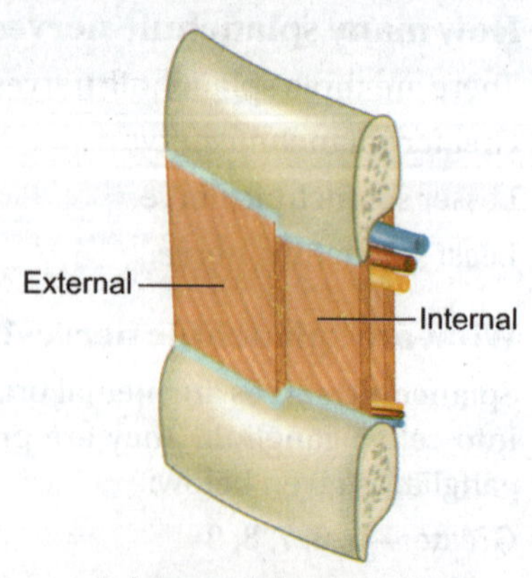

Intercostal space

External Intercostal Muscle

External intercostal muscle extends from the tubercle of the rib to the costochondral junction. Between the costochondral junction and sternum, it is replaced by membrane.

Internal Intercostal Muscle

Internal intercostal muscle extends from angle of rib to the lateral border of sternum. Fibers run downwards, backwards and laterally.

Transversus Thoracis

Transversus thoracis is made up of three parts:

1. Subcostalis—posterior part of lower intercostal space.
2. Intercostales intimi—confined to middle two fourth.
3. Sternocostalis—anterior parts of upper intercostal spaces.

Intercostal Nerves

Intercostal nerves are anterior rami of thoracic spinal nerve. Upper three intercostal nerves also supply the upper limb and lower five also supply the abdominal wall:

- T4, T5 and T6 are typical thoracic nerves
- T12 is also known as subcostal nerve
- They supply the muscles in the intercostal space, parietal pleura and periosteum of the rib.

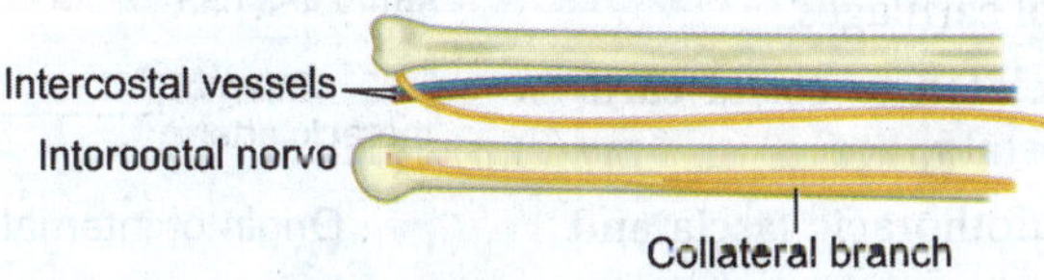

Intercostal nerve and vessels

Intercostal Arteries

- Each space has one posterior and two anterior intercostal arteries
- Posterior intercostal arteries are 11 in number
- First and second arteries arise from superior intercostal artery, which is a branch of costocervical trunk
- Descending aorta gives 3–11 branches
- Artery is accompanied by intercostal vein
- Anterior intercostal arteries arises from internal thoracic artery.

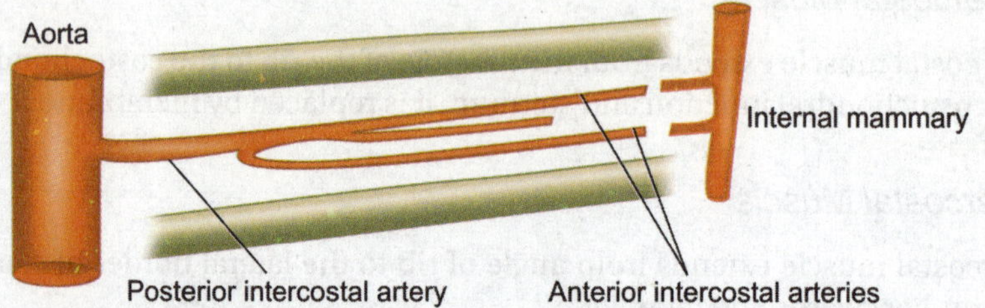

Intercostal artery

There are two anterior intercostal veins in upper nine spaces:

- Upper six drain into internal thoracic vein and remaining veins drain into musculophrenic vein
- Posterior vein drains into vertebral venous plexus.

Q. INTERNAL THORACIC ARTERY

Origin

Internal thoracic artery originates from the first part of subclavian artery opposite to the thyrocervical trunk.

Cause and Relations

- Internal thoracic artery runs vertically downward behind the sternal end of clavicle and costal cartilages
- It is anteriorly related to costal cartilages and intercostal space
- Posteriorly to endothoracic fascia and pleura.

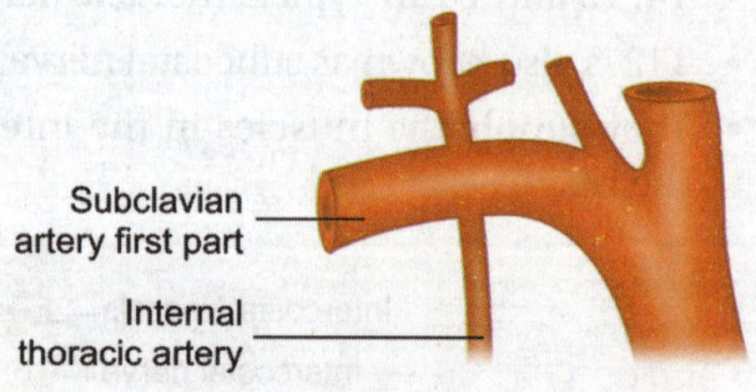

Origin of internal thoracic artery

Termination

- Internal thoracic artery terminates in sixth intercostal space into musculophrenic and superior epigastric
- The artery is accompanied by two venae comitantes.

Branches

- Pericardiophrenic
- Mediastinal arteries
- Anterior intercostal arteries

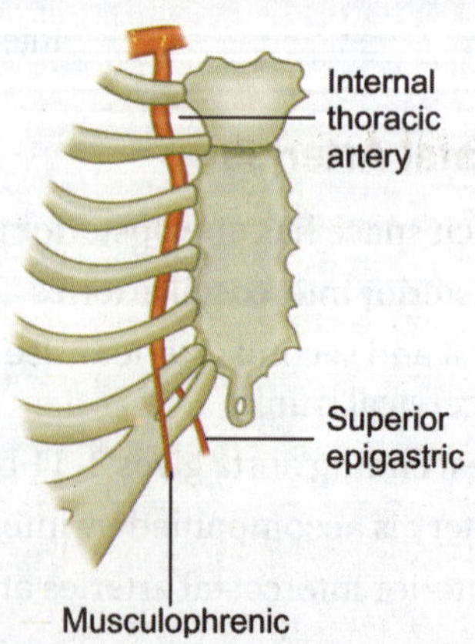

Internal mammary artery

- Superior epigastric
- Musculophrenic.

Applied Anatomy

Internal thoracic artery is used in bypass heart surgeries.

Q. PLEURAL RECESSES

Pleural recesses are the extra or reserve spaces of parietal pleura, which gives space for the lungs to expand.

Costodiaphragmatic Recess

- Costodiaphragmatic recess is a space located inferiorly between costal and diaphragmatic pleura
- It is across 8th to 10th ribs along the midaxillary line
- Approximately 5 cm in length.

Costomediastinal Recess

- Costomediastinal recess lies anteriorly behind the sternum and costal cartilages
- This recess is filled by lung, even during quiet breathing.

Applied Anatomy

These recesses get filled in cases of pleural effusion.

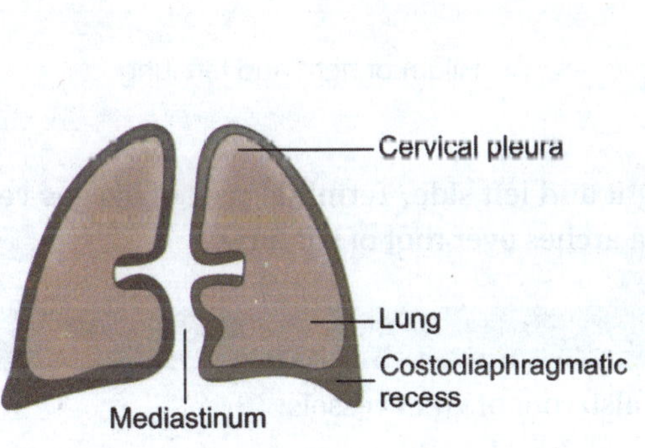

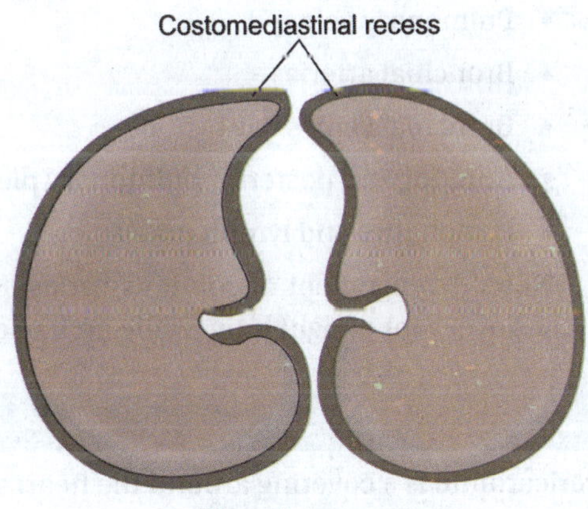

Pleural recesses

Q. MEDIASTINAL SURFACE OF LUNGS (DIAGRAM ONLY)

A. Right lung.

B. Left lung.

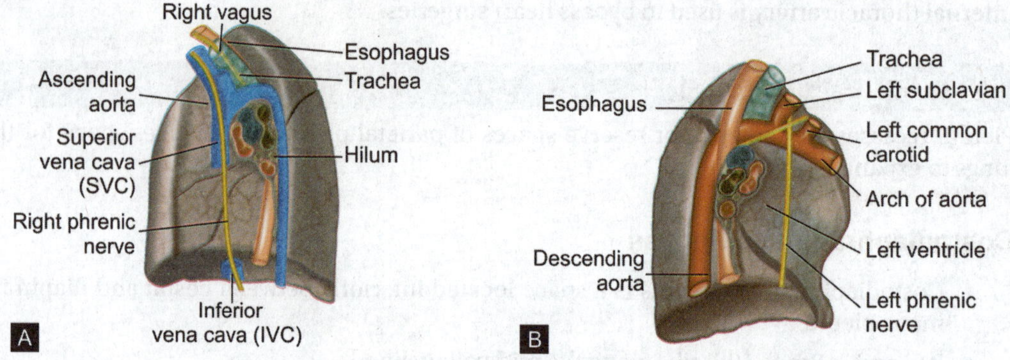

Mediastinal surfaces of lungs

Q. HILUM OF RIGHT AND LEFT LUNG

Hilum is a pedicle of lung, which connects the medial surface of lungs to the mediastinum. It lies against T5, T6, T7 vertebrae.

Contents

- Principal bronchus
- Pulmonary artery
- Pulmonary veins
- Bronchial arteries
- Bronchial veins
- Anterior and posterior pulmonary plexus
- Lymphatics and lymph nodes.

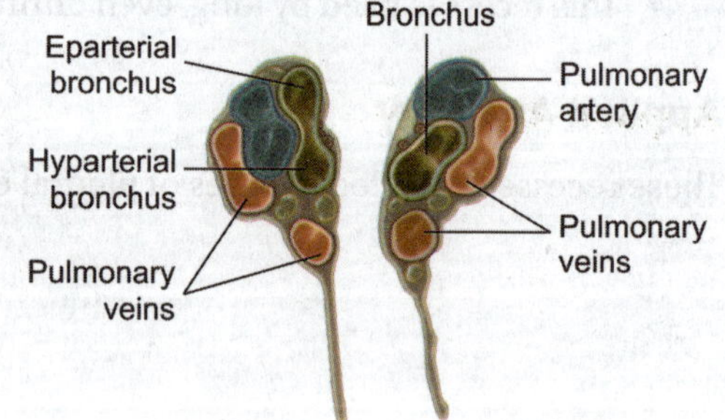

Hilum of right and left lung

Note: Arrangement of contents varies in right and left side. Terminal part of azygos vein arches over root of right lung, while arch of aorta arches over root of left lung.

Q. PERICARDIUM

Pericardium is a covering around the heart and also root of great vessels:

- It is located in the middle mediastinum
- It consists of fibrous and serous pericardium.

Fibrous Pericardium

- Fibrous pericardium is a fibrous tissue around the heart, it blends with the parietal layer of serous pericardium
- It is connected to sternum with sterno-pericardial ligaments
- Below, it fuses with central tendon of diaphragm and above with root of aorta.

Serous Pericardium

- Serous pericardium is thin, double-layered serous membrane
- Outer layer is parietal layer, which fuses with fibrous pericardium and inner layer is visceral layer.

Applied Anatomy

Pericardial effusion occurs in between the parietal and visceral layer of serous pericardium.

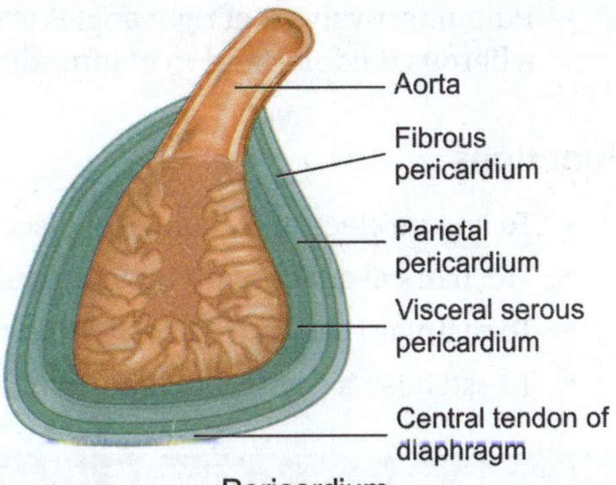

Pericardium

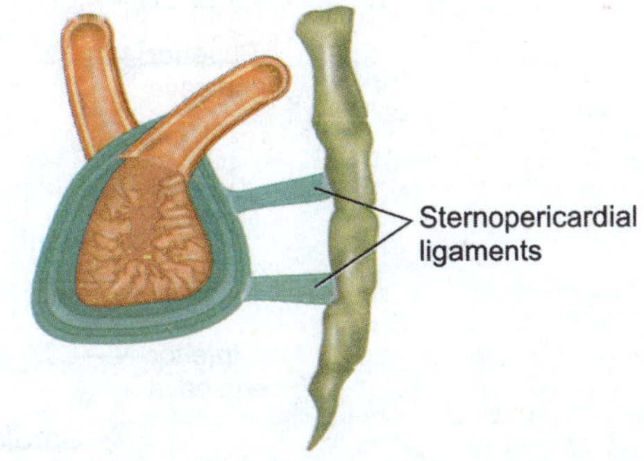

Q. FIBROUS SKELETON OF HEART

Fibrous skeleton of heart lies roughly at the same plane of coronary sulcus, i.e. ventricular base and atrioventricular inflow and arterial outflow. It is a complex framework of dense collagen with intervening membrane. It is a deformable continuum.

Components

- Mitral annulus
- Tricuspid annulus
- Aortic valve annulus
- Pulmonary valve annulus.

Directions

- Mitral and tricuspid valve annuli are in one plane, i.e. coplanar
- Aortic valve annulus faces upwards, forwards and anterosuperior, right of mitral orifice

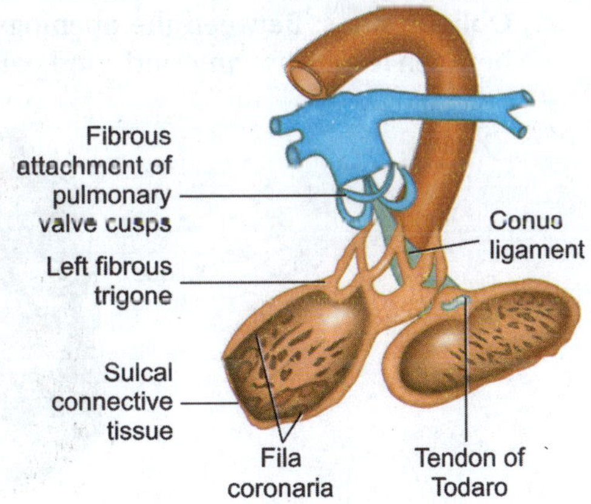

Fibrous skeleton of heart

- Pulmonary valve is at right angles to aortic valve. The only connection is conus ligament, a fibrous tendon (tendon of infundibulum).

Functions

- To ensure electrophysiological discontinuity except through conducting system
- Mechanical attachment for ventricular myocardium
- To maintain cardiac portion within the pericardium
- To establish a stable, but deformable base for valvular attachments.

Q. CARDIAC SILHOUETTE (DIAGRAM ONLY)

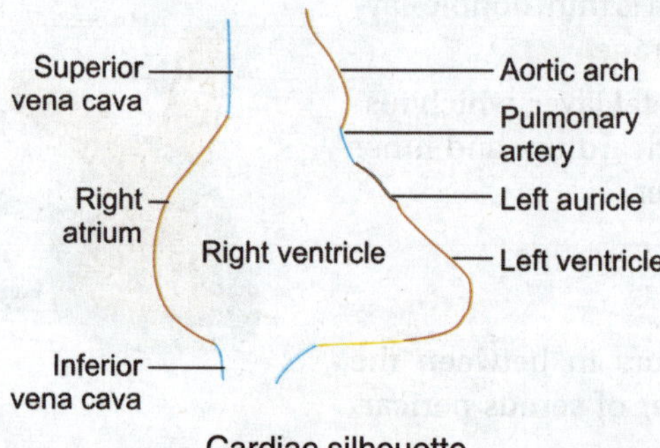

Cardiac silhouette

Q. SINUSES OF PERICARDIUM

There are two sinuses of pericardium, namely transverse and oblique:

1. **Transverse sinus:** Passage between arterial end and venous end is the transverse sinus. It lies between ascending aorta and pulmonary trunk in front and superior vena cava (SVC) and left atrium behind.

2. **Oblique sinus:** Between the openings of pulmonary veins is the oblique sinus. It lies between left atrium anteriorly and parietal pericardium posteriorly.

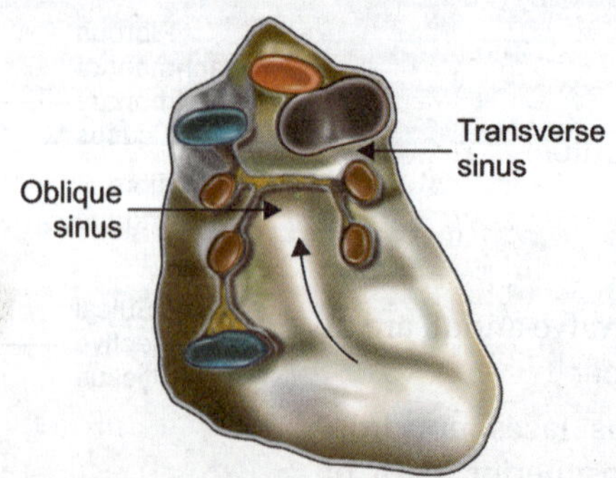

Sinuses of pericardium

Q. INTERIOR OF RIGHT ATRIUM

Interior of right atrium has three parts:

- Smooth posterior part
- Rough anterior part
- Septal wall.

Smooth Posterior Part Features

1. Right atrium is the receiving chamber of the heart. Thus, it has openings of superior and inferior vena cava, coronary sinus and openings of venae cordis minimi.
2. Just below the opening of SVC, there is a projection—intervenous tubercle of Lower.

Rough Anterior Part Features

There is vertical crest diagonally below sulcus terminalis known as crista terminalis from where horizontal muscular ridges run on the internal surface of right atrium known as musculi pectinati.

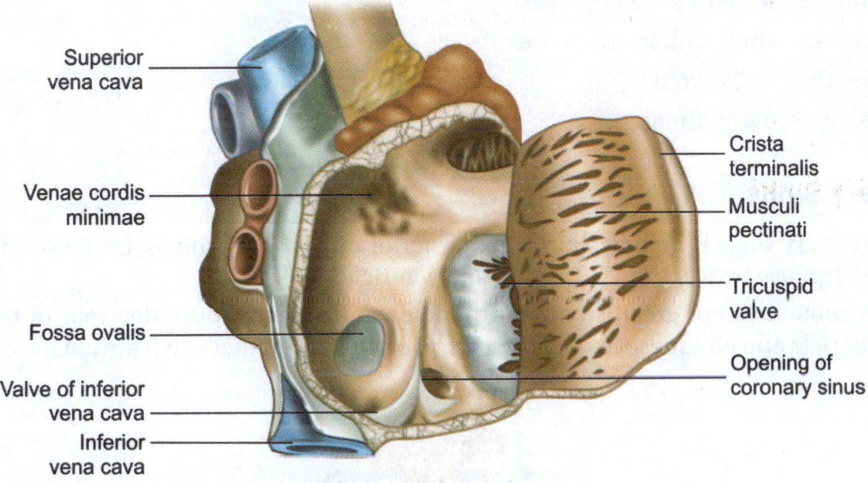

Interior of right atrium

Septal Wall Features

- Fossa ovalis—remnant of septum primum
- Annulus ovalis—remnant of septum secundum
- Remains of foramen ovale.

All of the above are embryonic remnants.

Q. SURFACE PROJECTION OF HEART VALVES (DIAGRAM ONLY)

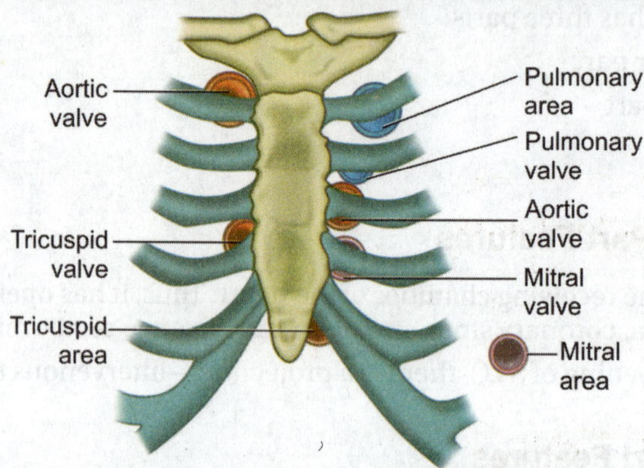

Surface projection of heart valves

Q. VEINS OF THE HEART

Veins draining the heart are grouped as:

- Coronary sinus with its tributaries
- Anterior cardiac vein
- Venae cordis minimae.

Coronary Sinus

1. Coronary sinus is oblong sinus lying posterior on coronary sulcus, i.e. atrioventricular (AV) groove between left (L) atrium and ventricle.

2. Its tributaries are great, small and middle cardiac veins, posterior vein of the (left) ventricle and oblique vein of left atrium. All veins except that of left atrium have valves:

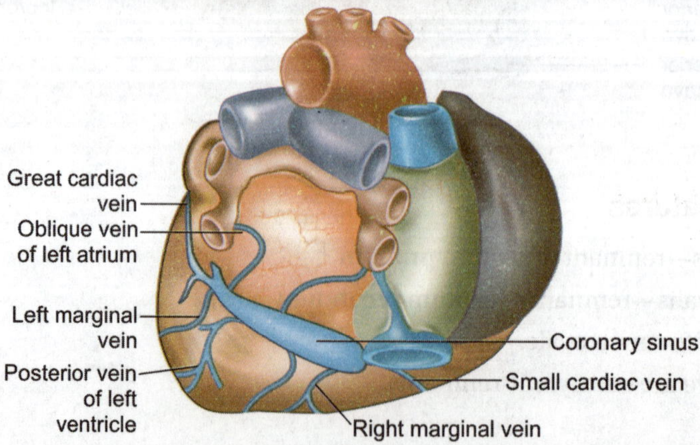

Venous drainage of heart

- Great cardiac vein begins at the cardiac apex and ascends in anterior interventricular sulcus; and it receives blood from left atrium and both ventricles
- Small cardiac vein lies in posterior atrioventricular sulcus, receives blood from posterior part of right atrium and ventricle
- Middle cardiac vein is present in posterior interventricular sulcus
- Oblique vein of left atrium is continuous above with the ligament of left vena cava.

Anterior Cardiac Vein

- Anterior cardiac vein drains the anterior part of right atrium. Right marginal vein courses around the inferior margin draining adjacent parts of left ventricle.

Venae Cordis Minimae

- Venae cordis minimae directly open into right atrium.

Q. CARDIAC PLEXUS

Nerve plexus around the heart is made up of sympathetic and parasympathetic nerve. Depending upon its location, it is classified into superficial and deep plexus.

Superficial Cardiac Plexus

- Superficial cardiac plexus is located in front of arch of aorta
- It is formed by superior cervical cardiac branch of left sympathetic chain and inferior cervical cardiac branch of left vagus.

Deep Cardiac Plexus

- Deep cardiac plexus is located over bifurcation of trachea
- It is formed by cardiac nerves of cervical and thoracic ganglia.

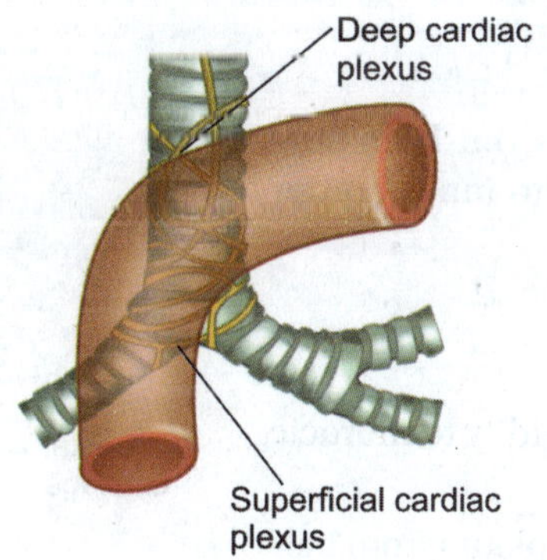

Cardiac plexus

Q. CONSTRICTIONS OF ESOPHAGUS (DIAGRAM ONLY)

Esophagus has four constrictions as shown in the figure.

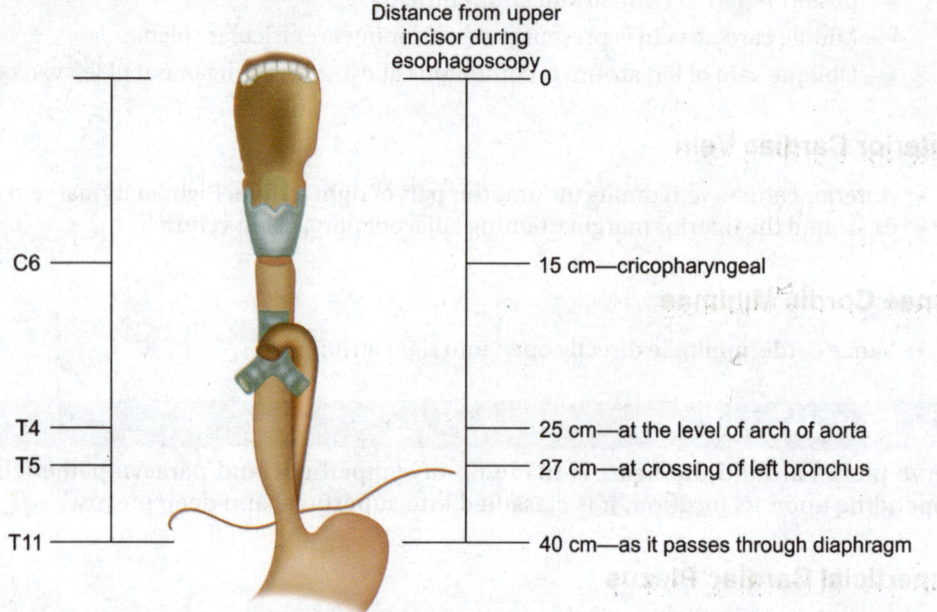

Constrictions of esophagus

Q. SIBSON'S FASCIA

Sibson's fascia is suprapleural membrane. The cervical pleura rises to the neck of first rib, around 4 cm above the level of sternal end of first costal cartilage.

It is protected externally by scalene muscles and lined internally by dense fascia, i.e. the suprapleural membrane.

Attachments

- Sibson's fascia spreads out from seventh cervical vertebra to inner border of first rib.

Functions

- Sibson's fascia gives rigidity to thoracic inlet
- It prevents the cervical pleura from ballooning in and out during respiration.

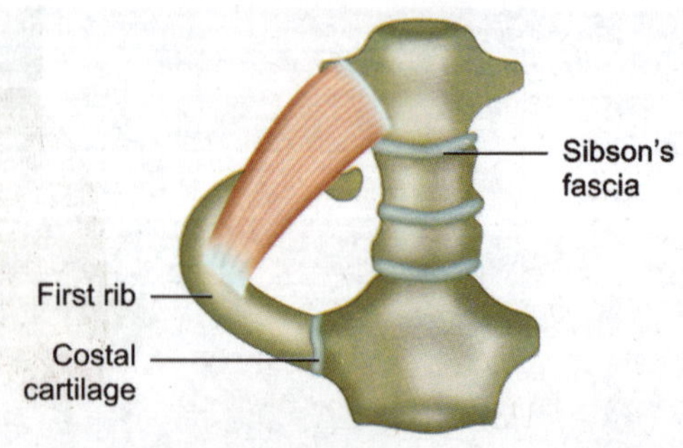

Sibson's fascia

Q. TRIANGLE OF KOCH

Triangle of Koch is located in the interior of right atrium.

Boundaries

Boundaries exist between the base of tricuspid valve's septal leaflet, anteromedial margin of coronary sinus orifice and collagenous subendocardial tendon of Todaro.

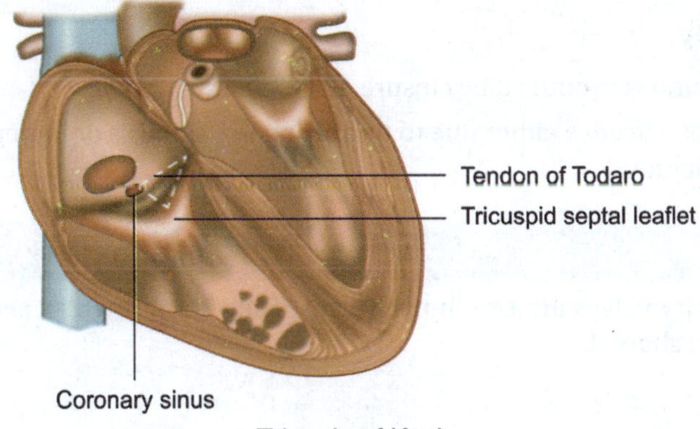

Triangle of Koch

Importance

Triangle of Koch is the site of AV node and associated juxta nodal bundles.

Q. ATRIOVENTRICULAR VALVES (AV)

There is one pair of atrioventricular (AV) valve, i.e. right and left. Right AV valve is tricuspid valve and has three cusps. Left AV valve is bicuspid valve and has two cusps. It is also known as mitral valve.

Structure

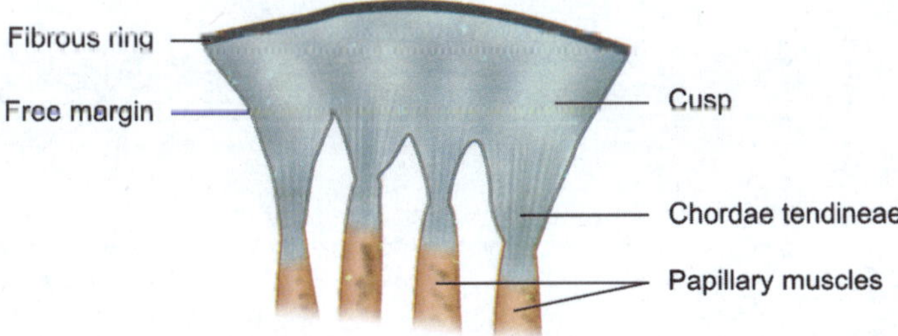

Structure of atrioventricular (AV) valve

Parts

- Fibrous ring
- Cusp has smooth atrial surface and rough ventricular surface
- Free and attached margins
- Free margin gives attachment to chordae tendineae, which in turn is attached to papillary muscle.

Applied Anatomy

- First heart sound is produced by closure of AV valves
- Valves may get defective either due to narrowing, i.e. stenosis or imperfect closure giving rise to regurgitation.

Q. SEMILUNAR VALVES

Aortic and pulmonary valves are semilunar valves. They are termed as semilunar, since the cusps are half-moon shaped.

Structure

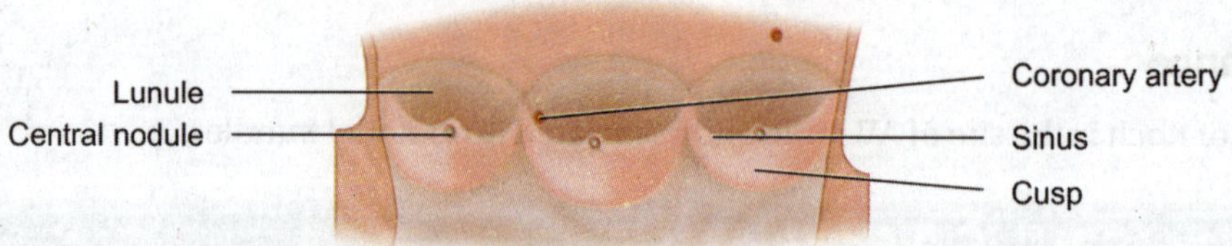

Structure of semilunar valve

- Fibrous ring is absent
- Cusps are directly attached to vessel wall
- Free margin has a nodule in the center and flimsy side margin is known as lunule.

Long Questions

Key long questions

- Diaphragm
- Azygos vein
- Bronchopulmonary segments
- Mediastinum
- Thoracic duct
- Arterial supply to heart

Q. DISCUSS DIAPHRAGM UNDER FOLLOWING HEADINGS: PARTS, APERTURES, NERVE SUPPLY, DEVELOPMENT AND APPLIED ANATOMY.

Diaphragm is a musculotendinous partition, which separates thorax from abdomen.

Parts

- Central tendon
- Costal part
- Sternal part
- Lumbar part (lumbocostal arches and crura).

Apertures

Large Apertures

1. Aortic opening:
   - Lies at T12
   - Aorta, thoracic duct and azygos vein pass through this opening.

2. Esophageal opening:
   - Lies at T10
   - Esophagus, vagus nerves and esophageal branches of (L = left) gastric artery and vein pass through it.

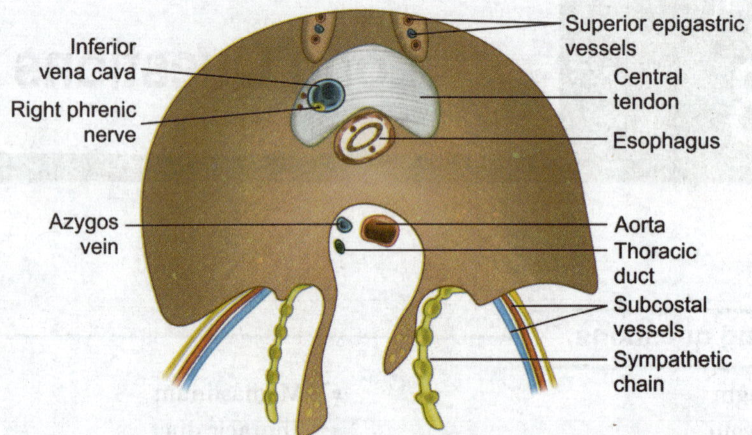

Structures piercing the diaphragm

3. Vena caval opening:
   - Lies at T8
   - It transmits inferior vena cava and branches of left phrenic nerve.

Mnemonics	Structures
"Voice	T8: Inferior **V**ena cava
Of	T10: **O**esophagus (esophagus)
America"	T12: **A**orta

Small Aperture

1. Superior epigastric vessels pass between xiphoid process and 7th costal cartilage. This gap is known as Larry's space or foramen of Morgagni.
2. Musculophrenic vessels pierce the diaphragm at 8th or 9th costal cartilage.
3. Greater and lesser splanchnic nerves piercing the crura.
4. Openings for small veins are common in central tendon.

Structures closely related to diaphragm are:
- Sympathetic chain
- Subcostal vessels.

Nerve Supply

- Motor fibers travel in phrenic nerves
- Lower 6 or 7 intercostal nerves distribute sensory fibers to peripheral diaphragm.

Development

Following components contribute to the development:

- Septum transversum
- Pleuroperitoneal membranes
- Ventral and dorsal mesenteries of esophagus
- Mesoderm of body wall including mesoderm around dorsal aorta.

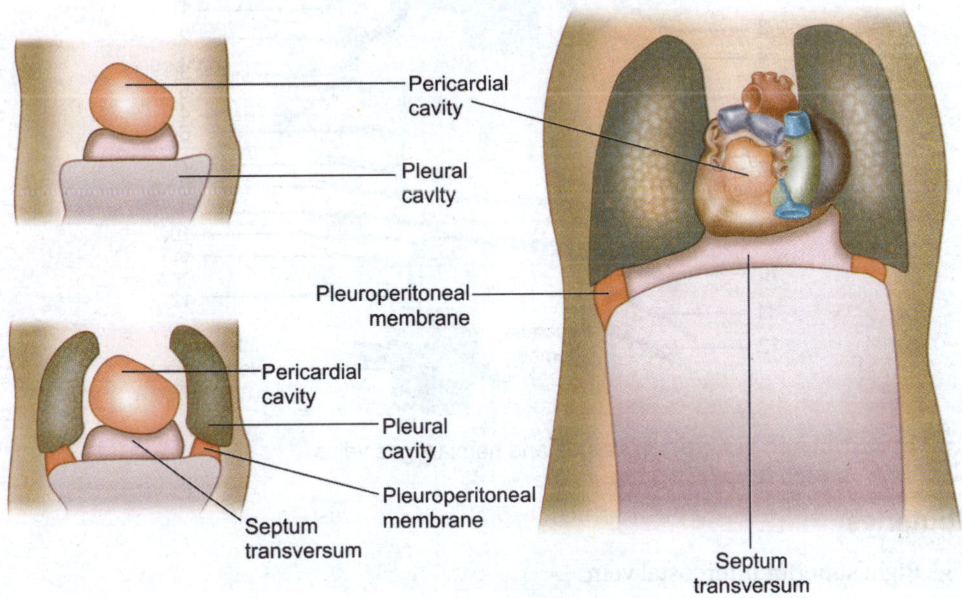

Development of diaphragm

Applied Anatomy

When abdominal organs, usually stomach herniate into thorax, i.e. diaphragmatic hernia.

Q. DESCRIBE AZYGOS VEIN IN DETAIL.

Azygos vein is large venous channel draining the thoracic wall and upper lumbar region. It is an important channel connecting superior vena cava to inferior vena cava.

Formation

Azygos vein is formed by union of right ascending lumbar vein with right subcostal vein.

Course

Azygos vein ascends upwards and enters the thorax by passing through aortic opening. Then it ascends upwards up to sternal angle, where it arches over the root of right lung. It terminates by joining the superior vena cava.

Relations

- Anteriorly—esophagus
- Posteriorly—lower eight thoracic vertebra, right posterior intercostal arteries
- To the left—thoracic duct, aorta.

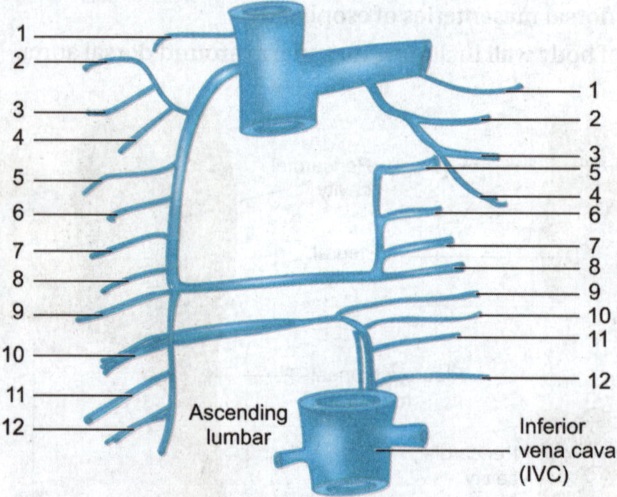

Azygos and hemiazygos veins

Tributaries

- Right superior intercostal vein
- Intercostal veins 4–11
- Hemiazygos vein
- Accessory hemiazygos vein
- Esophageal, mediastinal and pericardial veins.

Hemiazygos Vein

Hemiazygos vein is the mirror image of the lower part of azygos vein.

Formation: Hemiazygos vein is formed by the union of left subcostal vein and left ascending lumbar vein.

Course: Hemiazygos vein pierces the left crus of diaphragm and ascends on the left side of the vertebral column.

Termination: At T9, it turns to the right and joins azygos vein.

Tributaries: As follows:

- Left ascending lumbar vein
- Left subcostal vein
- Left posterior intercostal veins 9–11.

Accessory Hemiazygos Vein

Accessory hemiazygos vein is the mirror image of upper part of azygos vein.

Course: Accessory hemiazygos vein begins at the medial end of 4th and 5th intercostal space and descends on the left side of vertebral column.

Termination: Accessory hemiazygos vein turns to the right at T8.

Tributaries: Intercostal veins 5–8.

Applied Anatomy

In superior vena caval thrombosis, the blood from the upper limb and upper half of the body gets bypassed to inferior vena cava through azygos vein.

Q. DISCUSS BRONCHOPULMONARY SEGMENTS.

Each lung has 10 bronchopulmonary segments.

Peculiarities

- Each segment is an independent unit not merging with adjacent structures
- Each segment has its own bronchus, artery and vein
- Each segment has a constant disposition and relationship to the overlying ribs.

Right Lung

Upper Lobe

The upper lobe has three segments:

 1—Apical.

 2—Anterior.

 3—Posterior.

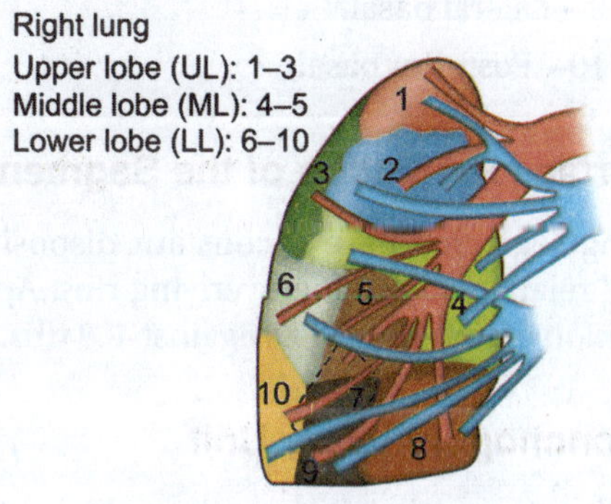

Bronchopulmonary segments of right lung

Middle Lobe

The middle lobe has two segments:

 4—Medial.

 5—Lateral.

Lower Lobe

The lower lobe has five segments:

 6—Apical.

 7—Medial basal.

8—Anterior basal.

9—Lateral basal.

10—Posterior basal.

Left Lung

Upper Lobe

The upper lobe has five segments:

1—Apical.

2—Anterior.

3—Posterior.

4—Superior lingular.

5—Inferior lingular.

Lower Lobe

The lower lobe has five segments:

6—Apical.

7—Medial basal.

8—Anterior basal.

9—Lateral basal.

10—Posterior basal.

Surface Projection of the Segments

Lung segments have a constant disposition and relationship to the overlying ribs. Apical portion of lower lobe lies against 4–8 ribs.

Bronchopulmonary Unit

Each segment has its own bronchial artery, terminal bronchiole and intersegmental vein.

Applied Anatomy

- Segmental architecture is by and large constant
- Infective or neoplastic processes are located to one or more segments
- Limited resection can be possible, i.e. lobectomy can be done in case of neoplasia restricted to one lobe.

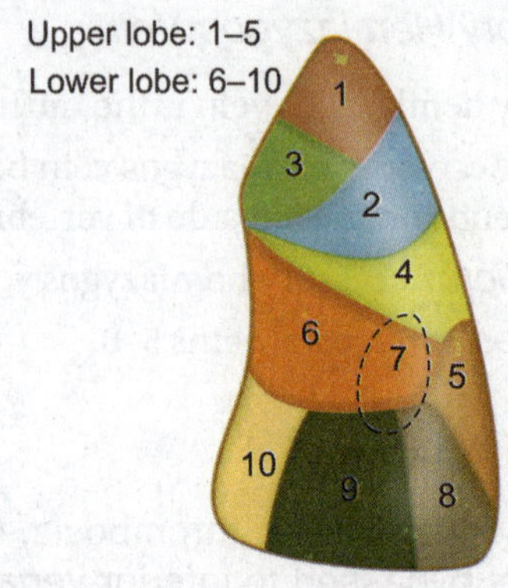

Bronchopulmonary segments of left lung

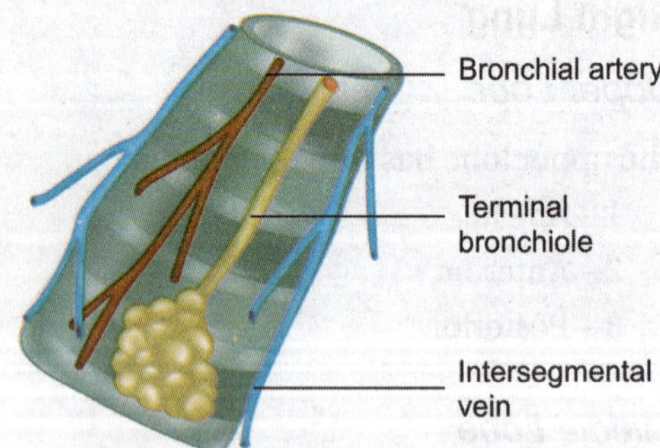

Contents of bronchopulmonary segment

Q. DISCUSS MEDIASTINUM.

Mediastinum is the median septum between the two lungs.

Boundaries

- Anteriorly: Sternum
- Posteriorly: Vertebral column
- Superiorly: Thoracic inlet
- Inferiorly: Diaphragm
- On each side: Pleura.

Subdivisions

An imaginary line passing through sternal angle divides the mediastinum into superior and inferior mediastinum.

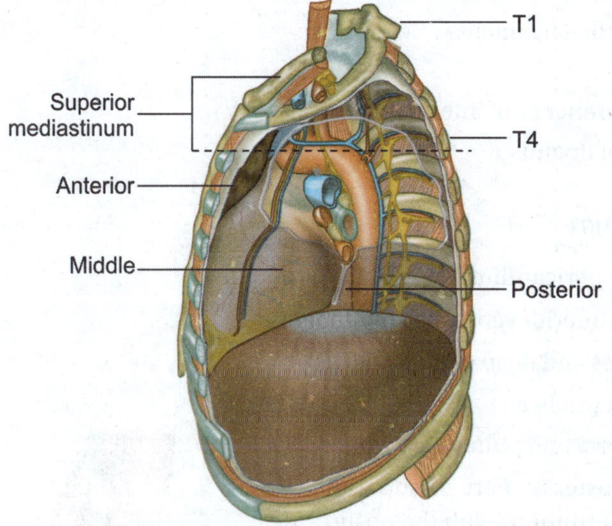

Mediastinum

Inferior mediastinum is subdivided into:

- Anterior
- Middle
- Posterior.

Contents of Superior Mediastinum

- Trachea
- Brachiocephalic vein
- Arch of aorta with its branches

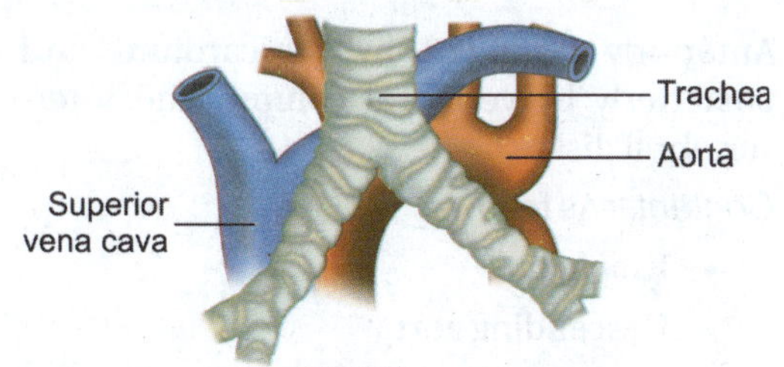

Contents of superior mediastinum

- Thymus
- Thoracic duct
- Lymph nodes.

Special Features

- Prevertebral fascia extends up to T4. Thus infection in the neck can track down to superior mediastinum
- Pretracheal fascia also extends up to superior mediastinum, where it blends with arch of aorta.

Anterior Mediastinum

Anterior mediastinum is a space between sternum in front and pericardium behind. It is continuous with the pretracheal space of the neck above.

Contents: As follows:

- Sternopericardial ligaments
- Lymph nodes
- Mediastinal branches of internal thoracic artery
- Lowest part of thymus.

Middle Mediastinum

- Heart with its pericardium
- Superior and inferior vena caval openings
- Phrenic nerves and deep cardiac plexus
- Bifurcation of trachea
- Ascending aorta and pulmonary trunk.

Structures in posterior part of superior mediastinum are continuous with the posterior mediastinum.

Posterior Mediastinum

Anteriorly bounded by pericardium and posteriorly by vertebral column and intervertebral disk.

Contents: As follows:

- Esophagus
- Descending aorta

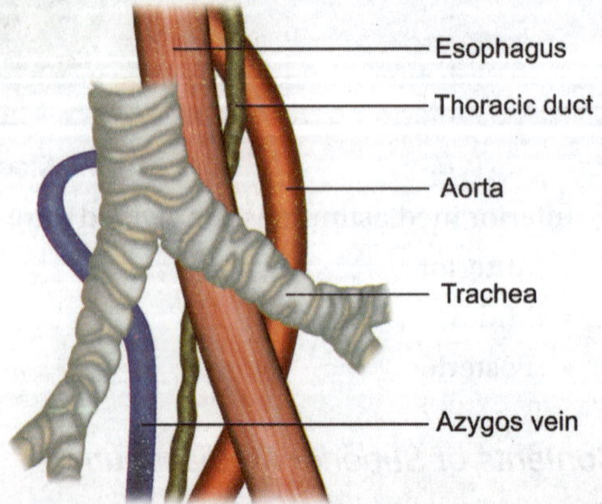

Contents of posterior mediastinum

- Azygos vein, hemiazygos vein, accessory hemiazygos vein
- Right and left vagi
- Splanchnic nerves
- Lymph nodes.

Applied Anatomy

Neck infections can track down from retropharyngeal space to posterior part of superior mediastinum.

Q. DISCUSS THORACIC DUCT.

Thoracic duct is the largest lymphatic channel extending from upper abdomen to the root of the neck. It is about 18 inches long.

Course

1. It begins from upper end of cisterna chyli and enters the thorax through the aortic opening.
2. Ascends through posterior mediastinum and crosses at the level of sternal angle to end at the junction of left subclavian vein with left internal jugular vein.

Relations

In Abdomen

Thoracic duct lies between azygos vein to the right and aorta to the left all throughout its course.

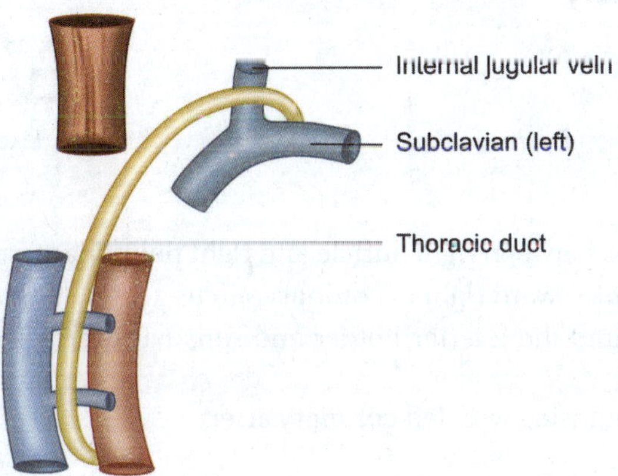

Thoracic duct course and termination

In Posterior Mediastinum

Anteriorly, it is related to esophagus and posteriorly related to vertebral column.

In Superior Mediastinum

To the right is esophagus and behind is vertebral column.

In the Neck

Thoracic duct forms an arch of 3–4 cm above the clavicle.

Tributaries

1. Receives lymph from both halves of the body below the diaphragm and left half above the diaphragm via left mediastinal trunk.
2. In thorax, it receives lymph vessels from posterior mediastinal nodes.
3. Efferent vessels from nodes in the neck forms left jugular trunk, those from the nodes in the axilla forms left subclavian trunk. These trunks drain into thoracic duct.

Applied Anatomy

While doing left side neck dissections, the surgeon should be cautious regarding thoracic duct, otherwise there could be lymphatic leak, which needs urgent exploration. On postoperative day one, presence of milky fluid in the drain suggests thoracic duct leak.

Q. DESCRIBE ARTERIAL SUPPLY TO HEART IN DETAIL.

Heart is supplied by two coronary arteries, which take origin from ascending aorta (coronary = crown like).

Right Coronary Artery

Origin

Anterior aortic sinus.

Like crown

Course

1. At its origin, it lies between right auricle and right pulmonary trunk.
2. It runs downwards toward right in coronary sulcus.
3. It then winds round the inferior border and runs backwards in the posterior coronary sulcus.
4. It ends by anastomosing with left coronary artery.

Branches

- Marginal
- Posterior interventricular
- Nodal
- Right atrial.

Areas Supplied

1. Right atrium.
2. Ventricles:
    a. Most of the right ventricle area except near anterior interventricular groove.

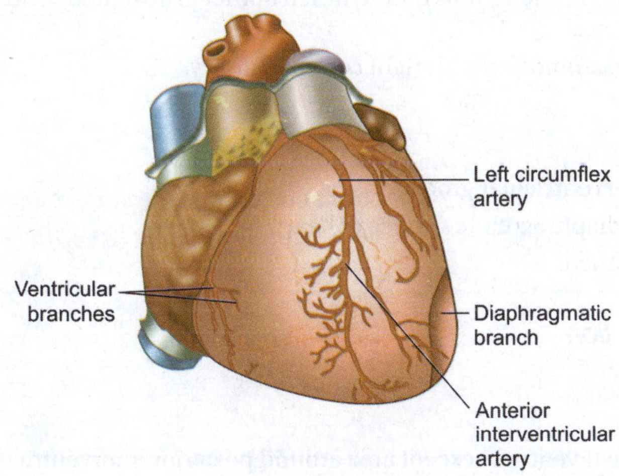

Anterior view

    b. Left ventricle near posterior interventricular groove.
    c. Posterior part of interventricular septum.
3. Most of the conducting system of heart.

Left Coronary Artery

Origin

Left posterior aortic sinus.

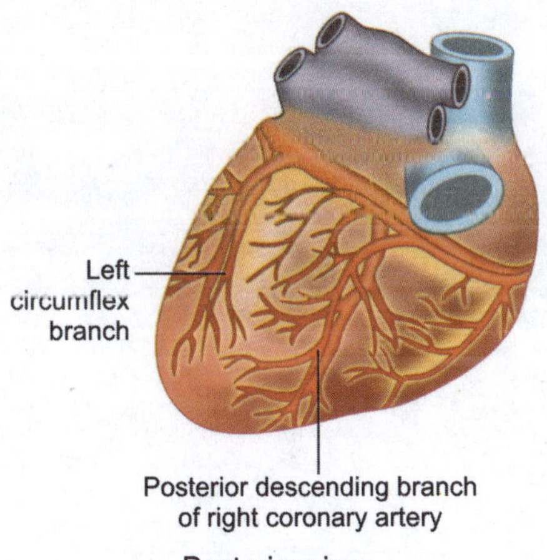

Posterior view

Course

1. At its origin, it lies between left auricle and left pulmonary trunk.
2. With a short course, it divides into anterior interventricular branch and left circumflex branch.
3. Left circumflex branch winds round the left border of heart and continues in left posterior coronary sulcus.
4. It ends by anastomosing with right coronary artery.

Branches

1. Anterior interventricular groove.
2. A branch to diaphragmatic surface of heart.
3. Left atrial branch.

Areas of Distribution

1. Left atrium.
2. Ventricles:
    a. Most of left ventricle except area around posterior interventricular groove.
    b. Small part of right ventricle adjoining anterior interventricular groove.
    c. Anterior part of interventricular septum.

Applied Anatomy

1. Left anterior descending artery is known as widow's artery as it commonly gets blocked.
2. To overcome a block in artery, a bypass surgery is undertaken.

Key Diagrams with MCQ Tips

Diagrams for

- Scalene tubercle
- Attachments of 12th rib
- Intercostal space
- Internal thoracic artery
- Hilum of right and left lung
- Mediastinal surfaces
- Cardiac silhouette
- Interior of right atrium
- Structures piercing the diaphragm
- Bronchopulmonary segments

Q. First rib

Ans.

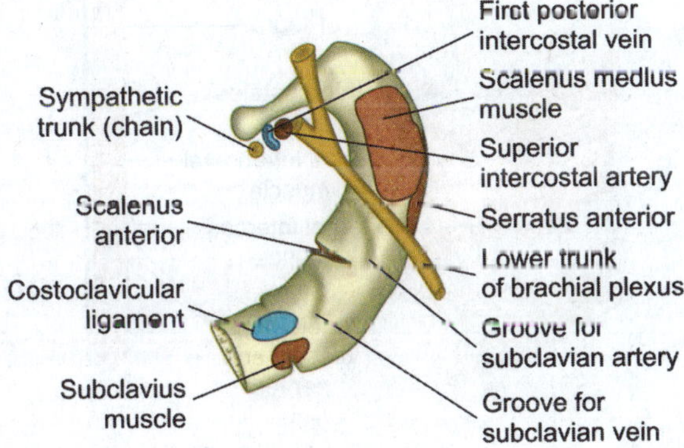

Scalene tubercle:

- Scalenus anterior muscle is attached
- Lower trunk of brachial plexus is related to first rib.

Q. Attachments of 12th rib

Ans. Please note that all the attachments can be asked in viva.

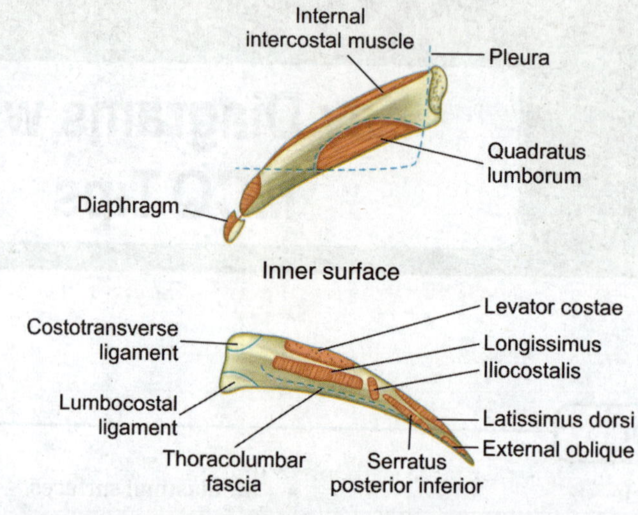

- Costal cartilage is hyaline cartilage.

Q. Intercostal space

Ans.

- There are 11 posterior intercostal arteries.

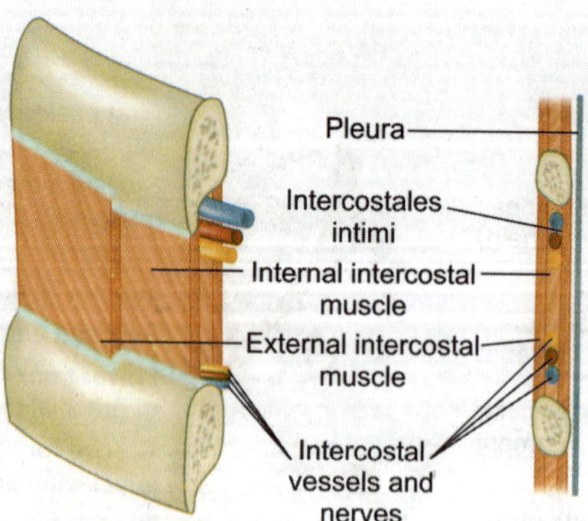

Q. Openings in diaphragm

Ans.	**Mnemonics**	**Structures**
	"Voice	T8: Inferior **V**ena cava
	Of	T10: **O**esophagus (esophagus)
	America"	T12: **A**orta

Q. Internal thoracic artery

Ans.

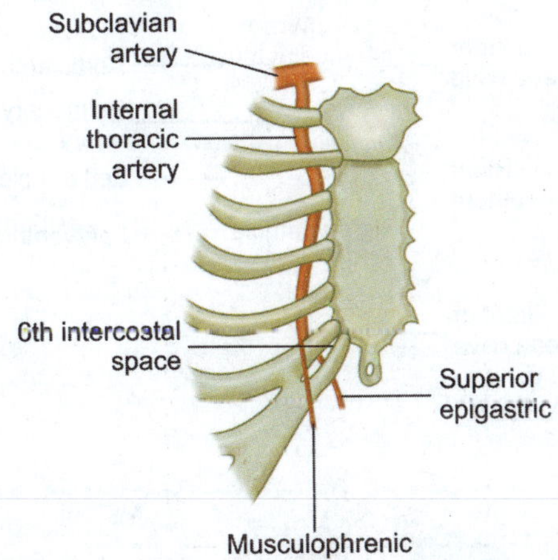

- Internal thoracic artery divides in sixth intercostal space
- Terminal divisions of internal thoracic artery are musculophrenic and epigastric.

Q. Hilum of right and left lung.

Ans.

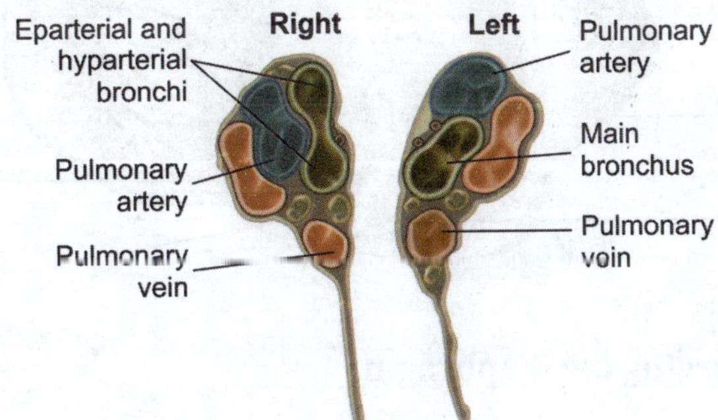

Q. Mediastinal surfaces of right and left lung.

Ans.

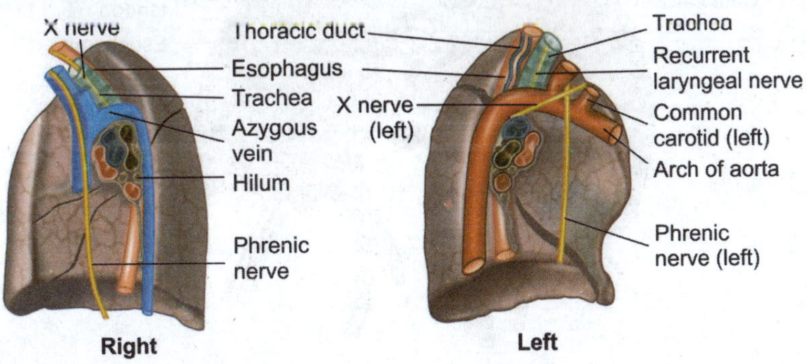

Q. Cardiac silhouette
Ans.

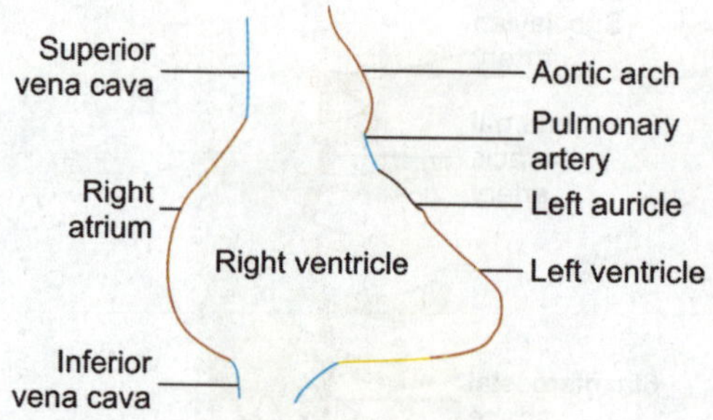

Q. Interior of right atrium
Ans.

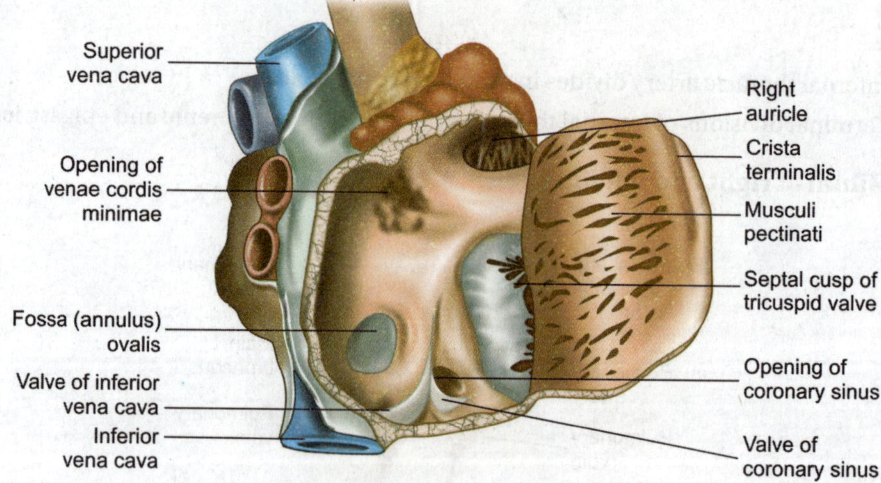

Q. Structures piercing the diaphragm.
Ans.

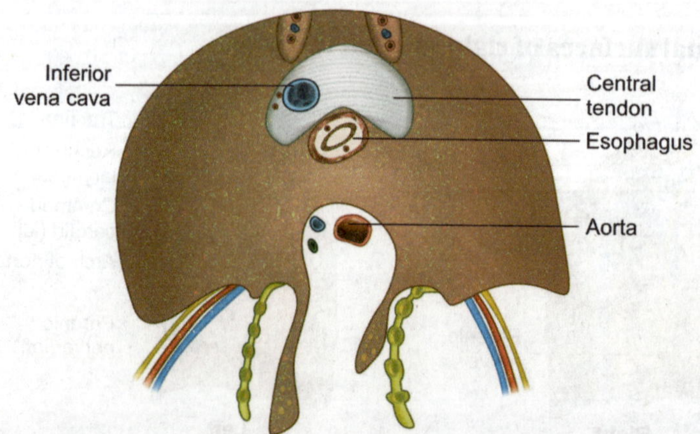

Q. Bronchopulmonary segments

Ans.

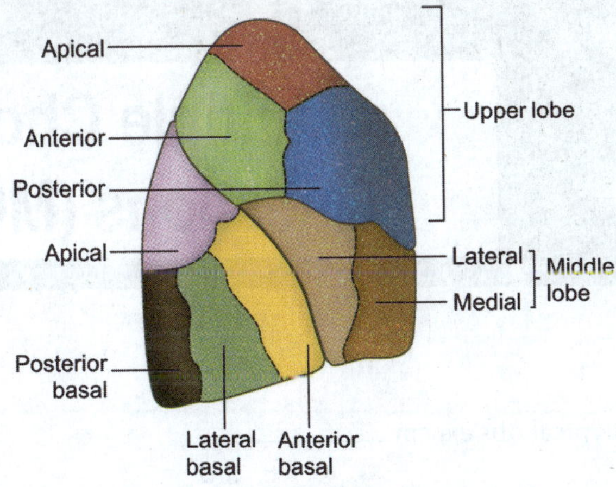

Right lung

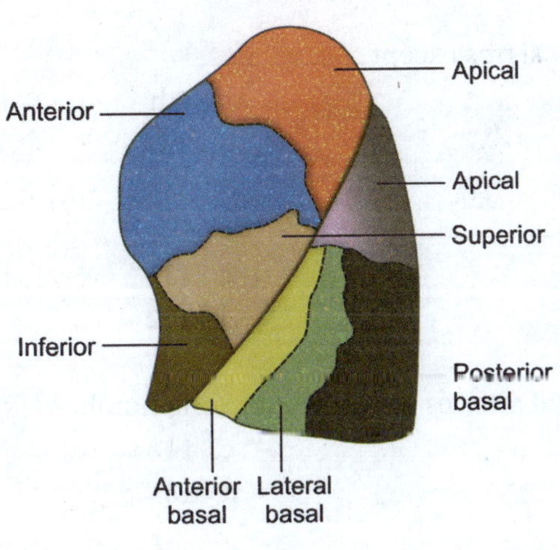

Left lung

Multiple Choice Questions (MCQs)

1. Following are atypical ribs except ____________
   a. 1st
   b. 2nd
   c. 3rd
   d. 12th

   Answer: c

2. Following are typical ribs except ____________
   a. 3rd
   b. 2nd
   c. 4th
   d. 7th

   Answer: b

3. Subcostal nerve is ____________
   a. T7
   b. T10
   c. T11
   d. T12

   Answer: d

4. Posterior intercostal arteries are ____________ in number.
   a. 10
   b. 12
   c. 11
   d. 13

   Answer: c

5. Internal mammary artery divides into terminal branches in the ____________ intercostal space.
   a. 5th
   b. 6th
   c. 4th
   d. 7th

   Answer: b

6. Hilum of lungs line against ____________ thoracic vertebrae.
   a. T3, T4, T5
   b. T4, T5, T6
   c. T5, T6, T7
   d. T6, T7, T8

   Answer: c

7. Left atrium is identified by the openings of ____________ veins.
   a. SVC
   b. IVC
   c. Pulmonary artery
   d. Pulmonary veins

Answer: d

8. Receiving chamber of the heart is ____________
   a. Left atrium
   b. Right atrium
   c. Right ventricle
   d. Left ventricle

Answer: b

9. Esophagogastric junction is at the level of ____________ vertebra.
   a. T8
   b. T9
   c. T10
   d. T11

Answer: d

10. Cricopharyngeal sphincter is ____________ from upper incisor.
    a. 15 cm
    b. 25 cm
    c. 27 cm
    d. 40 cm

Answer: a

11. Esophagus pierces the diaphragm ____________ from upper incisor.
    a. 15 cm
    b. 25 cm
    c. 27 cm
    d. 40 cm

Answer: d

12. Arch of aorta crosses the esophagus ____________ from upper incisor.
    a. 15 cm
    b. 25 cm
    c. 27 cm
    d. 40 cm

Answer: b

13. Left bronchus crosses the esophagus ____________ cm from the upper incisor.
    a. 15
    b. 25
    c. 27
    d. 40

Answer: c

14. Sibson's fascia is ____________
    a. Cervical fascia
    b. Investing layer
    c. Suprapleural membrane
    d. Pleura

Answer: c

15. The boundaries of triangle of Koch are all except ____________
    a. Posterolateral margin of coronary sinus orifice
    b. Anteromedial margin of coronary sinus orifice
    c. Tricuspid valve septal leaflet
    d. Tendon of Todaro

Answer: a

16. Aortic opening in the diaphragm is at the level of ___________ vertebra.
    a. T8
    c. T12
    b. T10
    d. L1

Answer: c

17. Esophageal opening is at the level of ___________ in diaphragm.
    a. T8
    c. T12
    b. T10
    d. L1

Answer: b

18. Inferior vena cava pierces the diaphragm at ___________ level.
    a. T8
    c. T12
    b. T10
    d. L1

Answer: a

19. Following structure passes through the Larry's space ___________
    a. Internal mammary vessels
    c. Inferior epigastric vessels
    b. Superior epigastric vessels
    d. Musculophrenic vessels

Answer: b

20. Azygos vein is formed by the union of ___________
    a. Intercostal vein with lumbar vein
    b. Renal vein with lumbar vein
    c. Ascending lumbar vein with right subcostal vein
    d. Ascending lumbar vein with left subcostal vein

Answer: c

21. Hemiazygos vein is formed by the union of ___________
    a. Right subcostal vein with left ascending lumbar vein
    b. Left subcostal vein with left ascending lumbar vein
    c. Left subcostal vein with right ascending lumbar vein
    d. Right subcostal vein with right ascending lumbar vein

Answer: b

22. Hemiazygos vein joins the azygos vein at ___________ level.
    a. T7
    c. T9
    b. T8
    d. T10

Answer: c

23. How many bronchopulmonary segments does each lung have?
    a. 8
    c. 10
    b. 9
    d. 11

Answer: c

24. Apical portion of lower lobe of lung lies against ___________ ribs.
    a. 3rd to 7th
    c. 7th to 11th
    b. 5th to 9th
    d. 4th to 8th

Answer: d

25. Prevertebral fascia extends up to ____________
    a. T1
    b. T2
    c. T3
    d. T4

    Answer: d

26. Thoracic duct enters the thorax through ____________ opening in the diaphragm.
    a. Aortic
    b. Vena caval
    c. Esophageal
    d. Foramen of Morgagni

    Answer: a

27. Thoracic duct is ____________ inches long.
    a. 15
    b. 18
    c. 20
    d. 25

    Answer: b

28. Thoracic duct lies in ____________ mediastinum in thorax.
    a. Anterior
    b. Posterior
    c. Superior
    d. Middle

    Answer: b

29. Right coronary artery takes origin from ____________
    a. Anterior aortic sinus
    b. Posterior aortic sinus
    c. Right (R) posterior aortic sinus
    d. Left (L) posterior aortic sinus

    Answer: a

30. Left coronary artery takes origin from ____________
    a. Anterior aortic sinus
    b. Posterior aortic sinus
    c. Right (R) Posterior aortic sinus
    d. Left (L) Posterior aortic sinus

    Answer: d

31. Widow's artery is ____________
    a. Right coronary artery
    b. Left anterior descending artery
    c. Left coronary artery
    d. Apical

    Answer: b

SECTION - V

HEAD AND NECK

Key Questions

Key questions

- Reid's baseline
- Frankfurt's plane
- Skull
- Vertex
- Bregma, lambda
- Parietal tuber, obelion
- Inion
- Nuchal line
- Superciliary arch
- Glabella
- Gonion
- Nasion, rhinion
- Antrum of Highmore
- Antral puncture
- Mental point
- Jugal point
- Zygomatic arch
- Articular tubercle
- Macewen's triangle
- Entomion
- Asterion
- Pterion
- Pterygopalatine fossa
- Sylvian point
- Vidian nerve
- Arnold's nerve (Alderman's nerve)
- Pharyngeal tubercle
- Pterygoid plate
- Nervous spinosus
- Gasserion ganglion
- Glossopharyngeal notch
- Frontal crest
- Cribriform plate
- Optic canal
- Superior orbital fissure
- Internal acoustic meatus
- Mandible
- Clavicle
- Cervical vertebra
- Skull
- Cephalic index
- Le Fort fractures
- Sella turcica
- Ethmoid bone

Contd...

Contd...

- FESS
- Maxilla
- Scalene triangle
- Joll's triangle
- Beahr's triangle
- Artery of epistaxis
- Goethe's ossicle

Q. What is Reid's baseline?

Ans. Reid's baseline is an imaginary horizontal line, joining the infraorbital margin to the center of external acoustic meatus (auricular point).

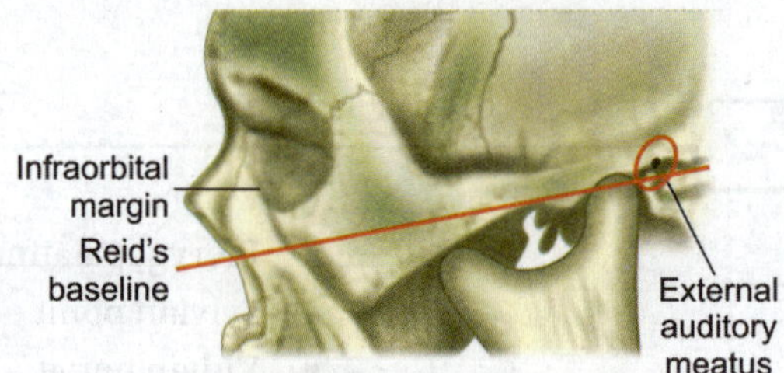

Reid's baseline

Q. What is Frankfurt plane?

Ans. Frankfurt plane is obtained by joining the infraorbital margin to the upper margin of external acoustic meatus.

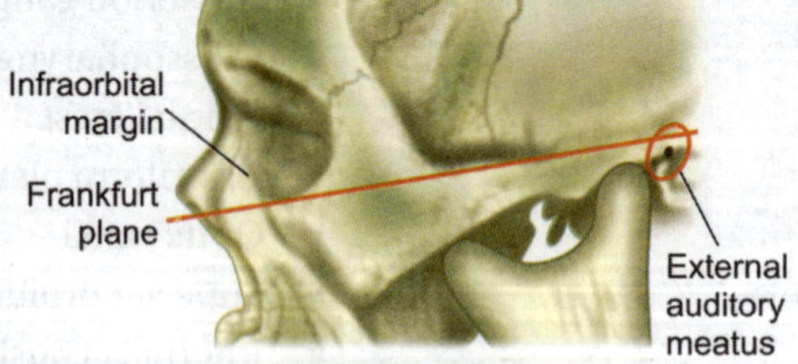

Frankfurt plane

Q. What do you understand by skull? Is cranium synonymous?

Ans. Skull is skeleton of head. Cranium is not synonymous to skull. Skull without mandible is known as cranium (skull = calvaria + facial skeleton with mandible).

Q. What is vertex?

Ans. Highest point on the sagittal suture is vertex.

Q. What is bregma? What is lambda?

Ans.

- Junction of coronal and sagittal suture is bregma
- Junction of lambdoid and sagittal suture is lambda.

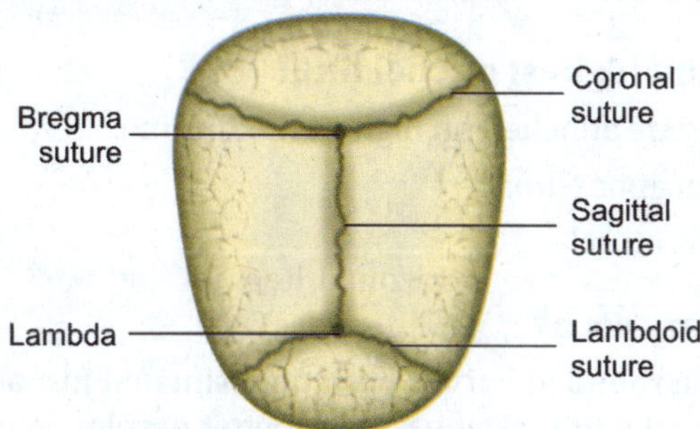

Q. What is parietal tuber? What is obelion?

Ans.

1. Parietal tuber is the area of maximum convexity of the parietal bone. This is the common site of fracture of skull bone.

2. Obelion is the point on sagittal suture between the two parietal foramina. Some believe that this is the site of pineal (third) eye.

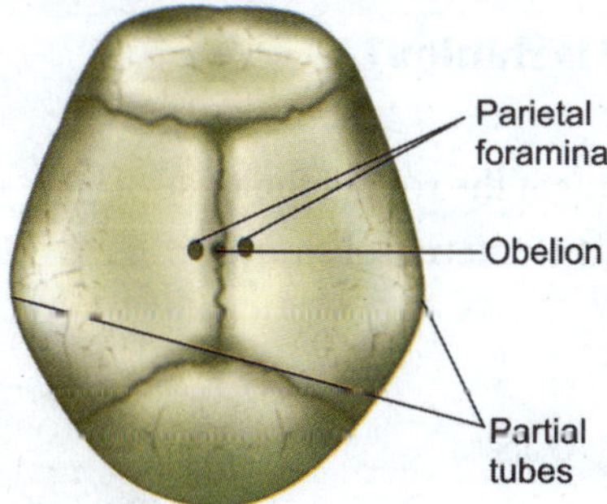

Q. What is attached to the temporal lines?

Ans. Epicranial aponeurosis and temporalis fascia is attached to the superior temporal line and temporalis muscle is attached to the inferior temporal line.

Q. What is inion?

Ans. The most prominent point on the external occipital protuberance is known as inion.

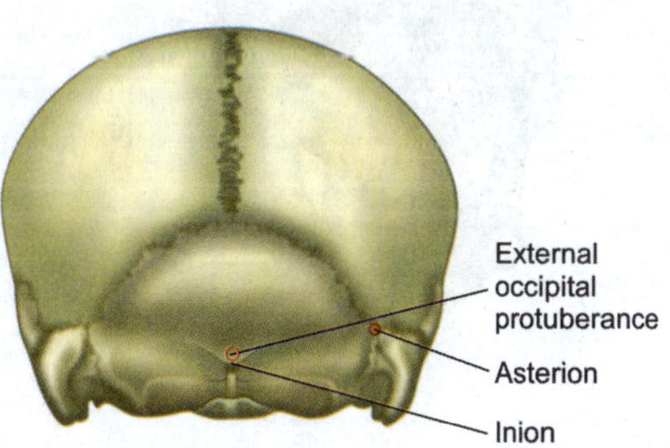

Q. What is attached to the superior nuchal line?

Ans. Superior nuchal line gives attachment to the following muscles:

- Medially—trapezius
- Laterally—sternocleidomastoid, splenius capitis.

Q. What is attached on highest nuchal line?

Ans. Following structures are attached on highest nuchal line:

- Medially—epicranial aponeurosis
- Laterally—occipitalis muscle.

Q. What is superciliary arch?

Ans. Superciliary arch is a rounded curved elevation, situated just above the medial part of each orbit. It overlies the frontal sinus and is better developed in males. Its medial part gives origin to corrugator supercilii muscle.

Q. What is glabella?

Ans. Glabella is the median elevation between the two superciliary arches.

Q. What is gonion?

Ans. The point on the angle of mandible is gonion.

Q. What is nasion? What is rhinion?

Ans.

- Nasion is the median point at the root of the nose
- Rhinion is the lower point of internasal suture.

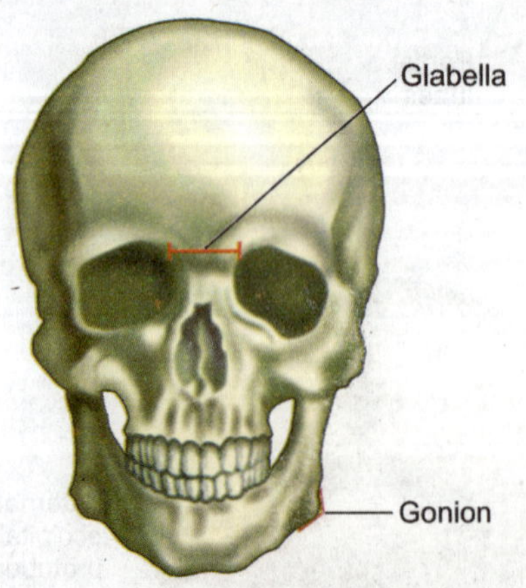

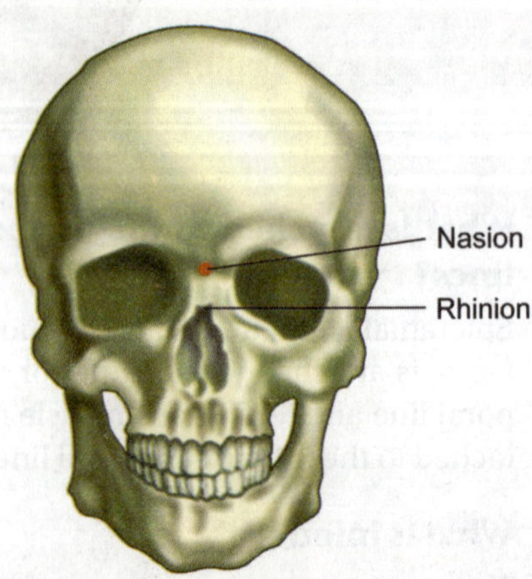

Q. What are the parts of maxilla?

Ans.

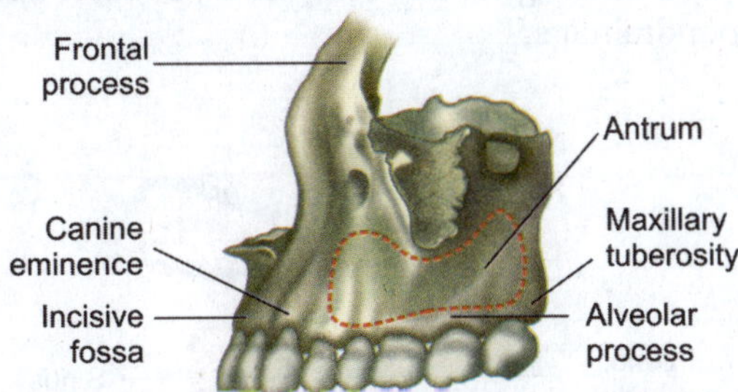

Q. Where is the maxillary ostium located?

Ans. Maxillary ostium is the opening of sinus, which is located in the posterior part of middle meatus, at a level higher than floor of the sinus (an unfavorable site for drainage).

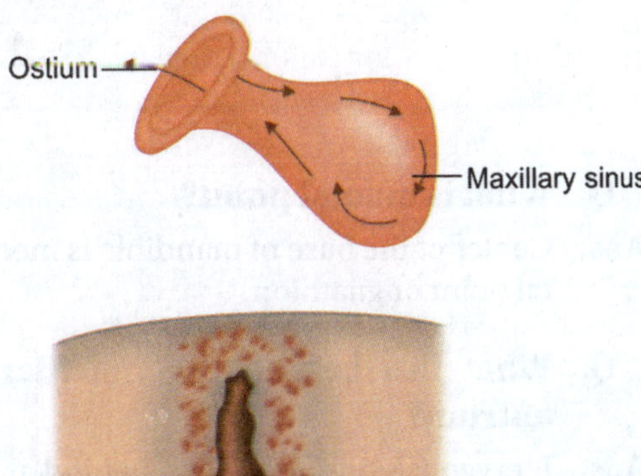

Q. What do you understand by sinus?

Ans. Sinus is a blind track leading from the surface down to the tissues.

Q. What is 'antrum of Highmore'? What are its features?

Ans. 'Antrum of Highmore' is maxillary sinus. Following are its features:

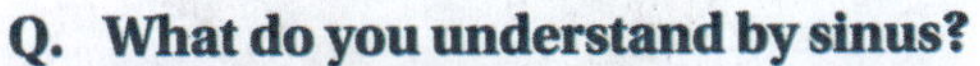

1. It is pyramidal in shape.
2. It is largest of all the sinuses.
3. It is approximately 15 cc in capacity.
4. Roof is formed by orbital surface of maxilla. Floor is formed by alveolar process of maxilla. Anterior wall is formed by body of maxilla. Posterior wall is a thin plate of bone separating it from pterygopalatine fossa.
5. Ostium lies in the posterior part of middle meatus, near the upper part of sinus cavity.
6. In 30%–40% cases, there is accessory ostia.

Q. What do you understand by fistula?

Ans. Fistula is a communicating track between two epithelial surfaces, commonly between a hollow viscus and skin or between two hollow viscera.

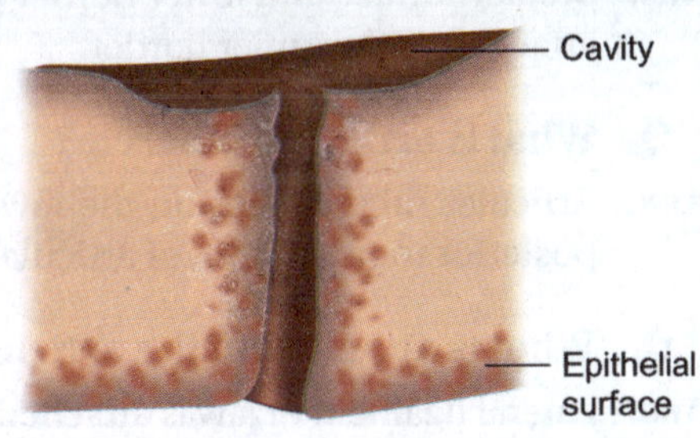

Q. What is antral puncture?

Ans. In cases of inadequate drainage of maxillary sinus, another opening is created in maxillary sinus for proper drainage.

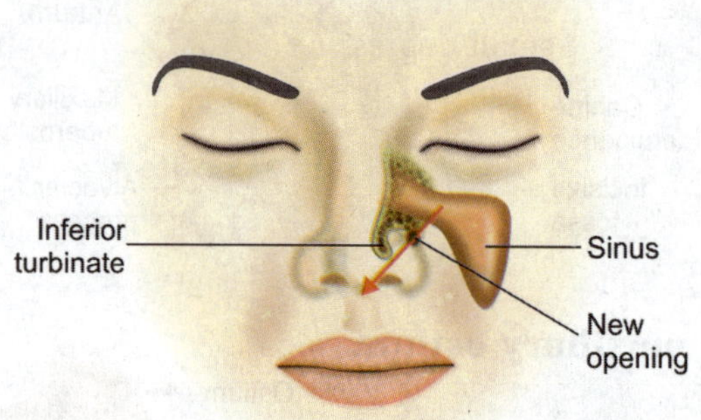

Q. What is mental point?

Ans. Center of the base of mandible is mental point or gnathion.

Q. What lies behind the maxillary antrum?

Ans. Pterygopalatine fossa lies behind the maxillary antrum (transantral approach).

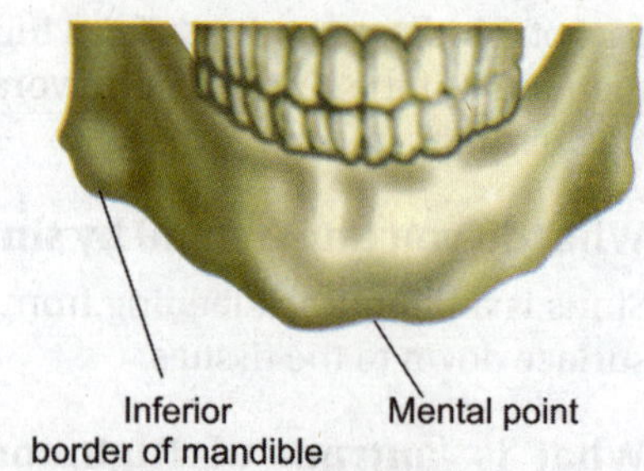

Q. What is jugal point?

Ans. Anterior end of the upper border of zygomatic arch is the jugal point.

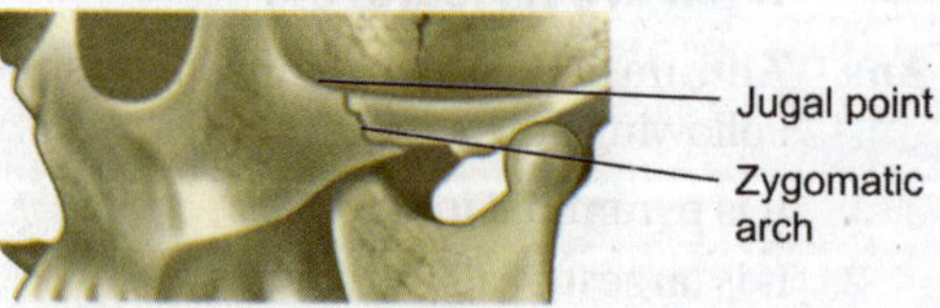

Q. How is zygomatic arch formed?

Ans. Zygomatic arch is formed by temporal process of zygomatic bone (1/3) and zygomatic process of temporal bone (2/3).

Q. What is attached to zygomatic arch (zygoma)?

Ans. Medial surface and lower border gives attachment to masseter and temporalis fascia is attached to the upper border.

Q. What is articular tubercle?

Ans. Articular tubercle lies on the lower border of zygoma, at the junction of anterior and posterior roots, in front of articular fossa.

Q. What is attached to the articular tubercle?

Ans. Lateral ligament of jaw is attached to the articular tubercle.

Q. What is auricular point?

Ans. The central point of external auditory meatus is auricular point through which Reid's baseline passes.

Q. What is suprameatal triangle (Macewen's triangle)?

Ans. Suprameatal triangle is a small depression posterosuperior to the external auditory meatus.

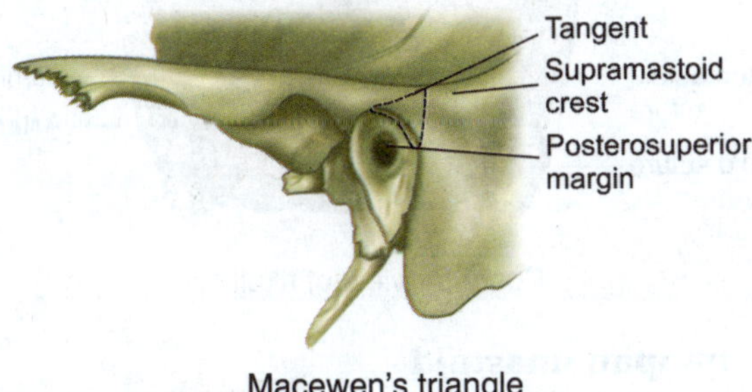

Macewen's triangle

It is bounded by:
- Supramastoid crest superiorly
- Posterosuperior margin of meatus anteriorly
- A tangent to posterior margin of meatus posteriorly.

Q. What is the importance of Macewen's triangle?

Ans. Macewen's triangle forms the lateral wall of mastoid antrum. The antrum lies below it (approximately 12–15 mm deep in adults and 1 mm deep in infants).

Q. What are the parts of temporal bone?

Ans. There are five parts of temporal bone:
- Mastoid
- Styloid
- Petrous
- Tympanic
- Squamous.

Q. When does the mastoid process ossify?

Ans. Mastoid process ossifies at the end of 2nd year.

Q. What is entomion?

Ans. Entomion is a point near the anterior part of parietomastoid suture.

Q. What is asterion?

Ans. The point, where parietomastoid, occipitomastoid and lambdoid sutures meet is asterion. It is the site of posterior fontanel in infants.

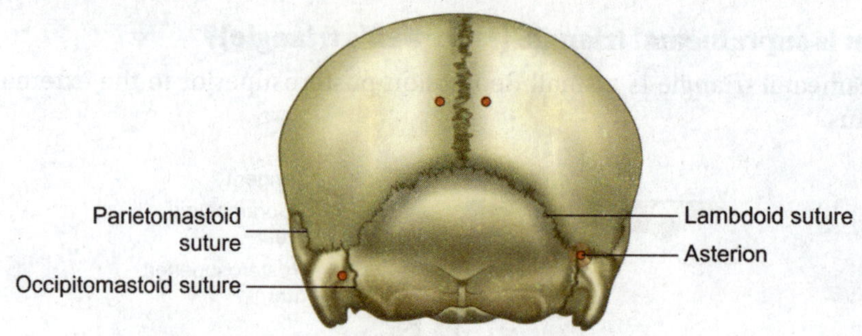

Posterior view of skull

Q. Where is the tympanomastoid suture located? What does it transmit?

Ans. Tympanomastoid suture is placed on the anterior aspect of the base of mastoid process. It transmits the auricular branch of vagus nerve (Arnold's or Alderman's nerve).

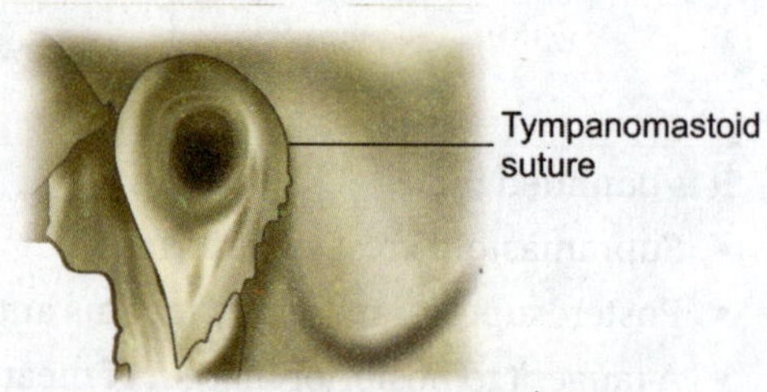

Q. What structures are attached to the styloid process?

Ans. Following structures are attached to the styloid process:

- Three muscles—stylohyoid, styloglossus, stylopharyngeus
- Two ligaments—stylohyoid, stylomandibular.

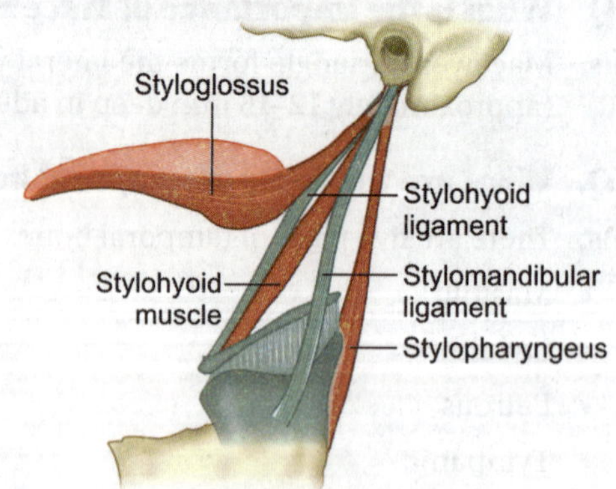

Q. What are the foramina in the roof of infratemporal fossa?

Ans. Roof is pierced by:

- Foramen ovale
- Foramen spinosum.

Q. What is pterion?

Ans. Pterion is an 'H'-shaped suture formed at the junction of frontal, parietal, sphenoid and temporal.

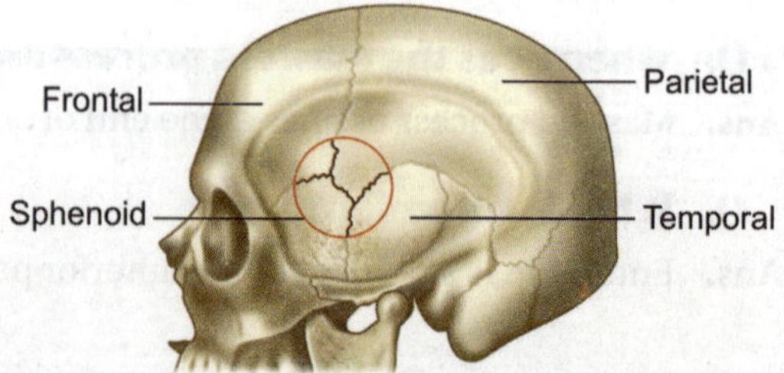

Q. What is the importance of pterion?

Ans. Following structures lie deep to pterion:

- Middle meningeal vein
- Anterior division of middle meningeal artery
- Stem of lateral sulcus of brain.

Q. What are the structures in pterygopalatine fossa?

Ans. Structures in pterygopalatine fossa are:

- Maxillary nerves and its branches
- Maxillary artery and its branches
- Fat
- Pterygopalatine venous plexus
- Vidian nerve.

Q. What is sylvian point?

Ans. Stem of lateral sulcus is sylvian point.

Q. What is Vidian nerve?

Ans. Also known as nerve of pterygoid canal. It is formed by the union of deep petrosal nerve with greater superficial petrosal nerve.

Q. Which ganglion is present on the roof of infratemporal fossa?

Ans. Otic ganglion.

Q. What is Arnold's nerve (Alderman's nerve)?

Ans. Auricular branch of vagus nerve is the Arnold's nerve (Alderman's nerve).

Q. Which muscle takes origin from posterior nasal spine?

Ans. Musculus uvulae muscle takes origin from posterior nasal spine.

Q. What is nervus spinosus?

Ans. Meningeal branch of mandibular nerve is known as nervus spinosus.

Q. Where is foramen of Vesalius located?

Ans. Foramen of Vesalius is located between foramen ovale and scaphoid fossa.

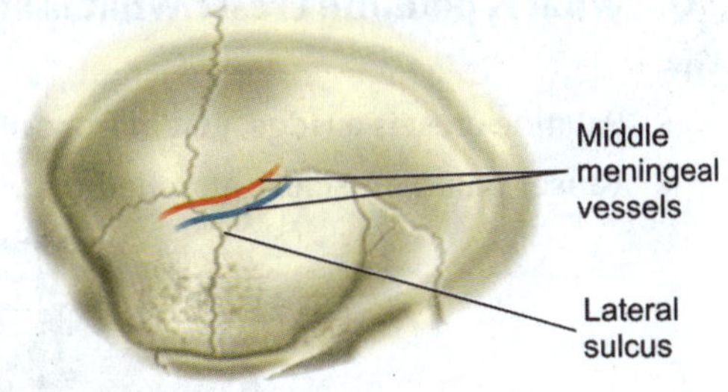

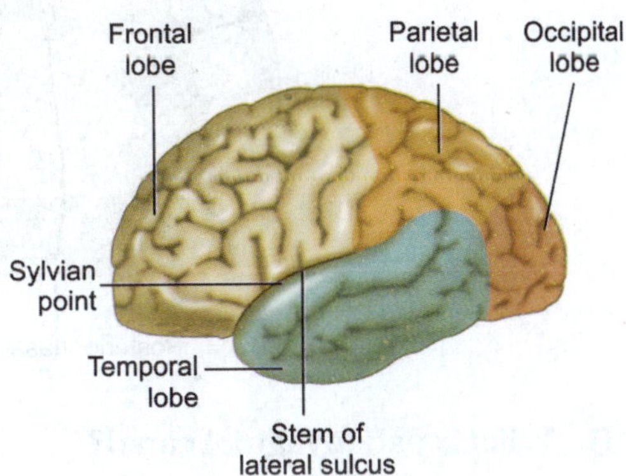

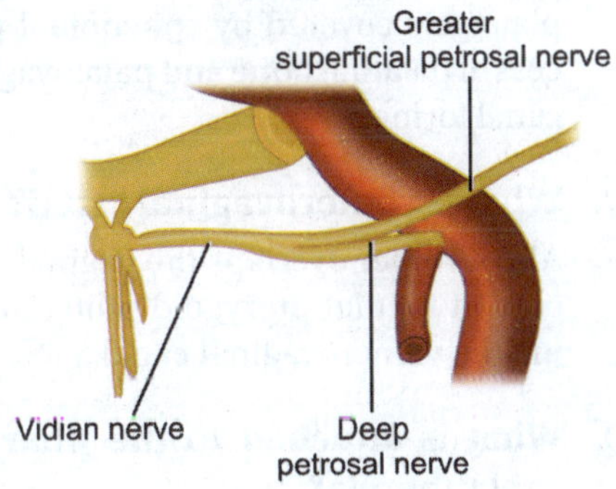

Q. What is palatine crest? What is attached to it?

Ans.

- Palatine crest is a ridge, just in front of posterior border of hard palate
- Tensor palati muscle is attached to it.

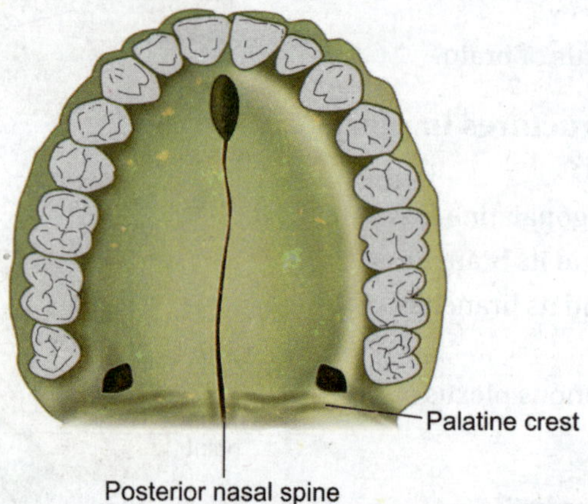

Q. What is palatovaginal canal?

Ans. Vaginal process of medial pterygoid plate gets covered by sphenoidal process of palatine bone and palatovaginal canal formed.

Q. What is vomerovaginal canal?

Ans. Ala of vomer overlaps the vaginal process of medial pterygoid plate, forming the vomerovaginal canal.

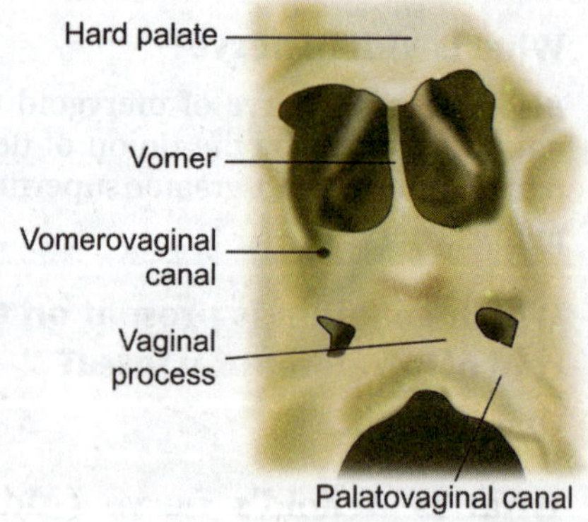

Q. What is attached to the pharyngeal tubercle?

Ans. Uppermost fibers of superior constrictor muscle are attached to pharyngeal tubercle.

Q. What are the attachments on medial pterygoid plate?

Ans. Following are the attachments on medial pterygoid plate:

- Pharyngobasilar fascia is attached to its whole length
- Scaphoid fossa gives origin to tensor palati muscle
- Upper part is notched by auditory tube.

Q. What is the importance of pterygoid hamulus?

Ans. Pterygoid hamulus is infractured during cleft palate surgery, to reduce the tension on suture line and relax the tensor palati muscle.

Q. What is attached to pterygoid hamulus?

Ans. Following is attached to pterygoid hamulus:

- Upper fibers of superior constrictor muscle
- Pterygomandibular raphe.

Q. What muscles are attached to lateral pterygoid plate?

Ans. Following structures are attached to lateral pterygoid plate:

- Lateral surface gives attachment to lateral pterygoid muscle
- Medial surface gives attachment to medial pterygoid muscle.

Q. Where is auditory tube lodged?

Ans. Auditory tube is lodged in sulcus tubae. Sulcus tubae is a groove between posteromedial margin of greater wing of sphenoid and petrous temporal bone.

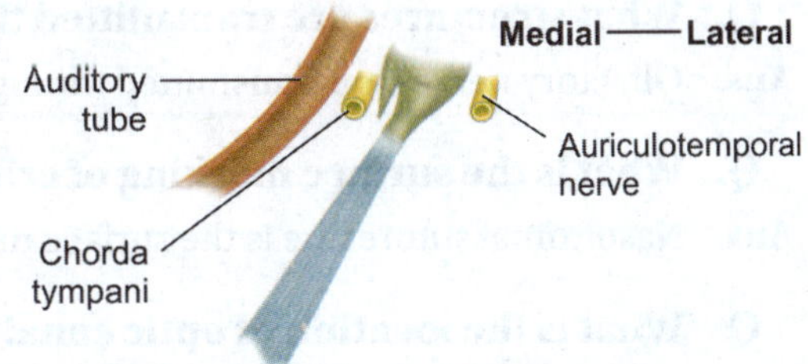

Q. What are the crucial relations of spine of sphenoid?

Ans. Spine of sphenoid is related laterally to auriculotemporal nerve and medially to chorda tympani nerve and auditory tube.

Q. What structures pass through foramen lacerum?

Ans. No significant structure passes through foramen lacerum.

Q. What is tegmen tympani?

Ans. Tegmen tympani is a thin plate of bone, forming the roof of middle ear.

Q. What ligaments are attached around foramen magnum?

Ans. Anterior and posterior atlanto-occipital membrane and alar ligament.

Q. What is Gasserian ganglion?

Ans. Trigeminal ganglion is Gasserian ganglion.

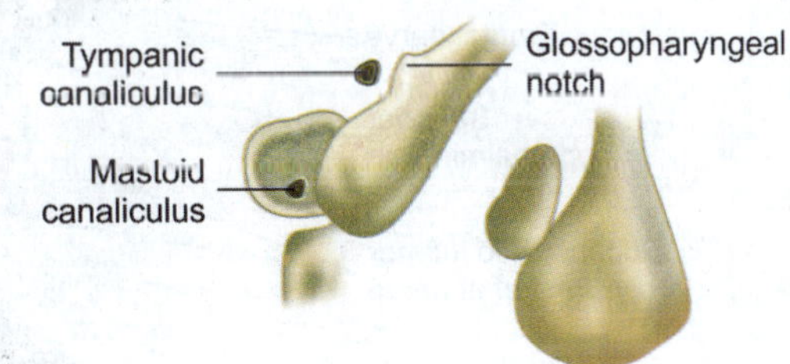

Q. What structure passes through mastoid canaliculus?

Ans. Auricular branch of vagus nerve passes through mastoid canaliculus.

Q. What structure passes through tympanic canaliculus?

Ans. Tympanic canaliculus transmits tympanic branch of IX cranial nerve.

Q. Where is the glossopharyngeal notch?

Ans. Glossopharyngeal notch is near the medial end of jugular foramen. It lodges the IX cranial nerve ganglion. At its apex, cochlear canaliculus opens and the perilymph drains through it into the subarachnoid space.

Q. What do the markings on the inner surface of vault signify?

Ans. Markings are produced by meningeal vessels, venous sinuses, arachnoid granulations and gyri.

Q. What is attached to the frontal crest?

Ans. Falx cerebri is attached to the frontal crest.

Q. What structures are transmitted through the cribriform plate?

Ans. Olfactory nerves are transmitted through the cribriform plate.

Q. What is the surface marking of cribriform plate?

Ans. Nasofrontal suture line is the surface marking of cribriform plate.

Q. What is the location of optic canal?

Ans. Optic canal is located between the two roots of lesser wing of sphenoid.

Q. Where is the superior orbital fissure located?

Ans. Superior orbital fissure is located between lesser and greater wings of sphenoid.

Q. Draw a neat labeled diagram of structures passing through the superior orbital fissure.

Ans.

Superior orbital fissure with its contents

Q. **Draw a neat labeled diagram of structures related to cavernous sinus.**

Ans.

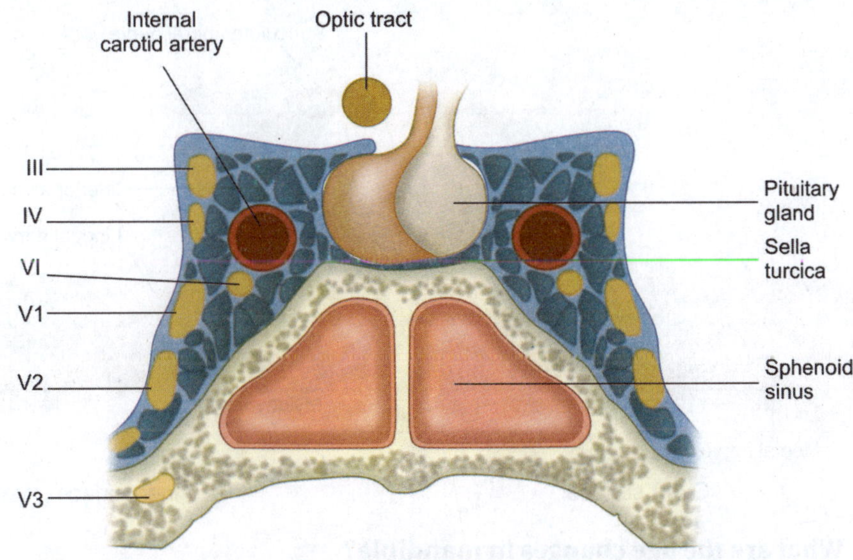

Cavernous sinus relations

Q. **Draw a neat labeled diagram of internal acoustic meatus.**

Ans.

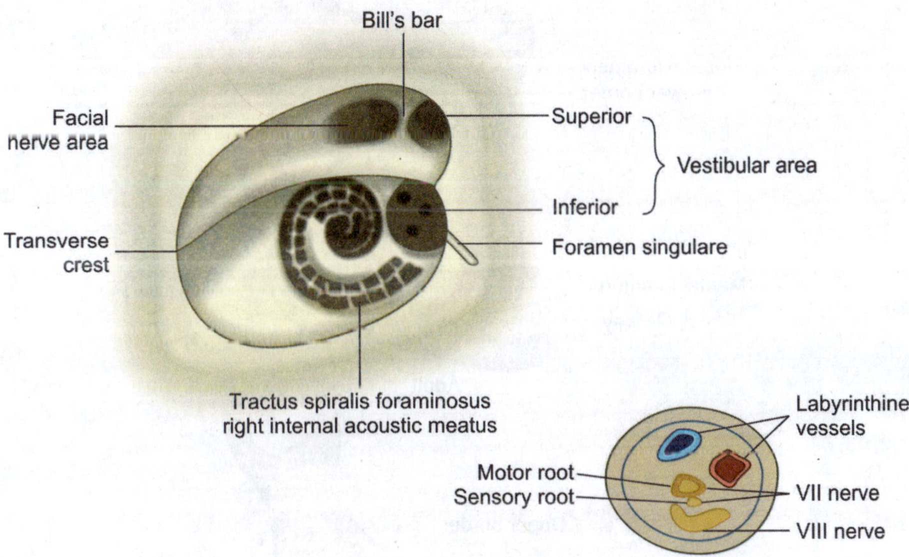

Q. **Which bone ossifies after clavicle?**

Ans. Mandible is the bone, which ossifies after clavicle.

Q.   What are the nerves related to mandible?

Ans.   Following nerves shown in figure are related to mandible.

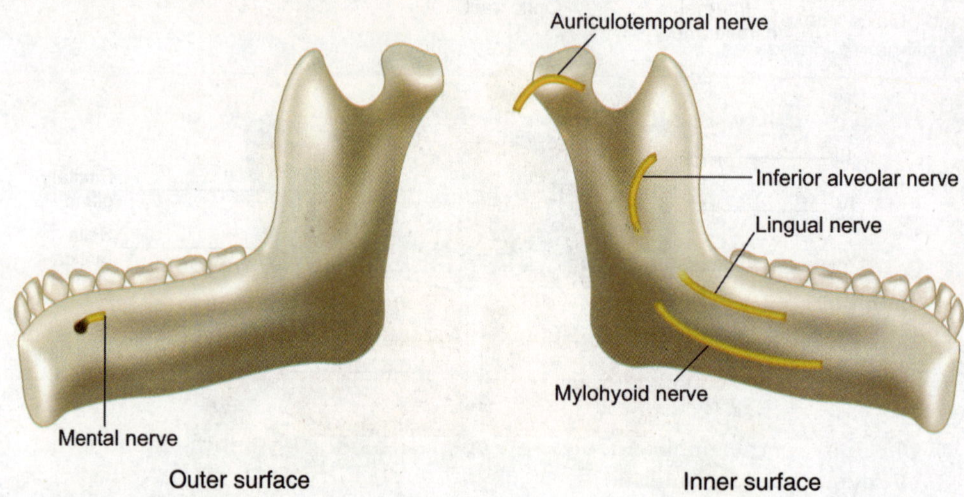

Q.   What are the age changes in mandible?

Ans.

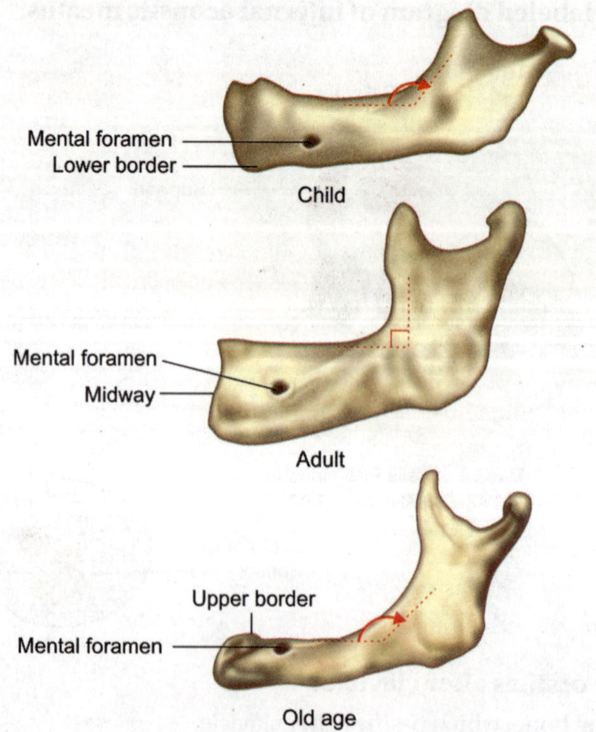

	Child	Adult	Old
Mental foramen site	Near the lower border	Midway	Near the upper border
Mandibular angle approximately in degrees	140	110	140

Q. Describe the ossification of mandible?

Ans. Ossification of mandible:

- Each half of mandible ossifies from a center appearing near mental foramen around 6th week
- Ossification progresses from the above primary center to form the body and ramus of mandible
- Later Meckel's cartilage around incisive foramen is surrounded and invaded by bone
- Secondary cartilage appears each for condylar process, anterior border of coronoid process
- One or two cartilaginous nodules appear on each side of symphysis menti, which ossify by 7th month of intrauterine life
- At birth mandible has two halves connected by fibrous tissue at symphysis menti
- Bony union begins below upwards during first year of life and completed by end of first year.

Q. How are the cervical vertebrae identified?

Ans. Cervical vertebrae are identified by the small size and presence of foramen transversarium.

Q. What is the other name of first cervical vertebra?

Ans. The first cervical vertebra is also known as atlas.

Q. What is the other name of second cervical vertebra?

Ans. Second cervical vertebra is also known as axis.

Q. Which vertebra is known as vertebra prominens?

Ans. The seventh cervical vertebra is known as vertebra prominens. Since, its tip can be felt through the skin at the lower end of nuchal furrow.

Q. What events occur at the transverse process of sixth cervical vertebra?

Ans. Following events occur at the transverse process of sixth cervical vertebra:

- First part of vertebral artery ends
- Second part of vertebral artery begins
- Pharynx continues as esophagus
- Larynx continues as trachea
- Jugular vein crosses and terminates in subclavian vein
- Middle cervical ganglion lies at this level.

Q. How does the cervical vertebra ossify?

Ans. A typical cervical vertebra ossifies from three primary centers and six secondary centers:

1. There are two primary centers for the two halves of neural arch and one for the centrum. They fuse by 1–3 years.

2. There are two secondary centers for annular epiphyseal disks, two for the transverse processes, two for the spine. All fuse by 25 years.

Q. How does a fetal skull differ from adult skull?

Ans. Fetal skull has following features:

- Skull is large in size
- Facial skeleton is small compared to the calvaria due to rudimentary status of facial bones and small size of sinuses
- Base of the skull is short
- Frontal and parietal tuber are prominent
- Glabella, superciliary arches and mastoid processes are not developed
- Stylomastoid foramen is exposed.

Q. What structure of fetal skull is of adult size?

Ans. Middle and internal auditory parts are of adult size in fetal skull.

Q. What is cephalic index?

Ans. Cephalic index expresses the shape of the head and is the proportion of breadth to the length of the skull.

$$\text{Cephalic index} = \frac{\text{Breadth} \times 100}{\text{Length}}$$

Q. When does the anterior fontanel close?

Ans. Anterior fontanel closes by 18th months (1½ year).

Q. When does the posterior fontanel close?

Ans. Posterior fontanel closes by 2–3 months.

Q. What is metopic suture?

Ans. When two halves of frontal bone fail to fuse in midline, a metopic suture develops, 3%–8% of individuals with racial variations have metopic suture.

Q. What is sella turcica?

Ans. The upper surface of the body of sphenoid is hollowed out in the form of Turkish saddle. This is known as sella turcica.

Q. What are Le Fort fractures? How are they classified?

Ans. Central variety of middle third facial fractures are Le Fort fractures.

There are three types of Le Fort fractures:

- Type 1— transverse fractures of maxilla involving palate only
- Type 2—fracture en bloc of palate and middle third of face
- Type 3—complete disruption of facial skeleton from the cranium.

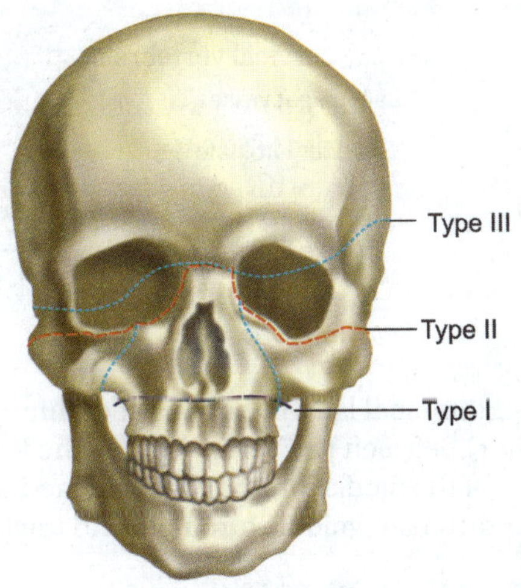

Le Fort fracture lines

Q. What is the status of paranasal sinuses at birth?

Ans. All the paranasal sinuses are rudimentary at birth except frontal, which is absent.

Q. How is the lateral wall of the nose divided?

Ans.

1. The lateral wall of the nose is divided by bony elevations namely superior, middle and inferior turbinates (conchae). Due to which the lateral wall space gets divided into superior, middle and inferior meatus below the respective turbinates.
2. Superior and middle conchae are parts of ethmoid bone.
3. Inferior conchae is a separate bone.

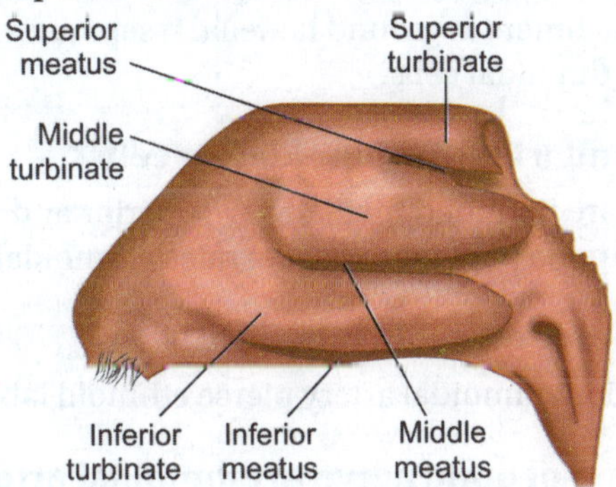

Lateral wall of nose

Q. What are the parts of ethmoid bone?

Ans. Ethmoid bone has a horizontal, perforated, cribriform plate, a median perpendicular plate and two lateral labyrinth.

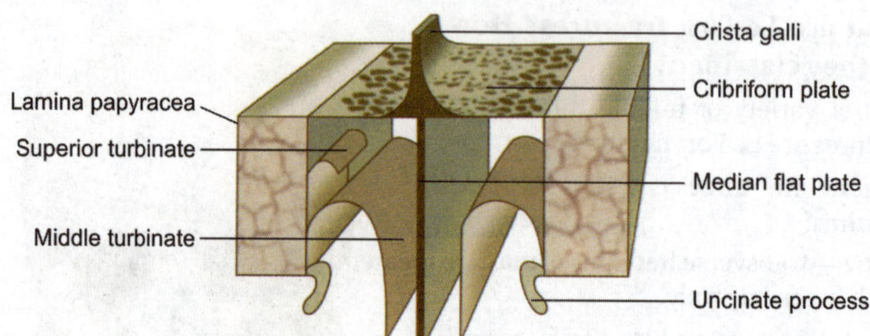

Ethmoidal labyrinths consist of thin-walled ethmoidal air cells (anterior, middle and posterior) between two vertical plate. The lateral vertical plate is lamina papyracea, which forms part of the medial orbital wall. The medial vertical plate forms part of lateral nasal wall. Superior turbinate, middle turbinate and uncinate process are parts of ethmoid bone.

Q. How is the middle turbinate attached?

Ans. Middle turbinate has three planes of attachment:

- Anterior attachment is in sagittal plane to frontonasal process of maxilla

- In coronal plane, it is attached to lamina papyracea

- Horizontally also, it is attached to lamina papyracea.

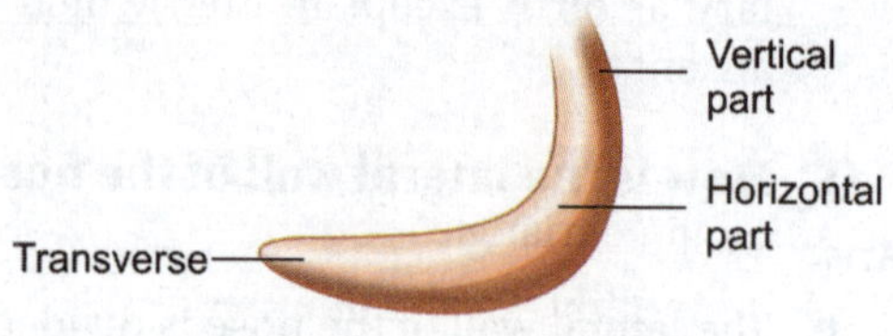

Parts of middle turbinate

Q. What is ground lamella (basal lamella)?

Ans. Middle turbinate turns laterally to get attached in coronal plane to the lamina papyracea. This area of attachment is ground lamella. It separates the anterior ethmoidal cells from the posterior ethmoidal cells.

Q. What are the boundaries of ethmoidal air cells?

Ans. Ethmoidal air cells are bounded medially by superior and middle turbinate, and laterally by paper-thin lamina papyracea. It separates ethmoidal air cells from orbit.

Q. Which arteries pierce ethmoid labyrinth?

Ans. Anterior and posterior ethmoidal artery pierce ethmoid labyrinth.

Q. What is the relation of optic nerve to ethmoidal arteries?

Ans. Anterior ethmoidal artery enters the orbit 4 cm behind the medial ligament of orbit and posterior ethmoidal artery is 2 cm behind anterior ethmoidal artery and optic nerve is just 1 cm or even less than 1 cm behind posterior ethmoidal artery.

Q. What is FESS?

Ans. FESS means functional endoscopic sinus surgery.

Q. What is osteomeatal complex?

Ans. The various openings in the middle meatus as seen endoscopically is known as osteo-meatal complex. It is divided into anterior and posterior parts by ground lamella.

Q. What are the age changes in maxilla?

Ans. At birth:

- Transverse and sagittal dimensions are greater than vertical (small body)
- Frontal process is prominent
- Alveoli reach the orbital floor
- Maxillary sinus is rudimentary.

In adults:

- Vertical dimension is greater than transverse and sagittal dimensions
- Maxillary sinus is well-developed.

In old age:

- Height reduces
- Alveolar process gets absorbed.

Q. What are the boundaries and contents of scalene triangle?

Ans. Scalene triangle is bounded by:

- Anteriorly—scalenus anterior
- Posteriorly—scalenus medius
- Base—subclavian artery
- Contents—trunks of brachial plexus.

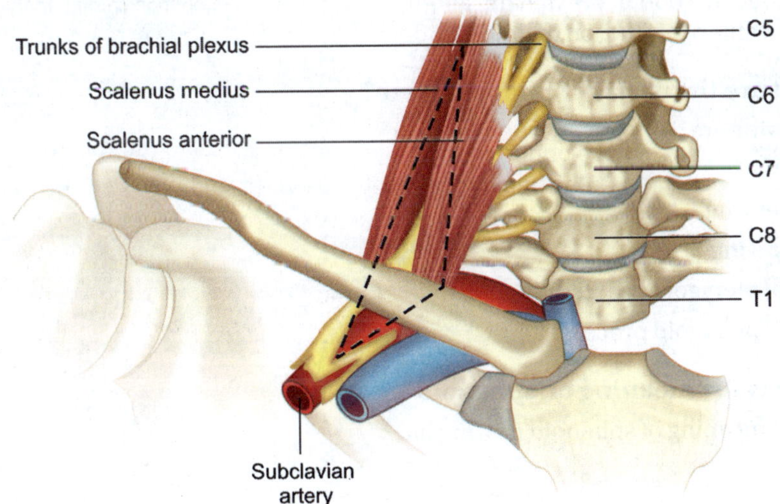

Q. What are the boundaries of Joll's triangle?

Ans. Following are the boundaries of Joll's triangle:

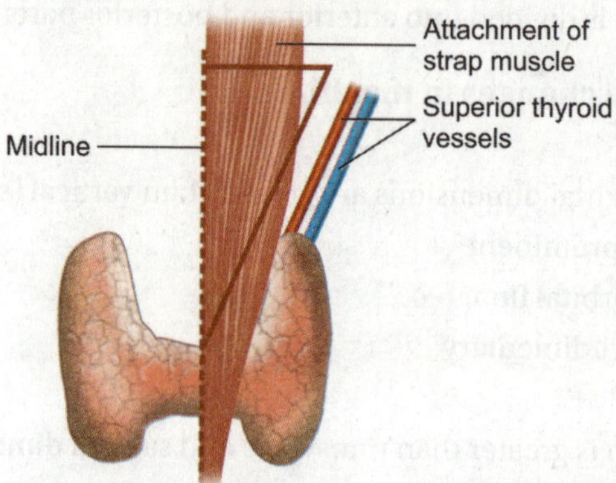

- Laterally—upper pole of thyroid with superior thyroid vessels
- Superiorly—attachment of strap muscles
- Medially—midline.

Q. What are the boundaries of Beahr's triangle?

Ans. Following are the boundaries of Beahr's triangle:

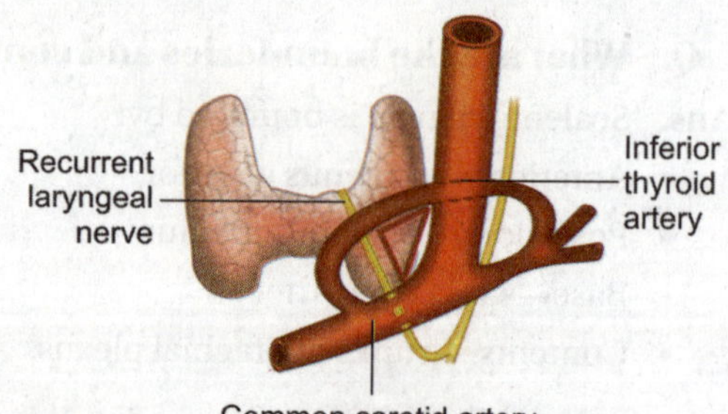

- Superiorly—inferior thyroid artery
- Medially—recurrent laryngeal nerve
- Laterally—common carotid artery.

Note: Surgeon should be vigilant about this triangle, while operating on thyroid gland.

Q. What are the parts of sphenoid bone?

Ans. Following are the parts of sphenoid bone:

- Body
- Greater wing
- Lesser wing
- Medial pterygoid process
- Lateral pterygoid process.

Q. What is the meaning of 'sphenoid'?

Ans. Literal meaning of sphenoid is 'wing like'.

Q. What are the parts of palatine bone?

Ans. Following are the parts of palatine bone:

- Horizontal plate
- Perpendicular plate
- Pyramidal process
- Orbital process
- Sphenoidal process.

Q. What are the parts of lacrimal bone?

Ans. Following are the parts of lacrimal bone:

- Lateral orbital surface
- Lacrimal crest
- Lacrimal hamulus
- Lacrimal fossa.

Q. Sphenopalatine notch is present on which bone?

Ans. Sphenopalatine notch is present on palatine bone between orbital and sphenoidal process.

Q. Which is the artery of epistaxis?

Ans. Sphenopalatine artery is the artery of epistaxis.

Q. What is Inca or Goethe's ossicle?

Ans. Goethe's ossicle is a sutural bone in lambda.

Q. Important foramina and its corresponding structures.

Ans.

Foramina	Structures
Anterior canal	Anterior ethmoidal artery, vein and nerve
Canaliculus innominatus	Lesser petrosal nerve
Carotid canal	Internal carotid artery with its venous and sympathetic plexus
Condylar canal	Emissary vein connecting sigmoid sinus to suboccipital venous plexus
Cochlear canaliculus	Aqueduct of cochlea
Foramen ovale (mnemonic MALE)	**M**—Mandibular nerve **A**—Accessory meningeal artery **L**—Lesser petrosal nerve **E**—Emissary vein (connecting cavernous sinus to pterygoid plexus of veins) anterior trunk of middle meningeal vein
Foramen spinosum	Middle meningeal artery meningeal branch of mandibular nerve (nervous spinosus)

Contd...

Contd...

Foramina	Structures
Foramen rotundum	Maxillary nerve
Foramen lacerum	Meningeal branch of ascending pharyngeal artery emissary vein from cavernous sinus (in fetal life only cartilage is present)
Foramen magnum	Lower part of medulla, tonsils of cerebellum, meninges, spinal accessory nerve, vertebral arteries with its sympathetic plexus, anterior and posterior spinal arteries, apical ligament of dens, membrana tectoria
Foramen of Vesalius	Emissary vein (connecting cavernous sinus to pterygoid plexus of veins)
Foramen cecum	A vein from the nose to the superior sagittal sin us
Foramina in cribriform plate	Olfactory nerves
Greater palatine foramen	Greater palatine artery and vein anterior palatine nerve
Hypoglossal canal	Hypoglossal nerve, ascending pharyngeal artery (meningeal branch), emissary vein connecting sigmoid sinus with internal jugular vein (IJV)
Internal acoustic meatus	Facial nerve, vestibulocochlear nerve, labyrinthine vessels
Inferior orbital fissure	Maxillary nerve
Jugular foramen	IX, X, XI cranial nerves; ascending pharyngeal and occipital arteries, (meningeal branch), internal jugular vein, inferior petrosal nerve
Lesser palatine foramen	Middle and posterior palatine nerves
Mastoid foramen	Meningeal branch of occipital artery, emissary vein (connecting sigmoid sinus with posterior auricular vein)
Mastoid canaliculus	Auricular branch of vagus nerve (Arnold's or Alderman's nerve)
Mental foramen	Mental artery, vein and nerve
Mandibular foramen	Inferior alveolar artery, vein and nerve
Optic canal	Optic nerve with it's meningeal sheath, ophthalmic artery
Parietal foramen	Emissary vein from superior sagittal sinus
Palatovaginal canal	Pharyngeal branch of maxillary artery, pharyngeal branch from pterygopalatine ganglion
Petrotympanic fissure	Chorda tympanic nerve, anterior tympanic artery
Posterior ethmoidal canal	Posterior ethmoidal artery and vein
Stylomastoid foramen	Facial nerve, stylomastoid branch of posterior auricular artery
Superior orbital fissure	Lacrimal nerve, frontal nerve, trochlear nerve, superior ophthalmic vein, meningeal branch of lacrimal artery, oculomotor nerve (upper and lower division), nasociliary nerve, abducens nerve, inferior ophthalmic vein
Supraorbital foramen	Supraorbital artery, vein and nerve
Tympanic canaliculus	Glossopharyngeal nerve (tympanic branch)
Vomerovaginal canal	Pharyngeal artery, vein and nerve

Short Notes

MUSCLE

- Facial muscles
- Sternocleidomastoid muscle
- Extraocular muscles
- Lateral pterygoid muscle
- Soft palate
- Constrictors of pharynx
- Scalenus anterior muscle
- Intrinsic muscles of larynx

NERVE

- Secretomotor pathway to parotid gland
- Secretomotor pathway to submandibular gland
- Secretomotor pathway to lacrimal gland
- Trigeminal ganglion
- Otic ganglion
- Pterygopalatine ganglion
- Stellate ganglion
- Submandibular ganglion
- Acoustic pathway
- Galen's anastomosis
- Frey syndrome

ARTERY

- Facial artery
- Vertebral artery
- External carotid artery
- Central artery of retina

VEIN

- Venous drainage of the face
- Internal jugular vein
- Cavernous sinus
- External jugular vein

Contd...

Contd...

LYMPH NODES

- Waldeyer's ring
- Superficial cervical lymph nodes
- Deep cervical lymph nodes
- Lymphatic drainage of tongue

JOINT

- Atlanto-occipital joint
- Atlantoaxial joint
- Sphenomandibular ligament
- Stylomandibular ligament

MISCELLANEOUS

- Auricle
- Formation of the triangles of the neck
- Carotid sheath
- Carotid triangle
- Falx cerebri
- Tentorium cerebelli
- Midline structures of the neck
- Superior orbital fissure
- Styloid apparatus
- Palatine tonsillar bed
- Auditory tube
- Nasal septum
- Cavity of larynx
- Tympanic membrane
- Prussak's pouch
- Eyeball
- Ear ossicles
- Neurobiotaxis
- Cochlear section
- Sclerocorneal junction

▶ MUSCLE

Q. FACIAL MUSCLES

Facial muscles differ from other skeletal muscles in following ways:

- Subcutaneous muscles
- Control the orifices on face (like sphincters)
- Have fine control on movement
- Exhibit facial expression
- Develop from second branchial arch.

Classification

Muscles around the eye:

- Orbicularis oculis
- Corrugator supercilii
- Levator palpebrae superioris.

Muscles around the mouth:

- Orbicularis oris
- Levator labii superioris alaeque nasi
- Levator labii superioris
- Levator anguli oris
- Zygomaticus major and minor
- Depressor anguli oris and labii inferioris
- Mentalis
- Risorius
- Buccinator.

Muscles around the nostril:

- Procerus
- Compressor naris
- Dilator naris
- Depressor septi
- Occipitofrontalis
- Platysma.

Nerve Supply

Facial nerve.

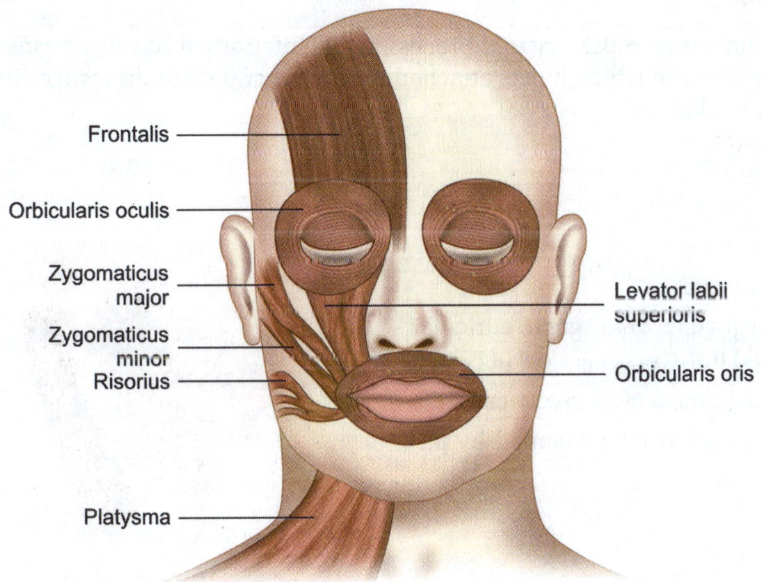

Facial muscles

Function

- Primarily regulates the facial openings
- Frontalis causes wrinkling of forehead
- Orbicularis oris—whistling
- Orbicularis oculis—helps in tight closure of eyes
- Platysma—draws the angle of mouth downwards.

Common Facial Expressions

- Smiling and laughing—zygomaticus major
- Sadness—levator labii superioris, levator anguli oris
- Grief—depressor anguli oris
- Frowning—corrugator supercilii and procerus.

Applied Anatomy

Facial nerve injury will affect facial muscles and lead to facial asymmetry.

Q. STERNOCLEIDOMASTOID MUSCLE

Sternocleidomastoid muscle is considered as a key muscle of the neck, surgically dividing the region into anterior triangle and posterior triangle.

Attachments

Superior attachment is to the mastoid process, while inferiorly it has two heads—clavicular and sternal by virtue of which it gets attached to clavicle and sternum respectively. Both attachments are tendinous.

Relations

Superficial

- Skin, platysma
- External jugular vein, great auricular nerve and transverse cervical nerve
- Superficial lamina of deep cervical fascia
- In upper part, it is overlapped by parotid gland.

Deep

- Great vessels of the neck (carotid sheath).

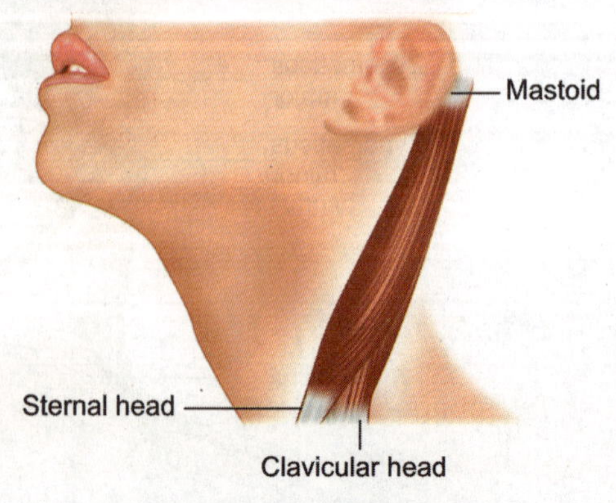

Nerve Supply

Accessory nerve and ventral rami of C2, C3, C4, spinal nerves.

Action

Acting alone, the muscle tilts the head toward the ipsilateral shoulder turning the face to opposite side.

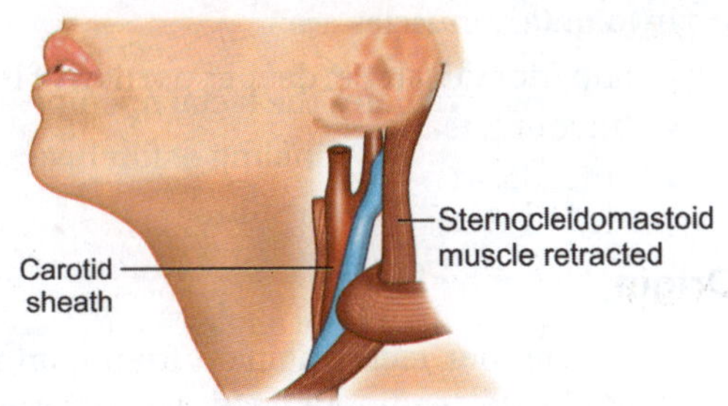

Applied Anatomy

Torticollis is due to permanent contraction of sternocleidomastoid.

Q. EXTRAOCULAR MUSCLES

There are seven voluntary and three involuntary extraocular muscles.

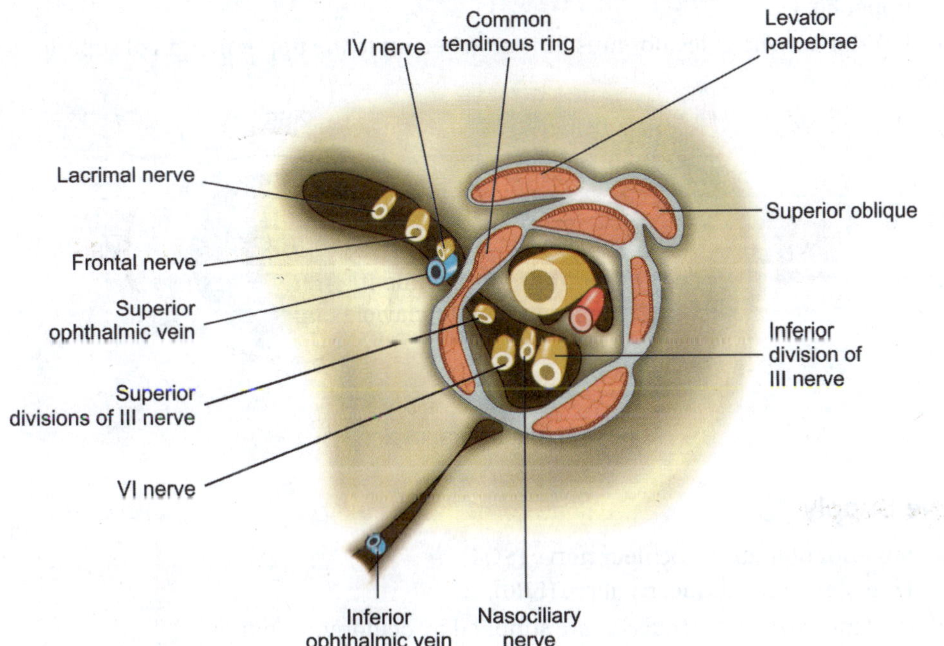

Voluntary muscles are:

- Four recti—superior, inferior, medial, lateral
- Two obliques—superior, inferior
- One—levator palpebrae superioris.

All have short tendons of origin and long tendons of insertion.

Involuntary muscles are:

- Superior tarsal (i.e. deeper portion of levator palpebrae superioris)
- Inferior tarsal
- Orbitalis.

Origin

1. All the four recti originate from common tendinous ring of Zinn. Lateral rectus has additional tendinous head, which arises from orbital surface of greater wing of sphenoid.
2. Superior oblique arises from body of sphenoid.
3. Inferior oblique arises from orbital surface of maxilla.

Insertion

- The recti are inserted into the sclera, a little posterior to the limbus on an average 6–7 mm
- The oblique are inserted on the sclera behind the equator of eyeball
- Superior lamella of levator muscle is inserted into anterior surface of tarsus and skin of upper lid
- Inferior lamella of levator muscle is attached on to the upper margin of superior tarsus.

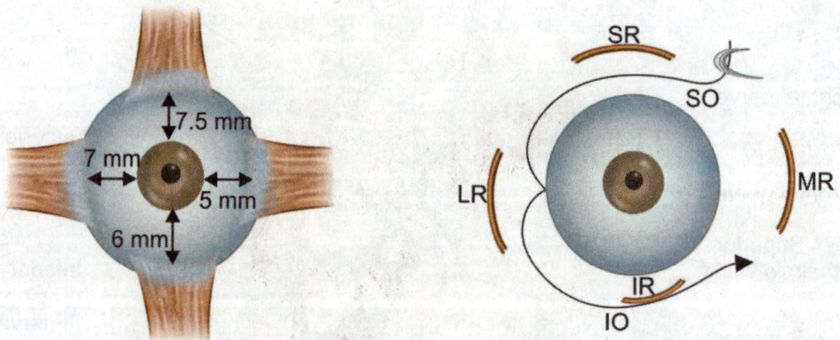

Extraocular muscles

Nerve Supply

- Superior oblique—trochlear nerve (SO4)
- Lateral rectus—abducens nerve (LR6).

Rest all the extraocular muscles are supplied by oculomotor nerve.

Action

Movements occur around:

- Transverse axis—elevation and depression
- Vertical axis—medial and lateral rotation
- Anteroposterior axis—intorsion and extortion.

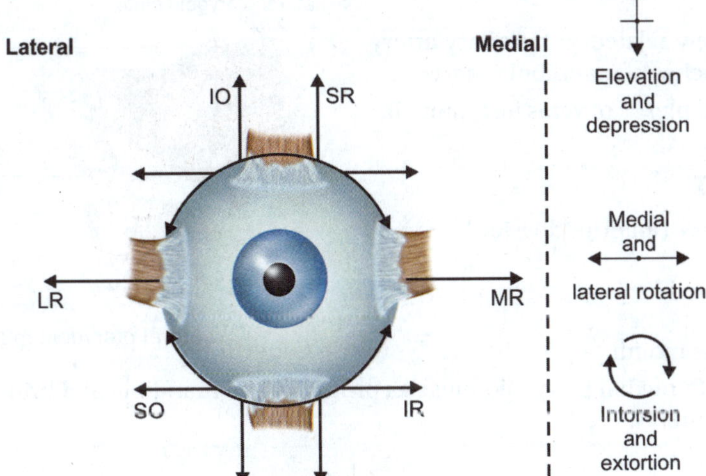

Movements can be best demonstrated on ball:

- Superior rectus—upward rotation, medial rotation, intorsion
- Medial rectus—medial rotation
- Inferior rectus—downward rotation, medial rotation, extortion
- Lateral rectus—lateral rotation
- Superior oblique—downward rotation, lateral rotation, intorsion
- Inferior oblique—upward rotation, lateral rotation, extortion.

Applied Anatomy

- Paralysis of extraocular muscles causes squint
- Nystagmus is characterized by involuntary, rhythmic, oscillatory movements.

Q. LATERAL PTERYGOID MUSCLE

Lateral pterygoid muscle is a muscle of mastication, which divides the maxillary artery into three parts.

Attachments

From

- Upper head—infratemporal surface and greater wing of sphenoid
- Lower head—lateral surface of lateral pterygoid plate.

To

- Pterygoid fovea
- Articular disk and capsule of temporomandibular joint.

Relation

- It is closely related to maxillary artery and branches of mandibular nerve
- Pterygoid plexus of veins lie around it.

Nerve Supply

Mandibular nerve (anterior division).

Action

- Opens the mouth
- Along with medial pterygoid muscles protrudes the mandible and brings about grinding movements.

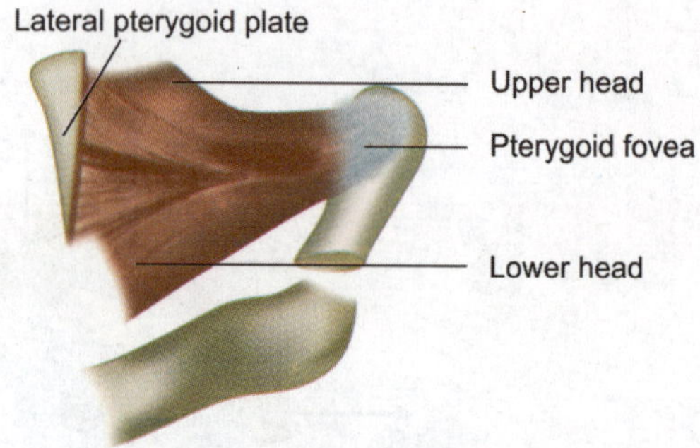

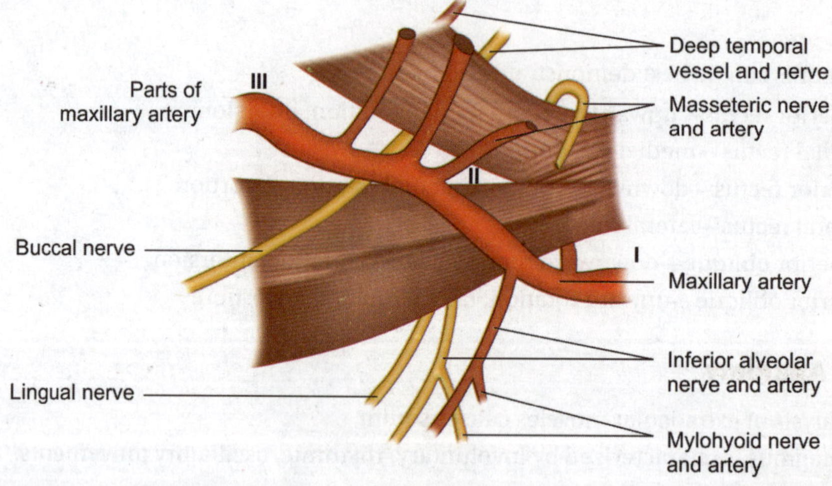

Q. SOFT PALATE

Soft palate is movable, muscular fold separating the nasopharynx from oropharynx. It is made up of:

- Tensor palati
- Levator palati
- Musculus uvulae
- Palatopharyngeus
- Palatoglossus.

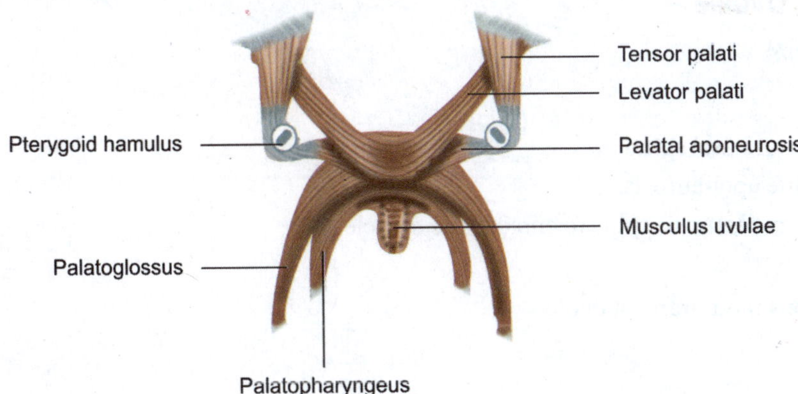

Tensor Palati

Attachments

From

- Auditory tube (lateral side) sphenoid (scaphoid fossa, spine and greater wing)
- The muscle forms a tendon, which winds around pterygoid hamulus.

To

- Hard palate (posterior border and inferior surface).

Action

- Tightens soft palate
- Opens auditory tube.

Levator Palati

Attachments

From

- Inferior surface of petrous temporal and auditory tube
- Upper part of carotid sheath.

Muscle enters pharynx by passing over the upper border of superior constrictor.

To

- Upper surface of palatine aponeurosis.

Action

- Elevates soft palate
- Opens auditory tube.

Musculus Uvulae

Attachments

From

- Posterior nasal spine
- Palatine aponeurosis.

Palatine aponeurosis splits to enclose the muscle.

To

- Mucous membrane of uvula.

Action

Pulls up the uvula.

Palatopharyngeus

Attachments

From

- Hard palate (posterior border)
- Palatine aponeurosis.

Muscle has two fasciculi—anterior and posterior.

To

- Lamina of thyroid cartilage
- Median raphe of pharynx.

Action

Pulls up and shortens pharynx during swallowing.

Palatoglossus

Attachments

From

- Palatine aponeurosis (oral surface).

Descends in palatoglossus arch.

To

- Side of tongue.

Action

Pulls up root of the tongue and closes the oropharyngeal isthmus.

Nerve Supply

All the muscles of soft palate are supplied by pharyngeal plexus except tensor palati muscle, which is supplied by mandibular nerve.

Applied Anatomy

- Diphtheria may produce paralysis of soft palate resulting in regurgitation of fluids, nasal intonation and flattening of palatal arch
- Oral cavity in a newborn should be carefully examined otherwise a soft palate cleft may be missed easily.

Q. CONSTRICTORS OF PHARYNX

Pharynx is a muscular tube made up of three muscles. They are:

- Superior constrictor
- Middle constrictor
- Inferior constrictor.

Superior Constrictor

Attachments

From

- Pterygoid hamulus, medial pterygoid plate
- Pterygomandibular raphe
- Mylohyoid line
- Side of tongue.

To

- Pharyngeal tubercle and raphe.

Middle Constrictor

Attachments

From

- Stylohyoid ligament
- Lesser and greater horn of hyoid bone.

To

- Pharyngeal raphe.

Inferior Constrictor

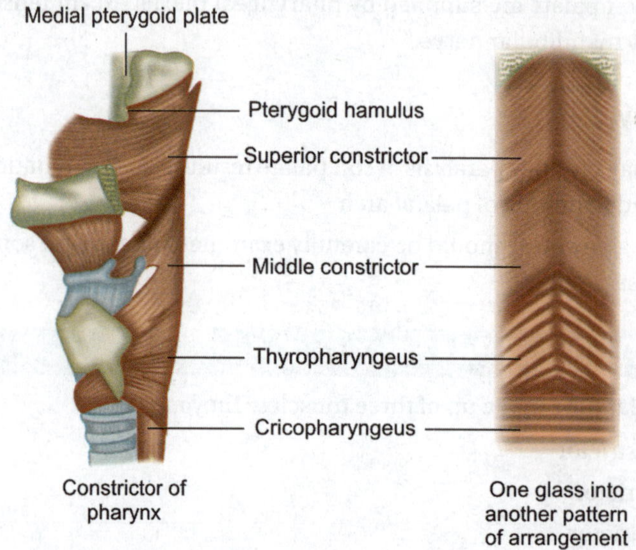

Attachments

From

- Oblique line of thyroid cartilage (thyropharyngeus)
- Side of cricoid (cricopharyngeus).

Inferior constrictor has two parts thyropharyngeus and cricopharyngeus.

To

- Pharyngeal raphe.

Action

All the constrictors help in deglutition.

Nerve Supply

All the constrictors are supplied by pharyngeal plexus.

Applied Anatomy

1. The lower part of thyropharyngeus is a single sheet of muscle, not overlapped internally by middle constrictor. This part is limited below by cricopharyngeal sphincter. This weak area is known as Killian's dehiscence. Pharyngeal diverticulum is an outpouching of this dehiscence.
2. Paralyses of constrictors lead to dysphagia.

Q. SCALENUS ANTERIOR MUSCLE

Scalenus anterior muscle is a key muscle of the lower part of posterior triangle of the neck.

Attachments

From

- Anterior tubercles of transverse processes of 3, 4, 5, 6 cervical vertebra.

To

- Scalene tubercle of first rib.

Relations

Anteriorly:

- Phrenic nerve
- Prevertebral fascia.

Nerve Supply

Ventral rami of C4, C5, C6 nerves.

Action

- Flexion and rotation of cervical spine
- Elevates first rib during inspiration.

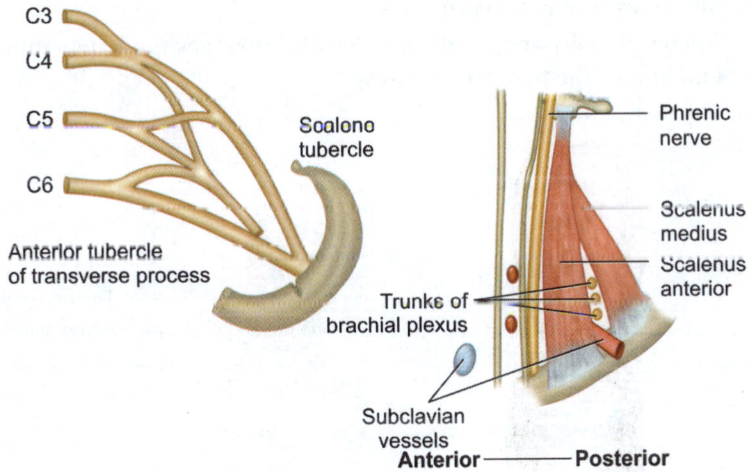

Scalenus anterior (muscle relations)

Q. INTRINSIC MUSCLES OF LARYNX

These are the muscles whose attachments are within the cartilages of larynx.

Following are the intrinsic muscles of larynx:

- Cricothyroid
- Posterior cricoarytenoid
- Lateral cricoarytenoid
- Transverse arytenoid
- Oblique arytenoid and aryepiglottic
- Thyroarytenoid, vocalis and thyroepiglottic.

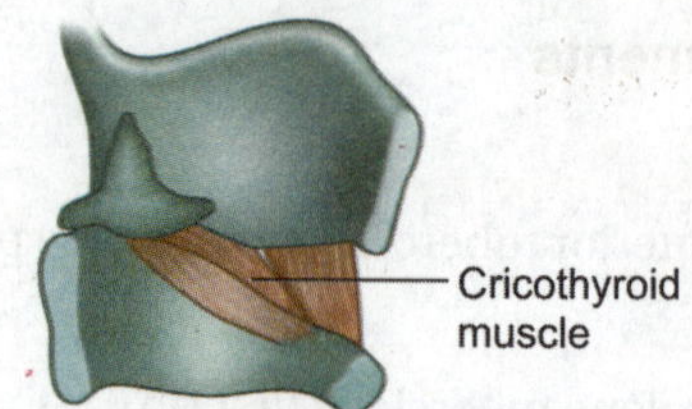

Attachments

Name of the muscles itself denotes its attachments.

Arytenoid is the key cartilage to receive muscular attachments. It has a vocal process and a muscular process.

Nerve Supply

All intrinsic muscles of larynx are supplied by recurrent laryngeal nerve except cricothyroid, which supplied by external laryngeal nerve.

Action

1. Cricothyroid—tensor of vocal cord.
2. Posterior cricoarytenoid—opens the glottis; it is known as the 'safety muscle of larynx' because it maintains the patency of airway:

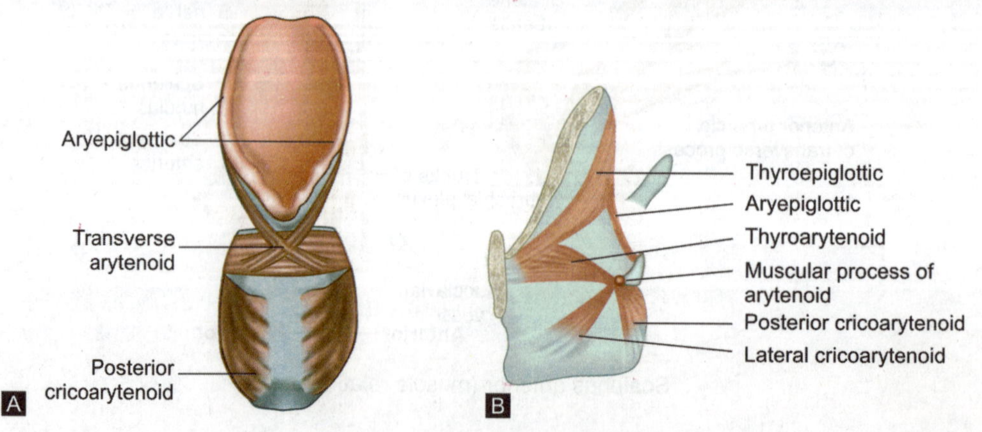

Intrinsic muscles of larynx

- Lateral cricoarytenoid—close the glottis
- Transverse arytenoid—close the glottis
- Oblique arytenoid and aryepiglottic—close the inlet of larynx
- Thyroarytenoid, vocalis—relax the vocal cord.

Applied Anatomy

- External laryngeal nerve injury will result in loss of tension of vocal cord giving rise to weak voice
- Laryngeal nerve injuries could be due to different causes like infection (diphtheria), cancer, diabetes.

▶ NERVE

Q. SECRETOMOTOR PATHWAY TO PAROTID GLAND.

Following is the secretomotor pathway to parotid gland:

$$\text{Inferior salivatory nucleus}$$
$$\downarrow$$
$$\text{Tympanic branch of IX cranial nerve}$$
$$\downarrow$$
$$\text{Tympanic plexus}$$
$$\downarrow$$
$$\text{Lesser petrosal nerve}$$
$$\downarrow$$
$$\text{Otic ganglion}$$
$$\downarrow$$
$$\text{Auriculotemporal nerve}$$
$$\downarrow$$
$$\text{Parotid gland}$$

Q. SECRETOMOTOR PATHWAY TO SUBMANDIBULAR GLAND.

Following is the secretomotor pathway to submandibular gland:

$$\text{Superior salivatory nucleus}$$
$$\downarrow$$
$$\text{Sensory root of VII nerve}$$
$$\downarrow$$
$$\text{Chorda tympani nerve}$$
$$\downarrow$$
$$\text{Lingual nerve}$$
$$\downarrow$$
$$\text{Submandibular ganglion}$$
$$\downarrow$$
$$\text{Submandibular gland}$$

Q. SECRETOMOTOR PATHWAY TO LACRIMAL GLAND.

Following is the secretomotor pathway to lacrimal gland:

$$\text{Lacrimatory nucleus}$$
$$\downarrow$$
$$\text{Sensory root of VII nerve}$$
$$\downarrow$$
$$\text{Geniculate ganglion}$$
$$\downarrow$$
$$\text{Greater petrosal nerve}$$
$$\downarrow$$
$$\text{Nerve of pterygoid canal}$$
$$\downarrow$$
$$\text{Pterygopalatine ganglion}$$
$$\downarrow$$
$$\text{Zygomatic nerve}$$
$$\downarrow$$
$$\text{Zygomaticotemporal nerve}$$
$$\downarrow$$
$$\text{Communicating branch to lacrimal nerve}$$
$$\downarrow$$
$$\text{Lacrimal gland}$$

Q. TRIGEMINAL GANGLION

Trigeminal ganglion is also known as semilunar or Gasserian ganglion. This is the sensory ganglion of V cranial nerve, which is homologous with the dorsal root ganglion.

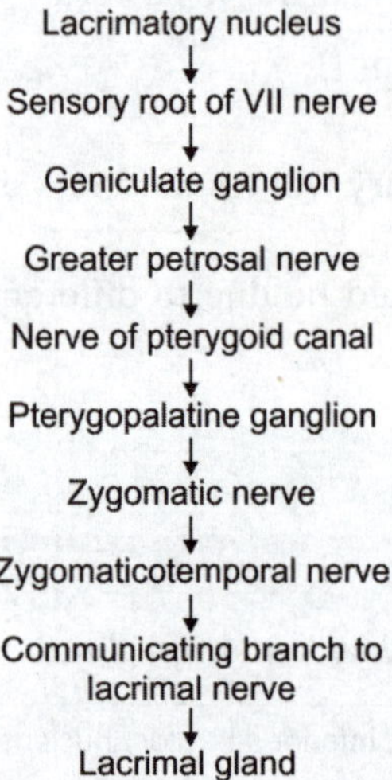
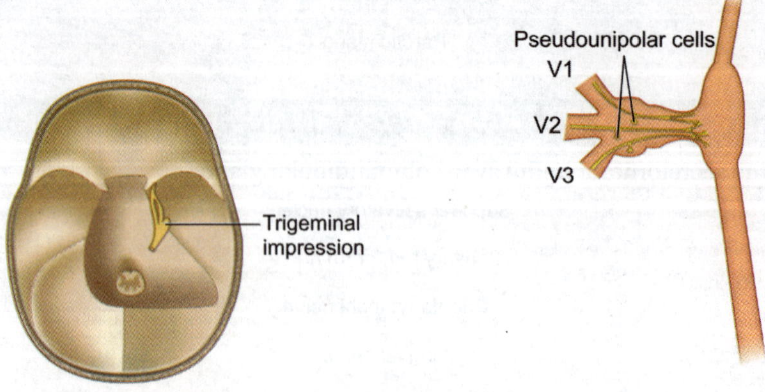

Trigeminal ganglion

Location

The ganglion lies on trigeminal impression, which is on the anterior surface of the apex of petrous temporal bone. It is enclosed in a dural pocket known as Meckel's cave.

Ganglion comprises of pseudounipolar cells, central processes of which form sensory root, which is attached to pons and peripheral processes form the three principal divisions of the trigeminal nerve (ophthalmic, maxillary, mandibular).

Relations

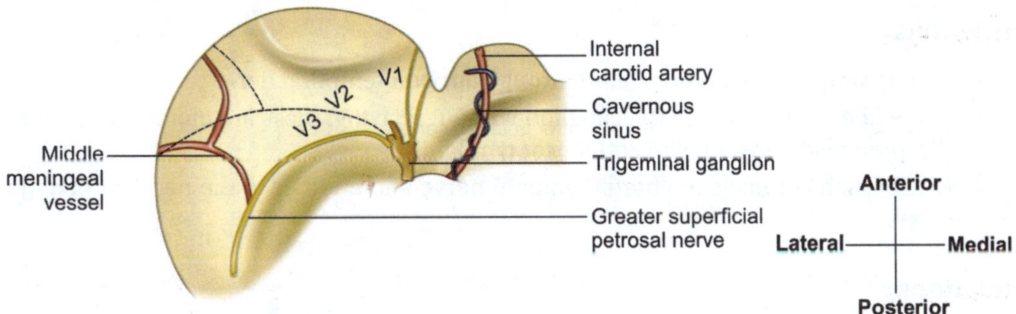

- Medially—internal carotid artery
- Laterally—middle meningeal artery
- Superiorly—parahippocampal gyrus
- Inferiorly—motor root of V cranial nerve.

Arterial Supply

Ganglion is supplied by adjacent arteries, i.e. internal carotid artery and middle meningeal artery.

Applied Anatomy

Ganglion lies at a depth of 5 cm from preauricular point, which needs to be approached in cases of intractable trigeminal neuralgia for injecting alcohol.

Q. OTIC GANGLION

Otic ganglion is peripheral parasympathetic ganglion, which serves to relay the secreto-motor fibers to parotid gland.

Located close to mandibular nerve, but functionally connected to IX cranial nerve.

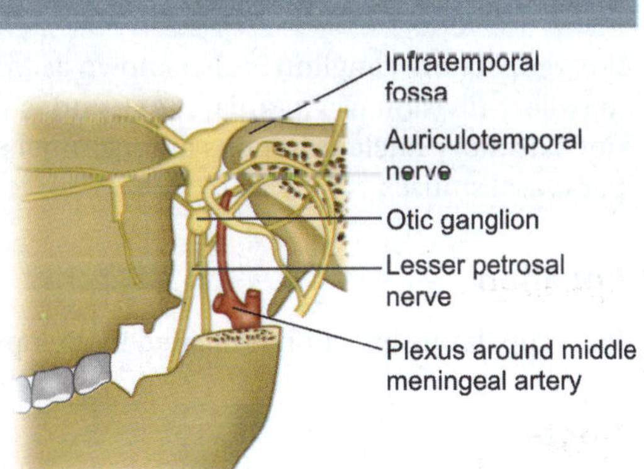

Size and Location

Otic ganglion is 2–3 mm in size and is located in infratemporal fossa, just below foramen ovale.

Connections

- Motor root of the ganglion is lesser petrosal nerve
- Sympathetic root is derived from the plexus on the middle meningeal artery
- Sensory root comes from auriculotemporal nerve.

Branches

- Mainly supplies the parotid gland through auriculotemporal nerve
- Some fibers only traverse the ganglion without relaying; these are motor nerves to medial pterygoid, tensor palati and tensor tympani
- One branch connects to chorda tympani nerve and another to the nerve of pterygoid canal.

Relations

- Laterally—mandibular nerve
- Medially—tensor palati muscle
- Posteriorly—middle meningeal artery
- Anteriorly—medial pterygoid muscle.

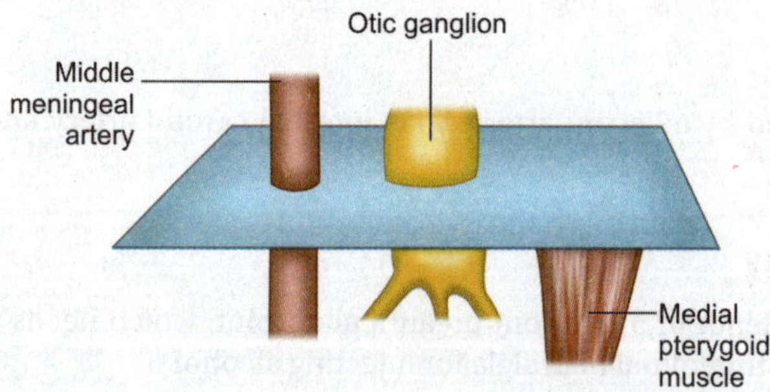

Q. PTERYGOPALATINE GANGLION

Pterygopalatine ganglion is also known as Meckel's ganglion. This ganglion is connected with maxillary division of V cranial nerve and is the parasympathetic relay station between superior salivatory nucleus in pons and lacrimal gland and mucous glands of the palate, nose and paranasal sinuses.

Location

Pterygopalatine ganglion is located in the upper part of pterygopalatine fossa.

Roots

1. Motor roots: The fibers leave the brainstem in nervus intermedius join the VII nerve and deviate from the geniculate ganglion as greater superficial petrosal nerve.

2. **Sympathetic roots:** The cell bodies are in superior cervical ganglion from which nerve fibers pass to the internal carotid plexus. It leaves the plexus as deep petrosal nerve and joins the greater superficial petrosal nerve to form nerve of pterygoid canal (Vidian nerve).

3. **Sensory root:** Comes from maxillary nerve.

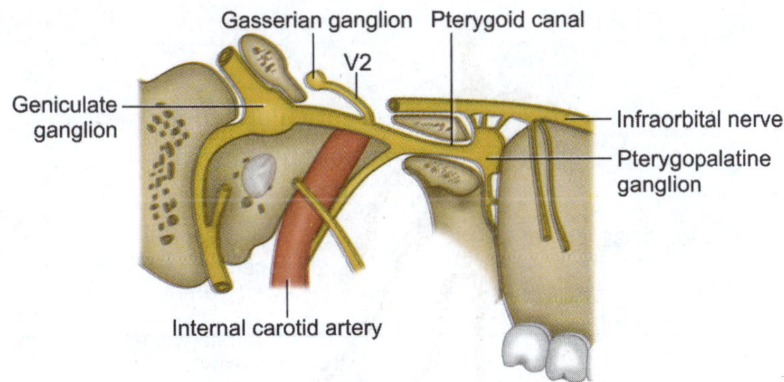

Connections of pterygopalatine ganglion

Branches

Branches to lacrimal gland through zygomaticotemporal branch of maxillary nerve and lacrimal branch of ophthalmic nerve:

- Orbital branches to periosteum of orbit
- Palatine nerves to the roof of mouth, soft palate, tonsil and nasal mucosa
- Nasal branches to anterior part of hard palate
- Pharyngeal branch to nasopharynx.

Q. STELLATE GANGLION

Stellate ganglion is a large ganglion formed by the fusion of lower two cervical segmental ganglion with first thoracic ganglion.

When not receiving contribution from thoracic mass it is known as inferior cervical ganglion.

Relations

- Stellate ganglion lies behind vertebral artery between first rib and transverse process of C7
- It is separated from cervical pleura by suprapleural membrane.

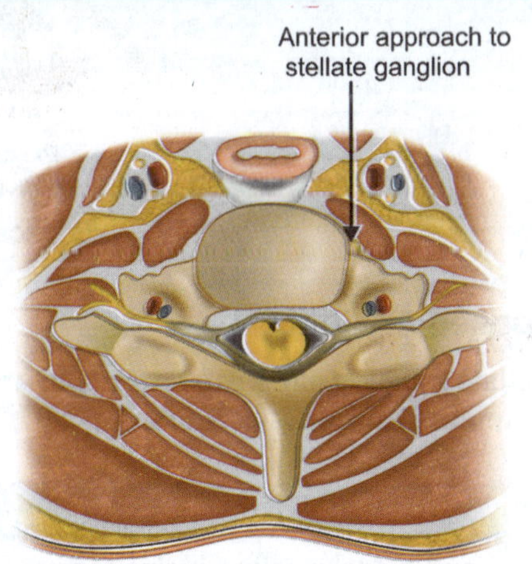

Branches

- It gives rise to gray rami communicantes to C7, C8, T1
- Contributes to the plexus around the subclavian artery and sympathetic supply to head and neck.

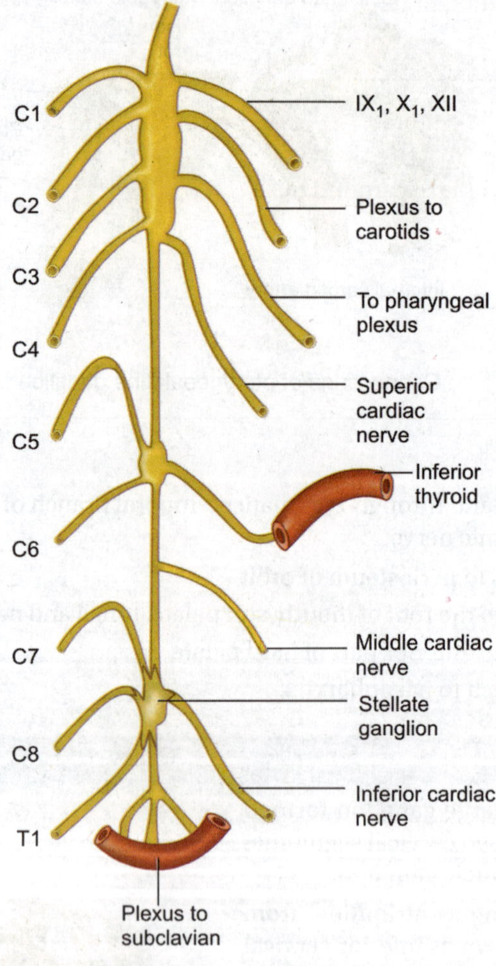

Cervical sympathetic chain

Applied Anatomy

Stellate ganglion block can be given by anterior approach. Stellate ganglion block will produce temporary Horner's syndrome.

Q.   SUBMANDIBULAR GANGLION

Submandibular ganglion is size of pinhead. It is situated on outer surface of hyoglossus muscle; suspended from lingual nerve.

Relations

- Lateral—submandibular gland
- Medial—hyoglossus muscle
- Above—lingual nerve
- Below—submandibular duct.

Roots

- Motor from chorda tympani
- Sensory from lingual
- Sympathetic from plexus around facial artery.

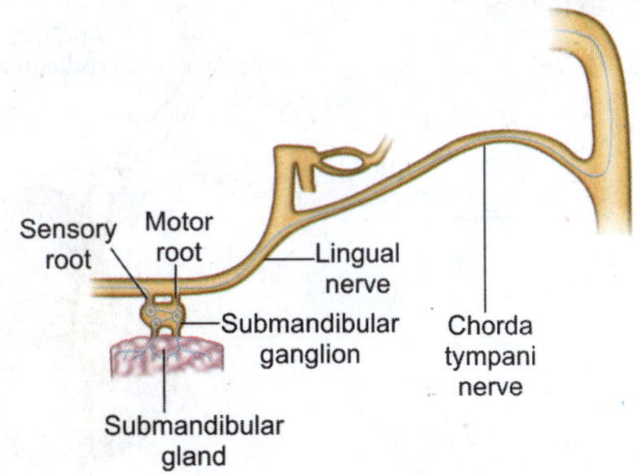

Branches

Submandibular ganglion hangs from the lingual nerve by two filaments and distributes fibers to submandibular gland and duct, to the sublingual gland, to the mucous membrane of mouth and tongue.

Q. ACOUSTIC PATHWAY

Acoustic pathway is as follows:

Auditory receptors
(hair cells of organ of
Corti in cochlea)
↓
Spiral ganglion
↓ Central processes
Coohloar nuoloi
↓
Trapezoid body
↓
Superior olivary complex
↓
Lateral lemniscus
↓
Nucleus of lateral lemniscus
↓
Inferior colliculus
↓
Medial geniculate body
↓ Auditory radiations
Auditory cortex

Acoustic pathway

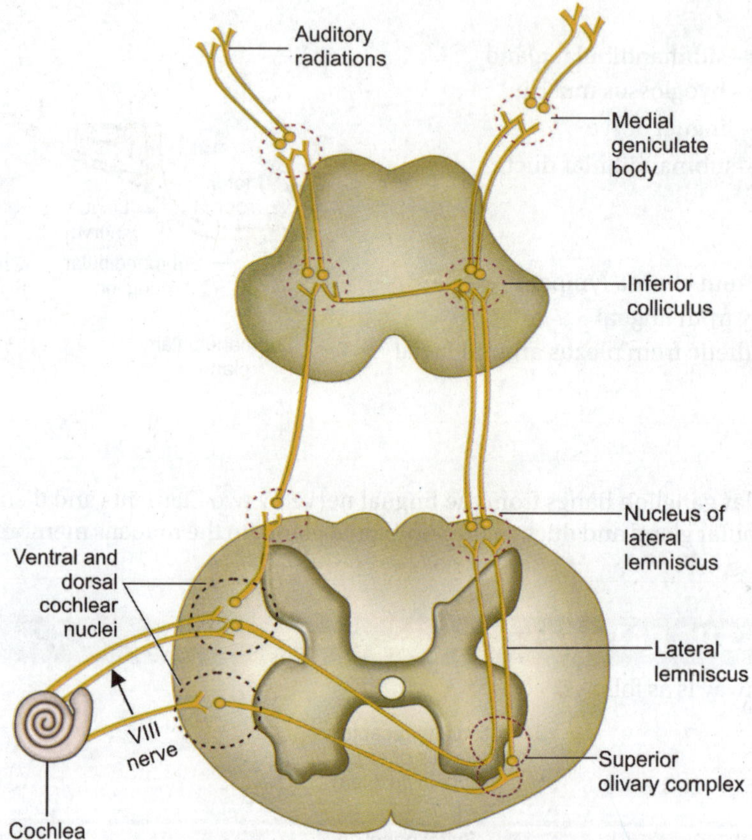

Acoustic pathway diagram

Applied Anatomy

BERA means brainstem evoked response audiometry wherein electrical responses in cochlear nuclei and central connections are recorded for early detection of deafness.

Seven waves are recorded in BERA. It is a non-invasive technique to detect the integrity of auditory pathway.

Waves	Site
I	Vestibulocochlear nerve
II	Cochlear nuclei
III	Superior olivary complex
IV	Lateral lemniscus
V	Inferior colliculus
VI	Medial geniculate body
VII	Auditory radiations

Q. GALEN'S ANASTOMOSIS

The internal branch of superior laryngeal nerve ends by anastomosing with an ascending branch of recurrent laryngeal nerve. This loop is Galen's anastomosis and is purely sensory.

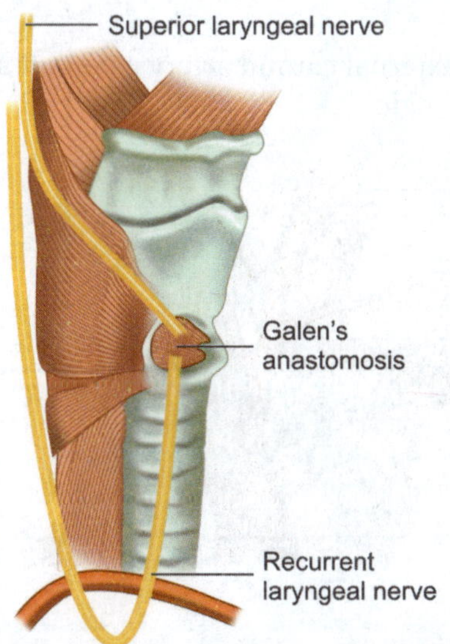

Q. FREY SYNDROME

Frey syndrome is also known as auriculo-temporal nerve syndrome. In this condition, there is redness and sweating of the skin over the parotid region, while having food.

It follows parotid surgeries or temporo-mandibular joint surgeries or direct injury.

Anatomical Basis of Frey Syndrome

After injury, during regeneration auriculo-temporal nerve gets aberrantly connected to branches from superior cervical ganglion, i.e. a parasympathetic nerve gets connected to sympathetic nerve.

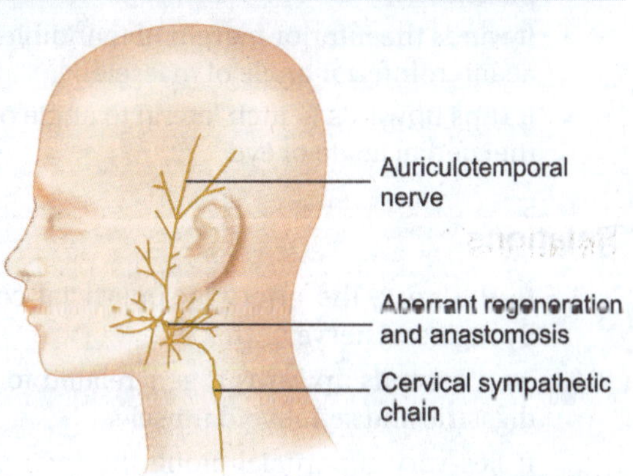

Thus, whenever parasympathetic component, i.e. secretomotor pathway gets stimulated during mastication sympathetic fibers also gets stimulated. Hence, the patient complains of sweating and redness on face, while chewing.

▶ ARTERY

Q. FACIAL ARTERY

Facial artery is one of the tortuous artery of the body others being uterine artery, lingual artery and splenic artery. It is tortuous to adapt to the movements of pharynx during swallowing and on the face to adapt to the movements of mandible, lips and cheeks.

Origin

Facial artery is a branch of external carotid artery given off above the tip of greater horn of hyoid bone in the carotid triangle.

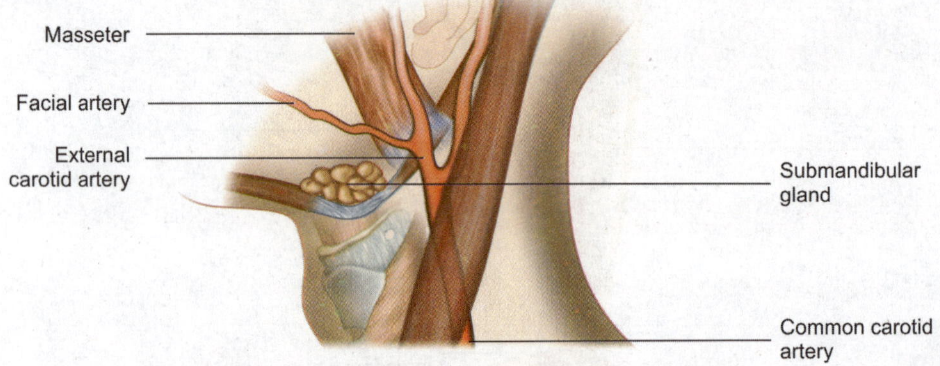

Course and Termination

- From its origin it arches upwards and forms a loop around the submandibular gland posteriorly
- It winds the inferior margin of mandible after crossing the submandibular region to lie, at anteroinferior angle of masseter
- It runs upwards ½ inch lateral to angle of mouth, by the side of the nose to terminate at the medial angle of eye.

Relations

1. In the neck, the artery is superficial covered only by skin, platysma and crossed by hypoglossal nerve.
2. As it ascends upwards it gets related to submandibular gland posteriorly, lies deep to digastric and stylohyoid muscle.
3. It lies very superficial along the inferior border of mandible, where it can be easily palpated.
4. On the face it is covered by skin, fat of the cheek and facial muscles. Buccinator and levator anguli oris lie deep to it.
5. At its termination, it lies embedded in levator labii superioris alaeque nasi.
6. The facial vein lies posterior to the artery and has a straight course, while the branches of the facial nerve cross over the artery.

Branches

The branches of facial artery can be broadly divided into cervical and facial.

Cervical	Facial
Ascending palatine	Inferior labial
Tonsillar	Superior labial
Glandular	Lateral nasal
Submental	

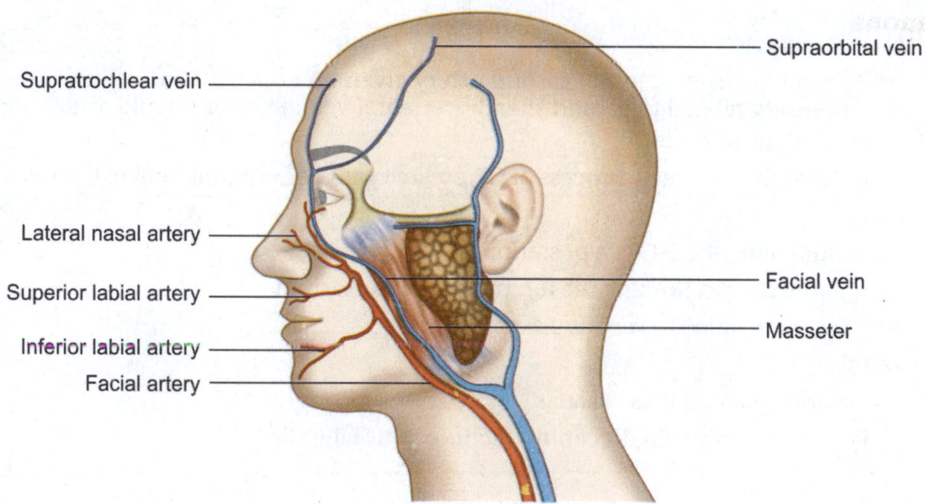

Applied Anatomy

- Rich vascularity of face causes blushing
- Wounds of the face bleed profusely, but also heal rapidly due to rich blood supply of the face.

Q. VERTEBRAL ARTERY

Vertebral artery is one of the principal arteries supplying the brain.

Origin

Vertebral artery is a branch of first part of subclavian artery.

Course

Vertebral artery is divided into following four parts:

- Part I—from its origin to C6
- Part II—from C6 to C1 is transverse process
- Part III—it lies on the posterior arch of atlas in suboccipital triangle
- Part IV—it extends from suboccipital triangle to lower border of pons.

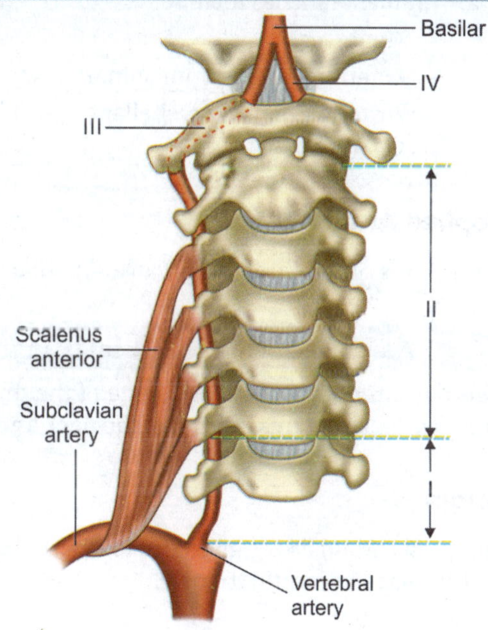

Relations

- Part I:
  - Anteriorly related to carotid sheath, vertebral vein, inferior thyroid artery, thoracic duct on the left side
  - Posteriorly transverse process of C7, stellate ganglion, ventral rami of C7, C8.
- Part II:
  - Ventral rami of C2–C6 lie posterior to the artery
  - II part traverses through the foramina transversarium
  - It is accompanied by venous plexus.
- Part III:
  - Anteriorly lateral mass of atlas
  - Posteriorly semispinalis capitis, rectus capitis lateralis.
- Part IV:
  - It ascends in front of the root of hypoglossal nerve.

Branches

Branches of vertebral artery can be broadly divided into cervical and cranial branches:

1. Cervical branches are divided into:
   - Spinal supplying the spinal cord
   - Muscular supplying the muscles of suboccipital triangle.
2. Cranial branches include:
   - Meningeal
   - Anterior and posterior spinal
   - Posterior inferior cerebellar
   - Medullary.

Applied Anatomy

Thrombosis of vertebral artery causes medial medullary syndrome.

Q. EXTERNAL CAROTID ARTERY

External carotid artery (ECA) is one of the terminal branches of common carotid artery and supplies the structures in front of the neck and face.

Origin

Common carotid artery gives rise to external carotid artery at the level of upper border of thyroid cartilage in carotid triangle.

Course and Relations

- From its origin it runs upwards under the cover of sternocleidomastoid and crossed superficially by VII and XII cranial nerves
- Above it lies within the parotid gland sandwiched between retromandibular vein and facial nerve
- It terminates behind the neck of the mandible into superficial temporal and maxillary arteries.

Mnemonics	Branches
Sister	Superior thyroid
Lucy's	Lingual
Powdered	Posterior auricular
Face	Facial
Often	Occipital
Attracts	Ascending pharyngeal
Medical	Maxillary
Students	Superficial temporal

Anterior	Posterior	Terminal
• Superior thyroid • Lingual	• Occipital • Posterior auricular • Facial	• Maxillary • Superficial temporal

- Superior thyroid branch is given off just below the level of greater cornu of hyoid bone
- Lingual branch is given off opposite to the tip of greater cornu of hyoid bone
- Facial branch is given off just above the tip of greater cornu of hyoid bone
- Occipital and posterior auricular branches are related to posterior belly of digastric.

Applied Anatomy

The ECA ligation is done in cases of severe tonsillar bleeding and severe epistaxis.

Q. CENTRAL ARTERY OF RETINA

Central artery of retina is a classic example of end artery.

Origin

Central artery of retina is a branch of ophthalmic artery.

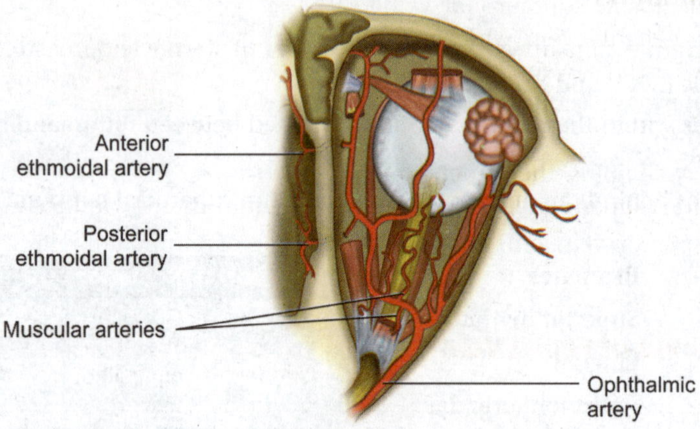

Course and Relations

- It is the first and small branch of ophthalmic artery, which begins below the optic nerve and is within its dural sheath
- About 1.25 cm behind the eye it enters the nerve and then lies at the inferomedial surface and runs toward the retina.

The central retinal artery occupies the aperture in lamina cribrosa.

Branches

Central retinal artery divided into two equal branches—superior and inferior, which further divide into superior and inferior nasal, and superior and inferior temporal branches. The arteries supply the respective quadrants of retina.

Applied Anatomy

- Central retinal vessels can be visualized by doing ophthalmoscopy
- Blockage in the retinal artery causes loss of vision, since it is an end artery.

▶ VEIN

Q. VENOUS DRAINAGE OF THE FACE (DANGER AREA OF FACE).

Lower part of nose, philtrum and upper lip are considered as the 'danger area of face' because infections in these regions lead to cavernous sinus thrombosis.

Anatomical Basis

Venous blood of the face finally drains into cavernous sinus. Following is the venous drainage of the face.

- Supratrochlear and supraorbital vein unite to form angular vein, which continues below as facial vein, to join below with anterior division of retromandibular vein

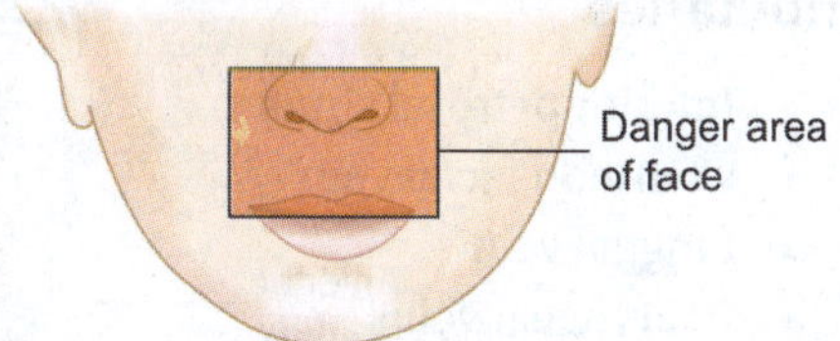

- Maxillary vein joins the superficial vein to form retromandibular vein, which divides into anterior and posterior
- Posterior auricular vein joins the posterior division of retromandibular vein to form external jugular vein.

Deep Connections of Facial Vein

- It communicates with superior ophthalmic vein through supraorbital vein
- Deep facial vein drains into pterygoid plexus of veins, which in turn drains into cavernous sinus.

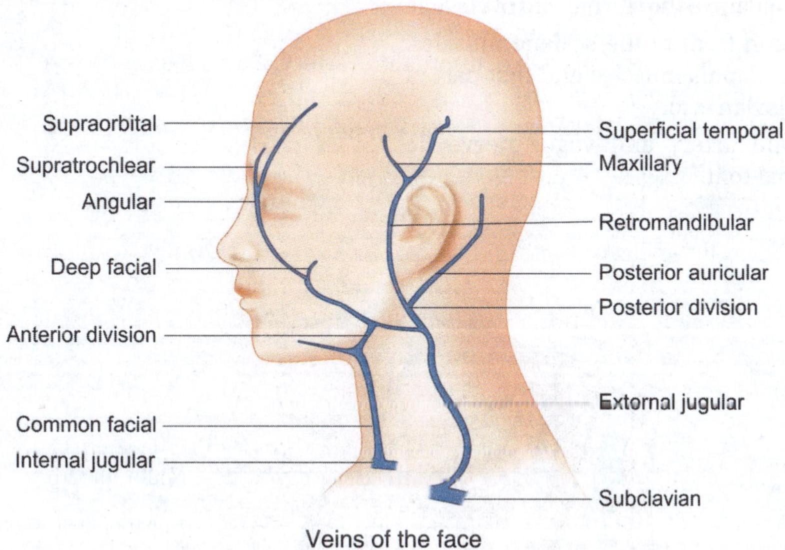

Veins of the face

Applied Anatomy

Furunculosis in the danger area of face should be treated aggressively with antibiotics to avert cavernous sinus thrombosis.

Q. INTERNAL JUGULAR VEIN

Internal jugular vein (IJV) is the prime venous channel in the neck within the carotid sheath.

Origin

Internal jugular vein is the direct continuation of sigmoid sinus at the jugular foramen. The origin is marked by 'superior bulb', which lies in the jugular fossa.

Tributaries

- Inferior petrosal sinus
- Common facial vein
- Lingual vein
- Pharyngeal veins
- Superior thyroid vein
- Middle thyroid vein
- Thoracic duct
- Oblique jugular vein.

Course and Relations

- Internal jugular vein courses vertically downwards behind the sternocleido-mastoid up to the sternal end of clavicle
- It lies in front of the scalene muscles, rectus capitis muscles and first part of subclavian artery
- Carotid artery and vagus nerve lie medial to it.

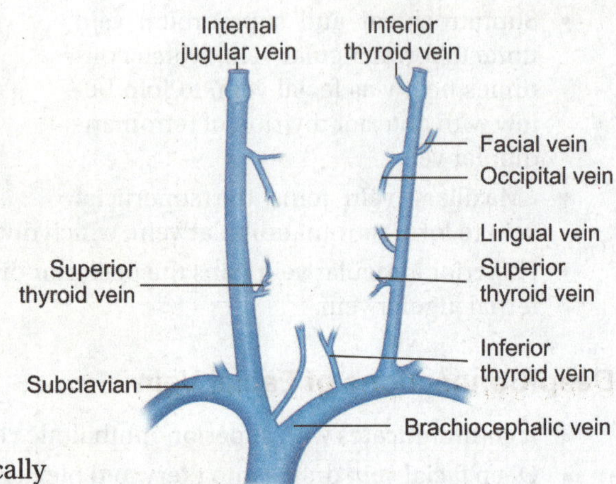

Tributaries of internal jugular vein

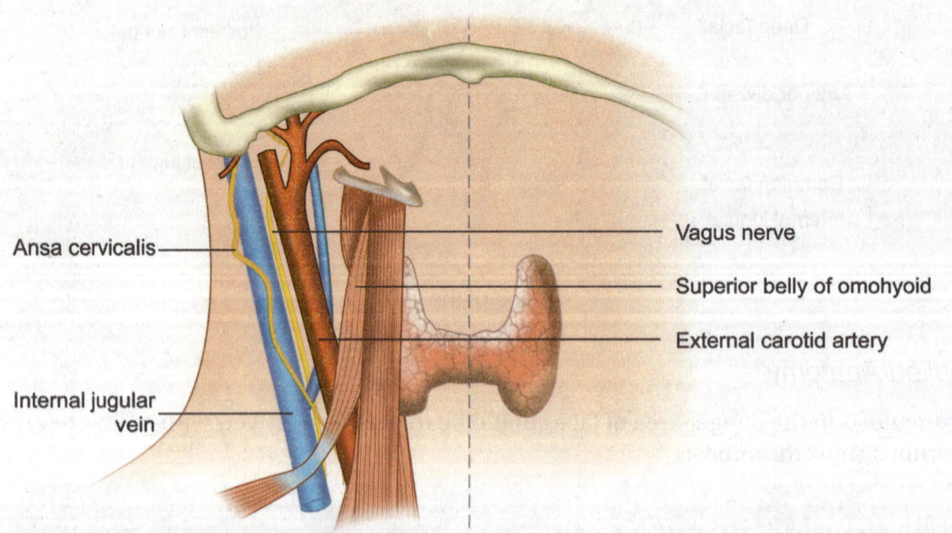

Termination

Internal jugular vein terminates behind the sternal end of clavicle by joining the subclavian vein to form brachiocephalic vein. It is marked by 'inferior bulb'.

Applied Anatomy

- It is used for recording venous pulse tracings
- In cardiac failure IJV is markedly dilated and engorged
- Jugular venous thrombosis may occur secondary to sigmoid sinus thrombosis in ear infections
- In radical neck dissection IJV is removed along with sternocleidomastoid and XI cranial nerve.

Q. CAVERNOUS SINUS (DIAGRAM ONLY)

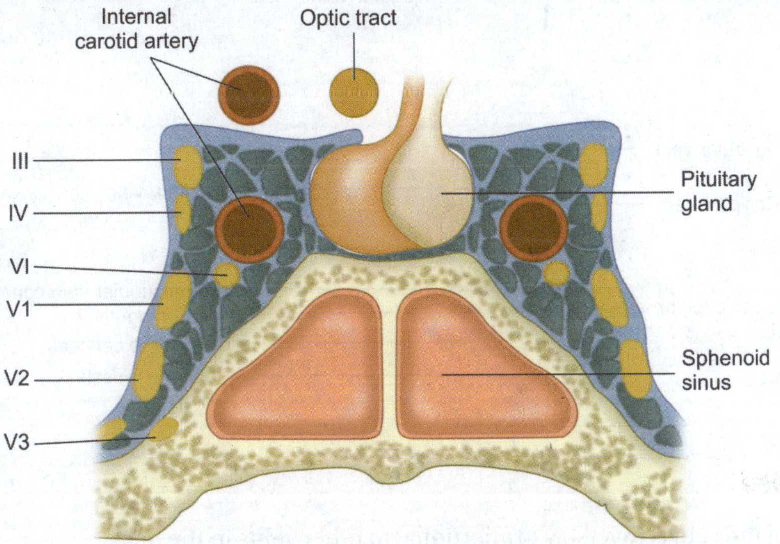

Cavernous sinus relations

Q. EXTERNAL JUGULAR VEIN

External jugular vein (EJV) by, and large drains the scalp and the face.

Formation

External jugular vein is formed by the union of posterior division of retromandibular vein and posterior auricular vein near the mandibular angle.

Course and Relations

- It runs obliquely and superficial to sternocleidomastoid up to the subclavian triangle to end in subclavian vein
- It is covered by skin, superficial fascia and platysma and lies in front of deep cervical fascia
- It lies parallel with the great auricular nerve, ascending posterior to its upper half.

Tributaries

- Retromandibular vein
- Posterior auricular vein
- Posterior external jugular vein
- Transverse cervical vein
- Suprascapular vein
- Anterior jugular vein
- Internal jugular vein
- Occipital vein (sometimes).

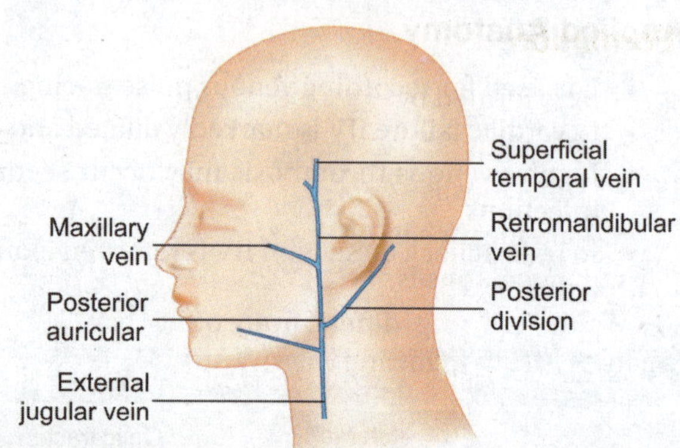

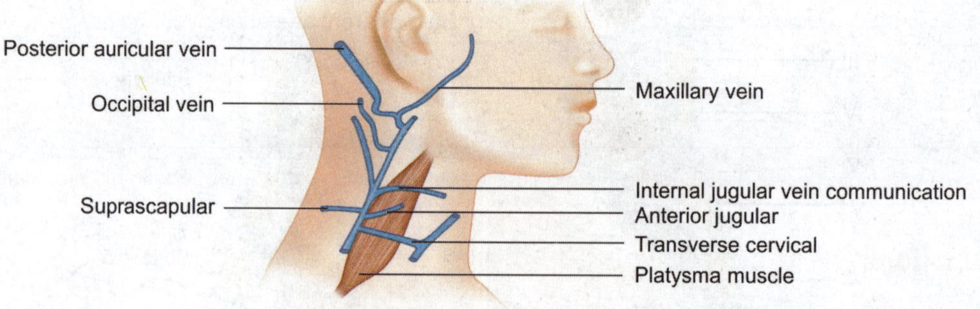

Peculiarities

- Size of the vein is inversely proportional to other veins in the neck
- It has valves at its termination into subclavian vein
- It is dilated 4 cm above the clavicle and is known as sinus
- The valves do not prevent regurgitation.

Applied Anatomy

- EJV gets distended by expiring against resistance (Valsalva maneuver)
- Division of EJV may give rise to air embolism and death, since the vein lies outside the axillary sheath and prevented from retraction.

▶ LYMPH NODES

Q. WALDEYER'S RING

Waldeyer's ring is an aggregation of lymphoid tissue at the junction of upper respiratory and upper digestive tract.

Formation

The ring is formed by:

- Adenoids
- Tubal tonsils
- Palatine tonsils
- Lingual tonsils.

Waldeyer's ring differs from other lymphatic tissue in following ways:

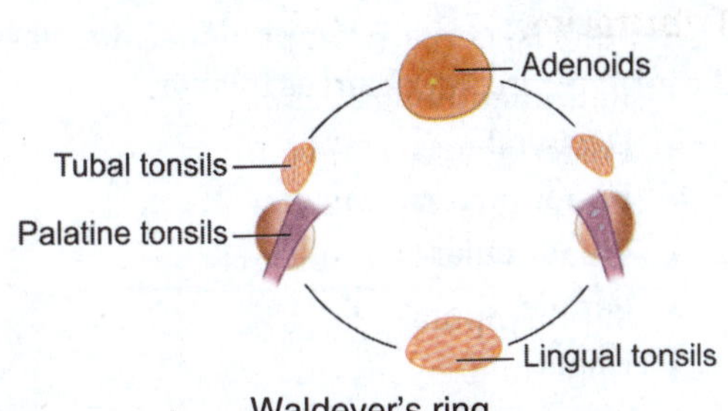

Waldeyer's ring	Lymph nodes
Situated at the junction of upper aerodigestive tract	Grouped according to the region
No afferent channels	Both afferent and efferent channels
No capsule	Capsulated
Crypts present	Crypts absent
Growth curve present	Growth curve absent
No division into cortex and medulla histologically	Divided into cortex and medulla histologically

Functions

- Helps in maintaining body immunity
- Protects the lower respiratory tract.

Q. SUPERFICIAL CERVICAL LYMPH NODES.

There are approximately 800 lymph nodes in the body out of which 300 are in the neck.

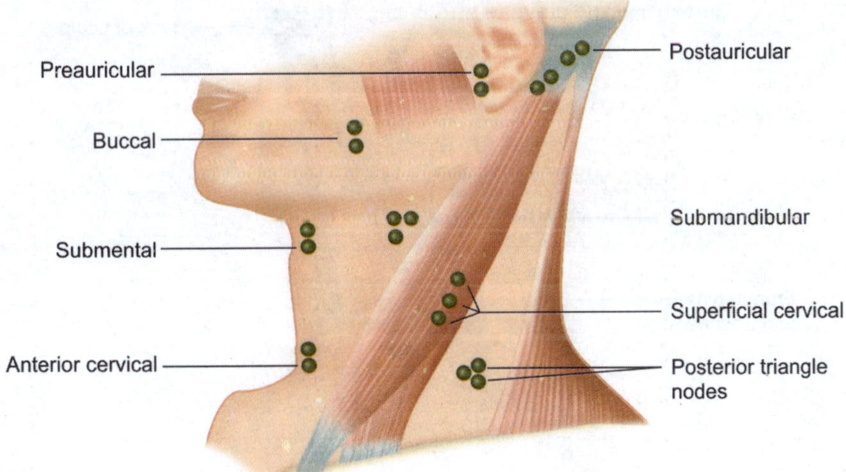

Grouping of cervical lymph nodes

Superficial cervical lymph nodes are classified according to the region they are present in the form of circular chain as follows:

- Occipital
- Posterior auricular
- Preauricular
- Parotid
- Facial
- Submandibular
- Submental
- Superficial cervical
- Anterior cervical.

Drainage Area

1. Occipital drains the back of the scalp.
2. Posterior auricular drains the temporal region, back of the pinna, external auditory meatus.
3. Preauricular drains the outer side of pinna and side of scalp.
4. Parotid nodes located in the substance of the gland drain the eyelids, front of scalp, external auditory meatus and tympanic cavity, while the nodes deep to the gland drain the nasopharynx and nose.
5. Superficial facial nodes receive lymph from conjunctiva, eyelids, nose and cheek. Deep facial nodes drain the temporal fossa, infratemporal fossa, back of the nose and pharynx.
6. Submandibular nodes drain the side of the nose, cheek, angle of eye and mouth, upper lip, gums and side of tongue.
7. Submental nodes drain the central part of the lower lip and floor of the mouth.

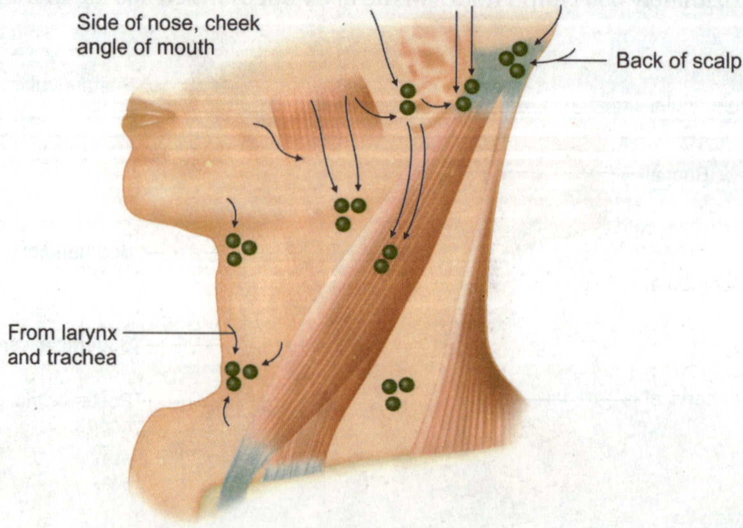

Drainage areas of cervical lymph nodes

8. Superficial cervical nodes drain the parotid region and the lower part of the ear.
9. Anterior cervical nodes drain the larynx and thyroid.

All the superficial lymph nodes drain into deep cervical lymph nodes.

Applied Anatomy

1. Malignancies are staged according to the involvement of the lymph nodes.
2. In radical neck dissections lymph nodes are cleared according to the level of involvement. Following are the levels of lymph nodes:
   - Level I—submental and submandibular nodes
   - Level II—upper cervical nodes
   - Level III—middle cervical nodes
   - Level IV—lower cervical nodes
   - Level V—posterior triangle nodes
   - Level VI—pretracheal and prelaryngeal nodes
   - Level VII—mediastinal nodes.

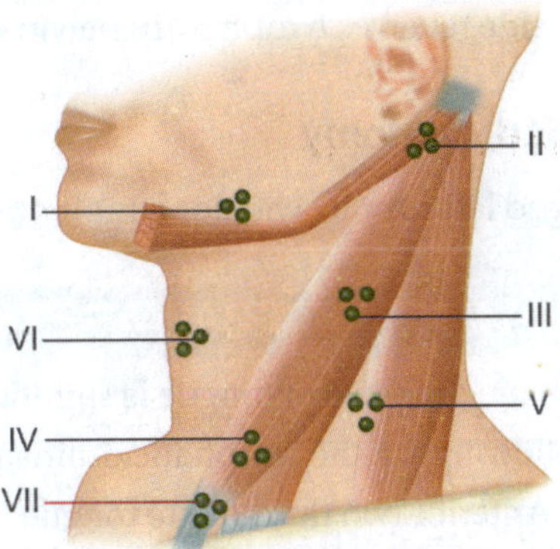

Levels of lymph nodes (surgically)

Q. DEEP CERVICAL LYMPH NODES.

All the deep cervical lymph nodes receive lymph from superficial cervical lymph nodes.

Location

Deep cervical lymph nodes form a vertical chain along the internal jugular vein.

Classification

Deep cervical lymph nodes are grouped as jugulodigastric, jugulo-omohyoid and supraclavicular lymph nodes.

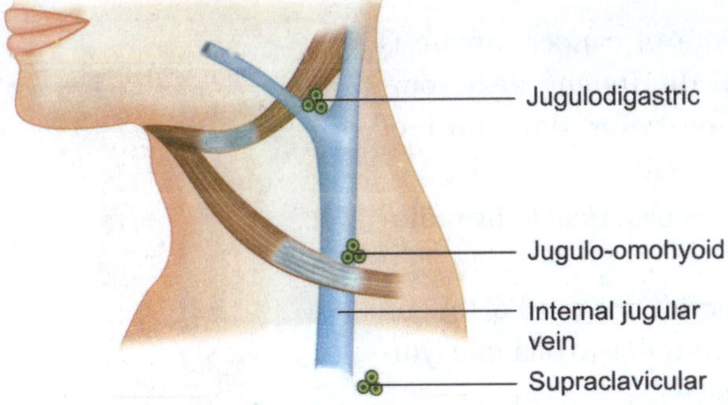

Deep cervical lymph nodes

Drainage Area

- Jugulodigastric nodes mainly drain the tonsils
- Jugulo-omohyoid mainly drains the tongue
- Supraclavicular lymph nodes receive the lymph from preceding nodes. Additionally, left side receives lymph from pelvic viscera (ovaries, testis) and breast.

Applied Anatomy

Enlarged left supraclavicular lymph nodes are known as Virchow's nodes.

Q. LYMPHATIC DRAINAGE OF TONGUE.

Lymphatic drainage of tongue is significant since cancer tongue is common in India.

Following are the lymphatic drainage of tongue:

- Anterior two third of the tongue (both halves) drains into submandibular nodes
- Tip of the tongue drains into submental nodes
- Posterior one third of the tongue drains into jugulo-omohyoid nodes bilaterally.

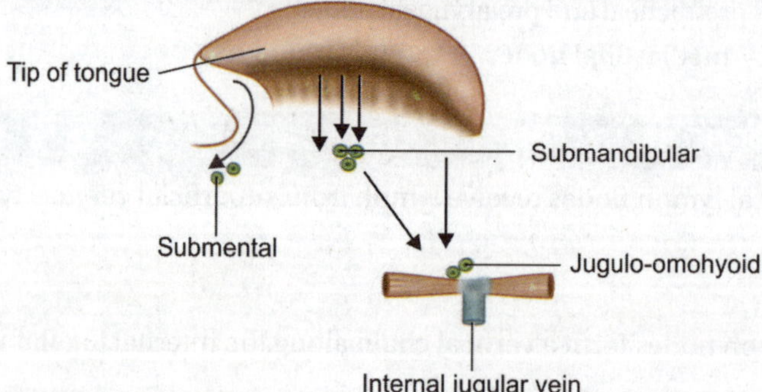

All the lymph from the tongue finally drains into jugulo-omohyoid node. Hence, it is known as lymph node of the tongue.

Applied Anatomy

- Commonest site of cancer tongue is lateral side of the tongue next common site is posterior one third of tongue
- Cancer tongue is best treated by radiotherapy
- Cancer of posterior one third of tongue is more dangerous due to bilateral lymphatic drainage.

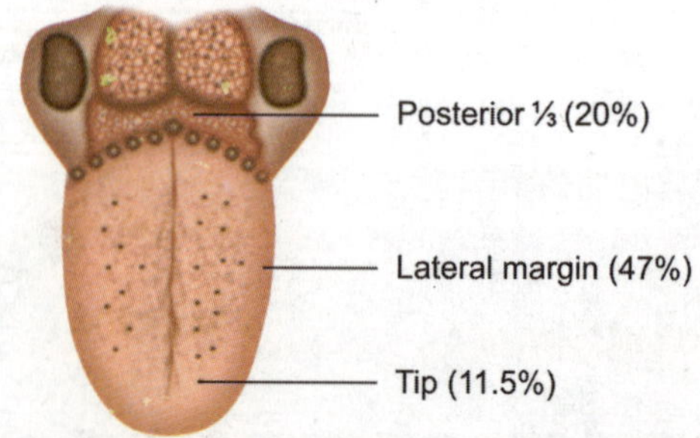

▶ JOINT

Q. ATLANTO-OCCIPITAL JOINT

Types of atlanto-occipital joint synovial joint, ellipsoid variety.

Articular Surfaces

- From above—occipital condyles
- From below—superior articular facets of atlas vertebra.

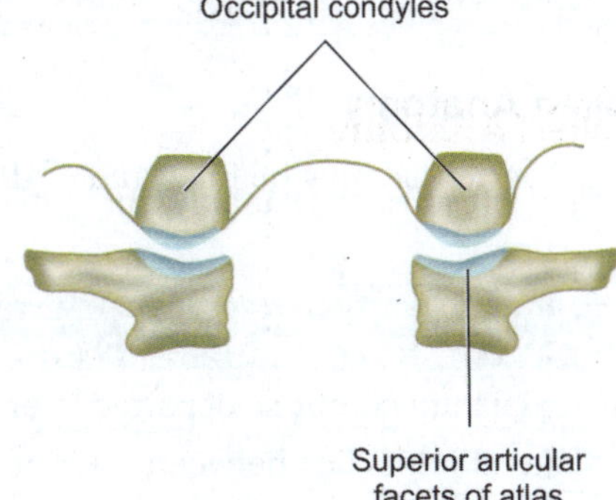

Ligaments

Fibrous capsule: It surrounds the articular surfaces. It is thick posterolaterally and thin anteromedially.

Anterior atlanto-occipital membrane: It extends from anterior margin of foramen magnum above to the upper border of anterior arch of atlas. It is reinforced anteriorly by anterior longitudinal ligament.

Posterior atlanto-occipital membrane: It extends from posterior margin of foramen magnum above to the upper border of posterior arch of atlas.

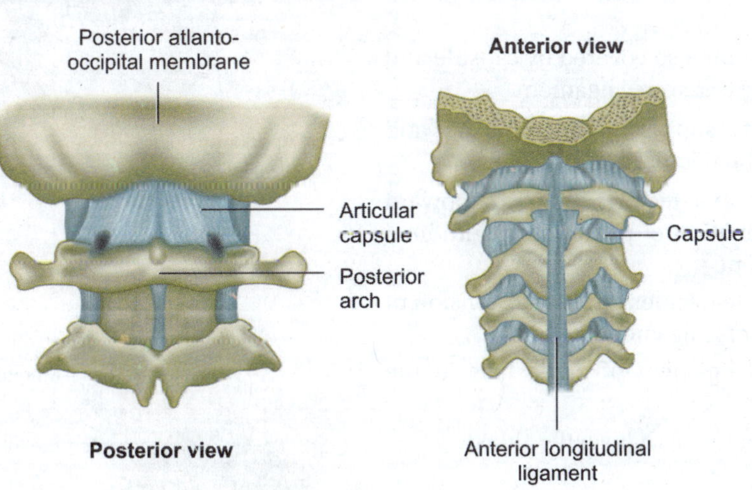

Nerve Supply

First cervical spinal nerve.

Blood Supply

Vertebral artery.

Action

'Yes' movement, i.e. flexion and extension occurs at this joint:

- Flexion—longus capitis, rectus capitis anterior
- Extension—rectus capitis posterior major and minor, superior oblique, semispinalis capitis, splenius capitis.

Applied Anatomy

Cervical vertebrae may be fractured or dislocated by a fall on the head with acute flexion of neck.

Q. ATLANTOAXIAL JOINT

Atlantoaxial joint comprise of paired lateral joints and a median single joint:

1. Lateral joints lies between inferior facets of atlas and superior facets of axis; they are plane joints.
2. Median joint lies between the dens, anterior arch and transverse ligament of atlas.

Ligaments

Lateral joint is covered by capsule all over, anterior longitudinal ligament and ligamentum flavum.

Median joint also covered by capsule and reinforced by transverse ligament.

Ligaments supporting atlantoaxial and atlanto-occipital joints are:

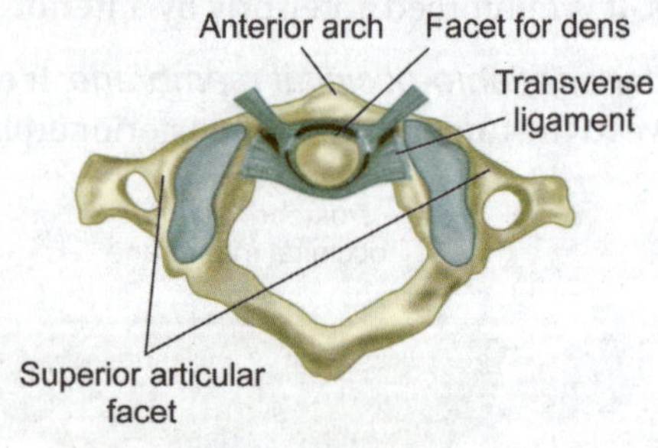

1. Membrana tectoria: It is an upward continuation of posterior longitudinal ligament.
2. Cruciate ligament: It is an extension of transverse ligament.
3. Apical ligament of dens: It is in the center.
4. Alar ligament: It is on the sides.

Nerve Supply

First and second cervical spinal nerve.

Blood Supply

Vertebral artery.

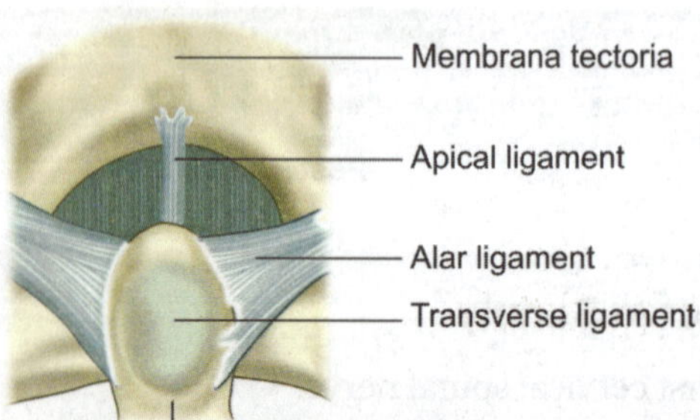

Atlantoaxial joint

Action

'No' movement, i.e. rotatory movements occurs at these joints. Rotatory movements are brought about by obliquus capitis inferior, rectus capitis posterior major and splenius capitis.

Applied Anatomy

- Death by hanging is due to dislocation of dens following rupture of transverse ligament
- Neck abscesses can cause attritional changes in transverse ligament causing dislocation of atlas or axis (Grisel's syndrome)
- Cervical spondylosis leads to degenerative changes in intervertebral disk, causing disk prolapse.

Q. SPHENOMANDIBULAR LIGAMENT

Sphenomandibular ligament is an accessory ligament of temporomandibular joint. It is a remnant of Meckel's cartilage.

Attachments

- Above: Spine of sphenoid
- Below: Lingula of mandibular foramen.

Relations

- Laterally: Lateral pterygoid, auriculotemporal nerve, maxillary artery, inferior alveolar nerve and vessels
- Medially: Medial pterygoid, chorda tympani nerve, pharynx.

It is pierced by mylohyoid nerve and vessels.

Q. STYLOMANDIBULAR LIGAMENT

Stylomandibular ligament is also an accessory ligament of temporomandibular joint. It represents the thickened portion of deep cervical fascia.

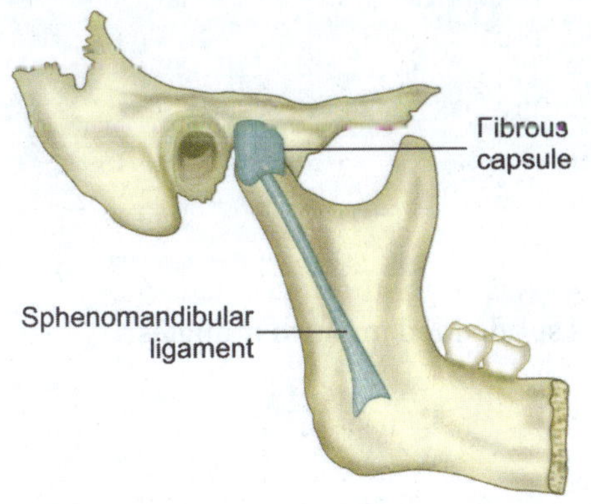

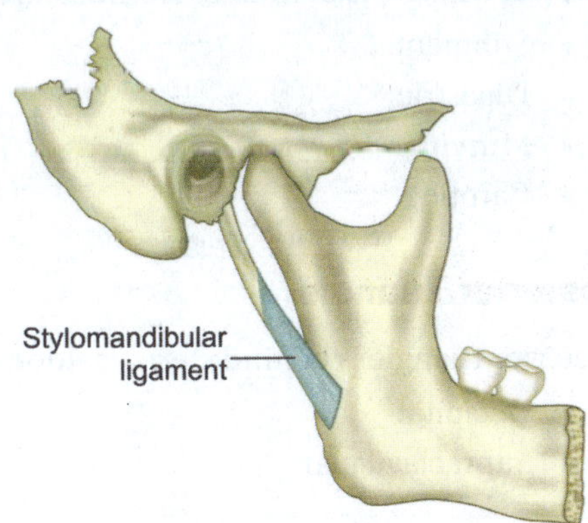

Attachments

- Above—lateral surface of styloid process
- Below—ramus of mandible.

▶ **MISCELLANEOUS**

Q. AURICLE (DIAGRAM ONLY)

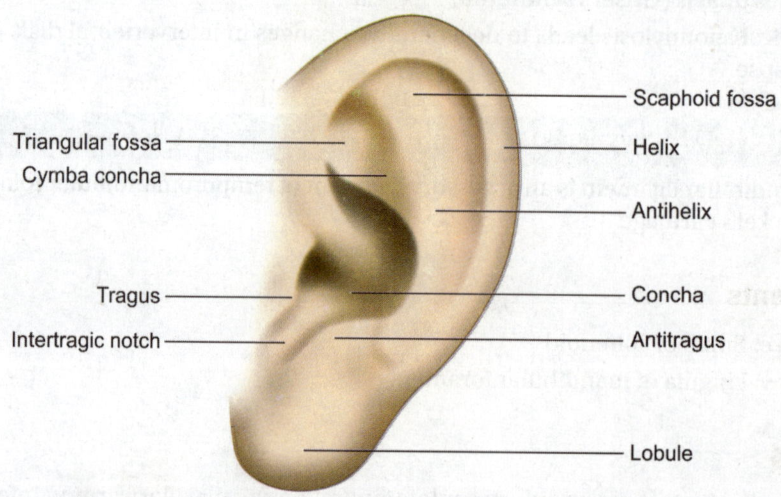

Q. FORMATION OF THE TRIANGLES OF THE NECK.

For study purposes, the neck region is divided into triangular areas. Sternocleidomastoid is the key muscle of the neck region dividing it into anterior and posterior triangles.

Anterior Triangle

Anterior triangle is in front of sternocleidomastoid and subdivided into four triangles:

- Submental
- Digastric
- Muscular
- Carotid.

Posterior Triangle

Posterior triangle is behind sternocleidomastoid and subdivided into two triangles:

- Occipital
- Supraclavicular.

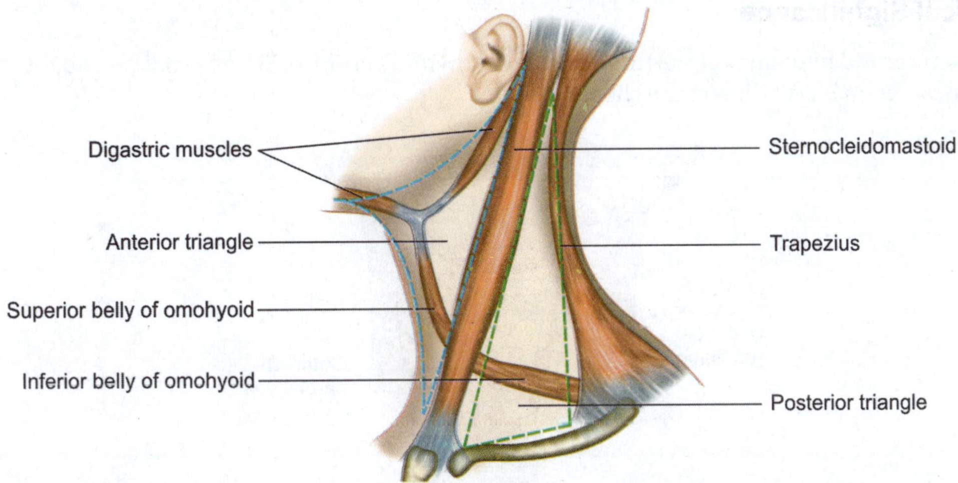

Q. CAROTID SHEATH

Carotid sheath is a condensation of fibroareolar tissue around the great vessels of the neck. It is derived from all the three layers of deep cervical fascia (investing layer, pretracheal layer and prevertebral layer).

Contents

Carotid sheath encloses the following structures:
- Common carotid artery with its bifurcation
- Internal jugular vein
- Vagus nerve.

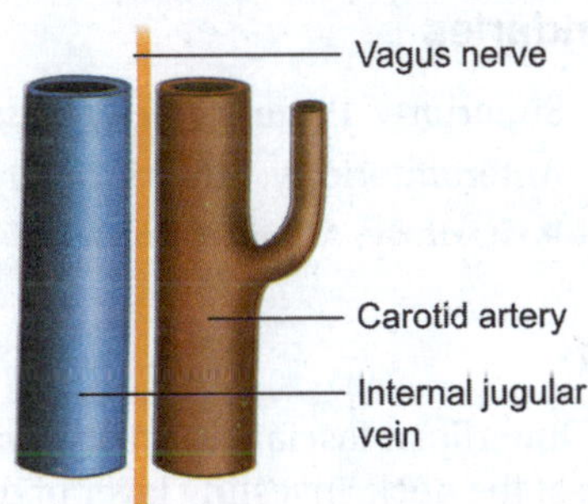

Relations

- Anteriorly—ansa cervicalis
- Posteriorly—sympathetic chain.

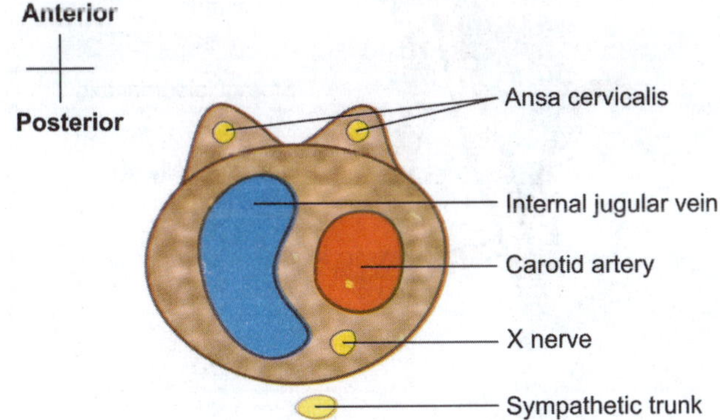

Surgical Significance

Common carotid bifurcates at the upper border of thyroid cartilage. For external carotid artery ligation, surgeon has to dissect the sheath.

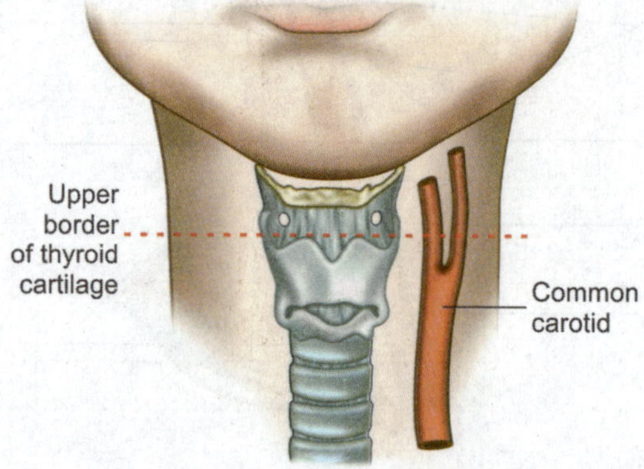

Q. CAROTID TRIANGLE

Carotid triangle is an area on the lateral side of the neck.

Boundaries

- Superiorly: Posterior belly of digastric
- Anteroinferiorly: Superior belly of omohyoid
- Posteriorly: Anterior border of sternocleidomastoid.

Roof

Skin, superficial fascia with platysma, cervical branch of facial nerve, transverse cutaneous nerve of the neck. Investing layer of deep cervical fascia.

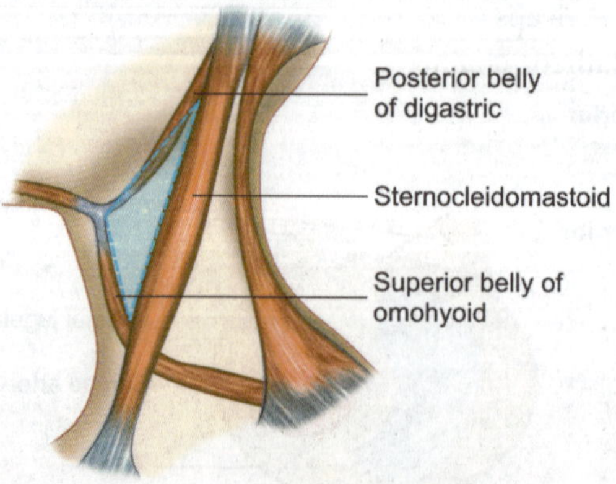

Floor

Constrictors of pharynx. Thyrohyoid membrane and muscle, hyoglossus muscle.

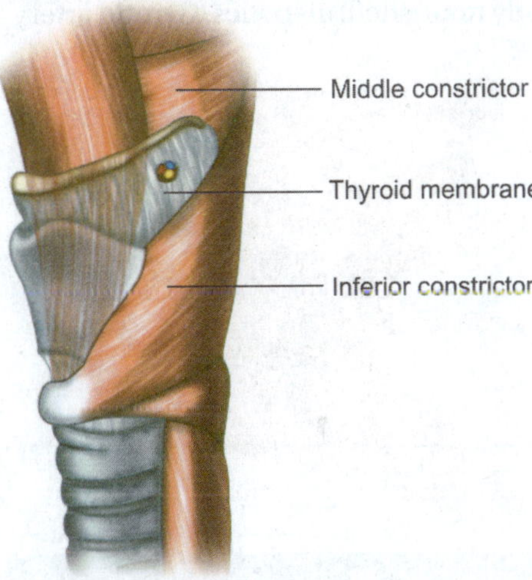

Floor of carotid triangle

Contents

Carotid artery with bifurcation and its five branches (facial, lingual, ascending pharyngeal, superior thyroid, occipital).

Internal jugular vein with its tributaries (common facial vein, superior thyroid vein and lingual vein) and X, XI, XII nerves.

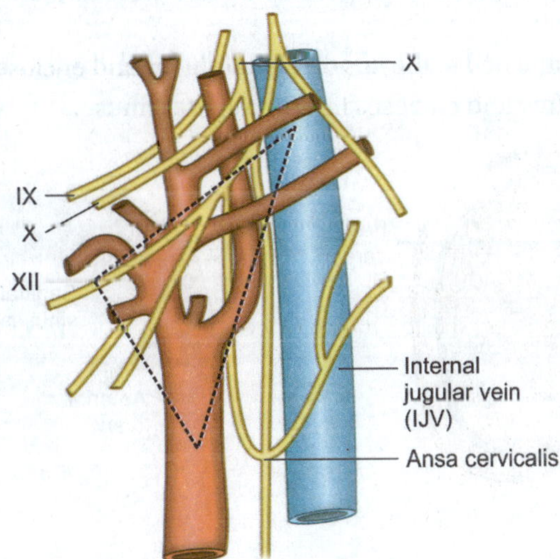

Surgical Significance

Carotid artery should be protected in any patient whose skin wound is likely to get infected; like in patients who are poorly nourished, diabetics. Carotid artery can be protected by rotating the levator scapulae muscle.

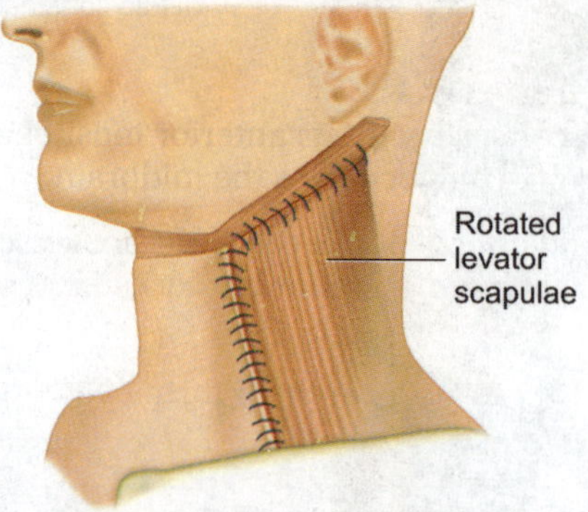

Q. FALX CEREBRI

Meningeal layer of dura mater folds within the cranial cavity and divides it into different chambers. Falx cerebri is one of the folds, which lies in median longitudinal fissure and divides the cranial cavity in two halves between the two cerebral hemispheres.

Attachments

- Anterior end is attached to crista galli
- Posterior end is broad and is attached along the median plane to the upper margin of tentorium cerebelli
- Upper margin is attached to the lips of sagittal sulcus and encloses superior sagittal sinus
- Lower margin is free and encloses inferior sagittal sinus.

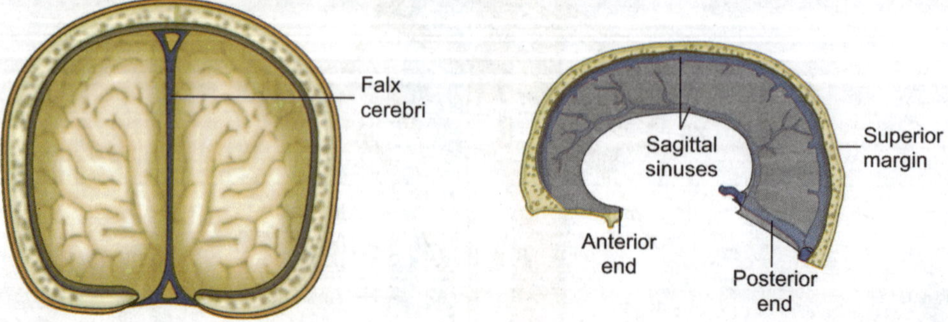

Relations

Surfaces are related to cerebral hemispheres.

Q. TENTORIUM CEREBELLI

Tentorium cerebelli is a tent-shaped fold of dura mater covering the posterior cranial fossa. It separates the cerebellum from occipital lobes of cerebrum. It divides the cranial cavity into supratentorial and infratentorial compartments.

Attachments

Anterior margin: Is free and concave, with its anterior most end attached to anterior clinoid process. It bounds tentorial notch and occupies the midbrain.

Outer margin: It is convex and attached to the lips of transverse sulcus of occipital bone and posteroinferior angle of parietal bone, superior border of petrous temporal bone and to posterior clinoid process.

Inferior layer: This layer of tentorium cerebelli forms an extra recess over the trigeminal impression known as Meckel's caves.

Surfaces

- Superior surface is convex and sloping. Along the line of attachment of falx cerebri it encloses straight sinus
- Inferior surface is concave
- At the junction of free and attached margins, it is pierced by III and IV cranial nerves.

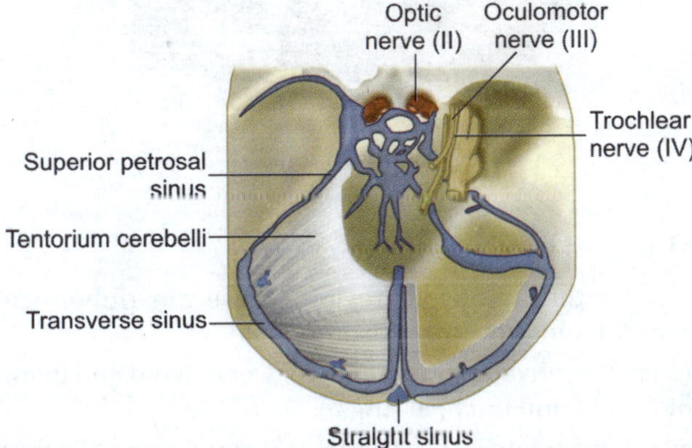

Applied Anatomy

Lesions in the infratentorial compartment should be attended at the earliest, as it may cause pressure on the brainstem and coning of medulla causing death.

Q. MIDLINE STRUCTURES OF THE NECK.

Midline structure is the central region, extending from the chin to the sternum. Midline structures of the neck can be divided into suprahyoid and infrahyoid regions.

Peculiarities

Skin covering this region is freely movable over deeper structures:

- Superficial fascia: It contains platysma, anterior jugular vein, lymph nodes and transverse cutaneous nerve
- Deep fascia: It is a single layer, up to cricoid, but below cricoid it splits to form suprasternal space of Burns.

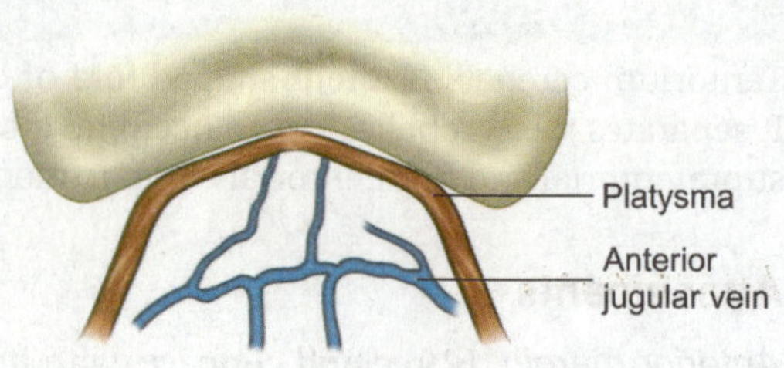

Suprahyoid Region

Suprahyoid region has mylohyoid muscle, forming the oral diaphragm and on either sides are the anterior bellies of digastric.

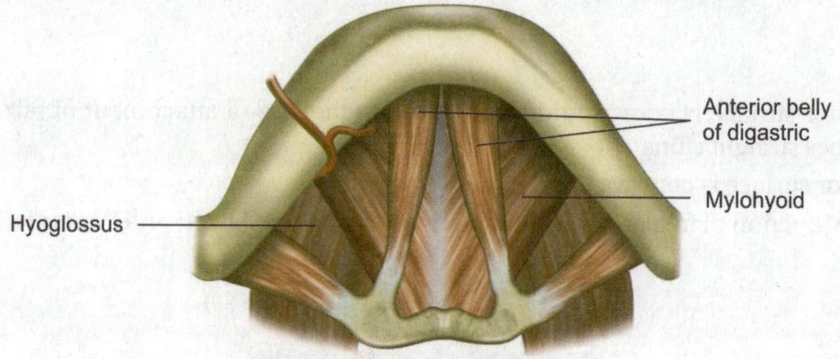

Suprahyoid region

Infrahyoid Region

1. Strap muscles cover the infrahyoid region. These are ribbon-like muscles namely, thyrohyoid, sternothyroid, sternohyoid, omohyoid.
2. Deep structures are thyrohyoid membrane, between hyoid and thyroid cartilage, cricoid cartilage, thyroid gland and tracheal rings.
3. Superior laryngeal vessels and internal laryngeal nerve pierce the thyrohyoid membrane.
4. Cricothyroid is the deep muscle in midline, which is the tensor of vocal cord.

Applied Anatomy

- Common midline swellings are thyroid enlargement known as goiter. Other swellings are thyroglossal cyst, lymph node enlargement, etc.
- Tracheostomy is a lifesaving procedure done about two finger breath above jugular notch.

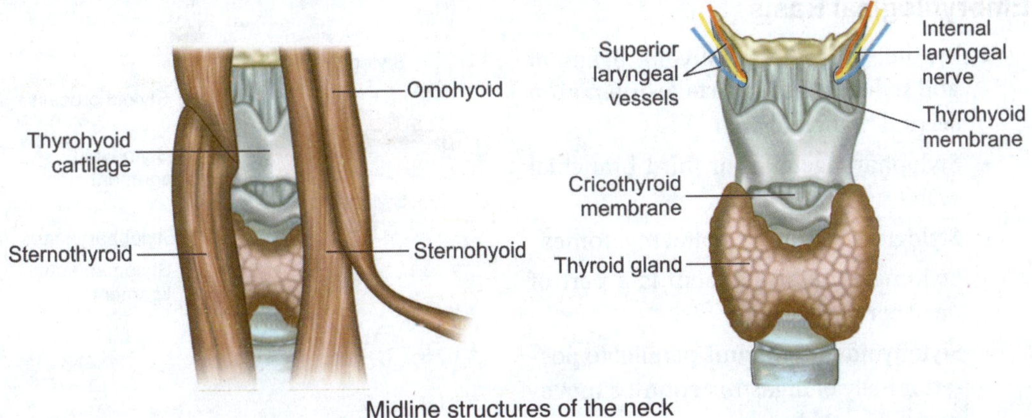

Midline structures of the neck

Q. SUPERIOR ORBITAL FISSURE (DIAGRAM ONLY).

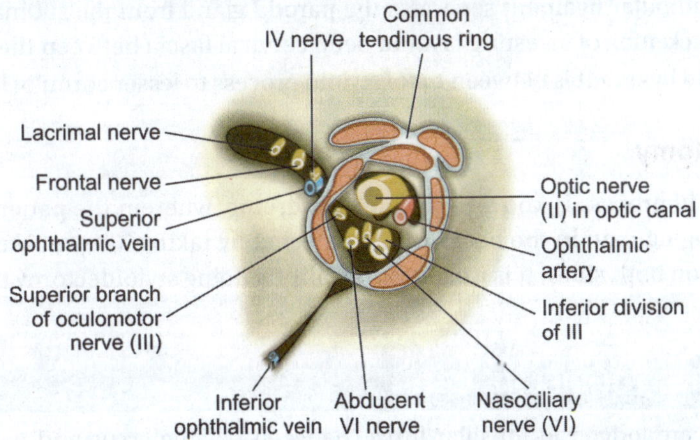

Q. STYLOID APPARATUS

Styloid process is slender bony projection from the temporal bone between parotid gland laterally and internal jugular vein (IJV) medially. Styloid process with its attachments is known as styloid apparatus.

Attachments

Styloid apparatus gives attachments to three muscles and two ligaments. These have diverse embryological origins.

Embryological Basis

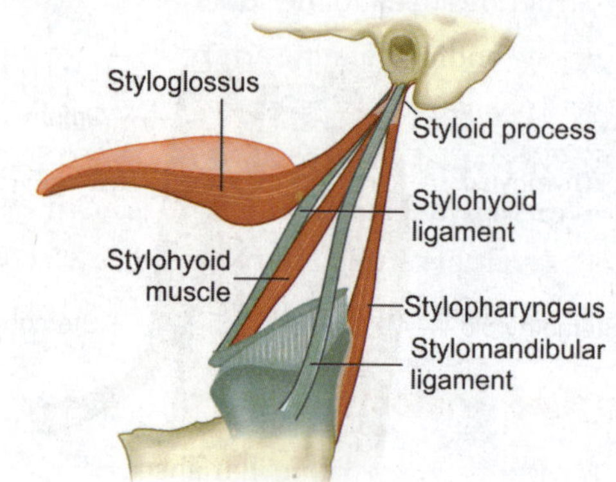

- Styloid process, stylohyoid ligament and stylohyoid muscle take origin from second branchial arch
- Stylopharyngeus from third branchial arch
- Styloglossus from occipital myotomes
- Stylomandibular ligament is a part of deep cervical fascia
- Stylohyoid muscle runs parallel to posterior belly of digastric; controls movement of hyoid bone
- Styloglossus muscle pulls the tongue upwards and backwards
- Stylopharyngeus muscle helps to lift the larynx during swallowing
- Stylomandibular ligament separates the parotid gland from the submandibular gland and its thickening of investing layer of deep cervical fascia between the two glands
- Stylohyoid ligament is between tip of styloid process to lesser cornu of hyoid bone.

Applied Anatomy

Elongated styloid process is known as Eagle's syndrome, wherein the patient presents with continuous nagging pain in the neck. This is detected by taking X-ray of skull and comparing the lengths on both sides. It is treated surgically by doing styloidectomy by transtonsillar approach.

Q. PALATINE TONSILLAR BED

Palatine tonsils are lodged in tonsillar fossa (between palatoglossus and palatopharyngeus muscles), which form the tonsillar bed.

Lateral surface of tonsil is separated from superior constrictor by lax connective tissue.

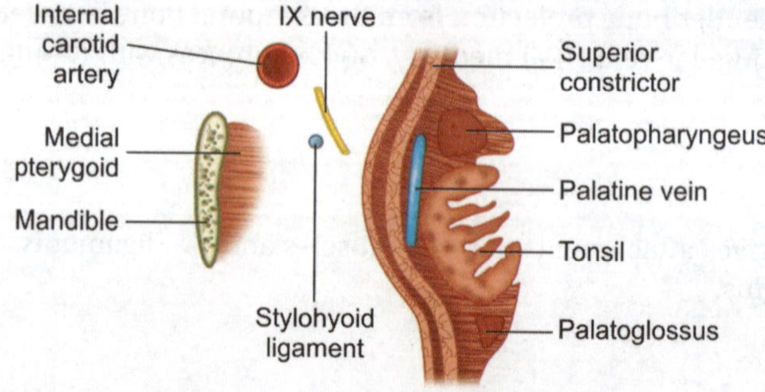

Tonsillar bed

Structures deep to the superior constrictor are:

- Ascending palatine artery
- Tonsillar artery
- IX cranial nerve
- Stylohyoid ligament
- Internal carotid artery (ICA) lies 2.5 cm behind and lateral to the tonsil
- Palatine vein.

Applied Anatomy

- Quinsy is a peritonsillar abscess
- Styloidectomy can be done through tonsillar fossa in cases of elongated styloid process
- Surgeon should remember the relation of internal carotid artery to tonsillar fossa, while doing tonsillectomy.

Q. AUDITORY TUBE (EUSTACHIAN TUBE)

Auditory tube is a cone-shaped passage connecting middle ear space with nasopharynx; lodged in sulcus tubae over the base of skull.

Gross Features

Auditory tube is about one and a half inch long and directed forwards and medially.

Parts

Auditory tube has two parts:

1. **Bony part**
   - Lateral end of bony part ends into anterior wall of middle ear cavity and medial end gives attachment to cartilaginous part
   - Superiorly it is related to tensor tympani, medially to carotid canal, laterally to chorda tympani and spine of sphenoid.
2. **Cartilaginous part**
   - It is a triangular part of cartilage, which curls to form superior and medial walls
   - Anterolaterally it is related to tensor palati, mandibular nerve and its branches, otic ganglion, chorda tympani, middle meningeal artery and medial pterygoid plate
   - Levator palati is attached to its inferior surface.

Blood Supply

Auditory tube receives arterial blood through ascending pharyngeal and middle meningeal artery and drains into pharyngeal plexus of veins.

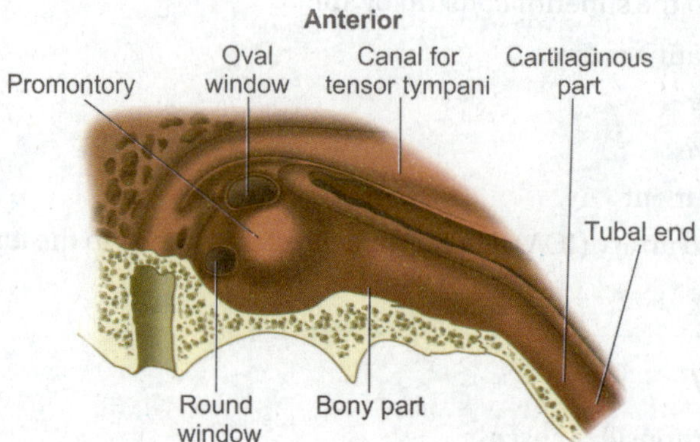

Auditory tube parts and middle ear connection

Nerve Supply

Pharyngeal plexus of nerves.

Function

Auditory tube maintains atmospheric pressure in the middle ear cavity. Thus, air pressure on both sides of tympanic membrane is equalized.

Applied Anatomy

- Inflammation of auditory tube secondary to common cold gives rise to middle ear effusion, which is common in children
- Throat infections may be transmitted by the tube to middle ear cavity causing otitis media.

Q. NASAL SEPTUM

Nasal septum is a median osseocartilaginous partition between the two halves of nasal cavity and is covered by mucous membrane.

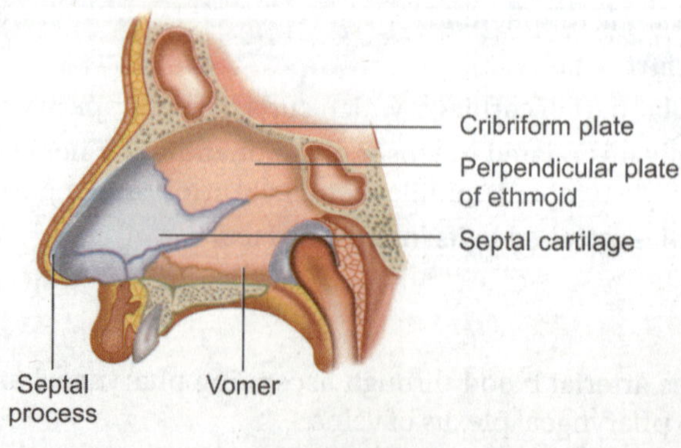

Nasal septum

Parts

Nasal septum is made up of three parts:

1. Bony components:
   - Vomer
   - Perpendicular plate of ethmoid.
2. Cartilaginous:
   - Septal cartilage
   - Septal process of inferior nasal cartilage.
3. Cuticular part:
   - Formed by fibrofatty tissue covered by skin
   - Nasal septum has four borders and two surfaces.

Borders

- Anterior
- Posterior
- Superior
- Inferior.

Surfaces

Right and left.

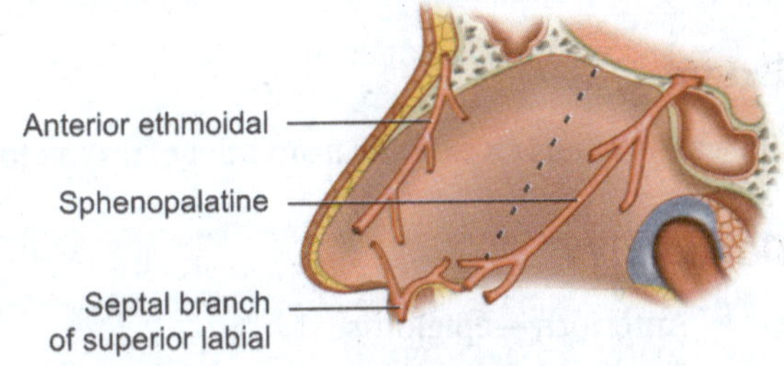

Blood supply of nasal septum

Blood Supply

1. Anterosuperior part is supplied by anterior ethmoidal artery and superior labial branch of facial artery.
2. Posteroinferior part is supplied by sphenopalatine artery.

Venous plexus is present over the lower part of septum, which drains into facial vein anteriorly and pterygoid plexus of veins posteriorly.

Nerve Supply

- Anterosuperior part is supplied by anterior ethmoidal nerve
- Posteroinferior part is supplied by nasopalatine branch of pterygopalatine ganglion.

Lymphatic Drainage

Anterior half to submandibular nodes, posterior half to retropharyngeal and deep cervical nodes.

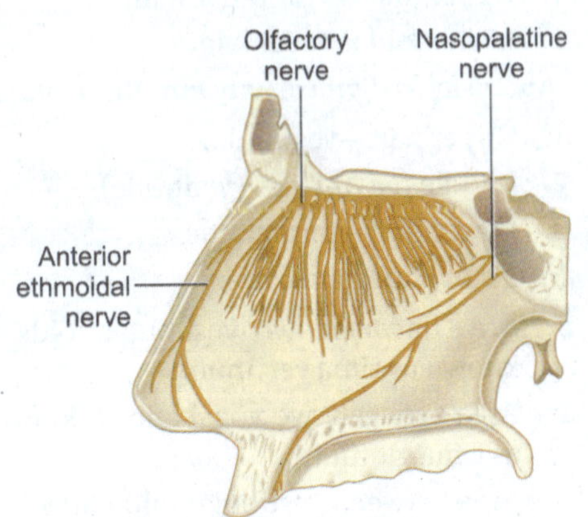

Nerve supply of nasal septum

Applied Anatomy

1. Nasal septum is deviated in most of the individuals. However, in few cases the septum is grossly deviated giving rise to symptoms of nasal obstruction and headache. This is known as deviated nasal septum (DNS) and it can be corrected by surgeries like septoplasty, submucous resection.
2. Anterior ethmoidal nerve syndrome is also known as Sludger's syndrome.
3. Little's area is a common site of bleeding through the nose. It is at the anteroinferior part of septum and contains anastomosis between septal ramus of superior labial branch, anterior ethmoidal artery, sphenopalatine artery and greater palatine artery.
4. Sphenopalatine artery is the artery of epistaxis.

Q. CAVITY OF LARYNX

The cavity of larynx is divided into compartments by mucosal folds as described below.

Extent

The cavity of larynx extends from inlet of larynx to lower border of cricoid cartilage.

Boundaries

- Anteriorly—epiglottis
- Posteriorly—interarytenoid fold of mucous membrane
- On each side—aryepiglottic fold.

Compartments

There are two folds of mucous membrane within the cavity of larynx:

1. Upper fold is vestibular fold.
2. Lower fold is vocal fold.

Above folds divide cavity into three parts:

1. Upper part—vestibule.
2. Middle part—sinus (ventricle).
3. Lower part—infraglottic.

Areas of importance are:

1. Area between two vestibular folds is known as rima vestibuli.
2. Area between two vocal folds is known as rima glottidis.
3. Area between vestibular fold and vocal fold is known as sinus of larynx.

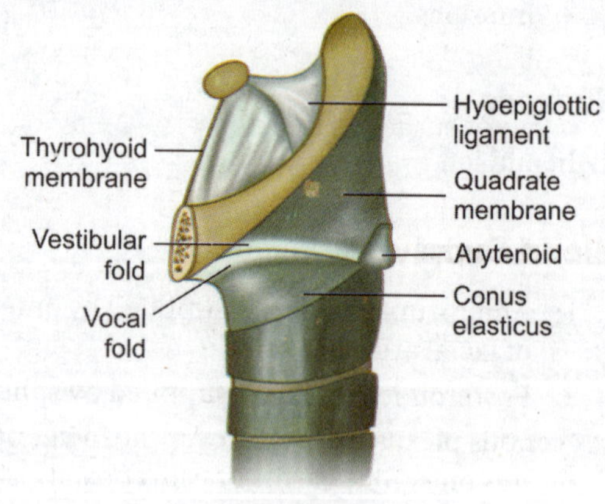

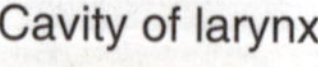

Cavity of larynx

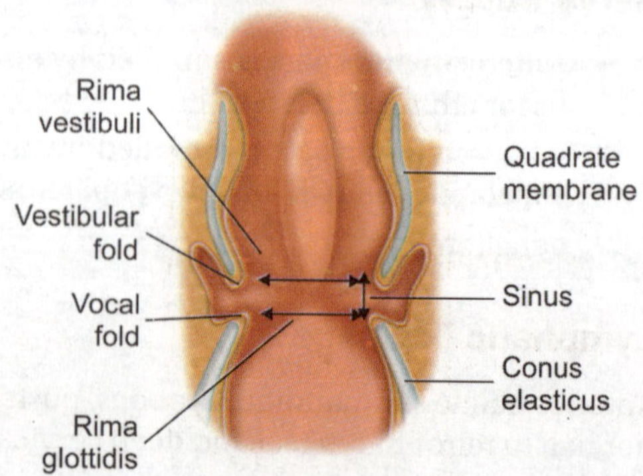

Applied Anatomy

Surgically the cavity of larynx is divided into supraglottic, glottic and infraglottic parts:

- Supraglottic—above the vestibular folds
- Glottic—between the vocal and vestibular fold
- Infraglottic—below vocal fold up to the level of cricoid cartilage.

Q. TYMPANIC MEMBRANE (EAR DRUM)

Tympanic membrane (TM) is a thin translucent partition between external acoustic meatus and middle ear.

Gross Anatomy

Tympanic membrane is oval in shape, 9 × 10 mm in size, placed obliquely at 55 degrees to the floor of meatus and facing downwards, forwards and laterally.

Circumference of TM is thickened forming the tympanic sulcus all around except superiorly, where it is deficient and attached to the notch of Rivinus. From the notch, two bands namely anterior and posterior malleolar folds arise to the lateral process.

Surfaces

- Outer surface is free and concave
- Inner surface is convex and provides attachment to the handle of malleus, the point of maximum convexity at the tip of handle is called umbo.

Parts

- Pars flaccida
- Pars tensa.

Layers

- Outer cuticular
- Middle fibrous
- Inner mucosal.

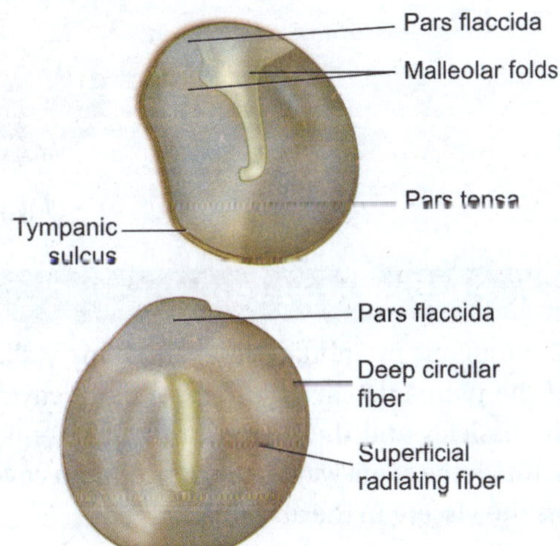

Tympanic membrane

Blood Supply

- Outer surface is supplied by deep auricular branch of maxillary artery
- Inner surface is supplied by anterior tympanic, a branch of maxillary artery and posterior tympanic, a branch of posterior auricular artery
- Blood drains into external jugular vein.

Lymphatic Drainage

To preauricular and retropharyngeal lymph nodes.

Nerve Supply

- Lateral surface in front supplied by auriculotemporal nerve and behind by auricular branch of vagus
- Medial surface is supplied by chorda tympani nerve.

Applied Anatomy

Myringotomy is a radial or curvilinear, incision taken on TM for middle ear effusion.

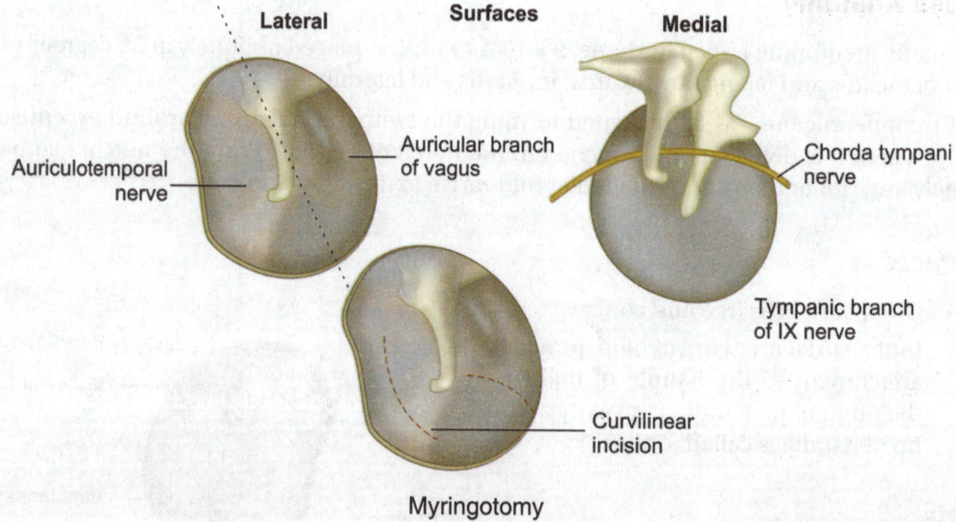

Q. PRUSSAK'S POUCH

The mucous membrane lines the bony walls of the tympanic cavity and extends to cover the ossicles and their supporting ligaments; in much the same way as the peritoneum covers the viscera in the abdomen.

The mucosal folds divide the middle ear space into compartments.

Prussak's pouch is a part of epitympanic region.

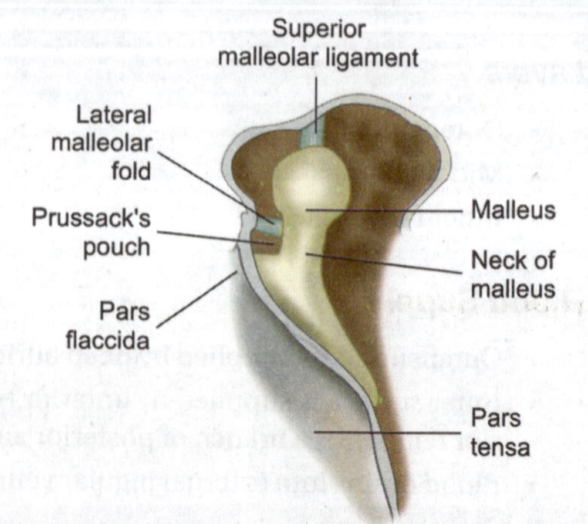

Boundaries

- Above—lateral malleolar fold

- Below—neck of malleus
- Laterally—pars flaccida.

Applied Anatomy

Unsafe middle ear disease begins from Prussak's pouch commonly.

Q. EYEBALL (DIAGRAM ONLY)

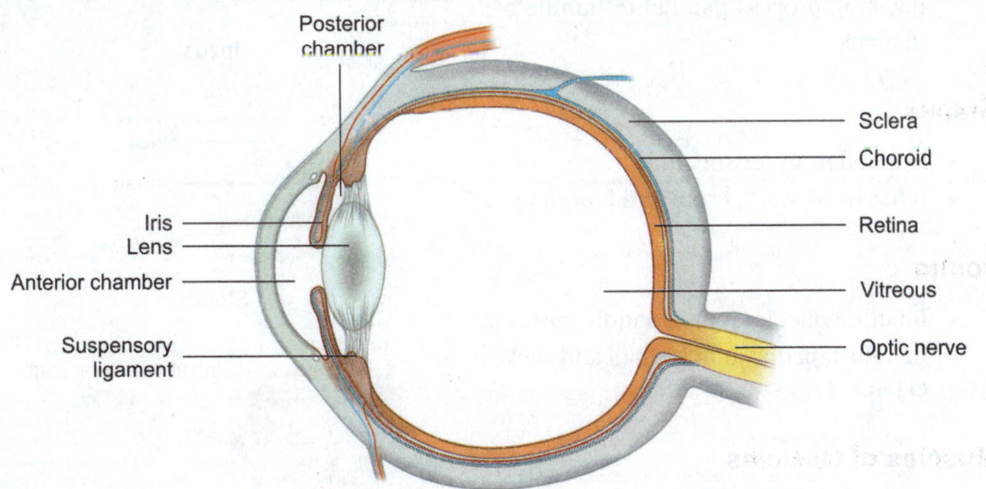

Q. EAR OSSICLES

Ear ossicles are the smallest bones in human body. There are three ossicles in the middle ear cavity namely malleus, incus and stapes.

Malleus

- Derived from Meckel's cartilage
- It is a largest ossicle located close to TM
- It has following parts—head, neck, anterior process and lateral process, and handle
- Head lies in attic and articulates posteriorly with incus
- Neck lies against pars flaccida and related medially to chorda tympani
- Anterior process has anterior ligament getting attached to petrotympanic fissure

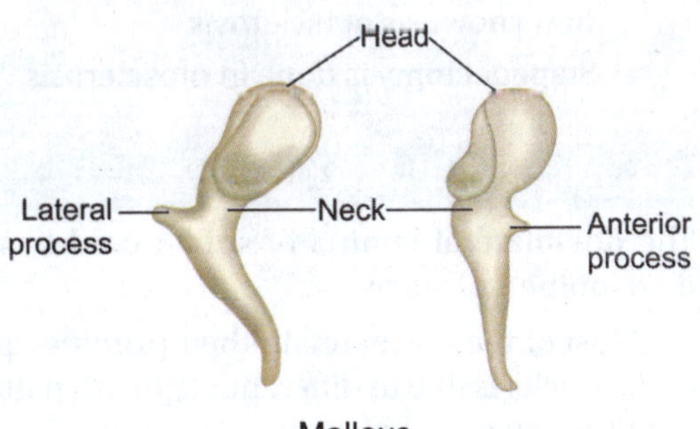

- Lateral process provides attachment to malleolar folds
- Handle extends downwards, backwards medially and is attached to TM. The point of attachment is known as umbo.

Incus

- Derived from second arch
- It has body, short process in fossa incudis, long process parallel to handle of malleus.

Stapes

- Derived from second arch
- It has head, neck, crura and footplate.

Joints

- Incudomalleolar joint is saddle joint
- Incudostapedial joint is a ball and socket joint.

Muscles of Ossicles

- Tensor tympani is a muscle for malleus, it arises from the walls of auditory tube and gets inserted into the upper part of handle of malleus
- Stapedius arises from pyramid and inserts on the neck of stapes.

Applied Anatomy

- Deafness behind intact TM may be due to ossicular chain fixity or stapes footplate fixation known as otosclerosis
- Stapedectomy is done in otosclerosis.

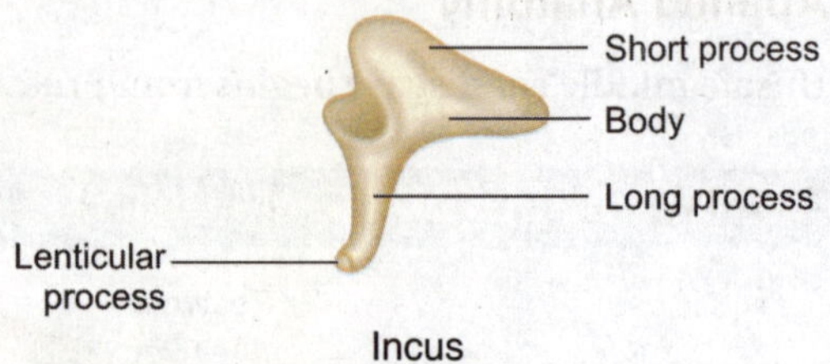

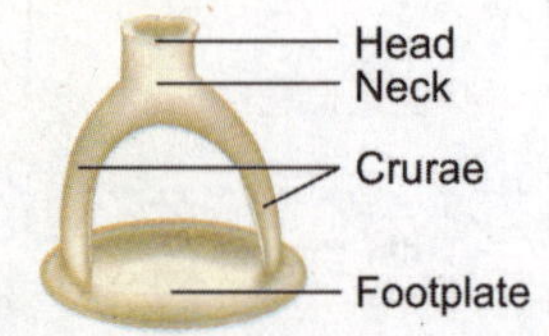

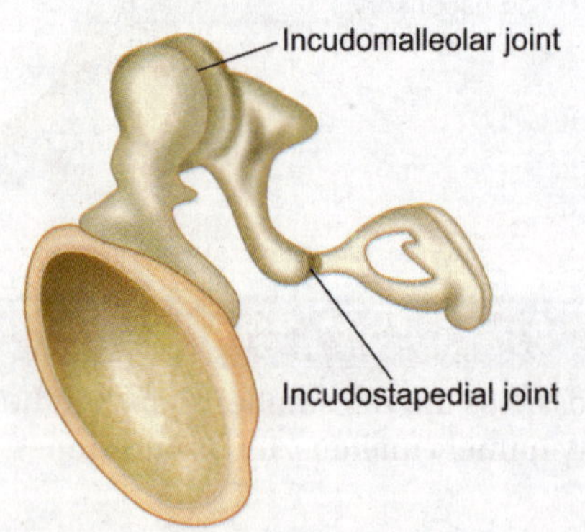

Q. NEUROBIOTAXIS

The dorsolateral lamina of spinal cord has specific locations of the nuclei within, in the developmental stage.

Most of the nuclei retain their primitive positions, but some move out. This displacement of the nuclei is due to differential growth patterns and by appearance and growth of neighboring fiber tracts and by active migration. This migration of nuclei in the direction of stimuli is known as neurobiotaxis like chemotaxis. Facial nerve nucleus and nucleus ambiguus assume different adult position by virtue of neurobiotaxis.

Q. COCHLEAR SECTION (DIAGRAM ONLY)

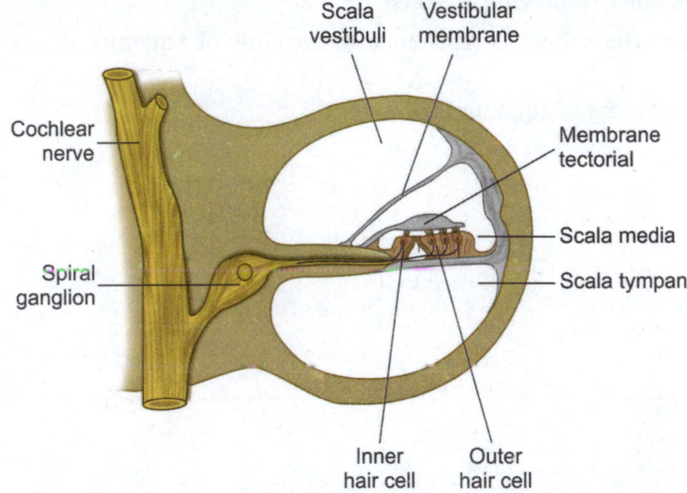

Q. SCLEROCORNEAL JUNCTION

The junction between sclera and cornea is the sclerocorneal junction, which is marked by canal of Schlemm.

Circulation of Aqueous Humor

The aqueous humor is secreted by ciliary process and it enters the posterior chamber. It then passes forward through the pupil to anterior chamber, where it leaves the eye by way of trabecular meshwork canal of Schlemm, aqueous veins and mixes with the blood in episcleral vessels.

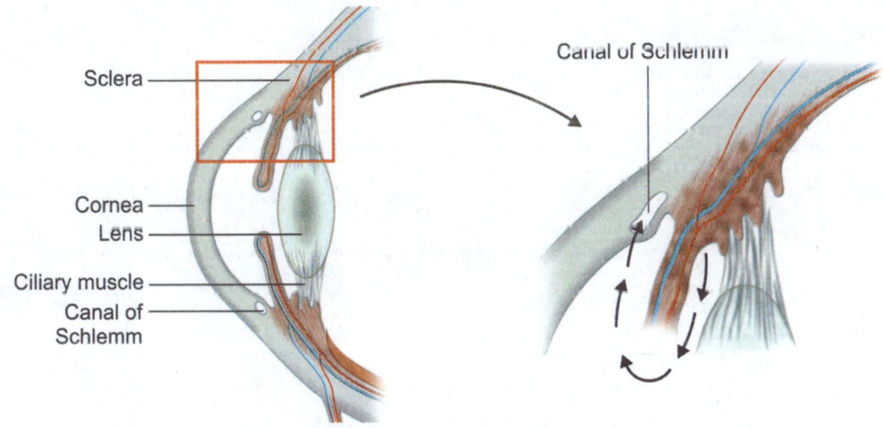

Circulation of aqueous humor

Applied Anatomy

Glaucoma occurs due to following reasons:

- Commonly, when there is resistance to the flow of aqueous at any level during its pathway
- Rarely, when more of aqueous is produced.

Long Questions

Key long questions

- Scalp
- Sensory innervation of face
- Components of lacrimal apparatus
- Arrangement of deep cervical fascia and neck spaces
- Posterior triangle of neck
- Suboccipital triangle of neck
- Venous sinuses
- Gross anatomy of parotid gland
- Cervical lymph nodes
- Facial nerve
- Muscles of mastication
- Mandibular nerve
- Maxillary artery
- Temporomandibular joint
- Gross anatomy of submandibular gland
- Gross anatomy of thyroid gland
- Larynx
- Relations of middle ear
- Lateral wall of nose, and its blood and nerve supply
- Pterygopalatine fossa
- Parathyroid glands
- Pharyngeal muscles
- Innervation of tongue
- Gross anatomy of pituitary gland
- Internal ear

Q. DESCRIBE 'SCALP' IN DETAIL. ADD A NOTE ON ITS APPLIED ANATOMY.

Soft tissues covering the upper part of skull form the scalp.

Boundaries

- Anteroposteriorly it extends between the supraorbital margin and external occipital protuberance and superior nuchal lines

- On either side, superior temporal lines form the boundary (thus forehead is included in scalp).

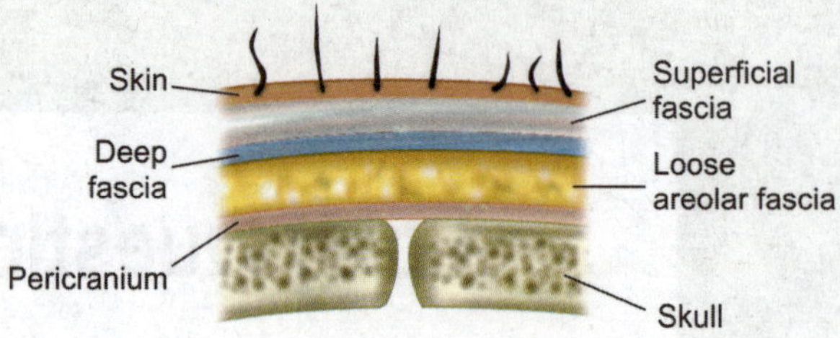

Layers

The following are the five layers:

1. Skin.
2. Superficial fascia.
3. Deep fascia (aponeurosis).
4. Loose areolar tissue.
5. Pericranium.

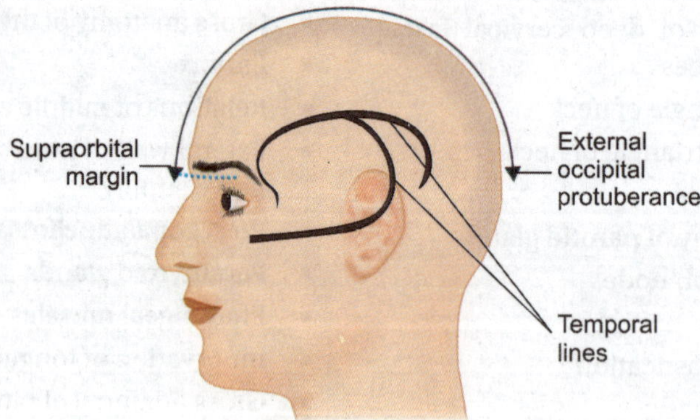

Extent of scalp

Here scalp stands for:

S—**S**kin

C—**C**onnective tissue

A—**A**poneurosis

L—**L**oose areolar tissue

P—**P**ericranium

Skin

- Thick and hairy
- It is adherent to epicranial aponeurosis through dense superficial fascia.

Superficial Fascia

- It is very fibrous and dense (central portion is more dense than periphery)
- Neurovascular bundle traverses this layer to reach the skin
- Occipitofrontalis muscle is present in this layer.

Deep Fascia

- It is adherent to the skin of scalp above, but freely movable from below
- It provides insertion for the occipitalis and temporalis muscle
- On each side it is attached to the superior temporal lines.

Loose Areolar Tissue

Extends anteriorly into the eyelids posteriorly to the superior nuchal lines and on each side temporal line.

Pericranium

Pericranium is loosely attached to the surface of the bone except at the suture lines, where it is firmly attached.

Blood Supply

Scalp has a rich blood supply derived from both internal and external carotid arteries (ICA and ECA):

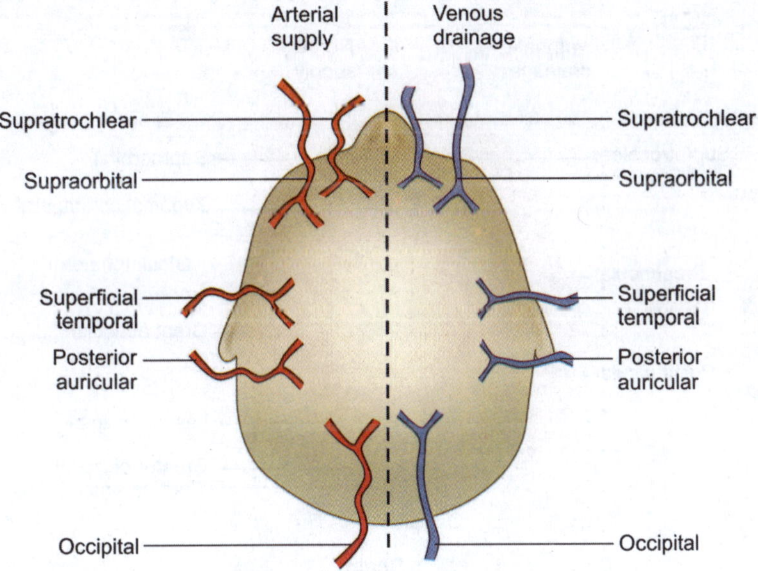

Blood supply of scalp

1. In front, scalp is supplied by:
- Supratrochlear
- Ophthalmic artery—a branch of ICA
- Supraorbital
- Superficial temporal—a branch of ECA.
2. From behind scalp is supplied by:
- Occipital—branches from ECA
- Posterior auricular.

Veins run close to the arteries and have the same nomenclature.

Lymphatic Drainage

Scalp drains anteriorly into preauricular lymph nodes and posteriorly into posterior auricular and occipital lymph nodes.

Nerve Supply

Scalp is supplied by three sets of nerves; they are V nerve, VII nerve and cervical plexus:

1. In front supplied by:
- Supratrochlear
- Supraorbital
- Zygomaticotemporal
- Auriculotemporal
- Temporal branch of VII nerve.

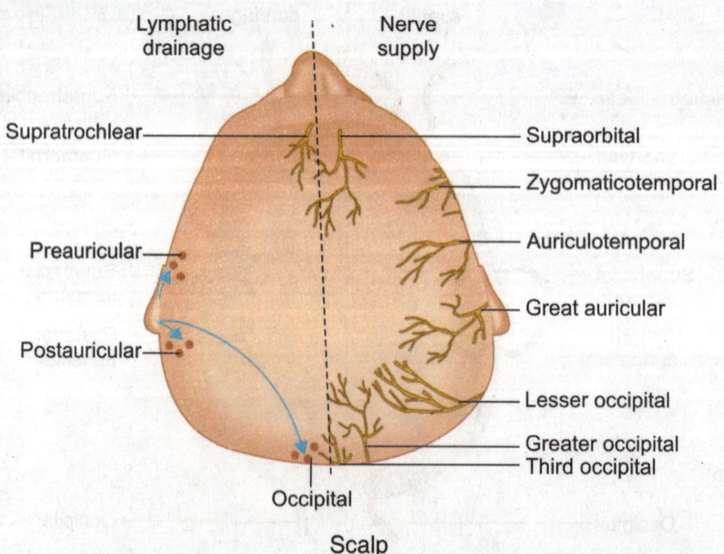

Scalp

2. From behind supplied by:
- Great auricular
- Lesser occipital
- Great occipital
- Third occipital
- Posterior auricular branch of VII nerve.

Applied Anatomy

1. Sebaceous cysts are very common in scalp.
2. In cases of head injury, scalp wounds bleed profusely because the fibrous nature of superficial fascia inhibits the injured blood vessels from retracting. Scalp also has rich blood supply.
3. Loose areolar layer (IV layer) of scalp is known as danger area of scalp, because infection from the scalp may traverse through the emissary vein to the cranial venous sinuses.
4. Hematoma in loose areolar layer may easily spread to the eyelids giving rise to the formation of black eye.
5. From the surgical standpoint, the skin, connective tissue, aponeurosis is intimately united and should be regarded as single layer attached to the bone posteriorly and skin anteriorly. One can easily peel off the first three layers from the pericranium with the intervening loose connective tissue in between.
6. Veins of the scalp are in subcutaneous plane and intravenous infusions can be given through them.

Q. DISCUSS SENSORY INNERVATION OF FACE.

Trigeminal nerve and cervical plexus carry the sensation from the face. It also supplies the nasal cavity, paranasal sinuses, eyeball, oral cavity, dura mater of anterior and middle cranial fossa. Trigeminal nerve has three divisions:
- Ophthalmic
- Maxillary
- Mandibular.

The above branches innervate the face.

Ophthalmic Division

Ophthalmic division gives five branches to supply upper part of face and scalp up to the vertex. The branches are:
- Supratrochlear
- Supraorbital
- Lacrimal

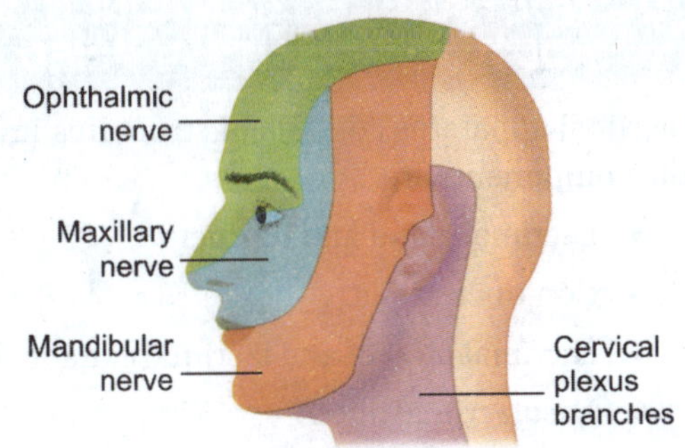

- External nasal
- Infratrochlear.

Maxillary Division

Maxillary division gives three branches to supply middle part of face. The branches are:

- Infraorbital
- Zygomaticofacial
- Zygomaticotemporal.

Mandibular Division

Mandibular division supplies the lower part of face. The branches are:

- Auriculotemporal
- Buccal
- Mental.

Cervical Plexus

The branches of cervical plexus supply the angle of jaw. The branches are:

- Great auricular nerve
- Transverse cutaneous nerve
- Lesser occipital nerve.

Applied Anatomy

1. Headache is a common symptom in common cold, sinusitis or dental caries by virtue of common innervation.
2. Trigeminal neuralgia (tic douloureux) is a condition, wherein patient complain of lancinating pain incited by trivial factors like washing the face.

Surgery is required in the form of thermocoagulation or cryotherapy or direct section of roots of V nerve.

Q. WHAT ARE THE COMPONENTS OF LACRIMAL APPARATUS? ADD A NOTE ON ITS APPLIED ANATOMY.

Lacrimal apparatus consists of structures involved in production and secretion of tear fluid. The components are:

- Lacrimal gland and its duct
- Conjunctival sac
- Lacrimal puncta and lacrimal canaliculi
- Nasolacrimal duct.

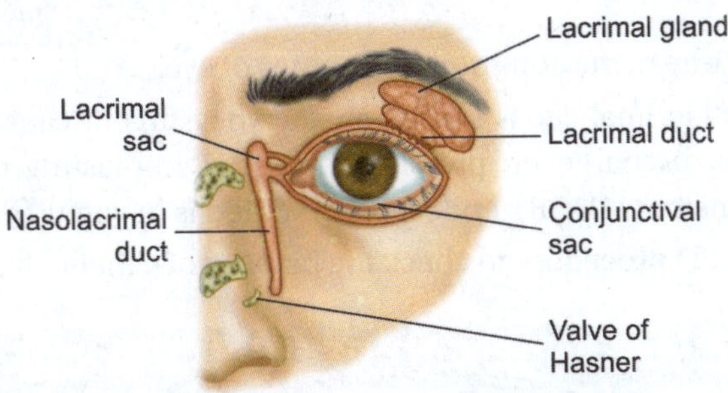

Components of lacrimal apparatus

Lacrimal Gland

Lacrimal gland is a serous, exocrine gland located in the lacrimal fossa. It is 'J' shaped, being indented by the tendon of levator palpebrae superioris muscle. Thus, it has two parts as orbital and palpebral. Ducts of the lacrimal gland open in the conjunctival sac. Gland is supplied by lacrimal nerve and lacrimal branch of ophthalmic artery.

Conjunctival Sac

Conjunctival sac is a mucous membrane covering the inner surface of eyelids (palpebral part) and front of the eyeball (orbital part):

- Palpebral part is thick, opaque and highly vascular
- Bulbar part has two parts—one covering the sclera, which is thick, transparent and loosely attached to eyeball and another covering the cornea, which is thin and firmly attached.

Ophthalmic artery and lacrimal artery supply the sac. Supratrochlear and supraorbital nerves supply the upper part and infraorbital nerve supply the lower part of eyelid.

Lacrimal Puncta and Canaliculi

Puncta is a small opening in the conjunctival sac, which leads into canaliculus. Canaliculus has a vertical and horizontal part, with the dilated part ampulla at the bend. Both the canaliculi open into lacrimal sac.

Lacrimal Sac

Lacrimal sac is a membranous sac, lodged in lacrimal groove just behind the medial palpebral ligament. It opens below into the nasolacrimal duct.

Nasolacrimal Duct

Nasolacrimal duct is membranous passage approximately 1.5 cm in length directed downwards, backwards and laterally and opens into inferior meatus and guarded by valve known as valve of Hasner.

Applied Anatomy

1. Conjunctivitis is one of the commonest diseases of eye.

2. Inflammation of lacrimal sac is known as dacryocystitis. It causes excessive watering of eyes and pus discharge on pressing the sac. Long-lasting ailment is treated by dacryocystorhinostomy (DCR), endoscopic method is in vogue (endoscopic DCR).

3. Syringing is an OPD procedure to check the patency of canaliculi and sac.

Q. DESCRIBE THE ARRANGEMENT OF DEEP CERVICAL FASCIA AND THE VARIOUS NECK SPACES.

Deep fascia of the neck has three layers:

- Investing layer
- Pretracheal layer
- Prevertebral layer.

Investing Layer

As the name suggests, it invests the structures on its way (resembles a polo neck T–shirt).

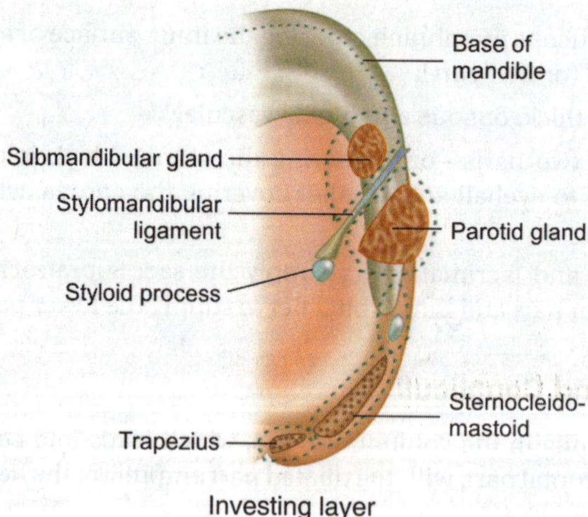

Attachments

- Superiorly—external occipital protuberance, superior nuchal line, mastoid process, base of mandible
- Inferiorly—spine of scapula, acromion process clavicle, manubrium
- Anteriorly—symphysis menti, hyoid bone
- Posteriorly—spine of C7 vertebra.

Special Features

- It forms two extra spaces, suprasternal and supraclavicular
- It forms two extra pulleys to bind the tendon of digastric and omohyoid
- It encloses two muscles, trapezius and sternocleidomastoid muscles
- It encloses two glands, parotid and submandibular gland.

Pretracheal Fascia

Pretracheal fascia encloses the thyroid gland.

Attachments

- Superiorly—hyoid bone, oblique line of thyroid cartilage and cricoid cartilage
- Inferiorly—it blends with adventitia of inferior thyroid veins and aorta
- On each side—it blends with carotid sheath.

Special Features

- On either side of the thyroid gland the fascia is thick, forming the so-called suspensory ligament of Berry
- Thyroid gland moves during deglutition by virtue of its attachment to hyoid bone, thyroid cartilage superiorly and inferiorly to the adventitia of great vessels.

Prevertebral Fascia

Prevertebral fascia lies in front of muscles of vertebra and forms the floor of posterior triangle of the neck.

Attachments

- Superiorly it is attached to the base of skull
- Inferiorly it is attached to the body of third and fourth thoracic vertebra
- On either side it is attached deep to trapezius.

Special Features

- It extends upto superior mediastinum
- Brachial plexus lies behind the fascia
- Subclavian artery is covered by fascia known as axillary sheath.

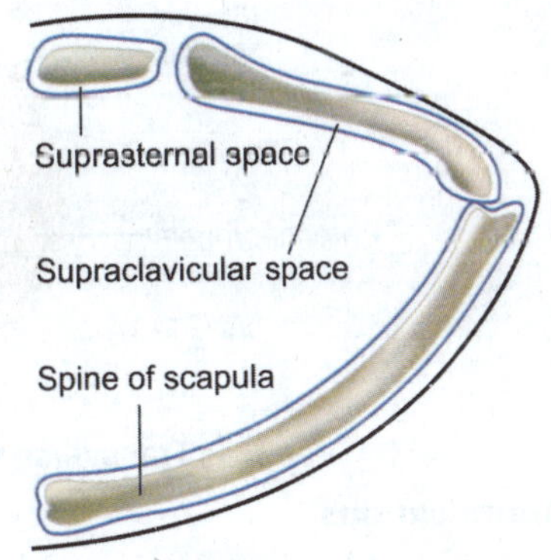

Investing layer of deep cervical fascia

Applied Anatomy

1. Parotitis is very painful because the parotid fascia is thick and unyielding in nature and also it sends thick septa into substance of gland.
2. Neck infections are very common; secondary to dental infections. Since the spaces are interconnected and extend up to mediastinum, a dental infection may spread into mediastinum and lead to death.
3. Division of external jugular vein may lead to air embolism and death, since vein lies outside the axillary sheath and prevented from retraction.

Neck Spaces

The arrangement of deep cervical fascia is such that it gives rise to 11 potential spaces. These spaces communicate with each other as a result of which infection in one space can spread to another. Few important spaces are discussed below.

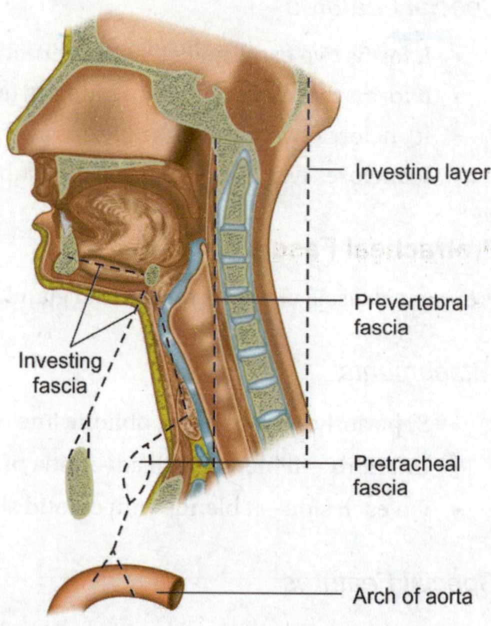

Layers of deep fascia of the neck

Parapharyngeal Space

Parapharyngeal space (lateral pharyngeal space, pterygomaxillary space, pterygopharyngeal space). This space is located above the hyoid bone (suprahyoid space). It extends from base of skull to lesser cornu of hyoid bone. Important posterolateral relation is carotid sheath.

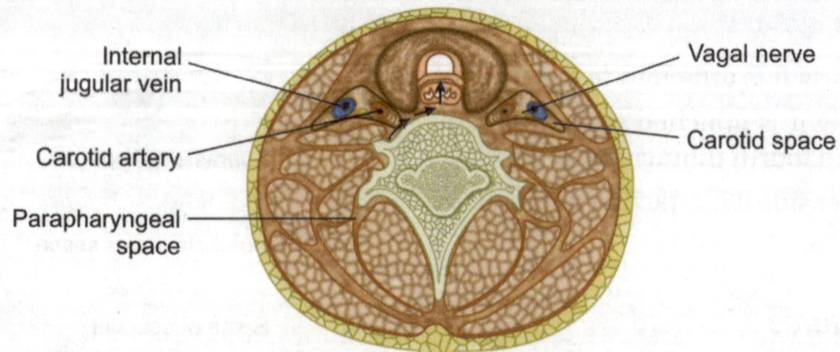

Transverse section of parapharyngeal space

Communications

- Anteriorly communicates with submaxillary and submandibular space
- Posteriorly communicates with retropharyngeal space and hence to prevertebral space.

Parotid Space

1. It lies between superficial and deep capsules of parotid gland.
2. The superficial capsule is thick and adherent to underlying parotid gland. There are multiple septae running from lateral capsule into gland itself. Medial capsule is thin and abuts around the lateral pharyngeal space.
3. Infection tends to spread medially into lateral pharyngeal space.

Submandibular Space

Mylohyoid muscle splits the submandibular space into sublingual and submaxillary.

Communications

Submandibular space communicates with parapharyngeal space.

Masticator Space

Masticator space is formed by splitting of superficial layers of deep cervical fascia. It encloses mandible and muscles of mastication.

Communications

Masticator space communicates superiorly with deep temporal space.

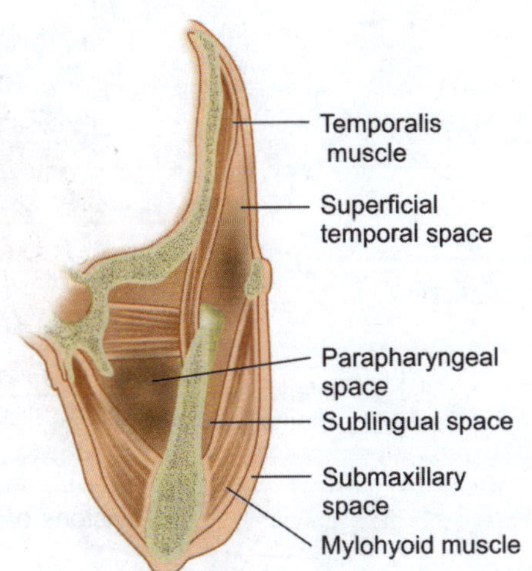

Retropharyngeal Space

1. It lies between prevertebral fascia and buccopharyngeal fascia. An ancillary portion of deep cervical fascia divides it into danger space, i.e. prevertebral space proper and retropharyngeal space.
2. It extends from skull to second thoracic vertebra, i.e. posterior mediastinum. It is divided into two lateral compartments by median raphe.

Communications

Retropharyngeal space communicates with prevertebral and parapharyngeal space.

Applied Anatomy

- Deep neck space infections are secondary to dental infections most commonly
- A neck infection can spread to mediastinum by virtue of its communications.

Q. WHAT ARE THE BOUNDARIES, FLOOR, ROOF AND CONTENTS OF POSTERIOR TRIANGLE OF NECK? WHAT IS ITS CLINICAL SIGNIFICANCE?

Divisions of Triangle of the Neck

Side of the neck is divided into anterior and posterior triangles by the key muscle—sternocleidomastoid. Area in front of it is anterior triangle and behind it is posterior triangle.

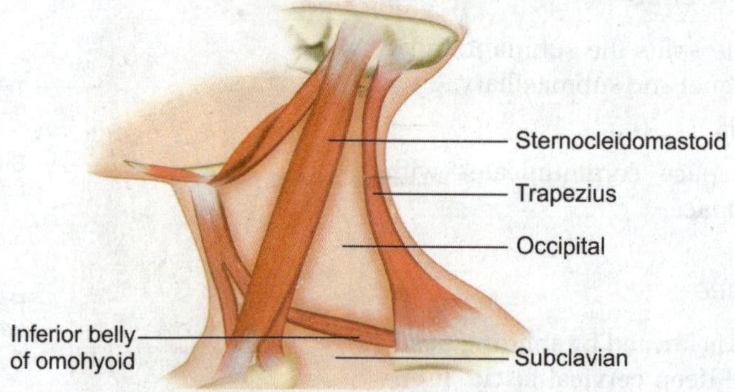

Divisions of triangles of the neck

Boundaries

- Anteriorly—posterior border of sternocleidomastoid
- Posteriorly—anterior border of trapezius
- Base—middle one-third of clavicle
- Apex—meeting of sternocleidomastoid and trapezius.

Roof

Roof is formed by the investing layer of deep cervical fascia. Following structures are present in the roof:

1. Nerves:
- Lesser occipital nerve
- Great auricular nerve
- Anterior cutaneous nerves
- Supraclavicular nerves.
2. Muscular arteries branching from suprascapular, transverse cervical, occipital.
3. Lymphatics.

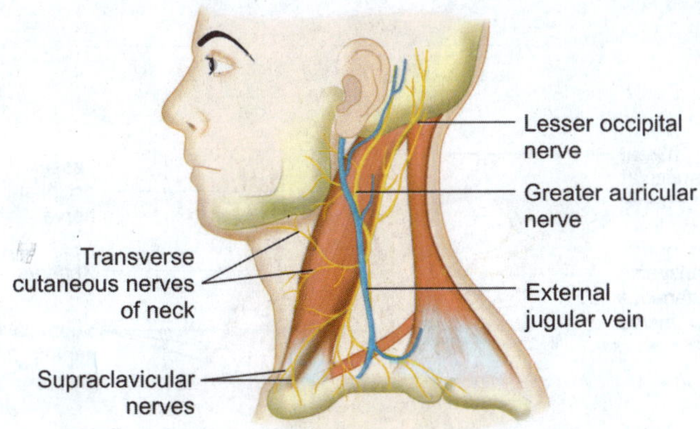

Nerves innervating the roof of posterior triangle

Floor

The floor is formed by muscles covered by prevertebral fascia. Following structures form the floor.

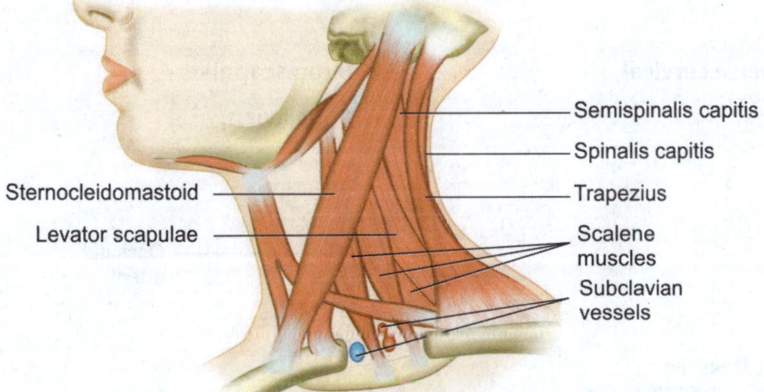

Muscles of the floor of posterior triangle

Muscles

- Semispinalis capitis
- Splenius capitis
- Levator scapulae
- Scalenus anterior

- Scalenus medius
- Scalenus posterior
- Serratus anterior.

Nerves

- Spinal accessory
- Nerve to trapezius
- Trunks of brachial plexus
- Suprascapular

- Nerve to subclavius
- Nerve to rhomboids
- Nerve to serratus anterior.

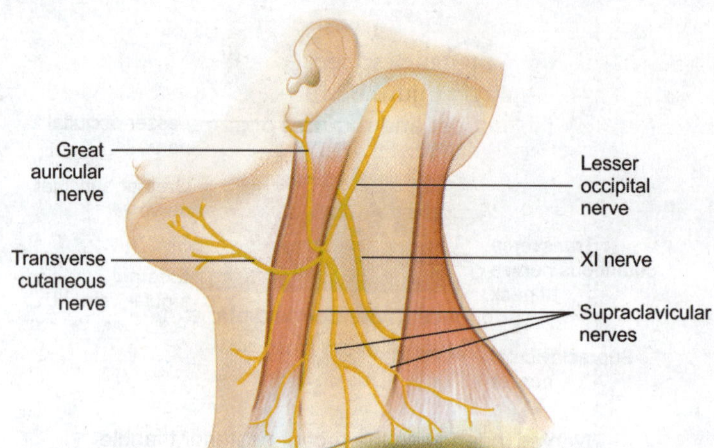

Nerves in posterior triangle

Vessels

- Transverse cervical
- Occipital
- Suprascapular
- Subclavian.

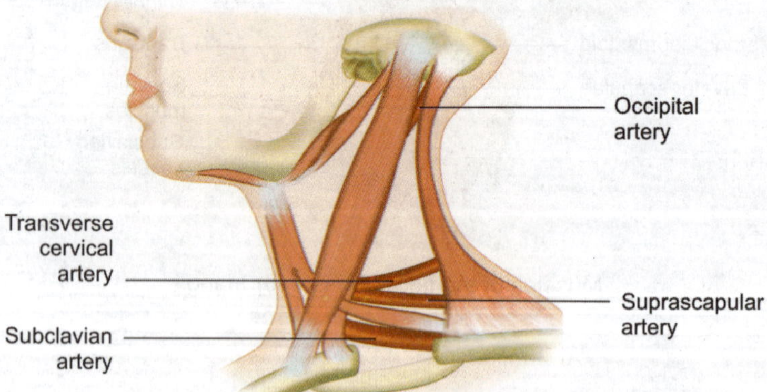

Vessels in posterior triangle

Lymph Nodes

- Posterior triangle nodes.

Applied Anatomy

1. Left-sided supraclavicular lymph nodes are enlarged in malignancies of stomach, testis known as Virchow's nodes.

2. Spasm of sternocleidomastoid is known as wryneck.
3. In neck dissections for malignancies, certain groups of lymph nodes are removed. Spinal accessory nerve may get injured, while removing the nodes. Injury to this nerve may lead to drooping of shoulder and requires postoperative rehabilitation.

Q. WHAT ARE THE BOUNDARIES, FLOOR, ROOF AND CONTENTS OF SUBOCCIPITAL TRIANGLE OF NECK? WHAT IS ITS CLINICAL SIGNIFICANCE?

Suboccipital triangle is a muscular space in the deepest plane of nape of the neck. To reach the triangle, one needs to expose the following layers from outside:

- Skin
- Superficial fascia
- Trapezius
- Splenius capitis
- Semispinalis capitis.

Boundaries

- Superomedially—rectus capitis posterior minor and major
- Superolaterally—superior oblique
- Inferiorly—inferior oblique.

Roof

- Semispinalis capitis medially
- Longissimus capitis laterally.

Floor

- Posterior arch of atlas
- Atlanto-occipital membrane.

Contents

- Dorsal ramus of C1
- Third part of vertebral artery
- Suboccipital plexus of veins.

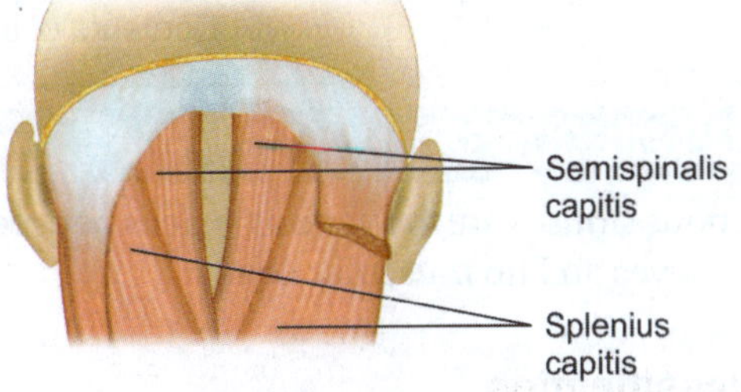

Muscles covering the suboccipital triangle

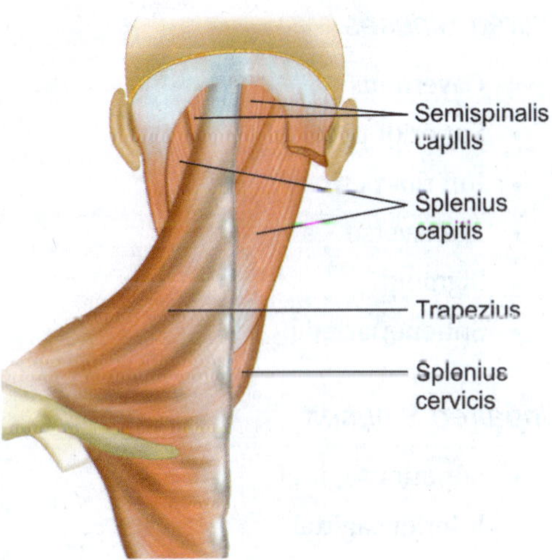

Suboccipital triangle

Surgical Significance

Posterior cranial fossa can be approached via suboccipital triangle for cisternal puncture.

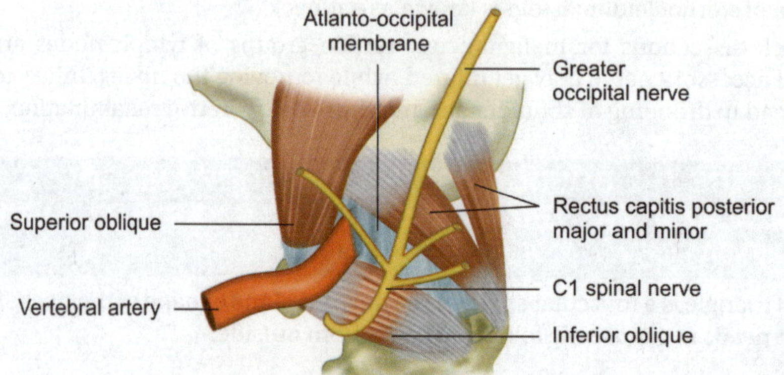

Contents of suboccipital triangle

Q. DISCUSS VENOUS SINUSES IN DETAIL.

Venous sinuses are the venous spaces between two layers of dura mater. Unlike veins they have no valves and no muscular coat.

Classification

Venous sinuses can be classified as paired and unpaired sinuses.

Paired Sinuses

- Cavernous
- Superior petrosal
- Inferior petrosal
- Transverse
- Sigmoid
- Sphenoparietal.

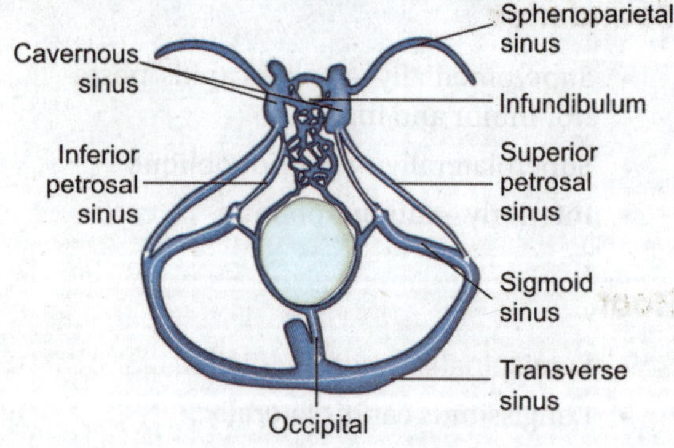

Paired venous sinuses

Unpaired Sinuses

- Superior sagittal
- Inferior sagittal
- Straight
- Occipital
- Anterior intercavernous
- Posterior intercavernous.

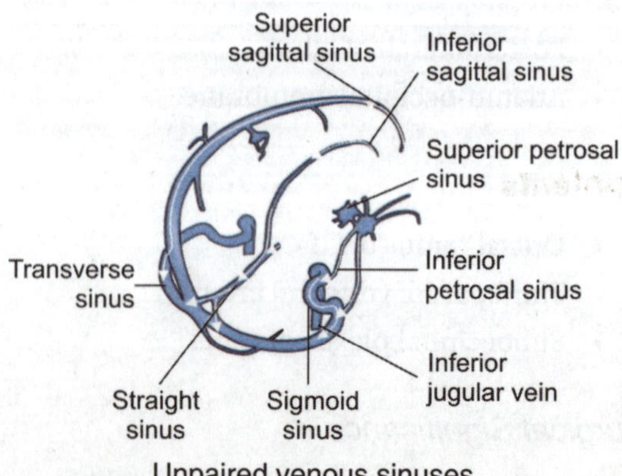

Unpaired venous sinuses

Arrangement of Sinuses and Drainage Pattern

Arrangement and drainage pattern is shown in the figure below.

Cavernous Sinus

Cavernous sinus is a large venous sinus located on either side of pituitary fossa, forming a very crucial location.

Extent: Anteriorly it extends up to the medial end of superior orbital fissure and posteriorly it extends up to the petrous temporal.

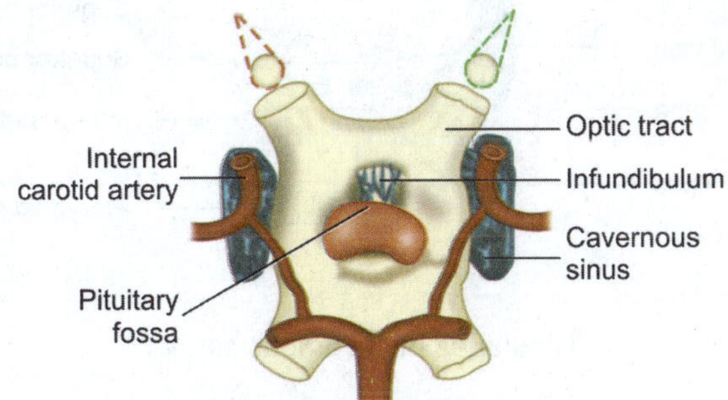

Cavernous sinus relations

Relations

- Superiorly—optic tract, internal carotid artery
- Inferiorly—foramen lacerum
- Medially—hypophysis cerebri and sphenoidal air sinus
- Laterally—temporal lobe
- Anteriorly—superior orbital fissure
- Posteriorly—apex of petrous temporal.

Structures in the lateral wall and the cranial nerves are shown in the figure below.

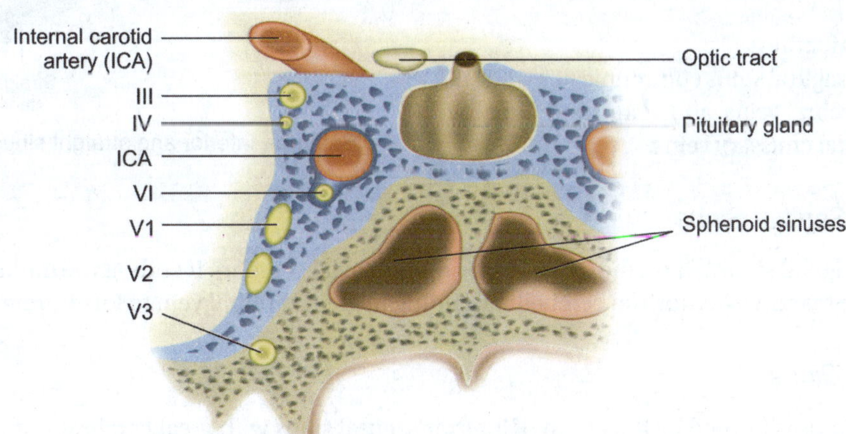

Cavernous sinus relations and nerve supply

Draining channels and communications of cavernous sinus

1. Cavernous sinus receives the superior ophthalmic vein, central vein of retina, inferior ophthalmic vein, sphenoparietal sinus.
2. It drains into transverse sinus, internal jugular vein, pterygoid plexus of veins, facial vein.
3. The two sinuses communicate with each other anteriorly and posteriorly.
4. All the communications are valveless and the blood can flow in either directions.

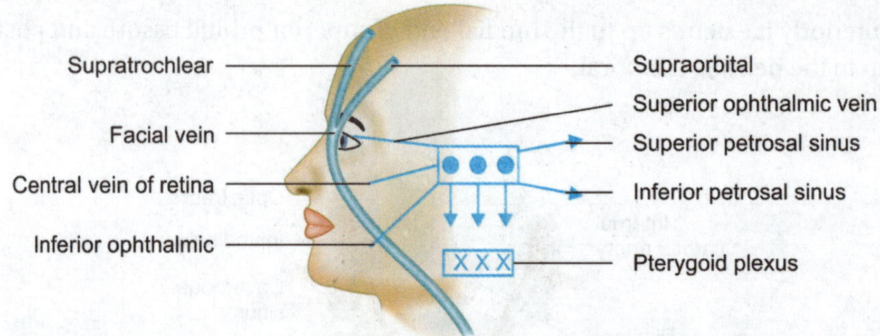

Tributaries of cavernous sinus

Superior Sagittal Sinus

Superior sagittal sinus is located on the superior border of falx cerebri.

Extent

Superior sagittal sinus begins at crista galli, here it communicates with veins of frontal sinus and veins of nose. It ends at internal occipital protuberance by turning to the right and becomes continuous as right transverse sinus.

Communications

Superior sagittal sinus communicates with superior cerebral veins, and veins from the nose and parietal emissary veins.

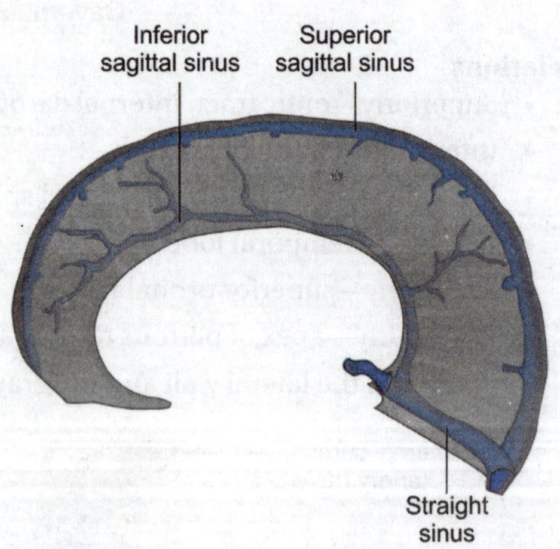

Superior, inferior and straight sinuses

Inferior Sagittal Sinus

Inferior sagittal sinus lies on the concave free margin of falx cerebri. It ends at the middle of anterior free margin of tentorium cerebelli by ending in great cerebral vein to form straight sinus.

Straight Sinus

Straight sinus is formed by the union of inferior sagittal sinus with great cerebral vein.

Transverse Sinus

Right transverse sinus is a continuation of superior sagittal sinus and left is the continuation of straight sinus.

Sigmoid Sinus

Sigmoid sinus is the continuation of transverse sinus and extends from posteroinferior angle of the parietal bone to the jugular foramen, where it continues as internal jugular vein.

Applied Anatomy

- Thrombosis (block) of sigmoid sinus occurs most commonly secondary to otitis media or mastoiditis
- Cavernous sinus thrombosis may occur secondary to infection in 'danger area of face'
- During mastoid operations one should not expose sigmoid sinus.

> **Q. DESCRIBE THE GROSS ANATOMY OF PAROTID GLAND, ITS RELATIONS, BLOOD SUPPLY, NERVE SUPPLY AND LYMPHATIC DRAINAGE. ADD A NOTE ON ITS APPLIED ANATOMY.**

Parotid gland is the largest of the salivary gland located below external acoustic meatus and between ramus of mandible and sternocleidomastoid.

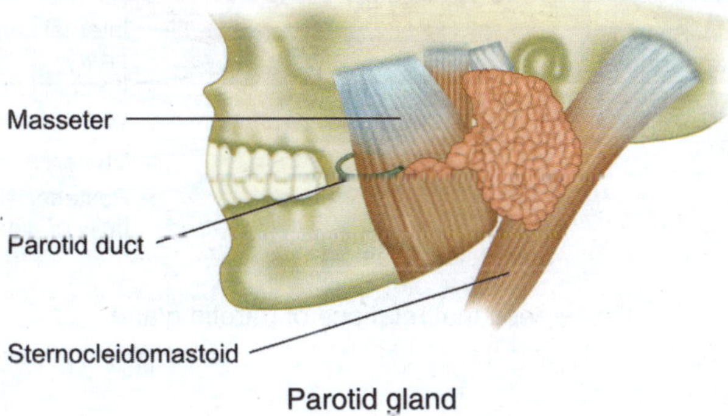

Parotid gland

Gross Features

Gland resembles inverted pyramid and has following parts:

- Apex
- Base
- Surfaces—superficial, anteromedial and posteromedial
- Borders—anterior, posterior, medial
- Parotid capsule—gland is covered by the investing layers of deep cervical fascia, which is thick and adherent.

Relations

Apex

Apex is related to posterior belly of digastic muscle cervical branch of VII nerve and retromandibular vein.

Base

Base lies just below external auditory meatus:

- Related to temporomandibular joint
- Superficial temporal vessels
- Auriculotemporal nerve.

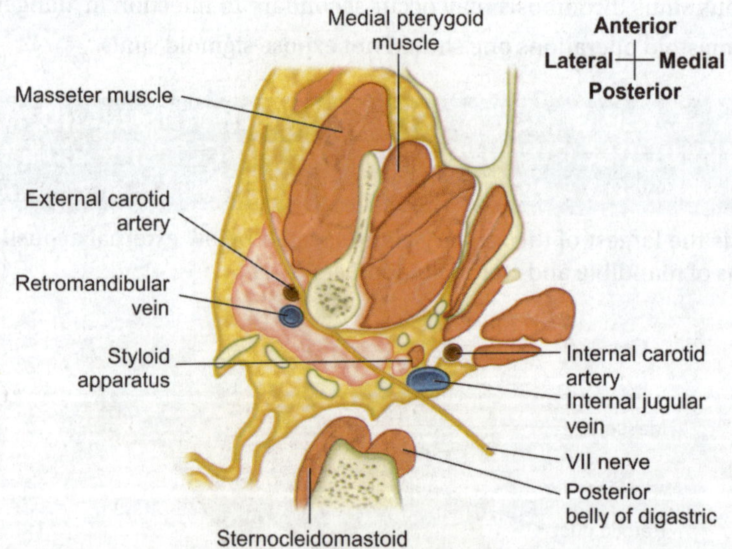

Cross-sectional relations of parotid gland

Surfaces

Superficial surface: It is covered with skin, superficial fascia, deep cervical fascia, lymph nodes.

Anteromedial surface: It is related to mandible and thus related to the muscles attached.

Posteromedial surface: It is related to mastoid and styloid process and thus the structures attached to it.

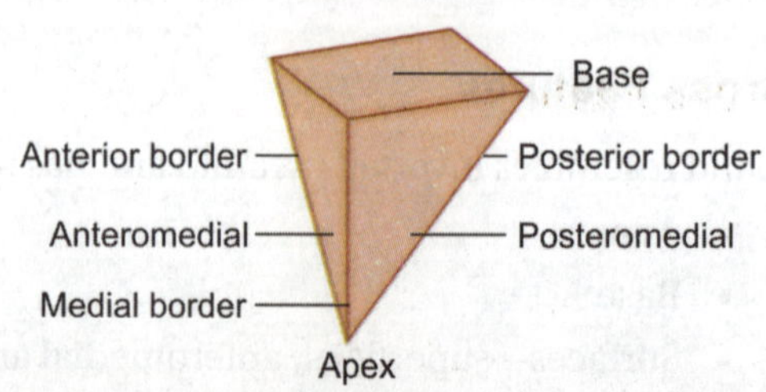

Surfaces of parotid gland (as seen from medial side)

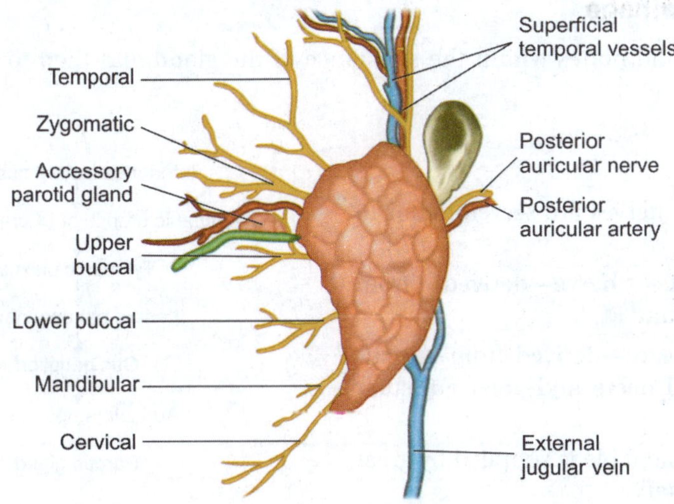

Neurovascular relations of parotid gland

Structures Within the Parotid Gland

The structures within the parotid gland are as follows:

- External carotid artery (it enters the gland through the posteromedial surface)
- Retromandibular vein
- Facial nerve.

Blood Supply

External carotid artery (ECA) and external jugular vein (EJV).

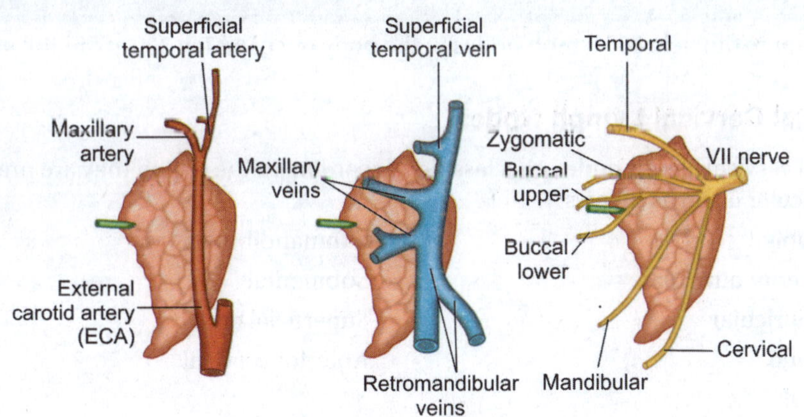

Structures piercing the parotid gland

Lymphatic Drainage

Drains into parotid nodes within the substance of the gland and then to the upper deep cervical nodes.

Nerve Supply

Parasympathetic nerves are secretomotor to gland:

- Sympathetic nerve—derived from plexus around ECA
- Sensory nerve—derived from auriculotemporal nerve and great auricular nerve
- Angle of mandible is supplied by great auricular nerve.

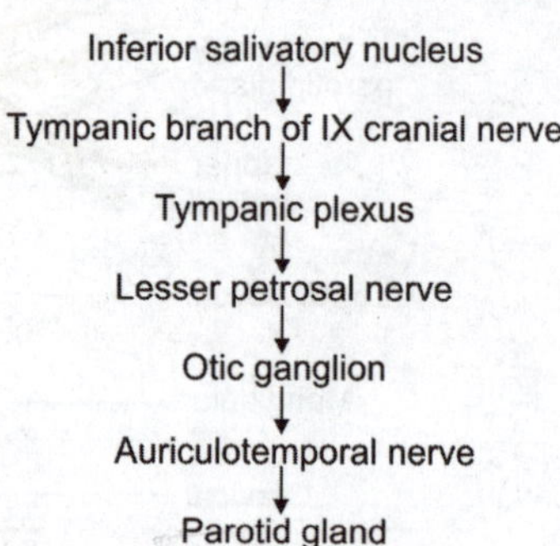

Applied Anatomy

- Parotid swellings, i.e. parotitis is extremely painful due to thick and adherent parotid fascia
- Conley's cartilaginous pointer—by pulling the pinna backwards, tragus points at a place from where the facial nerve is 1–1.5 cm deep
- Frey syndrome—in cases of injury to auriculotemporal nerve, the nerve grows aberrantly to anastomose with superior cervical ganglion fibers (it is an anastomosis between sympathetic and parasympathetic fibers).

In this condition, while chewing there is redness and sweating over the parotid region.

> **Q. DISCUSS CERVICAL LYMPH NODES AND ADD A NOTE ON ITS CLINICAL SIGNIFICANCE.**

There are approximately 800 lymph nodes in the body out of which 300 are in the neck.

Superficial Cervical Lymph Nodes

Superficial cervical lymph nodes are classified according to the region they are present in the form of circular chain as follows:

- Occipital
- Posterior auricular
- Preauricular
- Parotid
- Facial
- Submandibular
- Submental
- Superficial cervical
- Anterior cervical.

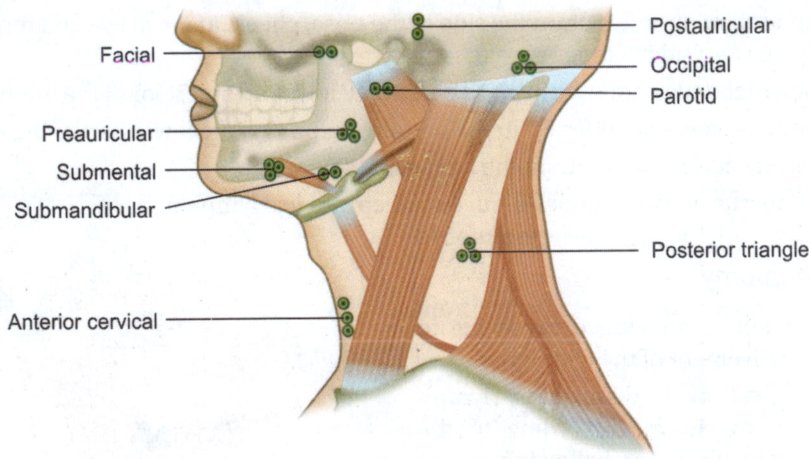

Superficial cervical lymph node grouping

Drainage Area

1. Occipital drains the back of the scalp.
2. Posterior auricular drains the temporal region, back of the pinna, external auditory meatus.

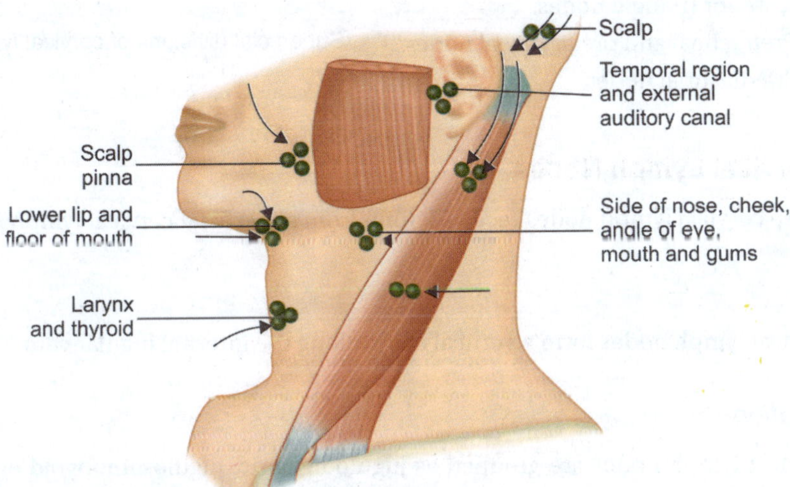

Drainage areas of superficial cervical lymph nodes

3. Preauricular drains the outer side of pinna and side of scalp.
4. Parotid nodes located in the substance of the gland drain the eyelids, front of scalp, external auditory meatus and tympanic cavity, while the nodes deep to the gland drain the nasopharynx and nose.
5. Superficial facial nodes receive lymph from conjunctiva, eyelids, nose and cheek. Deep facial nodes drain the temporal fossa, infratemporal fossa, back of the nose and pharynx.

6. Submandibular nodes drain the side of the nose, cheek, angle of eye and mouth, upper lip, gums and side of tongue.
7. Submental nodes drain the central part of the lower lip and floor of the mouth.
8. Superficial cervical nodes drain the parotid region and the lower part of the ear.
9. Anterior cervical nodes drain the larynx and thyroid.

All the superficial lymph nodes drain into deep cervical lymph nodes.

Applied Anatomy

1. Malignancies are staged according to the involvement of the lymph nodes.
2. In radical neck dissections, lymph nodes are cleared according to the level of involvement. Following are the levels of lymph nodes.

Level I: Submental and submandibular nodes.

Level II: Upper cervical nodes.

Level III: Middle cervical nodes.

Level IV: Lower cervical nodes.

Level V: Posterior triangle nodes.

Level VI: Pretracheal and prelaryngeal nodes.

Level VII: Mediastinal nodes.

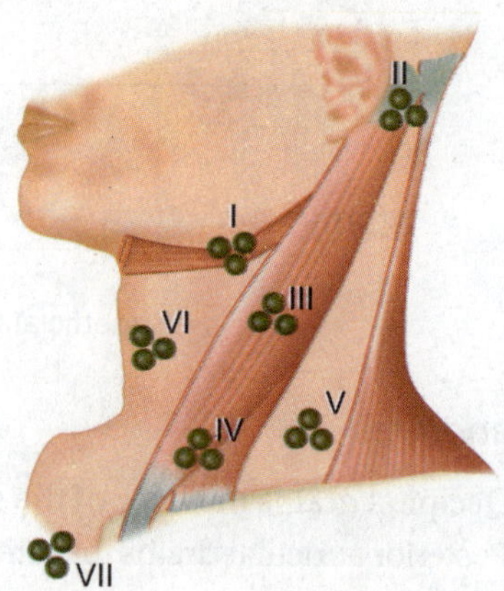

Superficial divisions of cervical lymph nodes

Deep Cervical Lymph Nodes

All the deep cervical lymph nodes receive lymph from superficial cervical lymph nodes.

Location

Deep cervical lymph nodes form a vertical chain along the internal jugular vein.

Classification

Deep cervical lymph nodes are grouped as jugulodigastric, jugulo-omohyoid and supraclavicular lymph nodes.

Drainage Area

1. Jugulodigastric nodes mainly drain the tonsils.
2. Jugulo-omohyoid mainly drains the tongue.
3. Supraclavicular lymph nodes receive the lymph from preceding nodes. Additionally, left side receives lymph from pelvic viscera (ovaries, testis) and breast.

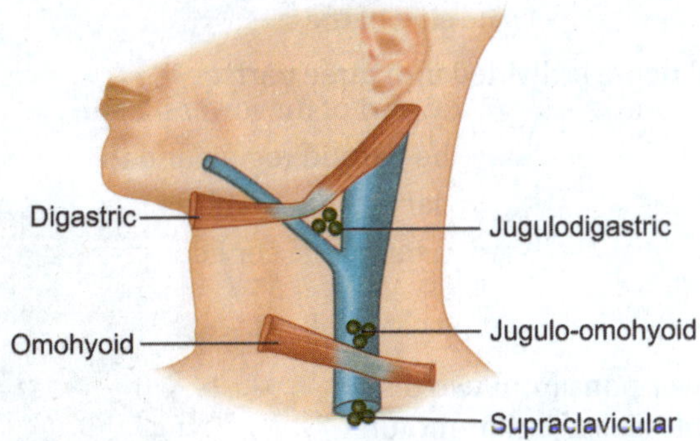

Applied Anatomy

Enlarged left supraclavicular lymph nodes are known as Virchow's nodes.

> **Q. DESCRIBE FACIAL NERVE IN DETAIL (FUNCTIONAL COMPONENTS NUCLEI, COURSE, BRANCHES AND APPLIED ANATOMY).**

Facial nerve is the VII cranial nerve, which supplies the muscles of the face, salivary glands (submandibular and sublingual) and lacrimal gland and carries sensation of taste from anterior two third of tongue.

Embryologically facial nerve is the nerve of second branchial arch.

Nuclei

There are four nuclei of facial nerve, located in lower pons are as follows:

- Motor nucleus
- Superior salivatory nucleus
- Lacrimatory nucleus
- Nucleus of tractus solitarius.

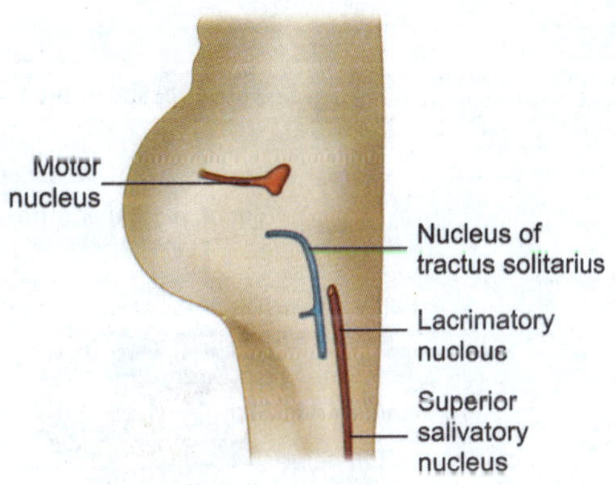

Nuclei of facial nerve in lower pons

Functional Components

- Special visceral afferent—for taste
- General visceral efferent—secretomotor for glands
- General somatic afferent—proprioception and general sensation from external auditory canal
- Branchial efferent—for facial muscles.

Course

The course of the facial nerve is divided into three parts:

- Intracranial
- Intrapetrous
- Extracranial.

Intracranial Part

The nerve begins at lower pons from two distinct roots—motor and sensory. The motor root winds the abducent nerve nuclei and emerges from lower border of pons to lie in the cerebellopontine angle.

It runs laterally and forwards to reach the internal acoustic meatus (IAM). In the meatus, motor root lies over the auditory nerve with intervening sensory root; accompanied by labyrinthine vessels.

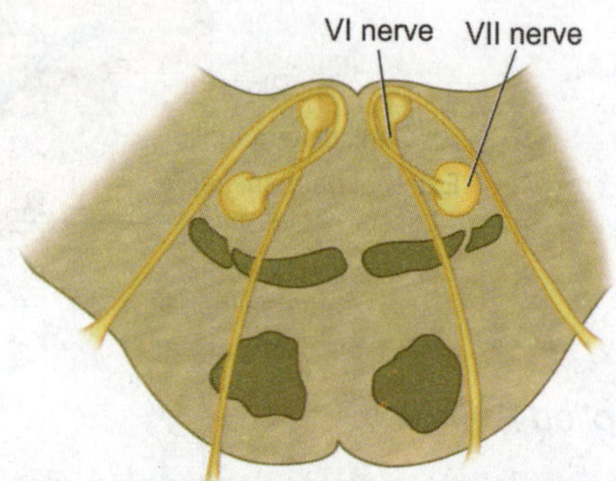

Transverse section at lower pons

Intrapetrous Part

In the intrapetrous part, the nerve runs in the bony canal known as fallopian canal with a sigmoid course. It has three parts:

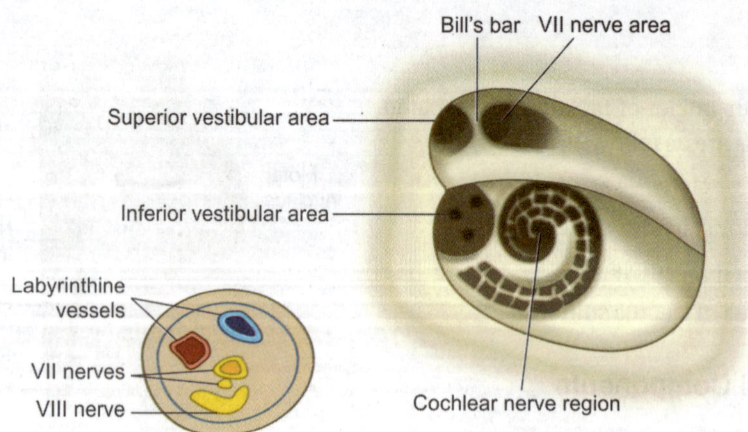

Internal acoustic meatus (IAM) with its structure

- One part is on top of vestibule—labyrinthine part—A
- Another part is closely related to the middle ear cavity—tympanic part—B
- The third part is vertically related to mastoid cavity—mastoid part—C.

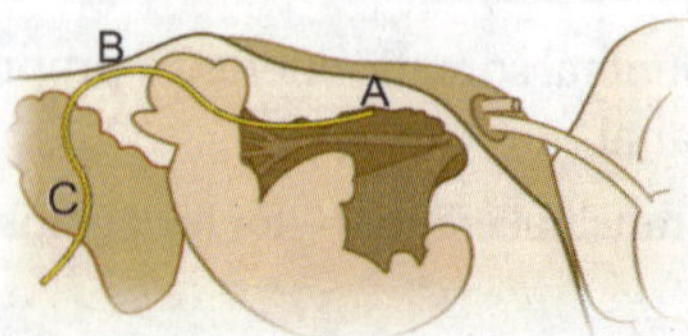

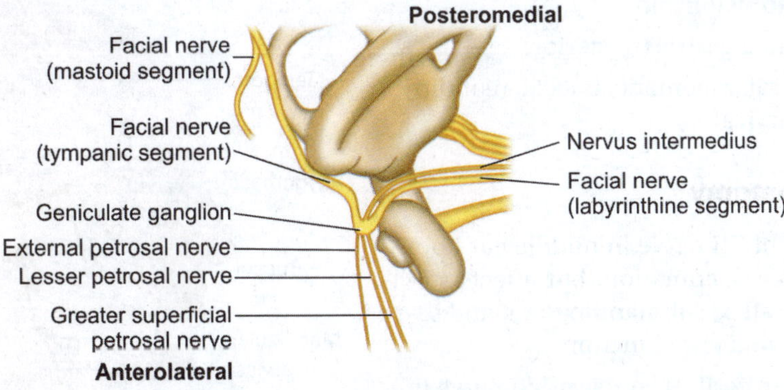

Intratemporal part of VII nerve

Extracranial Part

Extracranial part leaves the skull through stylomastoid foramen; crosses laterally the base of styloid process, enters the posteromedial surface of parotid gland, crosses the retromandibular vein and external carotid artery and divides behind the neck of mandible into five terminal branches.

Branches

- Greater superficial petrosal nerve
- Branch to stapedius
- Chorda tympani nerve
- Posterior auricular

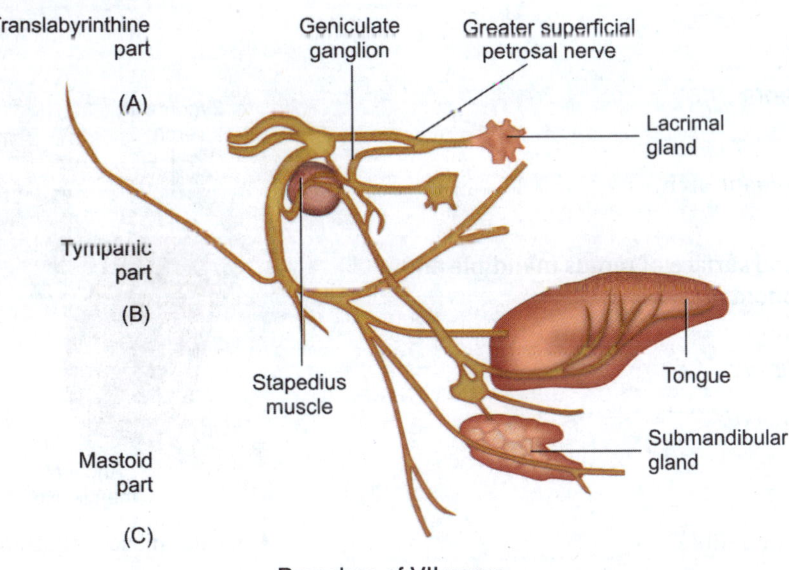

Branches of VII nerve

- Nerve to stylohyoid
- Nerve to digastric (posterior)
- Temporal, zygomatic, buccal, mandibular, cervical.

Applied Anatomy

- Lesion of VII nerve in middle ear does not affect lacrimation, but affects stapedial reflex, submandibular gland secretion and taste function
- Lesion in vertical course of VII nerve in mastoid segment, will cause decreased taste sensation and submandibular secretion however, lacrimation and stapedial reflex would be normal.

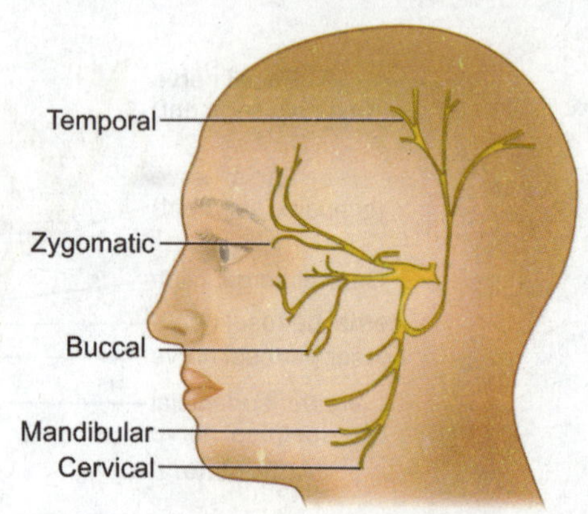

Extracranial branches of VII nerve

> **Q. WHAT ARE THE MUSCLES OF MASTICATION? DESCRIBE THEIR ATTACHMENTS, NERVE SUPPLY AND ACTION.**

There are four pairs of muscles of mastication, which bring about jaw movements. They are as follows:

- Masseter
- Temporalis
- Lateral pterygoid
- Medial pterygoid.

Masseter

Attachments

From

- Zygomatic arch.

To

- Lateral surface of ramus mandible and coronoid process.

Nerve Supply

Massetric nerve.

Action

Closes the mandible.

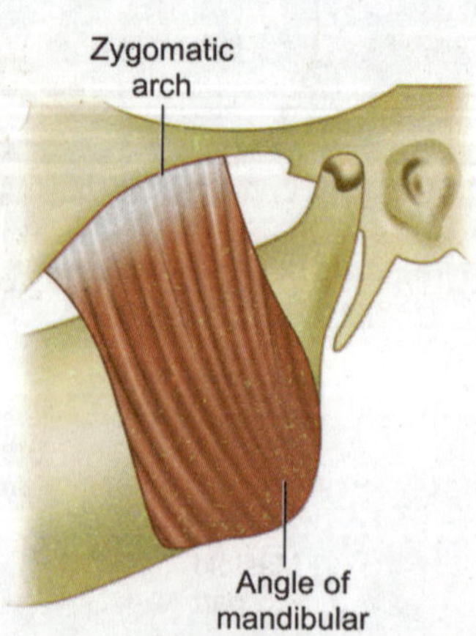

Masseter muscle attachment

Temporalis

Attachments

From

- Temporal fossa and temporalis fascia.

To

- Coronoid process of mandible.

Nerve Supply

Mandibular nerve.

Action

Closes the jaw, retracts the mandible behind and helps in side-to-side chewing movements.

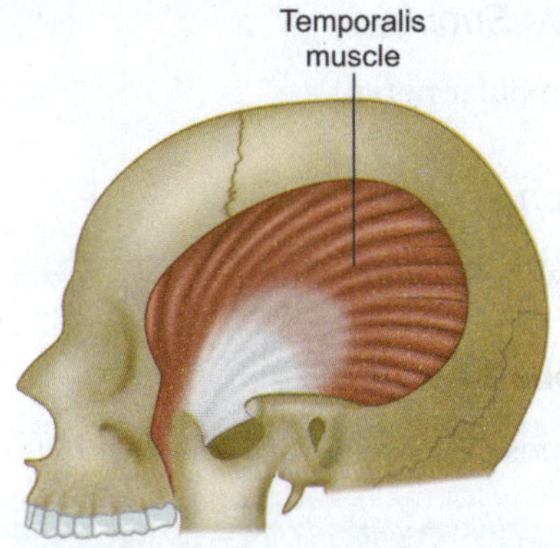

Temporalis muscle attachment

Lateral Pterygoid

Attachments

From

- Greater wing of sphenoid and lateral surface of lateral pterygoid plate.

To

- Pterygoid fovea, articular disk and capsule of temporomandibular (TM) joint.

Nerve Supply

Mandibular nerve.

Action

- Opens the mouth.

Medial Pterygoid

Attachments

From

- Tuberosity of maxilla medial surface of lateral pterygoid plate.

To

- Medial surface of angle and ramus of mandible.

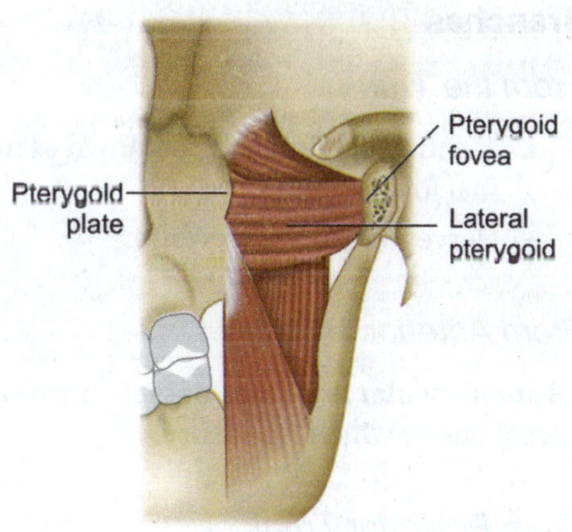

Pterygoid muscle

Nerve Supply

Mandibular nerve.

Action

Elevates the mandible.

Applied Anatomy

Trismus may occur due to fibrosis of muscles of mastication giving rise to dysphagia.

Q. DESCRIBE MANDIBULAR NERVE.

Mandibular nerve is largest of the three divisions of trigeminal nerve. It supplies teeth, gums, skin in temporal region, auricle, lower lip, lower part of face, muscles of mastication and mucosa of tongue and oral floor.

Roots

Mandibular nerve has two roots, i.e. sensory and motor.

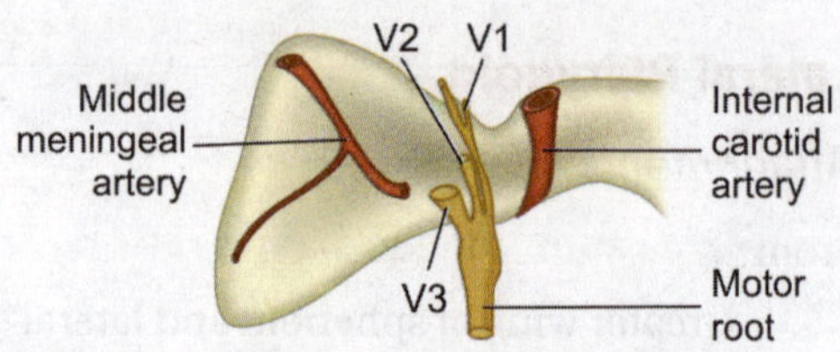

Root of mandibular nerve

Relations

- Motor root lies deep to sensory root
- Both unite just distal to foramen ovale
- After emerging from foramen ovale, the nerve lies between tensor veli palatini and lateral pterygoid muscle.

Branches

From the Trunk

- Meningeal branch (also known as nervous spinosus) supplies dura mater of middle cranial fossa
- Nerve to medial pterygoid.

From Anterior Trunk

All are muscular branches namely masseter, deep temporal, nerve to lateral pterygoid except buccal nerve, which is sensory.

From Posterior Trunk

- Auriculotemporal
- Lingual nerve

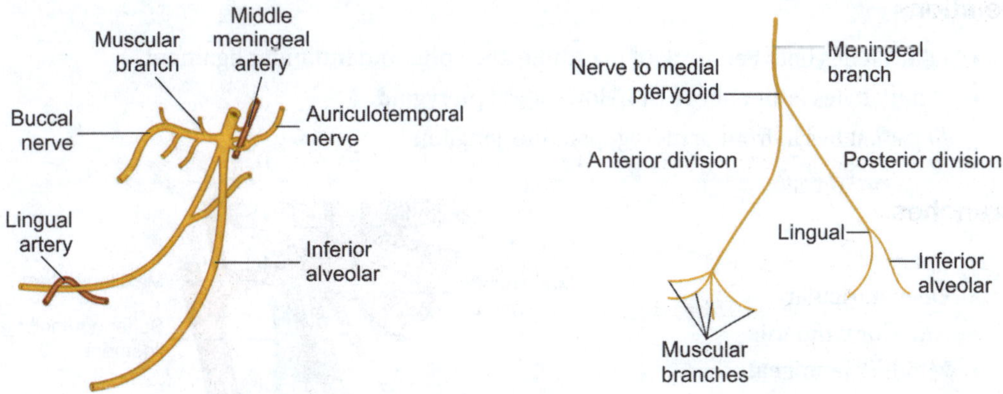

Branches of mandibular nerve

- Inferior alveolar.

Auriculotemporal nerve forms a loop around middle meningeal artery.

Applied Anatomy

In cases of cancer tongue, pain is referred to ear over the area of distribution of auriculotemporal nerve.

Q. WHAT IS THE ORIGIN, COURSE, RELATIONS AND BRANCHES OF MAXILLARY ARTERY. MENTION ITS SURGICAL IMPORTANCE.

Maxillary artery is one of the terminal branches of external carotid artery at the neck of the mandible.

Course

For simplicity, the artery is divided into three parts are as follows:

- *I part:* Horizontal part, which is proximal to lateral pterygoid
- *II part:* It lies sometimes superficial or deep to lateral pterygoid
- *III part:* It lies between the two head of lateral pterygoid muscle and enters pterygopalatine fossa through pterygopalatine fissure.

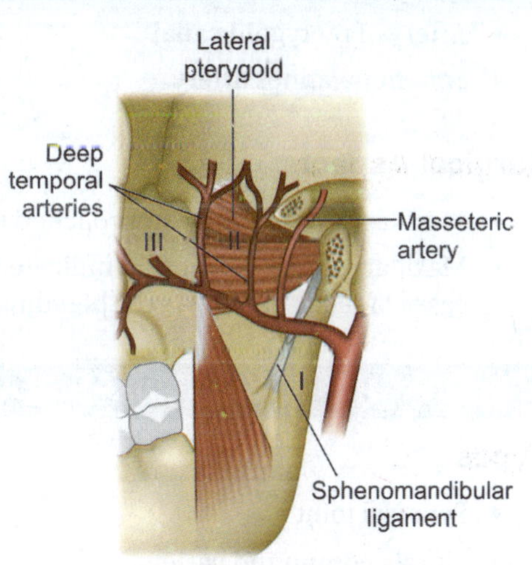

Parts of maxillary artery

Relations

- *I part:* It lies between neck of mandible and sphenomandibular ligament
- *II part:* It lies either above or below lateral pterygoid
- *III part:* It lies in front of pterygopalatine ganglion.

Branches

1. I part:
   - Deep auricular
   - Anterior tympanic
   - Middle meningeal
   - Accessory meningeal
   - Inferior alveolar.
2. II part:
   - Deep temporal
   - Pterygoid
   - Massetric
   - Buccal.
3. III part:
   - Posterior superior alveolar
   - Infraorbital
   - Greater palatine
   - Pharyngeal
   - Artery of pterygoid canal
   - Sphenopalatines artery.

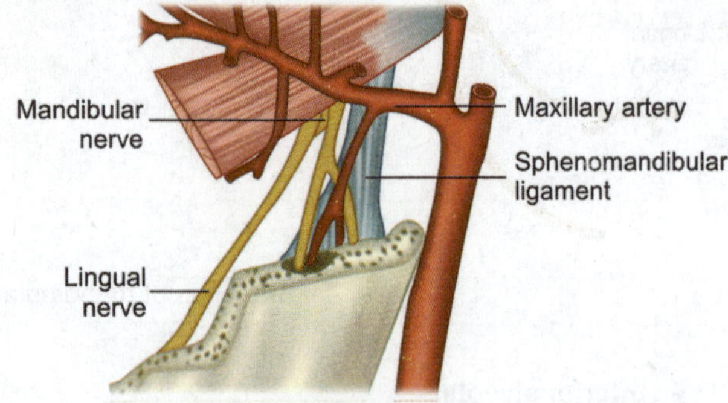

Maxillary artery

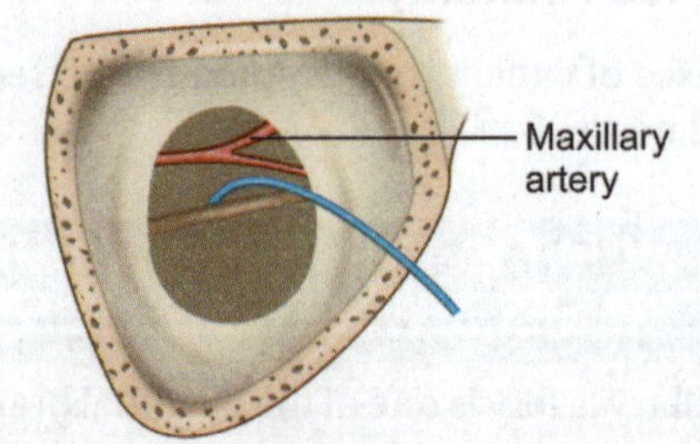

Transantral approach to maxillary artery

Surgical Aspects

- Maxillary artery can be approached transantrally
- Maxillary artery ligation is indicated in transantral approach to maxillary artery (tie) cases of recurrent epistaxis (bleeding through nose).

Q. DISCUSS TEMPOROMANDIBULAR JOINT IN DETAIL.

Types

- Synovial joint
- Simple compound variety.

Articular Surfaces

- Above—anterior part of mandibular fossa
- Below—head of mandible.

Ligaments

1. Fibrous capsule: It is attached above to the articular tubercle, around mandibular fossa and squamotympanic fissure, below to the posterolateral aspect of the neck of the mandible.
2. Articular disk: It is a fibrous plate dividing the joint into upper and lower compartment.
3. Sphenomandibular ligament: Attached superiorly to the spine of sphenoid and inferiorly to lingula of mandible. It is related laterally to lateral pterygoid muscle, auriculotemporal nerve, maxillary artery medially to medial pterygoid muscle and chorda tympani nerve.
4. Stylomandibular ligament: It is a thickened portion of deep cervical fascia. Temporomandibular joint is surrounded by parotid gland externally and internally related to spine of sphenoid.

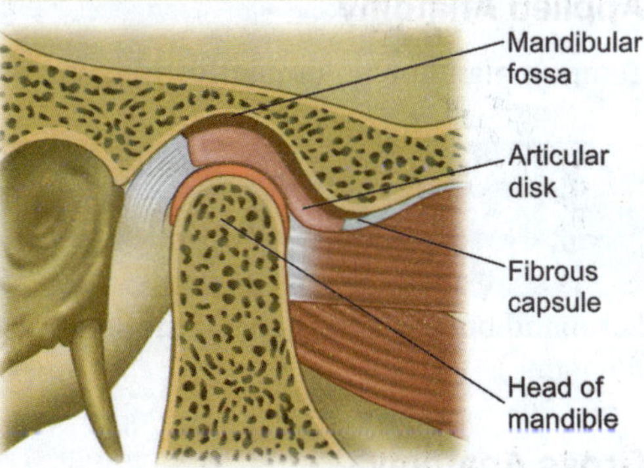

Articulating surfaces of temporomandibular joint

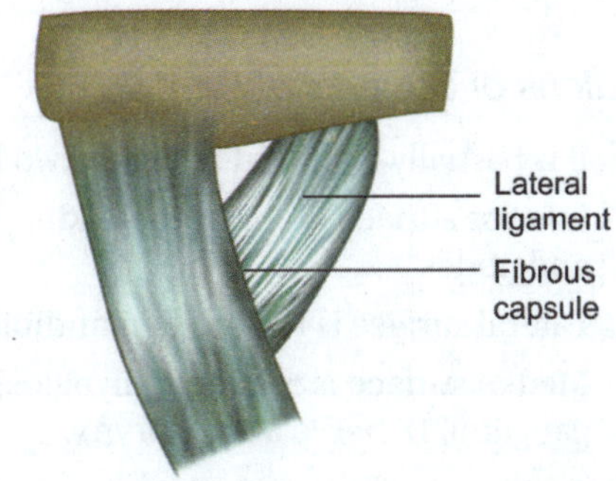

Ligaments of temporomandibular joint

Actions

- Depression is brought about by lateral pterygoid and other strap muscles assist depression
- Elevation is brought about by medial pterygoid, masseter and temporalis
- Protrusion is brought about by pterygoids
- Retraction is brought about by temporalis
- Side-by-side movement brought about by pterygoids.

Nerve Supply

- Auriculotemporal nerve
- Massetric nerve.

Blood Supply

Superficial temporal and maxillary artery.

Applied Anatomy

Temporomandibular joint arthritis may cause difficulty in opening the mouth, i.e. trismus.

> **Q. DESCRIBE THE GROSS ANATOMY OF SUBMANDIBULAR GLAND, ITS RELATIONS, BLOOD SUPPLY, NERVE SUPPLY AND LYMPHATIC DRAINAGE. ADD A NOTE ON ITS APPLIED ANATOMY.**

Submandibular gland is one of the serous salivary gland, located below the mandible (hence the name).

Gross Anatomy

Submandibular gland is divided into two parts by mylohyoid muscle—superficial part and deep part. It has medial, lateral and inferior surface.

Relations of Superficial Part

- It is partially enclosed between two layers of investing cervical fascia
- Inferior surface is covered by skin, platysma, cervical branch of facial nerve, facial vein and nodes
- Lateral surface is related to mandible
- Medial surface is related to hyoglossus and styloglossus, lingual nerve, submandibular ganglion, IX nerve and pharynx.

Relations of Deep Part

The deep part lies deep to mylohyoid muscle and superficial to hyoglossus. It continues anteriorly as Wharton's duct. Submandibular duct runs forwards on hyoglossus and opens on the floor of mouth.

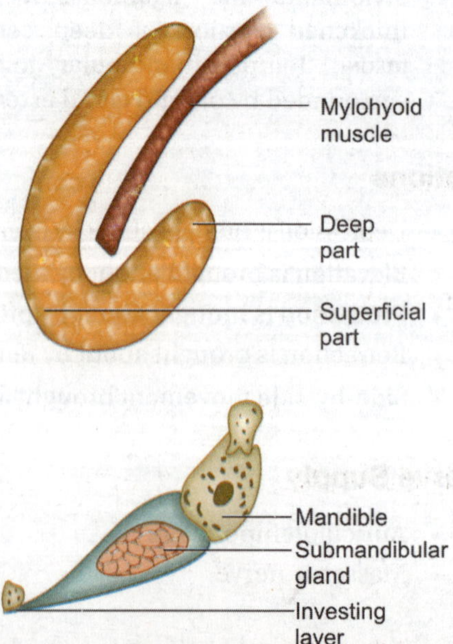

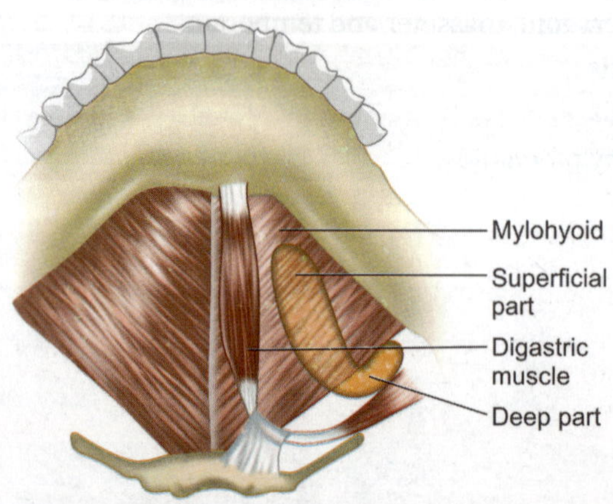

Deep fascia enclosing

Blood Supply

Submandibular gland is supplied by facial artery and drain in common facial vein. Lymphatics pass to submandibular nodes.

Nerve Supply

Chorda tympani nerve conveys secretomotor fibers, lingual nerve carries sensory fiber, sympathetic innervation comes from plexus around facial artery.

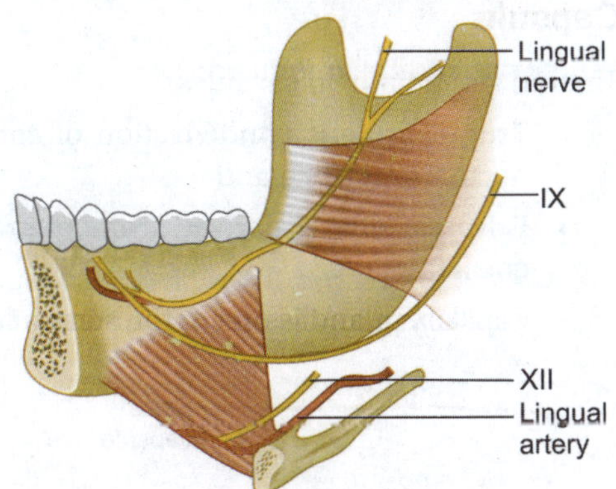

Deep part of submandibular gland

Secretomotor Pathway

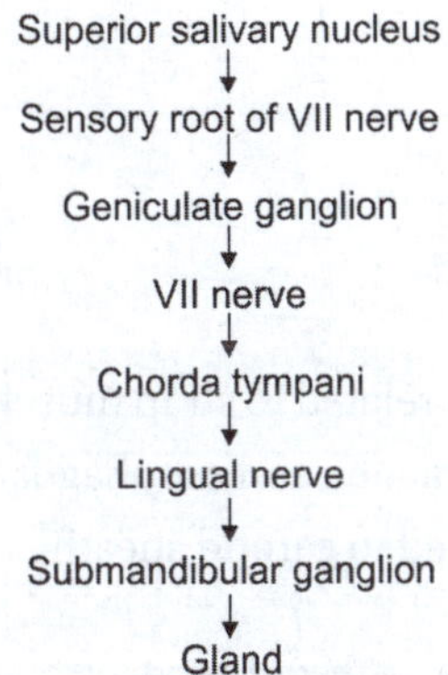

Applied Anatomy

- Submandibular gland is commonly excised in patients having calculi in submandibular duct
- It is palpable bimanually.

Q. DESCRIBE THE GROSS ANATOMY OF THYROID GLAND, ITS RELATIONS AND BLOOD SUPPLY. ADD A NOTE ON ITS APPLIED ANATOMY.

Thyroid gland is an endocrine gland, located in lower part of the neck. It undergoes physiological changes during pregnancy and menstruation.

Gross Anatomy

- It is butterfly-shaped gland, located against C5, C6, C7 vertebrae
- Gland weighs approximately 25 g
- Gland has two lobes connected by isthmus.

Capsule

Thyroid gland has two capsules:

- True capsule is condensation of connective tissue of gland
- False capsule is derived from pretracheal fascia
- Capillary plexus lies deep to true capsule.

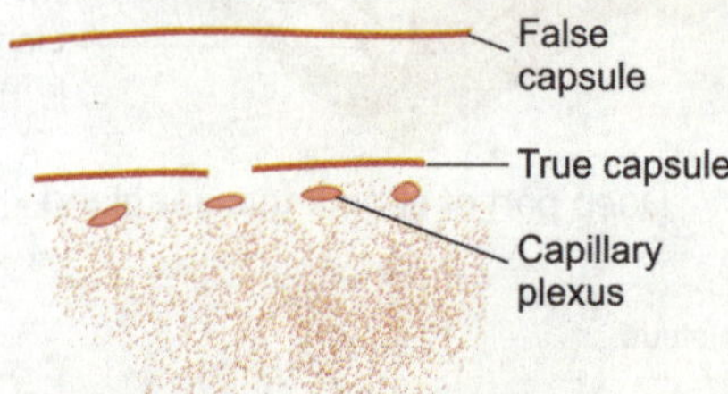

Capsule of thyroid gland

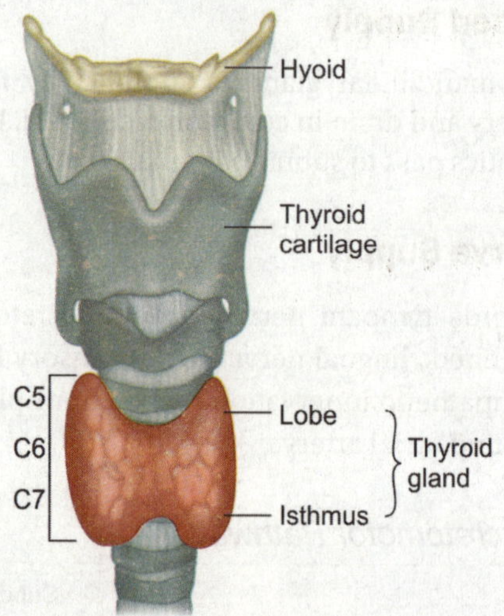

Location of thyroid gland

Relations

- Lateral surface of the lobes is related to strap muscles
- Medial surface is related to trachea and esophagus
- Posterolateral surface is related to carotid sheath.

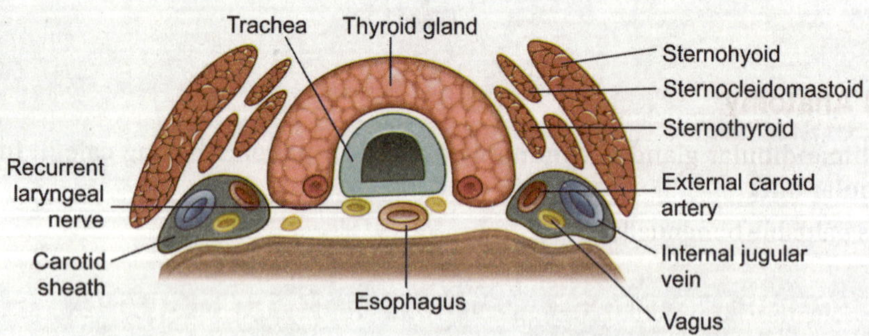

Transverse section showing relations of thyroid gland

Crucial Neurovascular Relations

1. External laryngeal nerve lies in close relation to superior thyroid artery, i.e. nerve and artery are away from each other close to the gland. So, artery should be ligated close to the gland.
2. Recurrent laryngeal nerve is related to inferior thyroid artery, i.e. nerve and artery (distance is more) distanced away from the gland. So, the artery should be ligated away from the gland.
3. Recurrent laryngeal nerve lies in the tracheoesophageal groove.

Blood Supply

1. Superior and inferior arteries supply the gland (sometimes thyroidea ima artery arises from brachiocephalic trunks).
2. It is drained by superior and inferior thyroid vein, which finally drains into internal jugular vein.

Applied Anatomy

- Enlargement of thyroid gland is known as goiter
- Hyperthyroidism and hypothyroidism are conditions associated with the functional status of the gland
- During thyroidectomy, surgeon needs to be cautious regarding the surgical relations of vessels, nerves and parathyroid glands
- Enlargement of thyroid can cause pressure symptoms on trachea and esophagus.

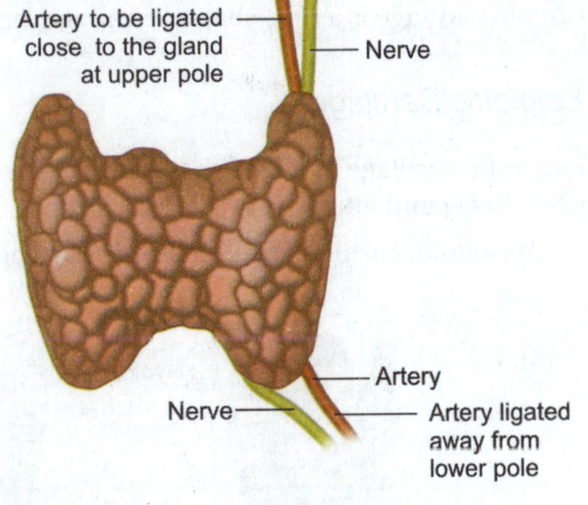

Q. DISCUSS LARYNX IN DETAIL.

Larynx is 'voice box', an organ, which produces voice, maintains the airway and acts as a guard for lower respiratory passage.

Gross Anatomy

Larynx is a midline structure in neck lying against C3, C4, C5, C6 vertebrae. In children and females it lies at a higher level. Differences between infant and adult larynx are shown in Table.

The framework of larynx is made up of cartilages and membranes connecting the cartilages.

Features	Infant	Adult
Position	C3, C4	C4, C6
Epiglottis	Folded and narrow	Leaf like
Narrowest part	Subglottis	Glottis
Cartilage	Soft	Rigid
Adam's apple	Less prominent	More prominent

Following forms the skeleton of larynx:

- Three unpaired cartilages—epiglottis, thyroid, cricoid
- Three paired cartilages—arytenoid, corniculate, cuneiform.

Thyroid Cartilage

Thyroid cartilage is a shield-like cartilage, splaying apart and forming a angular prominence in front of the neck as Adam's apple (more evident in males).

Cricoid Cartilage

Cricoid cartilage is a ring-shaped cartilage, narrow in front and broad behind.

Epiglottic Cartilage

Epiglottic cartilage is a leaf-shaped cartilage with upper free end projecting behind tongue, while lower end attached to thyroid cartilage.

Arytenoid, corniculate, cuneiform, cartilages are on the posterior aspect of larynx.

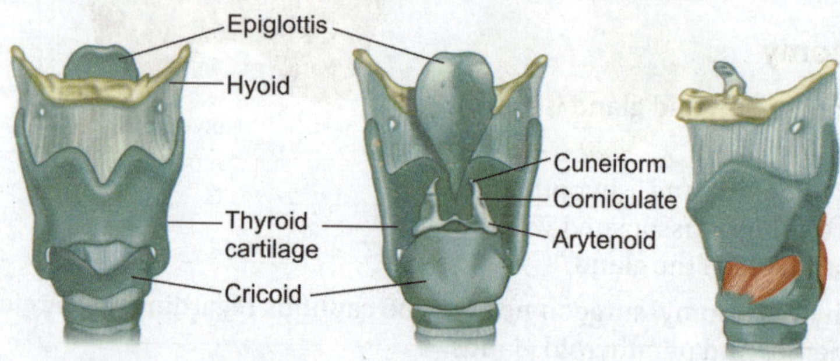

Laryngeal framework

Ligaments and Membranes

Ligaments connecting the adjacent cartilages are—thyrohyoid membrane, hyoepiglottic ligament.

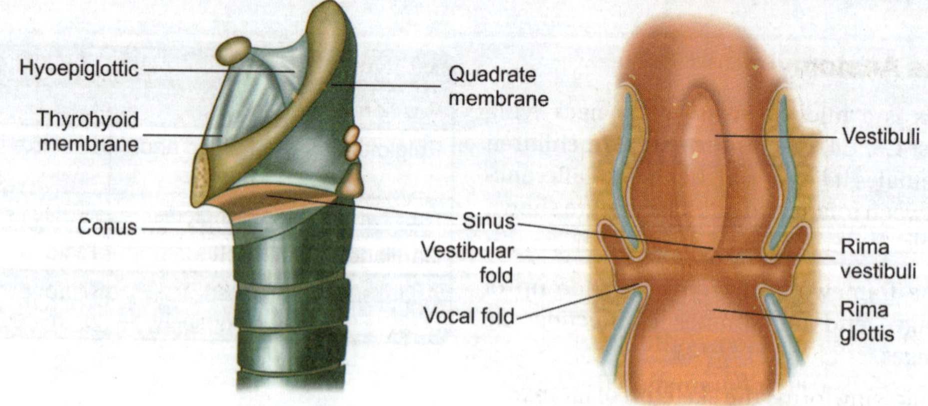

Interior of Larynx

Interior of larynx is lined by fibroelastic membrane, which is not continuous due to presence of 'sinus'. The membrane above the sinus is quadrate membrane and lower part is conus elasticus.

Muscles of Larynx

There are two varieties of muscles—the muscles within laryngeal framework are intrinsic muscles, while extrinsic muscles attach larynx to surrounding structures.

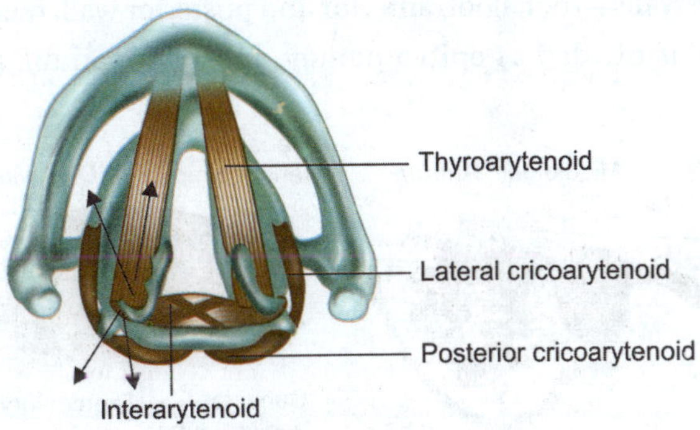

Intrinsic muscles of larynx

Salient Features

Name of the muscle depicts the attachment of the muscles. Cricothyroid is the only intrinsic muscle located on external surface. All the intrinsic muscles of larynx are supplied by recurrent laryngeal nerve except cricothyroid, which is supplied by external laryngeal nerve. Cricothyroid is the tensor of vocal cord. Posterior cricoarytenoid is the safety muscle of larynx.

Drainage

- Supraglottic larynx is drained by upper deep cervical lymph nodes
- Infraglottic larynx drained directly into pretracheal and prelaryngeal (delphian) nodes
- There are no lymphatics in vocal cords.

Applied Anatomy

- Cancer of larynx is very common in India due to tobacco chewing and smoking habits
- Carcinoma glottis is common in India, however cervical metastasis is rare
- Total laryngectomy is done in cases of cancer larynx
- Laryngitis is inflammation of larynx due to infection, swelling or trauma.

Q. WHAT ARE THE RELATIONS OF MIDDLE EAR? MENTION ITS SURGICAL SIGNIFICANCE.

Middle ear space is a narrow space situated in the petrous part of temporal bone.

Gross Anatomy

Tympanic cavity is a biconcave space with vertical and anteroposterior diameter of about 15 mm and transverse diameter of 2–6 mm.

Middle ear has six walls—roof, floor, anterior and posterior wall, medial and lateral wall.

Middle ear space is divided as epitympanum, mesotympanum, posterior tympanum, hypotympanum.

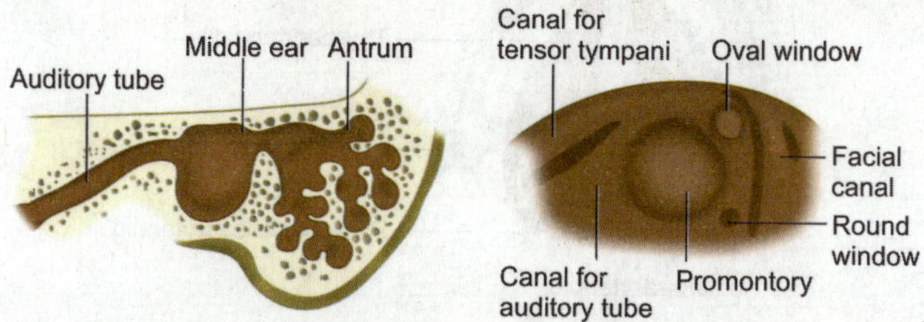

Communications and relations of middle ear

Relations

1. Roof is also known as tegmen tympani. It is a thin plate of bone separating middle ear cavity from cranial fossa.
2. Floor is related below to jugular bulb.
3. Lateral wall is formed mainly by tympanic membrane and partly above by bone (scutum).
4. Anterior wall has three important relations:
   a. Canal for tensor tympani.
   b. Eustachian tube orifice.
   c. Wall of carotid canal.

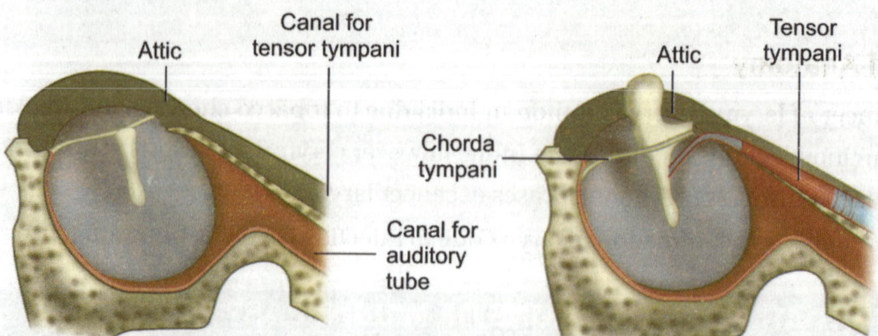

Inner side of tympanic membrane and anterior connections of middle ear cavity

5. Medial wall has following features:
   a. A bulge produced due to the basal turn of cochlea—promontory.
   b. Above and behind is fenestra ovalis (oval window) closed by footplate of stapes.

c. Above oval window is fallopian canal with facial nerve.

d. Below and behind is fenestra rotunda (round window) closed by secondary membrane.

6. Posterior wall: It presents an opening, which leads to mastoid antrum (aditus ad antrum).

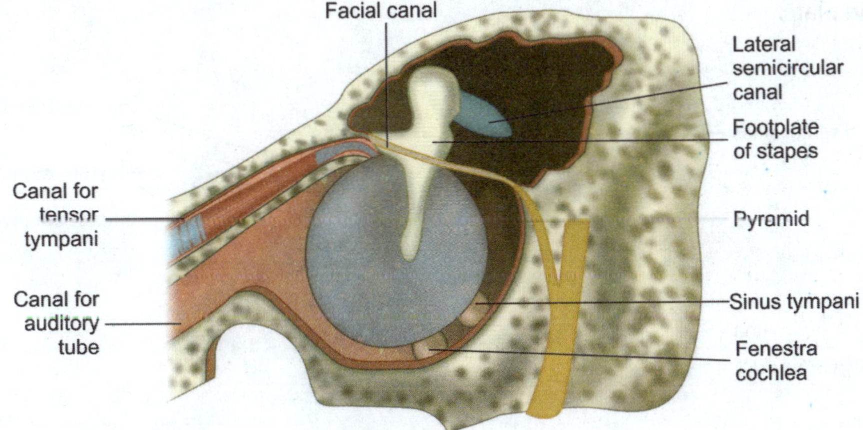

Applied Anatomy

The surgeon should be aware of the middle ear relations, while analyzing symptoms and operating on ear.

> **Q. DISCUSS LATERAL WALL OF NOSE, AND ITS BLOOD AND NERVE SUPPLY. ADD A NOTE ON ITS SURGICAL ANATOMY.**

Lateral wall of nose is an uneven area, which separates nose from orbit, maxillary sinus and nasolacrimal duct.

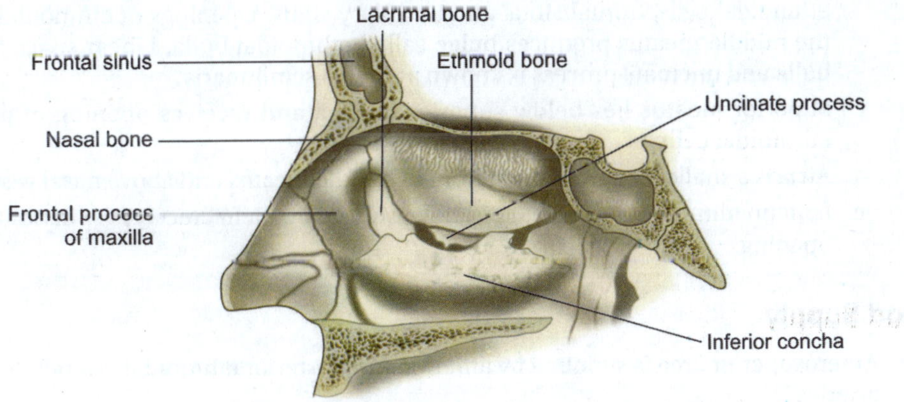

Bony framework of lateral wall of nose

Bony Skeleton of Lateral Wall

Bony skeleton is made up of (front to behind) nasal bone, frontal process of maxilla, lacrimal, ethmoid with superior and middle concha, perpendicular plate of palatine bone, medial pterygoid plate.

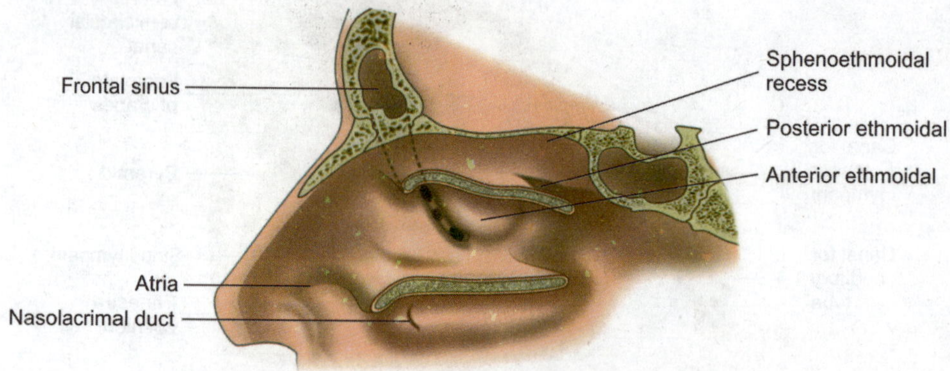

Lateral wall showing openings of sinuses

Features

1. Nasal conchae are shelf-like projections on lateral wall of nose:
   a. Superior and middle concha are parts of ethmoid bone.
   b. Inferior concha is a separate bone.
2. Meatus of nose—area below each concha is known as meatus:
   a. Inferior meatus is underneath inferior concha. Nasolacrimal duct opens in it.
   b. Middle meatus lies below middle concha. It presents openings of middle and ethmoidal cells, frontal sinus and maxillary sinus. Openings of ethmoidal cells in the middle meatus produces bulge called ethmoidal bulla. Linear space between bulla and uncinate process is known as hiatus semilunaris.
   c. Superior meatus lies below superior concha and receives opening of posterior ethmoidal cells.
   d. Atria is a shallow depression in front of middle meatus and above nasal vestibule.
   e. Sphenoethmoidal recess, space above superior concha, receives sphenoidal sinus opening.

Blood Supply

- Anterosuperior area is supplied by anterior and posterior ethmoidal arteries, and facial arteries
- Anteroinferior area is supplied by facial and greater palatine artery
- Posterosuperior quadrant by sphenopalatine artery
- Posteroinferior quadrant by greater palatine artery
- Veins drain into facial vein anteriorly and pterygoid plexus posteriorly.

Nerve Supply

- Anterosuperior quadrant is supplied by anterior ethmoidal nerve
- Anteroinferior quadrant by anterosuperior alveolar nerve
- Posterosuperior and posteroinferior quadrant by branches from pterygopalatine ganglion.

Lymphatics

Drain into submandibular nodes, retropharyngeal and deep cervical nodes.

Endoscopic Anatomy

Endoscopically middle meatus with the openings of sinuses is known as osteomeatal complex. It has two divisions—osteomeatal complex anterior and osteomeatal complex posterior.

Applied Anatomy

- Maxillary sinusitis is the commonest affection following common cold
- In antral puncture an accessory ostia is created at a lower level to improve the drainage of maxillary sinus
- Endoscopic sinus surgery involves improving drainage and aeration of sinuses by widening the natural ostia with the use of endoscopes.

> **Q. WHAT ARE THE BOUNDARIES, COMMUNICATIONS AND CONTENTS OF PTERYGOPALATINE FOSSA?**

Pterygopalantine fossa is cul-de-sac (blind sac) behind maxilla. This fossa serves as a distribution channel for nerves and vessels to face, nose and palate.

Boundaries

1. It lies between maxilla in front and pterygoid extension of sphenoid behind.
2. Laterally it is open.
3. Medially it is closed by vertical plate of palatine bone (the vertical plate of palatine bone bifurcates into short sphenoidal process and orbital process. The bifurcation is closed from above by body of sphenoid).

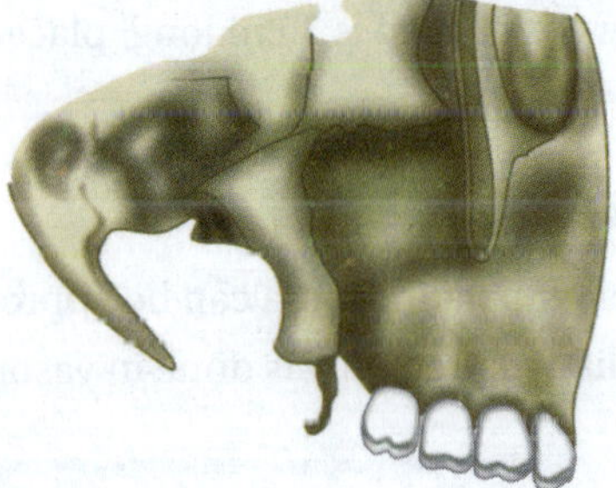

Communications

Pterygopalantine fossa opens into the apex of the orbit via inferior orbital fissure. It communicates medially into nasal cavity via sphenopalatine foramen and laterally through pterygomaxillary fissure to infratemporal fossa.

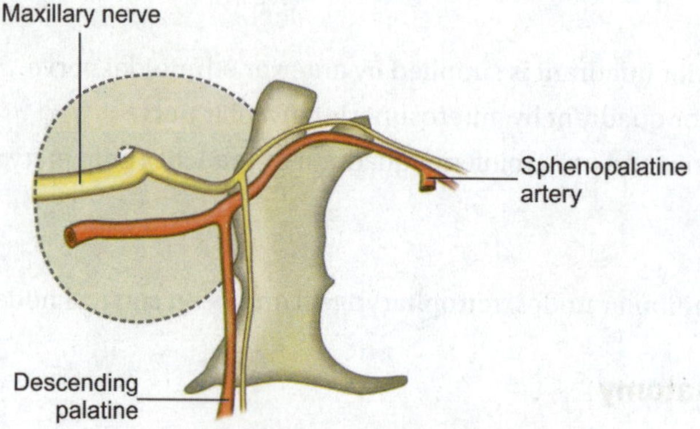

Pterygopalatine fossa with its contents

Contents

- Maxillary artery
- Maxillary nerve
- Pterygopalatine ganglion
- Vidian nerve
- Fat.

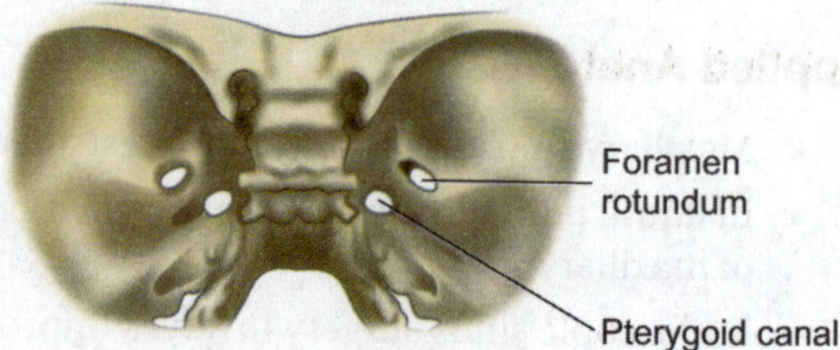

Foramen rotundum in pterygoid palatine fossa

Surgical Anatomy

1. In the sphenoid wall of fossa there are two foramen namely—foramen rotundum and pterygoid canal.
2. Foramen rotundum transmits maxillary nerves and marks the upper limit of dissection of pterygopalatine fossa.
3. Pterygoid canal is 1 cm long, placed anteroposteriorly and lies inferolateral to sphenoid sinus.

Applied Anatomy

- Pterygopalatine fossa can be approached transantrally
- Vidian neurectomy is done in vasomotor rhinitis.

Q. DISCUSS PARATHYROID GLANDS.

Parathyroid glands are endocrine glands in vicinity to thyroid gland. They may vary from two to six in number, but in 80% cases they are four in number. Total weight is 140 g.

Development

The upper parathyroid arise from fourth branchial pouch and come to lie in close association with the upper part of lateral lobes of thyroid. This position is constant.

Lower parathyroid are derived from third branchial pouch in association with thymus and descend with thymus and thus inferior parathyroid may be found anywhere from upper pole of thyroid to the mediastinum.

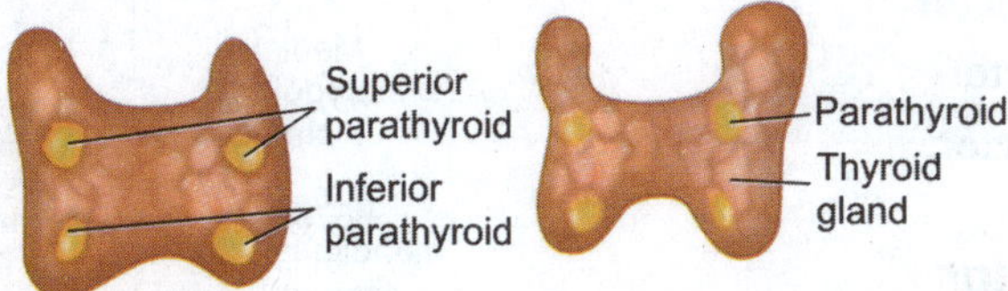

Gross Anatomy

- Glands are size of split pea
- Pink or brown in color, but covered by fat making them difficult to recognize
- Superior glands lie on the posterior surface of the middle third of thyroid gland, usually above inferior thyroid artery
- Inferior glands are found on posterior surface of thyroid gland within 1 cm of lower lobe of thyroid gland.

Parathyroid glands are located within the surgical false capsule of thyroid gland.

Blood Supply

- For upper parathyroid gland, artery comes from inferior thyroid artery
- For lower parathyroid gland, artery comes from either inferior thyroid artery or anastomosing artery joining superior and inferior thyroid artery.

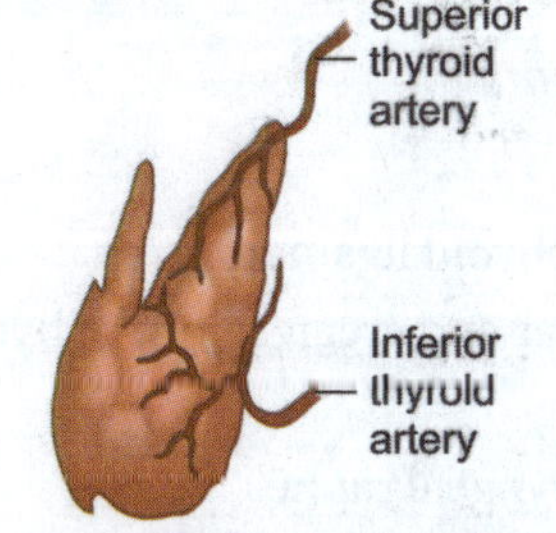

Blood supply of parathyroid gland

Endocrine Function

Parathyroid glands are controlled by calcium levels in the blood.

Parathormone is secreted by parathyroid glands and calcitonin is secreted by parafollicular cells of thyroid gland.

Applied Anatomy

- Lower parathyroid artery is a guide to the gland, if it lies below the lower margin of thyroid
- During thyroidectomy, parathyroid glands should be salvaged
- Parathyroid gland adenoma may cause hypercalcemia; it is surgically treated by excising the gland.

Q. DESCRIBE PHARYNGEAL MUSCLES WITH ITS APPLIED ANATOMY.

Pharynx is a muscular tube made up of three muscles:

- Superior constrictor
- Middle constrictor
- Inferior constrictor.

Superior Constrictor

Attachments

From

- Pterygoid hamulus, medial pterygoid plate
- Pterygomandibular raphe
- Mylohyoid line
- Side of tongue.

To

- Pharyngeal tubercle and raphe.

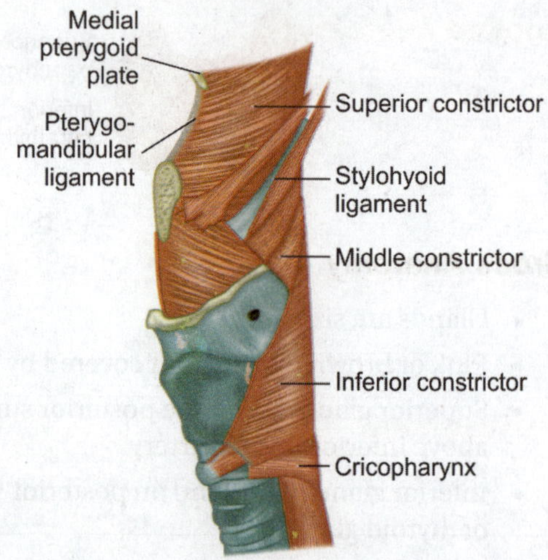

Pharyngeal musculature

Middle Constrictor

Attachments

From

- Stylohyoid ligament
- Lesser and greater horn of hyoid bone.

To

- Pharyngeal raphe.

Inferior Constrictor

Attachments

From

- Oblique line of thyroid cartilage (thyropharyngeus)
- Side of cricoid (cricopharyngeus).

Inferior constrictor has two parts—thyropharyngeus and cricopharyngeus.

To

- Pharyngeal raphe.

Action

All the constrictors help in deglutition.

Nerve Supply

All the constrictors are supplied by pharyngeal plexus.

Applied Anatomy

1. The lower part of thyropharyngeus is a single sheet of muscle, not overlapped internally by middle constrictor. This part is limited below by cricopharyngeal sphincter. This weak area is known as Killian's dehiscence. Pharyngeal diverticulum is an outpouching of this dehiscence.
2. Paralyses of constrictors lead to dysphagia.

Q. DISCUSS INNERVATION OF TONGUE AND ITS EMBRYOLOGICAL BASIS.

Development

- The tongue develops in relation to pharyngeal arches in the floor of developing mouth
- Medial most parts of mandibular arches proliferate to form two lingual swellings
- In between the lingual swelling is another swelling—tuberculum impar
- Another midline swelling appears in relation to II, III, IV arches called hypobranchial eminence
- Another two third of tongue is formed by fusion of tuberculum impar and lingual swelling, in relation to I arch
- Posterior one third of tongue develops from cranial part of hypobranchial eminence
- Posteriormost part is derived from IV arch.

With this embryological backdrop:

- Anterior two third is supplied by lingual nerve, branch of mandibular nerve and chorda tympani
- Posterior one third is supplied by IX nerve, which is nerve of arch III
- Posteriormost part by superior laryngeal nerve
- Muscles of tongue develop from occipital myotomes, supplied by XII nerve, which is the nerve of these myotomes.

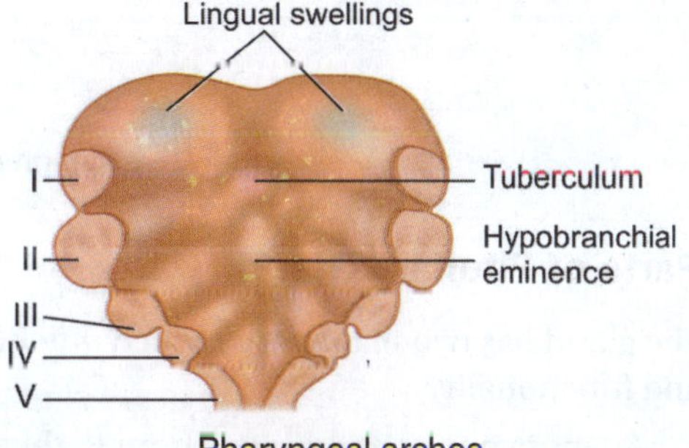

Applied Anatomy

- Taste is checked objectively by using galvanic current and subjectively by placing different solutions of salt, sugar

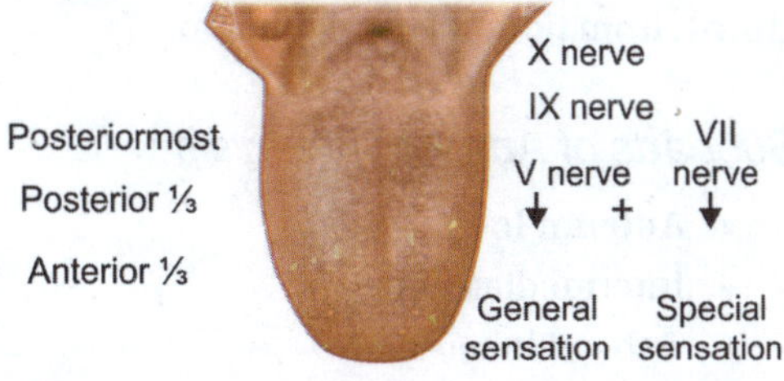

- In ear surgeries like tympanoplasty, chorda tympani may be stretched or severed giving rise to altered sensation or loss of taste.

Q. DESCRIBE THE GROSS ANATOMY OF PITUITARY GLAND, ITS RELATIONS AND BLOOD SUPPLY. ADD A NOTE ON ITS APPLIED ANATOMY.

Pituitary gland is also known as master gland since it produces trophic hormones, which control the secretions of other glands.

Location

Pituitary gland is lodged in pituitary fossa (sella turcica), which is roofed by diaphragma sella. Stalk of pituitary gland perforates the sella and is attached above to the third ventricle.

Dimension and Weight

Pituitary gland is 8 x 16 mm in dimensions and weighs around 500 g.

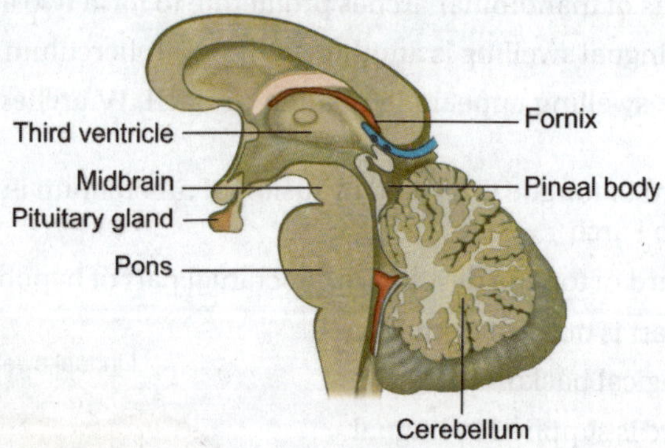

Location of pituitary gland

Parts of Pituitary Gland

The gland has two main parts, which differ from each other embryologically, morphologically and functionally.

Adenohypophysis develops from Rathke's pouch. Neurohypophysis develops as a down growth from floor of diencephalon.

Subparts of Adenohypophysis

- Anterior lobe
- Intermediate lobe
- Tuberal lobe.

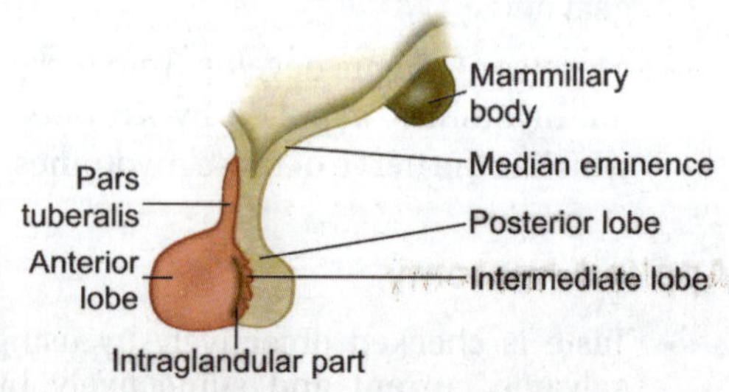

Parts of pituitary gland

Subparts of Neurohypophysis

- Posterior lobe
- Infundibular stem
- Median eminence.

Relations

- Superiorly—diphragma sella, optic chiasm
- Inferiorly—sphenoidal air sinus
- On each side—cavernous sinus.

Blood Supply

Arterial Supply

- Superior hypophyseal artery—branch of internal carotid artery
- Inferior hypophyseal artery—supplies the gland.

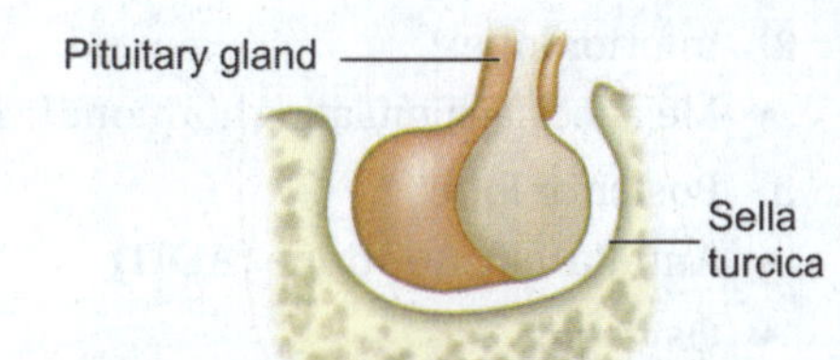

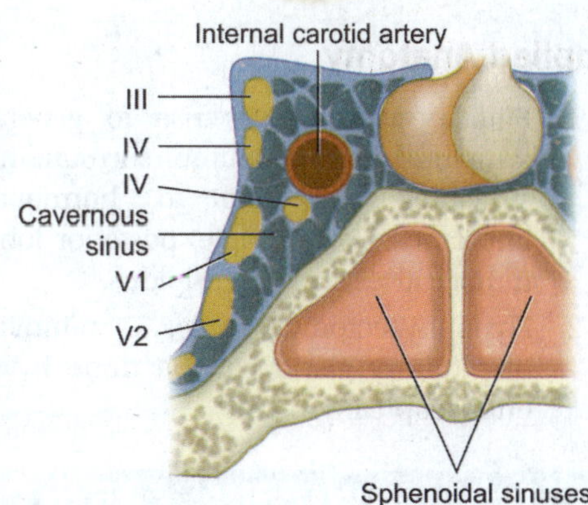

Relations of pituitary gland

Portal System

Anterior lobe is supplied by portal vessels arising from capillary tufts formed by superior hypophyseal artery.

Long portal vessels drain median eminence and infundibulum, short portal vessels drain lower infundibulum. Portal vessels carry the hormone-releasing factors.

Anterior lobe receives blood from portal system, while posterior lobe receives the blood from superior and inferior hypophyseal artery.

Blood supply of pituitary gland

Hormones Secretion

1. Anterior lobe:
- Growth hormone
- Lactogenic hormone
- Adrenocorticotropic hormone (ACTH)
- Thyroid-stimulating hormone (TSH), follicle-stimulating hormone (FSH), luteinizing hormone (LH).

2. Inferior lobe:
- Melanocyte-stimulating hormone (MSH).

3. Posterior lobe:
- Antidiuretic hormone (ADH)
- Oxytocin.

Applied Anatomy

1. Pituitary tumor gives rise to general symptoms due to pressure on surrounding structures and due to hormonal imbalance. For example, posterior lobe tumor causes diabetes insipidus.

2. Hypophysectomy, i.e. removal of pituitary gland can be done by transfrontal route or by transsphenoidal route, endoscopically.

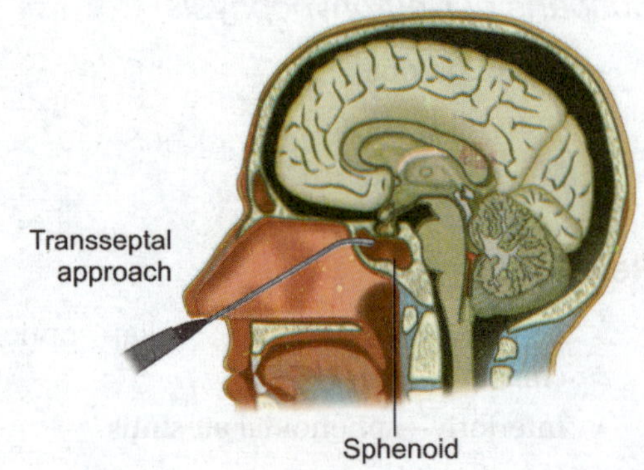

Hypophysectomy through transsphenoidal route

Q. DISCUSS INTERNAL EAR IN DETAIL.

Internal ear lies in the petrous part of temporal bone. It consists of bony labyrinth and membranous labyrinth.

The membranous labyrinth is filled with endolymph and surrounded by perilymph.

Bony Labyrinth

Bony labyrinth consists of the following:
- Cochlea
- Vestibule
- Semicircular canals.

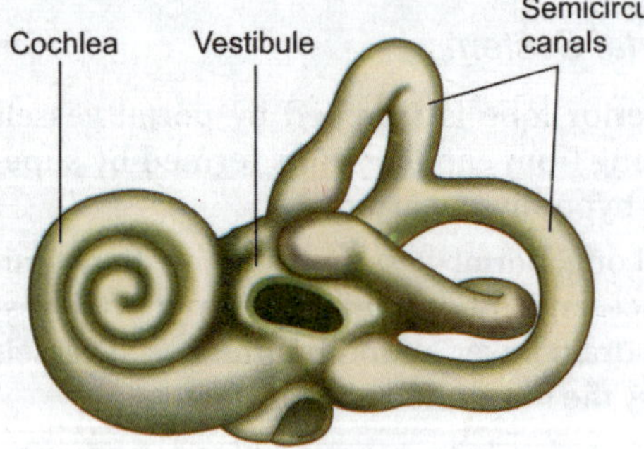

Bony labyrinth

Cochlea

Resembles shell of snail. The conical axis is known as modiolus around which cochlea makes two and half turns.

Spiral ridge of bone called spiral lamina projects from the modiolus and partially divides cochlea into scala vestibuli and scala tympani. Scala vestibuli and scala tympani communicate with each other at the apex by a small opening called helicotrema.

Vestibule

Vestibule is the central part of bony labyrinth and contains saccule and utricle.

Openings in vestibule:
- Lateral wall opens at fenestra vestibuli, which is closed by foot plate of stapes

- The semicircular canals open in the vestibuli posteriorly by five openings.

Medial wall:

- On the inner side of medial wall there is spherical recess for saccule and elliptical recess for utricle
- Medial to the medial wall is internal acoustic meatus.

Semicircular Canals

Semicircular canals are posterosuperior to vestibule and are at right angles to each other. Each canal has an dilated end known as ampulla. There are three semicircular canals namely superior and lateral and posterior.

Anterior canal of one side is in the same plane as the posterior canal of other side, i.e. parallel to each other, while lateral semicircular canals of both sides are in the same horizontal plane.

Membranous Labyrinth

Membranous labyrinth consists of:

1. Cochlear duct:
   a. It is a continuous closed cavity, which contains receptors for sound (organ of Corti).

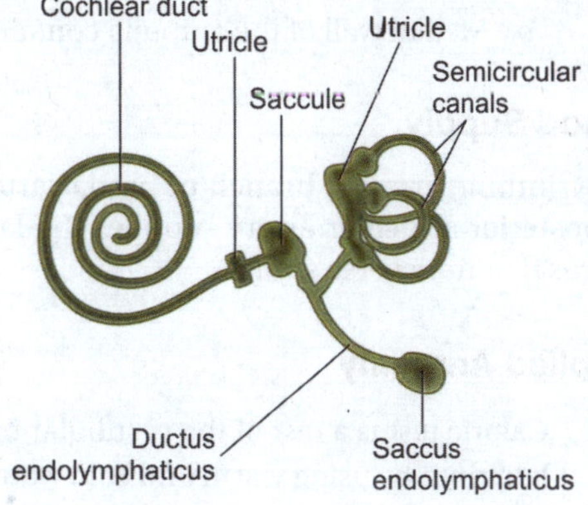

Membranous labyrinth of inner ear

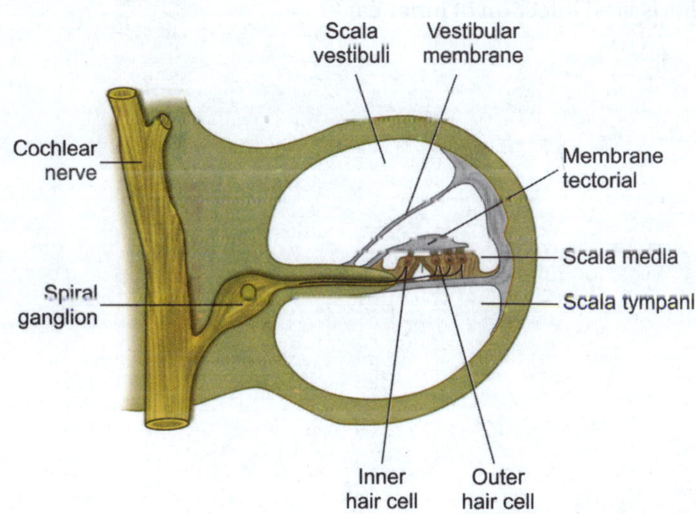

Cochlear duct section

   b. Cochlear duct lies between basilar membrane and vestibular membrane. The basilar membrane has the organ of corti, which consists of hair cells and supporting cells:

- Cochlear duct is connected to saccule by narrow ductus reuniens.

2. Saccule and utricle:

   a. Saccule lies in the anteroinferior part of vestibule.

   b. Utricle lies in the posterosuperior part of vestibule.

   c. Medial wall of saccule and utricle contains sensory organ (hair cell) known as macula.

3. Semicircular duct:

   a. The three ducts lie within the bony canals.

   b. Medial wall of the ampulla contains the sense organ and crista.

Blood Supply

Labyrinthine artery a branch of basilar artery and a small twig from stylomastoid branch of posterior auricular artery supplies the labyrinth. Labyrinthine vein drains into superior petrosal or transverse sinus.

Applied Anatomy

1. Caloric test is a test of the vestibular function based on the principle of stimulating the labyrinth by using warm and cold water.

2. Mènière's disease is characterized by periodic attacks of vertigo, tinnitus and sensorineural deafness. It is due to distension of endolymphatic sac; either due to excessive production of endolymph or inadequate drainage.

3. Labyrinthitis is viral infection of inner ear.

Key Diagrams with MCQ Tips

Diagrams for

- Scalp
- Sensory innervation of face
- Facial artery
- Danger area of face
- Triangles of the neck
- Carotid sheath
- Posterior triangle
- Suboccipital triangle
- Cavernous sinus
- Superior orbital fissure
- Extraocular muscles
- Midline structures of the neck
- Carotid triangle
- External carotid artery
- Parotid gland
- Muscles of mastication
- Lateral pterygoid muscle
- Sphenomandibular ligament
- Submandibular region
- Thyroid gland
- Cervical lymph nodes
- Styloid apparatus
- Tonsillar bed
- Lateral wall of nose
- Kiesselbach's area or Little's area
- Middle ear relations
- Internal acoustic meatus

Q. Scalp

Ans.

- Skin is thick and hairy
- Wounds of scalp bleed profusely because the torn vessels are prevented from retraction and scalp has rich blood supply
- Loose areolar tissue is the 'danger area of scalp' because infection from scalp can go to cranial venous sinus.

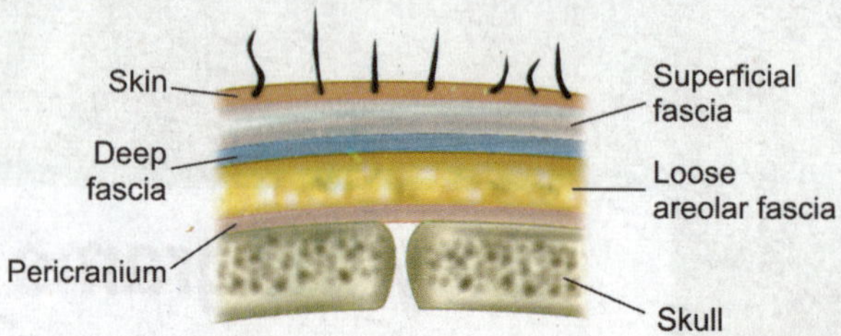

Q. Sensory innervation of face

Ans.

- Trigeminal nerve and cervical plexus innervate the face
- Trigeminal nerve also supplies nasal cavity, paranasal sinuses, eyeball, mouth cavity, supratentorial part of dura mater, lesion in any of the above may cause referred headache
- Angle of the jaw is supplied by great auricular nerve.

Q. Facial artery

Ans.

- Branch of external carotid artery given off in carotid triangle just above the tip of greater cornu of hyoid bone
- Tortuous artery (other, e.g. uterine artery, splenic artery).

Q. Danger area of face

Ans.

- Supraorbital and supratrochlear vein join to form angular vein

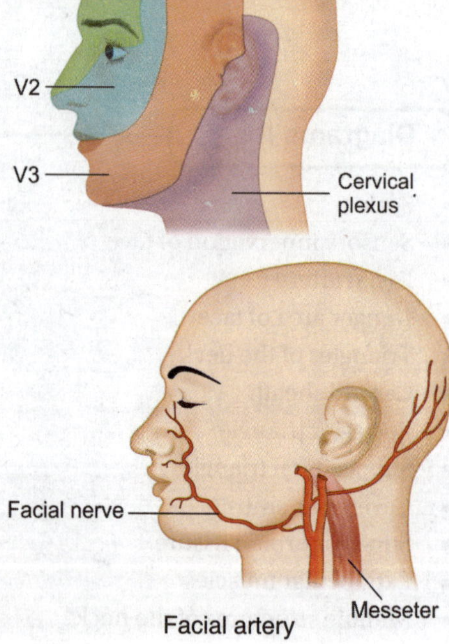

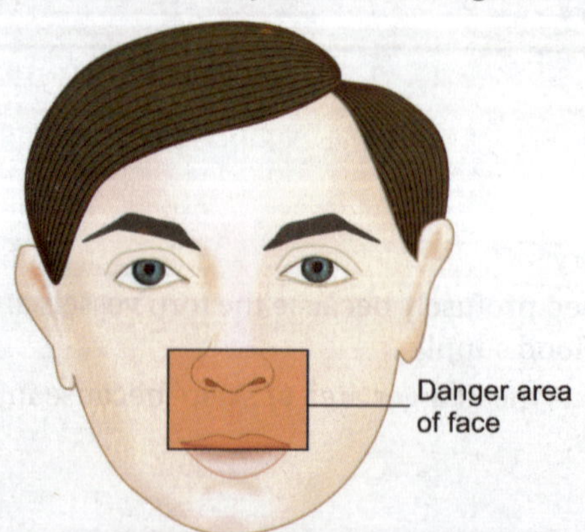

- Posterior division of retromandibular vein joins posterior auricular vein to form external jugular vein
- Deep facial vein and superior ophthalmic vein are deep connections of facial vein to cavernous sinus.

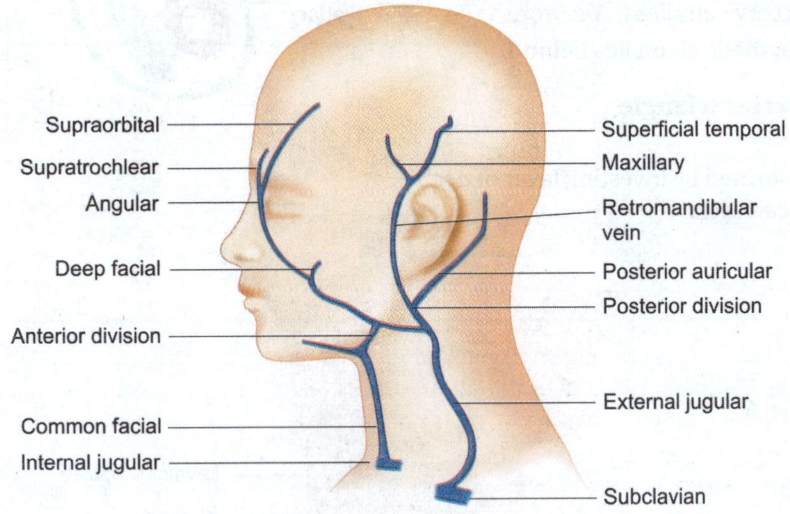

Venous drainage of face

Q. Triangles of the neck

Ans.

- Sternocleidomastoid is the key muscle of the neck
- Carotid sheath lies deep to sternocleidomastoid.

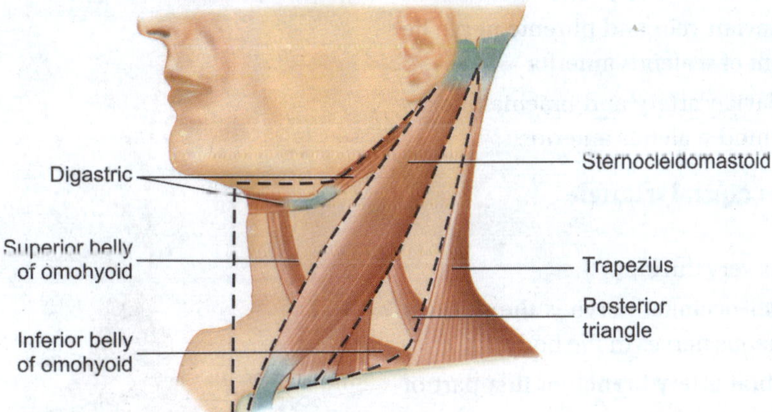

Q. Carotid sheath

Ans.

- Contains carotid arteries, internal jugular vein, vagus nerve
- Ansa cervicalis lies in the front
- Sympathetic chain lies behind.

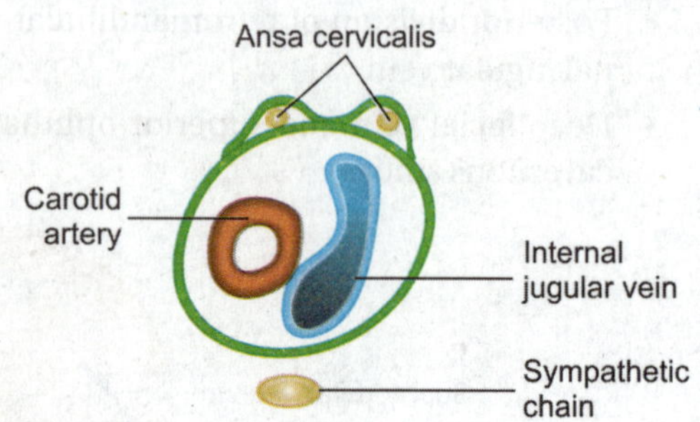

Q. Posterior triangle

Ans.

- Roof formed by investing layer of deep cervical fascia

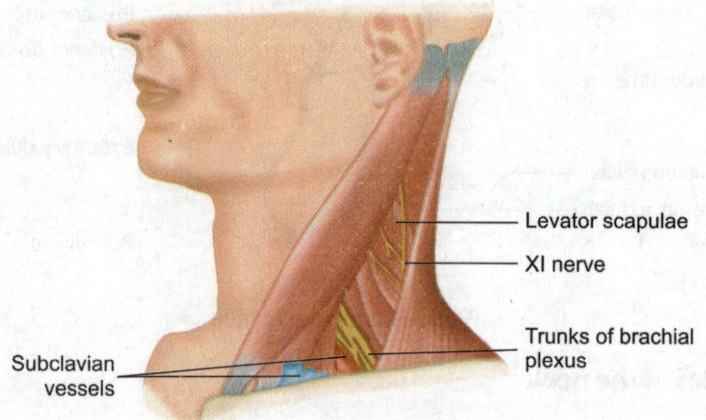

- Spinal accessory nerve lies on levator scapulae muscle
- Floor is covered by prevertebral layer of deep cervical fascia
- Subclavian vein and phrenic nerve lie in front of scalenus anterior
- Subclavian artery and brachial plexus lie behind scalenus anterior.

Q. Suboccipital triangle

Ans.

- Skin is very thick
- Greater occipital nerve is the thickest cutaneous nerves in the body
- Vertebral artery branch of first part of subclavian artery
- Third part of vertebral artery lies in suboccipital triangle.

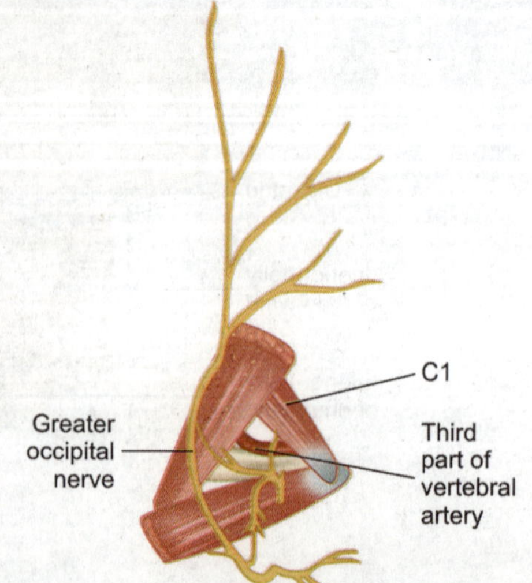

Q. Cavernous sinus

Ans.

- Lateral wall related to III, IV, V1, V2 cranial nerves
- V3 is away from lateral wall.

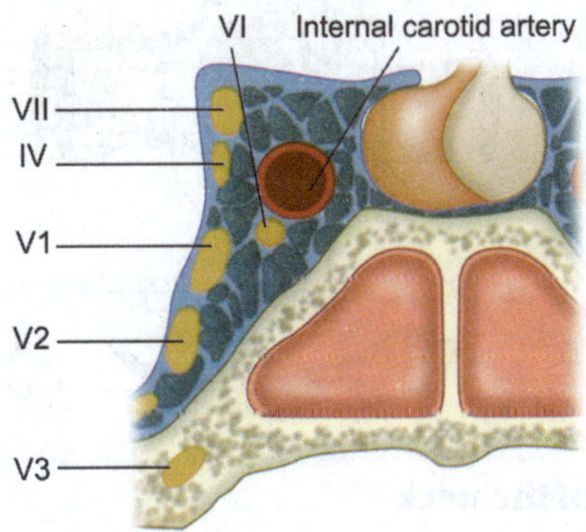

Q. Superior orbital fissure

Ans.

- Common tendinous ring divides it
- Nasociliary nerve lies in between upper and lower division of III nerve.

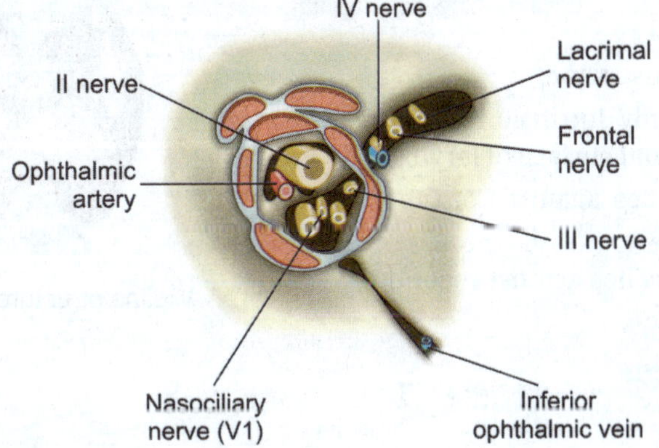

Q. Extraocular muscles

Ans.

- Superior oblique supplied by trochlear nerve (SO4)
- Lateral rectus supplied by abducent nerve (LR6)
- Upper division of III nerve supplies superior rectus, levator palpebrae superioris
- Lower division supplies inferior oblique, inferior rectus, medial rectus.

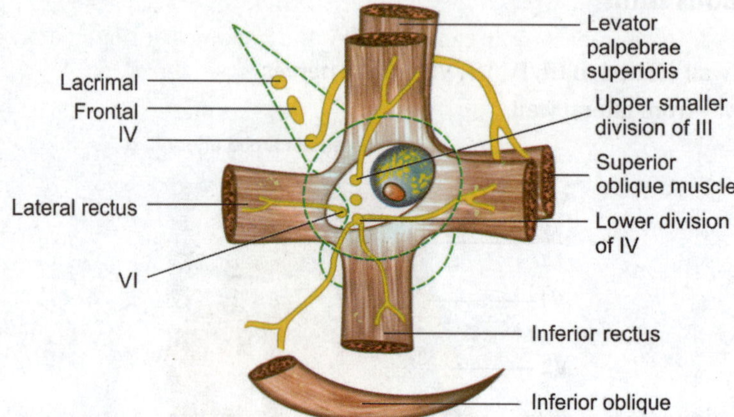

Q. Midline structures of the neck

Ans.

- Internal laryngeal nerve and superior laryngeal vessels pierce thyrohyoid membrane
- Oblique line on thyroid cartilage has:
    - Sternothyroid
    - Thyrohyoid
    - Inferior constrictor.
- Cricothyroid only intrinsic muscle of larynx on external surface of larynx
- Thyroid gland lies against C5, C6, C7 and T1 vertebra
- Thyroid isthmus lies against second to third tracheal rings.

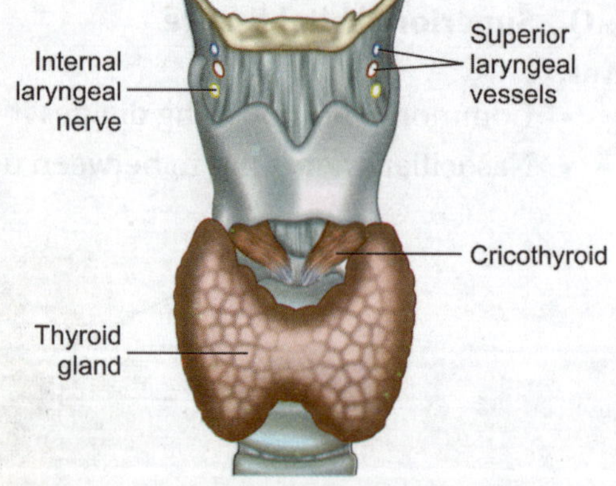

Midline structures of the neck

Q. Carotid triangle

Ans.

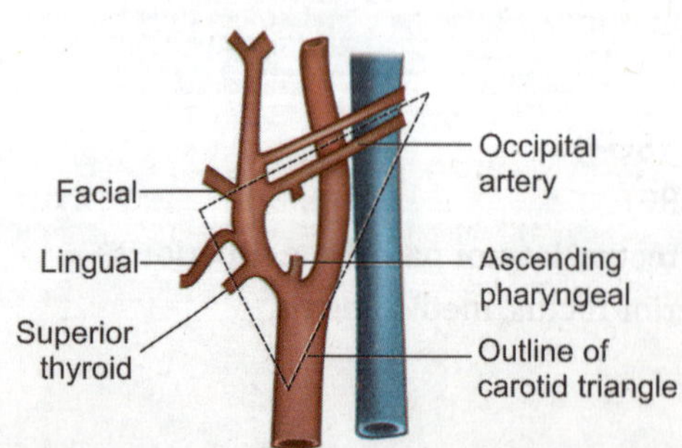

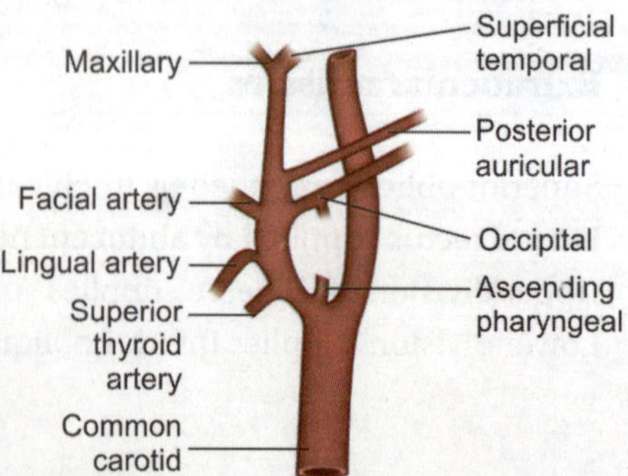

- Common carotid artery bifurcates at upper border of thyroid cartilage
- Terminal branches of external carotid artery and posterior auricular artery are not in the carotid triangle.

Q. External carotid artery

Ans.

- Has eight branches
- First anterior branch—superior thyroid, given off just below greater cornu of hyoid bone
- Lingual artery—given off at the level of greater cornu of hyoid bone
- Facial artery—given off just above greater cornu of hyoid bone
- Posterior auricular artery—given off just above the posterior belly of digastric
- Occipital artery—given off just below the posterior belly of digastric.

Mnemonic	Branches
"Sister	**Superior thyroid**
Lucy's	**Lingual**
Powdered	**Ascending pharyngeal**
Face	**Facial**
Often	**Occipital**
Attracts	**Posterior auricular**
Medical	**Maxillary**
Student"	**Superficial temporal**

Q. Parotid gland

Ans.

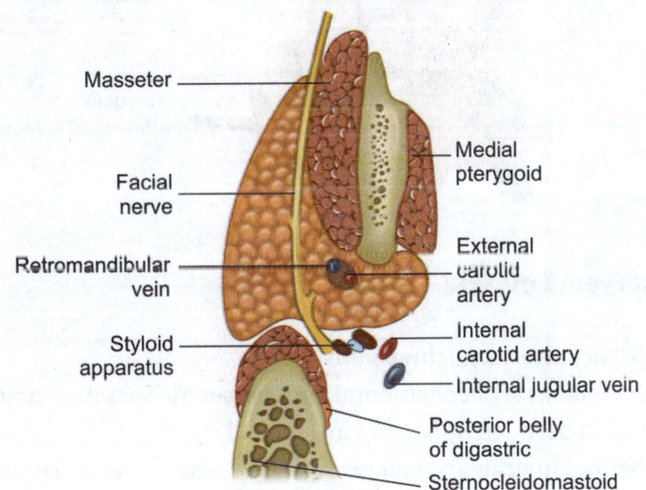

- Facial nerve surgically divides parotid gland into superficial and deep parts
- Facial nerve enters the gland through its posteromedial surface

- External carotid artery and retromandibular vein lie in the substance of parotid gland
- Secretomotor fibers of the gland relay in otic ganglion
- Postganglionic fibers pass through auriculotemporal nerve.

Q. Muscles of mastication

Ans.

- Masseter, temporalis, lateral pterygoid, medial pterygoid
- Develop from first branchial arch
- The nerve of the first arch is mandibular nerve
- Lateral pterygoid is the only muscle, which opens the mouth. Other muscles close the mouth.

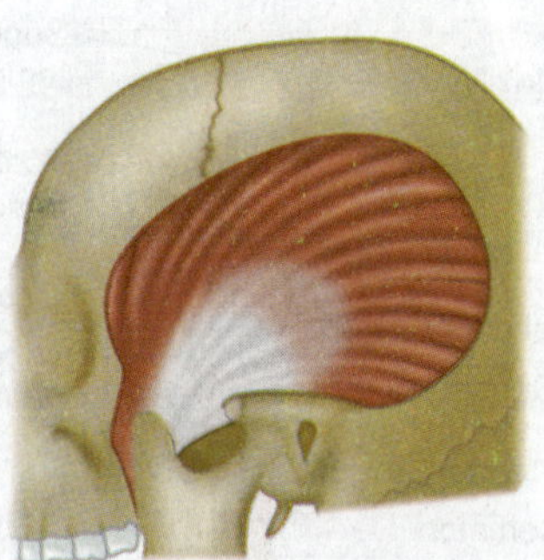

Temporalis muscle

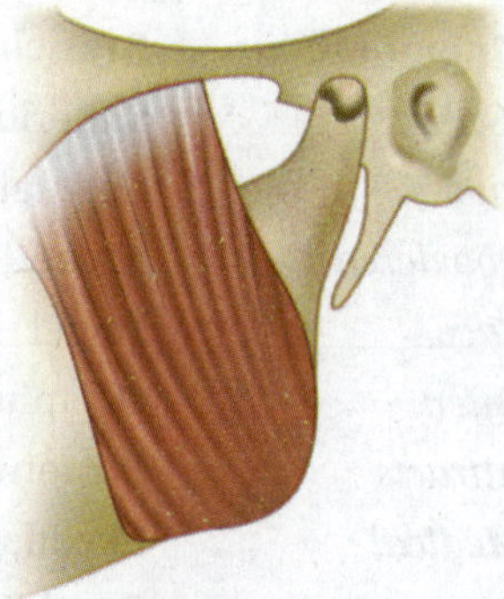

Masseter muscle

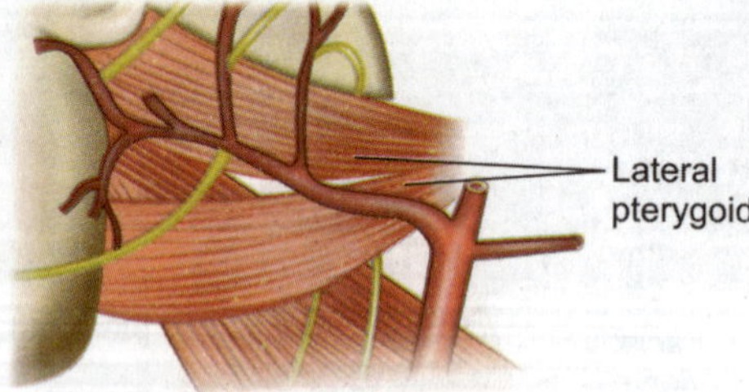

Q. Lateral pterygoid muscle

Ans.

- Divides maxillary artery into three parts
- Upper border related to deep temporal and masseteric vessels and nerves
- Buccal nerve lies between upper and lower head
- Lingual nerve and inferior alveolar nerve and vessels are related to inferior border.

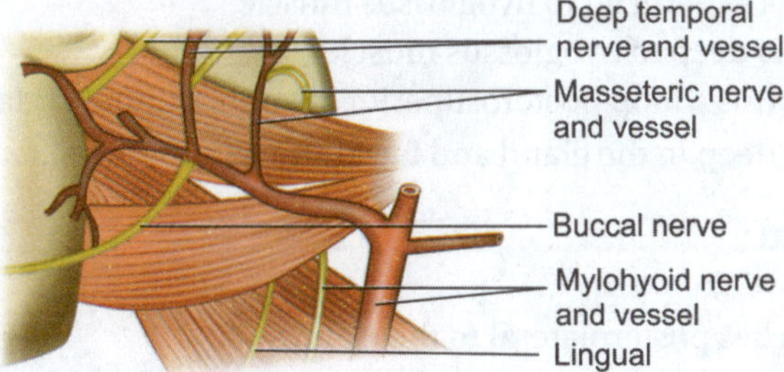

Q. Sphenomandibular ligament

Ans.

- Remnant of Meckel's cartilage
- Auriculotemporal nerve lies lateral
- Chorda tympani nerve lies medial
- Pierced by mylohyoid nerve and vessels
- Auriculotemporal nerve forms a loop around middle meningeal artery.

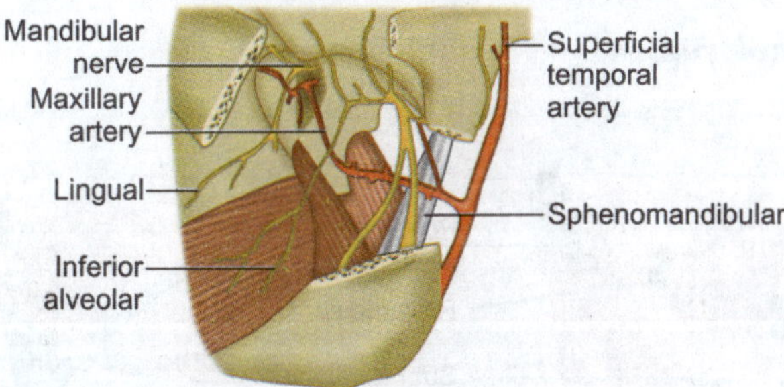

Q. Submandibular region

Ans.

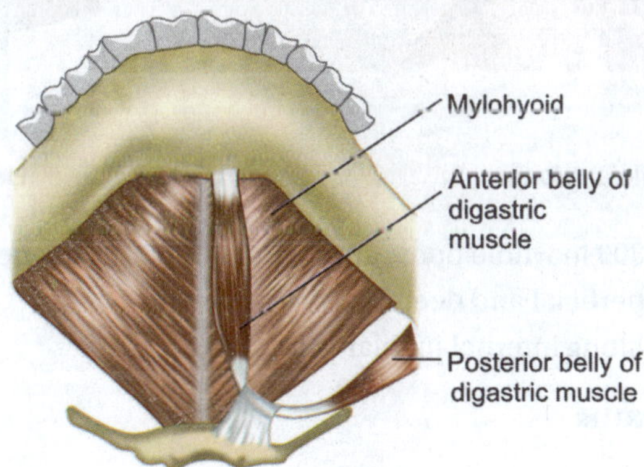

- Mylohyoid muscle is the oral diaphragm
- Lingual nerve winds around submandibular duct

- Lingual nerve is superficial to hyoglossus muscle
- Lingual artery is deep to hyoglossus muscle
- Facial artery forms a loop posterosuperior to submandibular gland
- Facial artery is deep to the gland and facial vein is superficial.

Q. **Thyroid gland**

Ans.

- Carotid sheath lies posterolateral to the gland
- Recurrent laryngeal nerve lies in the tracheoesophageal groove.

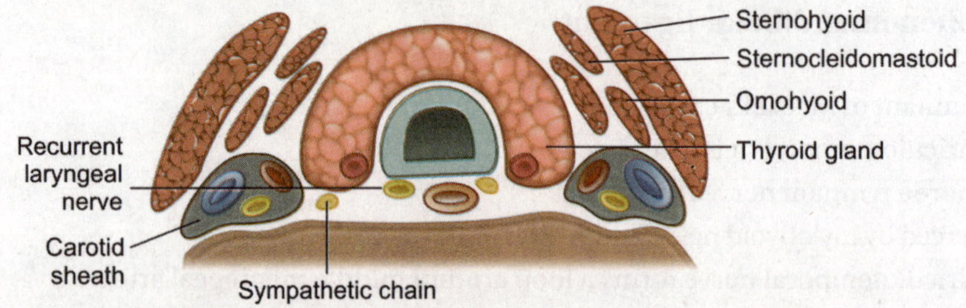

Q. **Cervical lymph nodes**

Ans.

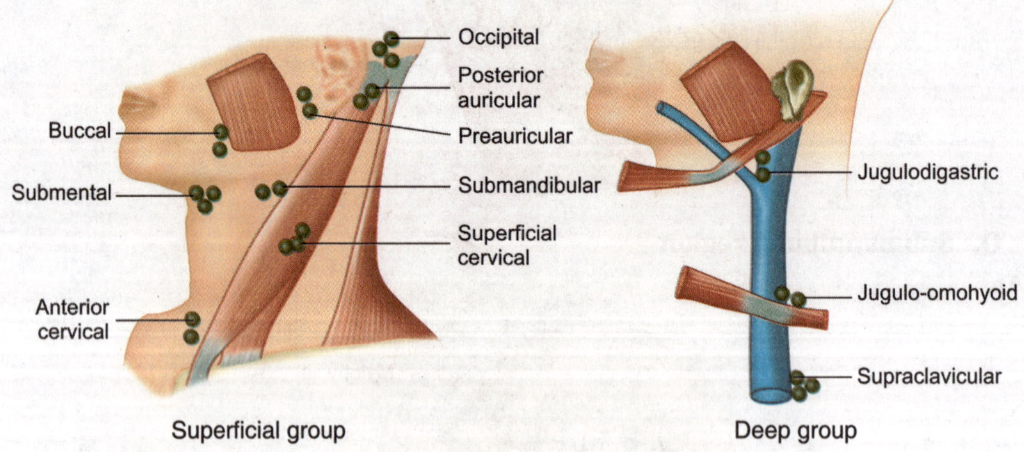

- Approximately 800 in whole body, approximately 300 in the neck
- Divided into superficial and deep
- Deep nodes lie along internal jugular vein.

Q. **Styloid apparatus**

Ans.

- Styloid process, stylohyoid ligament and muscle develop from second branchial arch
- Stylopharyngeus develops from third branchial arch and closely related to IX cranial nerve

- Styloglossus develops from occipital myotomes
- Stylomandibular ligament is a part of deep cervical fascia of the neck.

Q. Tonsillar bed

Ans.

- Superior constrictor muscle forms the floor
- Palatine vein is responsible for bleeding during tonsillectomy
- Internal carotid artery lies approximately 1 inch deep to tonsil.

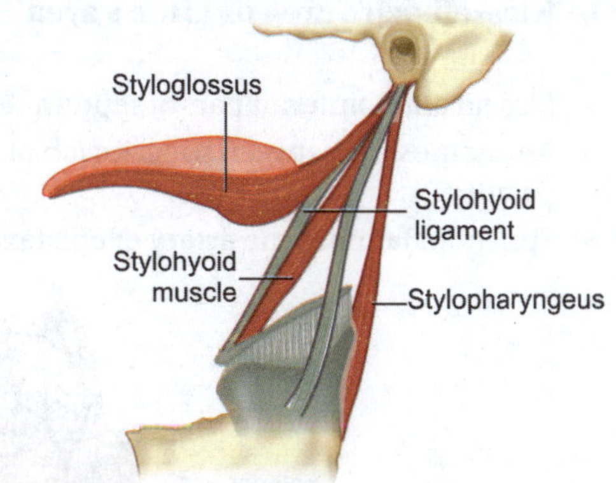

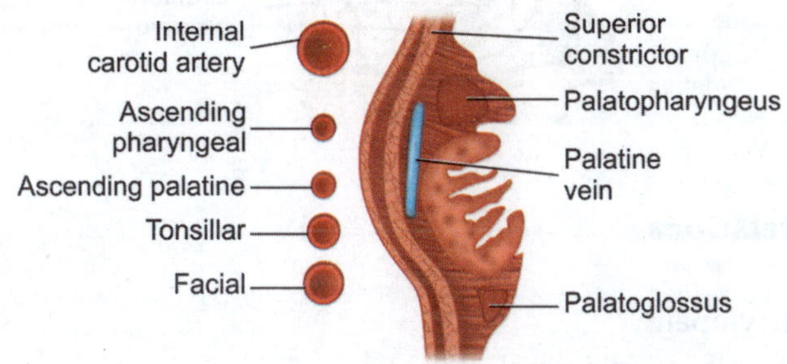

Q. Lateral wall of nose

Ans.

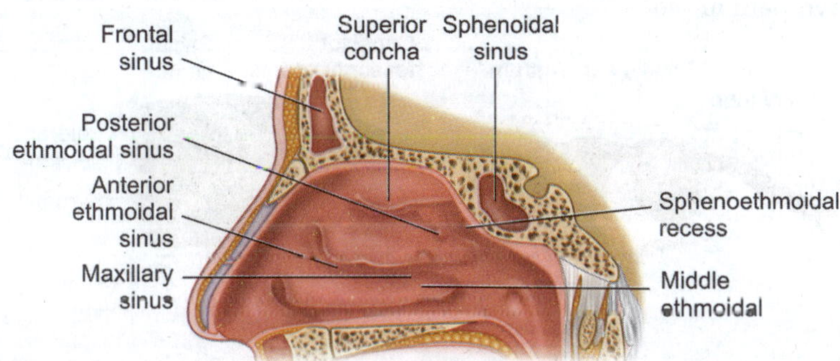

- Sphenoid sinus opens in sphenoethmoidal recess
- Frontal, anterior ethmoidal, maxillary, middle ethmoidal sinuses open in middle meatus
- Nasolacrimal duct opens in inferior meatus
- Posterior ethmoidal sinus opens in superior meatus.

Q. Kiesselbach's area or Little's area

Ans.

- Lies on anteroinferior part of septum
- Anastomosis is between superior labial, anterior ethmoidal, sphenopalatine and greater palatine
- Sphenopalatine is the artery of epistaxis.

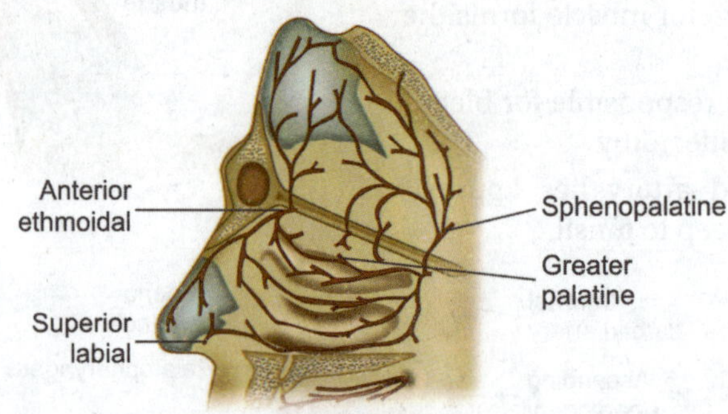

Q. Middle ear relations

Ans.

- Roof—tegmen tympani
- Floor—jugular bulb, carotid canal
- Anterior wall—canal for tensor tympani, opening of auditory tube, carotid canal
- Posterior wall—aditus to antrum, fossa incudis, pyramid, posterior canaliculus for chorda tympani nerve

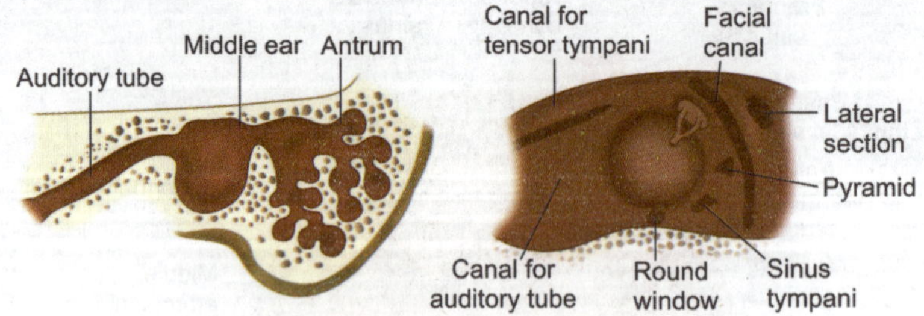

- Lateral wall—tympanic membrane, scutum
- Medial wall—promontory, fenestra vestibuli, facial canal, fenestra cochleae, sinus tympani, lateral semicircular canal.

Q. Internal acoustic meatus

Ans.

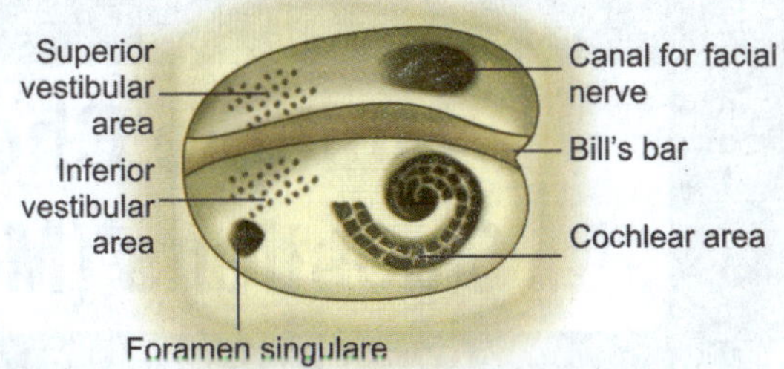

- Tympanic branch of glossopharyngeal nerve is known as Jacobson's nerve
- Internal laryngeal nerve lies in the floor of pyriform fossa.

Multiple Choice Questions (MCQs)

1. 'Danger layer' of scalp is ________
   a. Skin
   b. Superficial fascia
   c. Loose areolar tissue
   d. Pericranium

   Answer: c

2. Angle of the jaw is supplied by ________
   a. Greater occipital nerve
   b. Great auricular nerve
   c. Lesser occipital nerve
   d. Auriculotemporal nerve

   Answer: b

3. Facial artery is given off just above the level of ________
   a. Thyroid cartilage
   b. Hyoid bone
   c. Greater cornu of hyoid bone
   d. Lesser cornu of hyoid bone

   Answer: c

4. Deep connection of facial vein is through ________
   a. Posterior auricular vein
   b. Superior ophthalmic vein
   c. Inferior ophthalmic vein
   d. Common facial vein

   Answer: b

5. Key muscle in the neck is ________
   a. Sternocleidomastoid
   b. Trapezius
   c. Mylohyoid
   d. Omohyoid

   Answer: a

6. Oral diaphragm is ________
   a. Omohyoid
   b. Hyoglossus
   c. Digastric
   d. Mylohyoid

   Answer: d

7. Structure posterior to carotid sheath is ________
   a. Vagus nerve
   b. Sympathetic chain
   c. Ansa cervicalis
   d. Internal jugular vein

   Answer: b

8. Floor of the posterior triangle is covered by ______________
   a. Investing layer of deep fascia
   b. Pretracheal layer of deep fascia
   c. Prevertebral layer of deep fascia
   d. None

   Answer: c

9. Roof of posterior triangle of the neck is covered by ______________
   a. Prevertebral layer
   b. Pretracheal layer
   c. Investing layer
   d. All of the above

   Answer: c

10. Thickest cutaneous nerve in the body is ______________
    a. Ulnar nerve
    b. Saphenous nerve
    c. Peroneal nerve
    d. Greater occipital nerve

    Answer: d

11. Common carotid artery bifurcates at the level of ______________
    a. Cricoid cartilage
    b. Lower border of thyroid cartilage
    c. Upper border of thyroid cartilage
    d. Hyoid bone

    Answer: d

12. Phrenic nerve is anterior to the following muscle ______________
    a. Scalenus anterior
    b. Scalenus posterior
    c. Scalenus medius
    d. Levator scapulae

    Answer: a

13. Following nerves form the lateral relation of cavernous sinus except ______________
    a. III
    b. IV
    c. V
    d. VI

    Answer: d

14. Nasociliary nerve lies between the divisions of following cranial nerve in superior orbital fissure ______________
    a. IV
    b. VI
    c. III
    d. V

    Answer: c

15. Superior oblique muscle is supplied by ______________
    a. IV
    b. V
    c. III
    d. VI

    Answer: a

16. Lateral rectus is supplied by ______________
    a. IV
    b. V
    c. III
    d. VI

    Answer: d

17. Following structures pierce the thyrohyoid membrane _____________
    a. External laryngeal nerve and superior laryngeal vessels
    b. Internal laryngeal nerve and superior laryngeal vessels
    c. Internal laryngeal nerve and inferior laryngeal vessels
    d. External laryngeal nerve and inferior laryngeal vessels

Answer: b

18. All the intrinsic muscles of larynx are supplied by _____________
    except cricothyroid.
    a. External laryngeal nerve
    b. Recurrent laryngeal nerve
    c. Hypoglossal nerve
    d. Glossopharyngeal nerve

Answer: b

19. Cricothyroid muscle is supplied by _____________
    a. External laryngeal nerve
    b. Recurrent laryngeal nerve
    c. Hypoglossal nerve
    d. Glossopharyngeal nerve

Answer: a

20. Thyroid isthmus lies against _____________
    a. 2nd, 3rd tracheal rings
    b. 1st, 2nd tracheal rings
    c. 3rd and 4th tracheal rings
    d. 1st, 2nd and 3rd tracheal rings

Answer: a

21. First branch of the external carotid artery is _____________
    a. Superior thyroid
    b. Lingual
    c. Facial
    d. Occipital

Answer: a

22. Superior thyroid artery, a branch of external carotid artery is given off at the following level _____________
    a. Just below greater cornu of hyoid bone
    b. At the level of greater cornu of hyoid bone
    c. Just above the level of greater cornu of hyoid bone
    d. Not related to hyoid bone

Answer: a

23. Facial artery, a branch of external carotid artery is given off at the following level _____________
    a. Just above greater cornu of hyoid bone
    b. At the level of hyoid bone
    c. At the level of upper border of thyroid cartilage
    d. Just below greater cornu of hyoid bone

Answer: a

24. Lingual artery, a branch of ECA is given of at ____________
    a. Just above greater cornu of hyoid bone
    b. Just below greater cornu of hyoid bone
    c. At the level of greater cornu of hyoid bone
    d. At the level of upper border of hyoid cartilage

    Answer: c

25. Which nerve divides the parotid gland surgically into superficial and deep parts?
    a. V
    b. Vl
    c. Vll
    d. Vlll

    Answer: c

26. Facial nerve enters the parotid gland through following surface of parotid gland ____________
    a. Anteromedial
    b. Posteromedial
    c. Anterolateral
    d. Posterolateral

    Answer: b

27. Secretomotor pathway of parotid gland relays in the following ganglion ____________
    a. Submandibular ganglion
    b. Trigeminal ganglion
    c. Gasserian ganglion
    d. Otic ganglion

    Answer: d

28. All are the muscles of the mastication except ____________
    a. Lateral pterygoid
    b. Temporalis
    c. Mylohyoid
    d. Medial pterygoid

    Answer: c

29. Otic ganglion is located in ____________
    a. Pterygopalatine fossa
    b. Temporal fossa
    c. Infratemporal fossa
    d. Trigeminal impression

    Answer: c

30. All the muscles of mastication develop from ____________ branchial arch.
    a. I
    b. II
    c. III
    d. IV

    Answer: a

31. Nerve of first branchial arch is ____________
    a. Maxillary
    b. Mandibular
    c. Ophthalmic
    d. Glossopharyngeal

    Answer: b

32. The muscle, which opens the mouth is ____________
    a. Medial pterygoid
    b. Lateral pterygoid
    c. Masseter
    d. Temporalis

    Answer: b

33. The nerve in between the upper and lower head of lateral pterygoid muscle is
    ____
    a. Lingual nerve
    b. Inferior alveolar nerve
    c. Masseteric nerve
    d. Buccal nerve

    Answer: d

34. Following nerves are related to the lower border of lateral pterygoid muscle __________
    a. Masseteric nerve and lingual nerve
    b. Temporal nerve and inferior alveolar
    c. Lingual and inferior alveolar
    d. Masseteric and temporal nerve

    Answer: c

35. Sphenomandibular ligament is a remnant of __________
    a. Reichert's cartilage
    b. Meckel's cartilage
    c. Thyroid cartilage
    d. None

    Answer: b

36. Auriculotemporal nerve forms a loop around __________
    a. Maxillary artery
    b. Tympanic artery
    c. Lingual artery
    d. Middle meningeal artery

    Answer: d

37. The nerve winding the submandibular duct is __________
    a. Mylohyoid
    b. Buccal
    c. Lingual
    d. Facial

    Answer: c

38. Lingual artery is __________ to hyoglossus muscle.
    a. Superficial
    b. Deep
    c. Medial
    d. Lateral

    Answer: b

39. The facial artery forms a loop around the __________ aspect of submandibular gland.
    a. Inferior
    b. Superior
    c. Anterosuperior
    d. Posterosuperior

    Answer: d

40. Carotid sheath is __________ to thyroid gland.
    a. Lateral
    b. Medial
    c. Posterior
    d. Anterior

    Answer: a

41. Recurrent laryngeal nerve lies in __________
    a. Thyroid notch
    b. Oblique line of thyroid cartilage
    c. Tracheoesophageal groove
    d. Vocal fold

    Answer: c

42. All the muscles are attached on the oblique line of thyroid cartilage except _____________
    a. Sternothyroid
    b. Thyrohyoid
    c. Inferior constrictor
    d. Omohyoid

    Answer: d

43. There are approximately _____________ number of lymph nodes in the neck.
    a. 10
    b. 100
    c. 800
    d. 300

    Answer: d

44. Styloid process develops from _____________ branchial arch.
    a. I
    b. II
    c. III
    d. IV

    Answer: b

45. Stylopharyngeus muscle develops from _____________ branchial arch.
    a. I
    b. II
    c. III
    d. IV

    Answer: c

46. Nerve of III branchial arch is _____________
    a. X
    b. IX
    c. XI
    d. XII

    Answer: b

47. Styloglossus muscle develops from _____________
    a. Occipital myotomes
    b. II branchial arch
    c. III branchial arch
    d. None

    Answer: a

48. Stylomandibular ligament is a part of _____________
    a. Meckel's cartilage
    b. Superficial cervical fascia
    c. Deep cervical fascia
    d. Styloglossus muscle

    Answer: c

49. Muscle forming the floor of tonsillar bed is _____________
    a. Inferior constrictor
    b. Superior constrictor
    c. Palatoglossus
    d. Palatopharyngeus

    Answer: b

50. Internal carotid artery is _____________ inch deep to tonsil.
    a. 1/2
    b. 4
    c. 1
    d. 0.5

    Answer: c

51. All the sinuses open in the middle meatus except _____________.
    a. Frontal
    b. Maxillary
    c. Sphenoid
    d. Ethmoidal

    Answer: c

52. Following is known as artery of epistaxis _____________
    a. Greater palatine
    b. Superior labial
    c. Anterior ethmoidal
    d. Sphenopalatine

    Answer: d

53. Jacobson's nerve is _____________
    a. Auricular branch of vagus
    b. Auricular branch of IX nerve
    c. Tympanic branch of vagus
    d. Tympanic branch of IX nerve

    Answer: d

54. The nerve, which lies in the floor of pyriform fossa is _____________
    a. External laryngeal nerve
    b. Internal laryngeal nerve
    c. Recurrent laryngeal nerve
    d. Superior laryngeal nerve

    Answer: b

55. Auricular branch of vagus nerve is also known as _____________
    a. Arnold
    b. Jacobson's
    c. Gasserian
    d. Meckel's

    Answer: a

56. Reid's baseline is an imaginary horizontal line joining infraorbital margin to _____________
    a. Upper margin of external acoustic meatus (EAM)
    b. Lower margin of EAM
    c. Center of EAM
    d. Condyloid process of mandible

    Answer: c

57. Frankfurt plane is obtained by joining infraorbital margin to _____________
    a. Upper margin of EAM
    b. Lower margin of EAM
    c. Center of EAM
    d. Condyloid process of mandible

    Answer: a

58. Cranium is _____________
    a. Skull with mandible
    b. Skull without mandible
    c. Skull
    d. None of the above

    Answer: b

59. Bregma is _____________
    a. Junction of coronal and sagittal
    b. Junction of coronal and lambdoid
    c. Junction of parietomastoid and lambdoid suture
    d. Junction of sagittal suture to parietomastoid suture

    Answer: a

60. The fossa posterior to maxillary antrum is __________
    a. Temporal fossa
    b. Infratemporal fossa
    c. Pterygoid fossa
    d. Pterygopalatine fossa

    Answer: d

61. What is attached to the auricular tubercle?
    a. Fibrous capsule
    b. Anterior ligament of jaw
    c. Lateral ligament of jaw
    d. Medial ligament of jaw

    Answer: c

62. Macewen's triangle has following boundaries except __________
    a. Supramastoid crest
    b. Anterosuperior margin of meatus
    c. Posterosuperior margin of meatus
    d. Tangent to posterior margin of meatus

    Answer: b

63. All are the parts of temporal bone except __________
    a. Mastoid
    b. Pterygoid
    c. Petrous
    d. Tympanic

    Answer: b

64. Mastoid process ossifies by the end of __________
    a. 1st year
    b. 2nd year
    c. 3rd year
    d. 4th year

    Answer: b

65. Entomion is anterior part of __________
    a. Parietomastoid suture
    b. Sagittal suture
    c. Lambdoid
    d. Metopic suture

    Answer: a

66. The roof of infratemporal fossa has following foramina __________
    a. Foramen ovale and foramen rotundum
    b. Foramen ovale and foramen spinosum
    c. Foramen spinosum and foramen rotundum
    d. Foramen ovale and foramen lacerum

    Answer: b

67. Following nerve traverses the foramen rotundum __________
    a. Mandibular
    b. Maxillary
    c. Ophthalmic
    d. Masseteric

    Answer: b

68. The structures passing through foramen ovale are all except __________
    a. Mandibular nerve
    b. Lesser petrosal nerve
    c. Maxillary nerve
    d. Emissary vein

    Answer: c

69. Middle meningeal artery passes through following foramen _____________
    - a. Foramen spinosum
    - b. Foramen rotundum
    - c. Foramen ovale
    - d. Foramen lacerum

    Answer: a

70. Tympanic canaliculus transmits _____________ nerve.
    - a. X
    - b. XI
    - c. IX
    - d. XII

    Answer: c

71. A 45-year-old male met with road traffic accident (RTA), where he sustained head injury. The wound on the scalp was bleeding profusely.

    The anatomical basis for bleeding wound is _____________
    - a. Patient had thrombocytopenia
    - b. Patient had coagulation disorder
    - c. Blood vessels fail to retract into fibrous trabeculae of superficial fascia
    - d. Blood vessels lack tunica media

    Answer: c

72. A 65-year-old female diabetic patient developed a boil on the vestibule of nose. She gave history of fever and chills. Further investigations suggested that she developed cavernous sinus thrombosis.

    Anatomical basis of cavernous sinus thrombosis in 'danger area of face' is due to connection to cavernous sinus through _____________
    - a. Superior ophthalmic vein
    - b. Inferior ophthalmic vein
    - c. Facial vein
    - d. Maxillary vein

    Answer: a

73. While operating, a house surgeon is asked to retract sternocleidomastoid muscle. What structure lies below it, which house surgeon has to beware of _____________
    - a. Carotid sheath
    - b. Thyroid gland
    - c. External jugular vein
    - d. Subclavian artery

    Answer: a

74. Mother of a 3-year-old child complains of bleeding through the nose. On questioning the mother, history of the child putting fingers in the nose (nose picking) is elicited.

    The area traumatized is _____________
    - a. Posterosuperior part of nasal septum
    - b. Anteroinferior part of nasal septum
    - c. Lateral nasal wall
    - d. Vestibule of nose

    Answer: b

75. Mother of 7-year-old child complains of severe pain in the left ear of the child since 1 day. Mother said that she could see a boil in the ear. Anatomical basis for severe pain is _____________
    - a. Richly innervated
    - b. Tightly bound to perichondrium
    - c. Both a and b
    - d. None

    Answer: c

76. 25-year-old female complains of pain in left ear for 1 month on and off. On taking full history, she also complains of toothache. What is the anatomical link?
    a. Facial nerve
    b. IX nerve
    c. Auriculotemporal nerve
    d. X nerve

    Answer: c

77. While removing wax in 80-year-old male, he developed cough. This is due to stimulation of _____________ nerve.
    a. Arnold's nerve
    b. Jacobson's nerve
    c. IX nerve
    d. Nervus spinosus

    Answer: a

78. An intern during his ENT posting, when saw normal tympanic membrane (TM) through otoscope.
    i. The color of TM he appreciated was _____________
       a. Pink
       b. Gray
       c. White
       d. Pearl gray

       Answer: d

    ii. 'Cone of light' on TM, he appreciated was due to _____________
       a. Color of TM
       b. Light of otoscope
       c. Angulation of TM to horizontal
       d. None

       Answer: c

79. After thyroid surgery, the patient lost her voice due to injury of _____________ nerve.
    a. External laryngeal nerve
    b. Internal laryngeal nerve
    c. Recurrent laryngeal nerve
    d. Hypoglossal

    Answer: c

80. While operating on ear, the surgeon is close to oval window. What nerve lies in close relation to tympanic cavity?
    a. VI
    b. VII
    c. VII
    d. IX

    Answer: b

81. During tonsillectomy, there is an uncontrollable bleeding.
    i. The surgeon needs to tie (ligate) _____________ artery.
       a. Internal carotid
       b. External carotid
       c. Pharyngeal
       d. Lingual

       Answer: b

    ii. The level at which surgeon needs to take an incision to tie external carotid artery (ECA) is _____________
       a. Upper border of thyroid cartilage
       b. Lower border of thyroid cartilage
       c. At the level of cricoid cartilage
       d. At the level of jugular notch

       Answer: a

82. Bleeding from nose is profuse due to _______________
    a. Lack of tunica media in blood vessels
    b. Rich vascularity
    c. Lack of retraction
    d. All of the above

Answer: b

83. While operating on ear, the surgeon decides to do mastoidectomy (removal of antral cells). The surface landmark for the surgeon to do mastoidectomy is _____________
    a. Spine of Henle   c. Mastoid process
    b. Macewen's triangle   d. Supramastoid crest

Answer: b

84. The distance between the tympanic membrane and promontory is _____________
    a. 1 mm   c. 3 mm
    b. 2 mm   d. 4 mm

Answer: b

85. While removing tonsils (tonsillectomy), there was severe bleeding. This is due to _______________
    a. Facial artery   c. Pharyngeal vein
    b. Tonsillar artery   d. Palatine vein

Answer: d

86. Promontory in middle ear is due to _____________
    a. Facial canal   c. Tympanic plexus
    b. Basal turn of cochlea   d. Ossicles

Answer: b

87. All the germ layers contribute to the formation of _____________ structure.
    a. Stapes   c. Tympanic membrane
    b. External auditory canal   d. Incus

Answer: c

88. At birth, following structure is of adult size _____________
    a. Maxillary sinus   c. Frontal sinus
    b. Ear   d. Eustachian tube

Answer: b

89. Mother of 1-year-old child complains of small opening in front of both ears. It is likely to be _____________
    a. External auditory meatus   c. Preauricular sinus
    b. Sebaceous cyst   d. All of above

Answer: c

90. Inner ear is lodged in _____________ bone.

    a. Pterygoid
    c. Mastoid
    b. Petrous
    d. Tympanic

    Answer: b

91. A young male while playing on the ground had sustained blunt injury on head, half an hour back but continues to play. While playing he complains of headache and suddenly falls on the ground with loss of consciousness and hemiparesis.

    i. The ball would have hit _____________ region of temporal bone.

    a. Obelion
    b. Pterion
    c. Asterion
    d. Glabella

    Answer: b

    ii. The vessel that would have ruptured _____________

    a. Middle meningeal artery
    c. Middle meningeal vein
    b. Emissary vein
    d. Supraorbital vein

    Answer: a

92. Label the structures A, B, C, D in the following diagram.

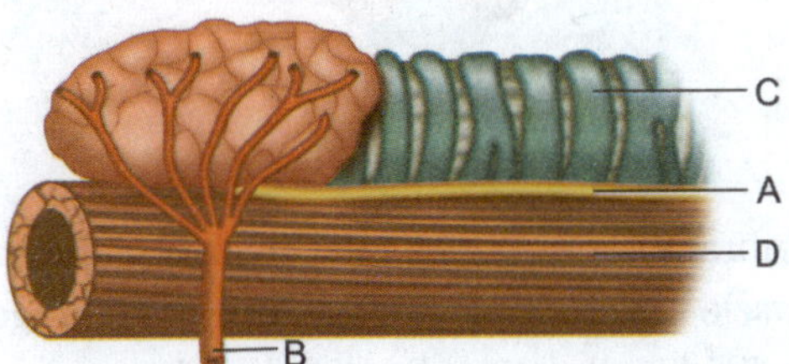

    Answer:

    A. Recurrent laryngeal nerve
    C. Trachea
    B. Inferior thyroid artery
    D. Esophagus

93. Identify the marked structure in the diagram of lymphatic drainage of breast.

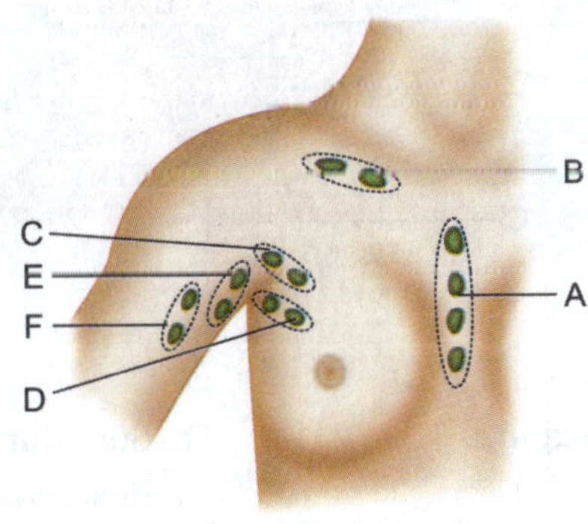

Answer:

A. Internal mammary
B. Apical
C. Central
D. Posterior axillary
E. Anterior axillary
F. Lateral

94. Label the midline structures of the neck.

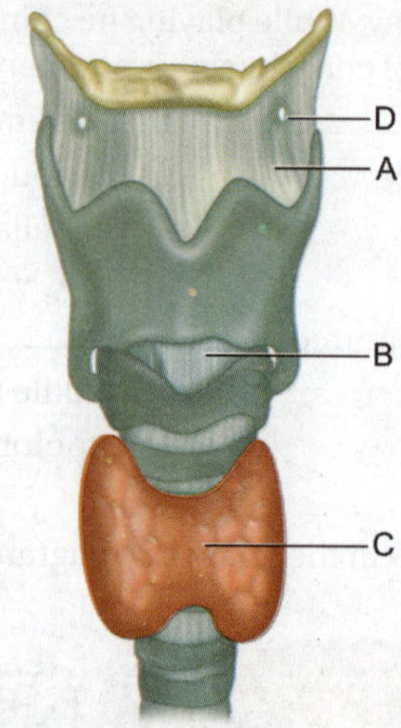

Answer:

A. Thyrohyoid membrane
B. Cricothyroid muscle
C. Thyroid gland
D. Superior laryngeal vessels

95. Identify the muscles dividing the triangles of the neck.

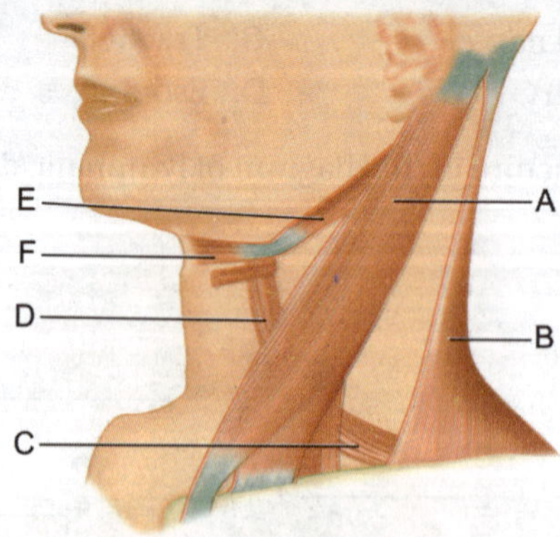

Answer:

A. Sternocleidomastoid
B. Trapezius
C. Inferior belly of omohyoid
D. Superior belly of omohyoid
E. Posterior belly of digastric
F. Anterior belly of digastric

96. Label the structures in the diagram.

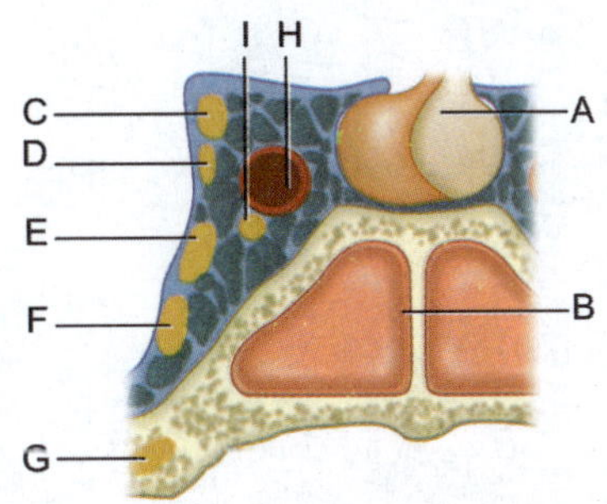

Answer:

A. Pituitary gland

B. Sphenoid sinus

C. III

D. IV

E. V1

F. V2

G. V3

H. Internal carotid artery

I. VI

97. Label the structures in the diagram.

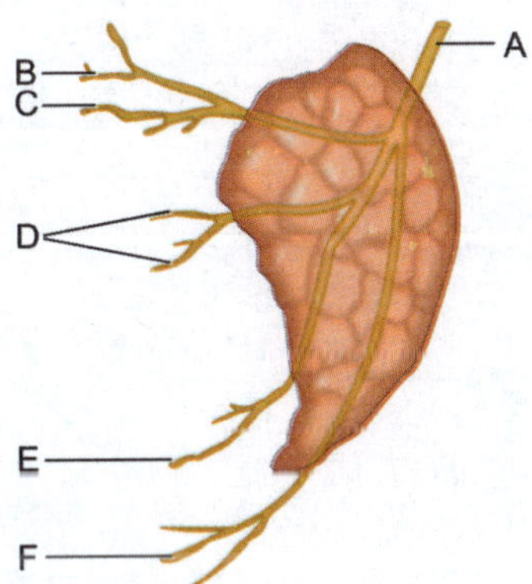

Answer:

A. Facial nerve

B. Temporal

C. Zygomatic

D. Buccal

E. Mandibular

F. Cervical

Facial nerve surgically divides the gland into superficial and deep parts.

SECTION - VI

NEUROANATOMY

Key Questions

Q. How is the nervous system classified?

Ans. The nervous system is classified as follows:

- Central nervous system (CNS)
- Peripheral nervous system (PNS).

Q. What are the parts of central nervous system?

Ans. The parts of CNS are brain (encephalon) and spinal cord (medulla spinalis).

Q. What is included in peripheral nervous system?

Ans. Peripheral nervous system includes following structures:

- 12 pairs of cranial nerves
- 31 pairs of spinal nerves.

Q. Is autonomic nervous system a part of CNS or PNS?

Ans. Autonomic nervous system by and large is considered as a separate functional unit. Since it is connected anatomically to CNS and PNS, it is included under both classifications.

Q. What are the subdivisions of brain?

Ans. The subdivisions of brain are:

- Cerebral hemispheres
- Brainstem
- Cerebellum.

Q. What are the parts of brainstem?

Ans. Following are the parts of brainstem:

- Diencephalon
- Mesencephalon (midbrain)
- Metencephalon (pons)
- Myelencephalon (medulla).

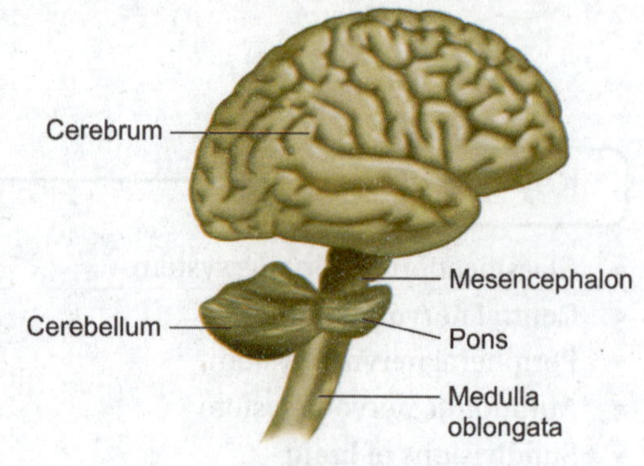

Parts of brain

Q. What is included in hindbrain?

Ans. Metencephalon (pons) and myelencephalon (medulla) together form hindbrain.

Q. What are the coverings of brain and spinal cord?

Ans. Three membranes surround the brain and spinal cord for protection, and support of these delicate structures. The membranes are as follows:

- Outer dura mater (pachymeninx)
- Middle arachnoid mater
- Inner pia mater.

Q. What are leptomeninges?

Ans. The pia mater and arachnoid mater together are known as leptomeninges.

Q. What are the layers of dura mater in the cranium?

Ans. The cranium dura has outer periosteal layer and inner meningeal layer. The meningeal layer gives rise to several folds (falx cerebri, tentorium cerebelli, falx cerebelli, diaphragma sellae), which divides the cranial cavity into compartments.

Q. Which main artery supplies blood to dura mater?

Ans. The middle meningeal artery, a branch of maxillary artery mainly supplies blood to dura mater. Middle meningeal artery enters the skull through foramen spinosum.

Q. Depict the covering of CNS.

Ans. Anesthetic drugs when injected in epidural space produce epidural anesthesia.

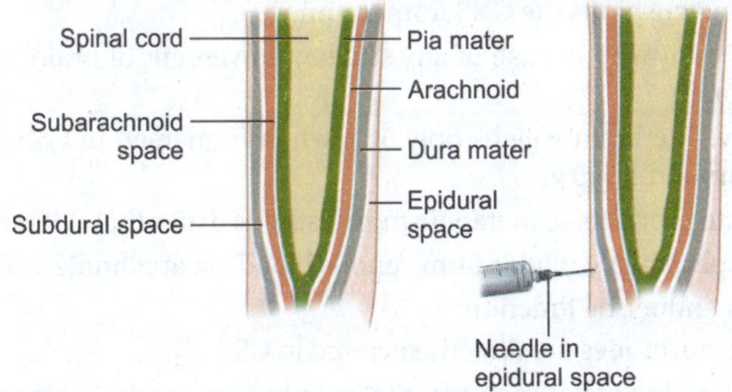

Coverings of CNS

Q. Discuss the normal cerebrospinal fluid (CSF) composition.

Ans. Following are the properties of normal CSF:

- Clear, colorless fluid
- By and large considered as ultrafiltrate of blood plasma
- Contains small quantities of protein and glucose
- Higher quantities of Na^+, Cl^- and Mg^{2+}
- Lower quantities of K^+, Ca^{2+}
- No cellular component.

Q. How is the CSF produced and what is its quantity?

Ans. About 70% of CSF is secreted by choroid plexus present in lateral ventricles, third and fourth ventricles. 30% of CSF is water produced due to metabolic reactions like oxidation of glucose.

- Total quantity of CSF is approximately 140 mL
- CSF production: 0.35 mL/min, 400–500 mL/24 hours.

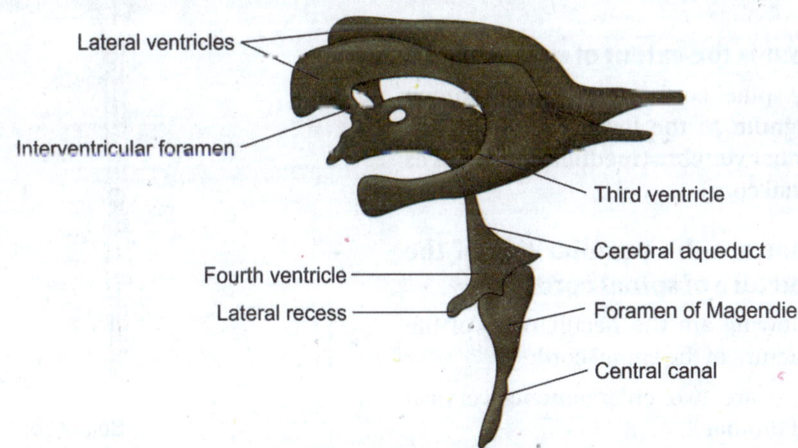

Ventricles of brain and choroid plexus

Q. What are the functions of CSF?

Ans. Following are the functions of the CSF:

- It protects and cushions the CNS from trauma
- By virtue of buoyancy in case of any sudden movement of brain, the CSF reduces the damage to brain
  - Buoyancy: The brain weighs only 50 g when immersed in CSF. The gross weight of brain is around 1,500 g.
- It clears waste products of metabolism, anesthetic drugs that diffuse in the brain
- It clears the particulate matter from venous blood via arachnoid villi
- Coordinates endocrine function
  - Releasing hormones are directly secreted in CSF.
- Influences function of neurons and glial cells by altering the ionic composition.

Q. What is choroid plexus?

Ans. Choroid plexus consist of single layer of folded cuboidal epithelium with a mesh of capillaries within it.

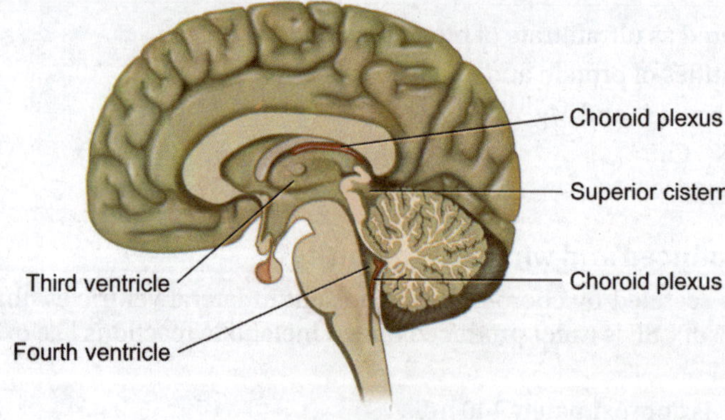

Q. What is the extent of spinal cord?

Ans. The spinal cord extends from foramen magnum to the lower border of first lumbar vertebra (medulla continues as spinal cord).

Q. What are the peculiarities of the structure of spinal cord?

Ans. Following are the peculiarities of the structure of the spinal cord:

- There are two enlargements cervical and lumbar

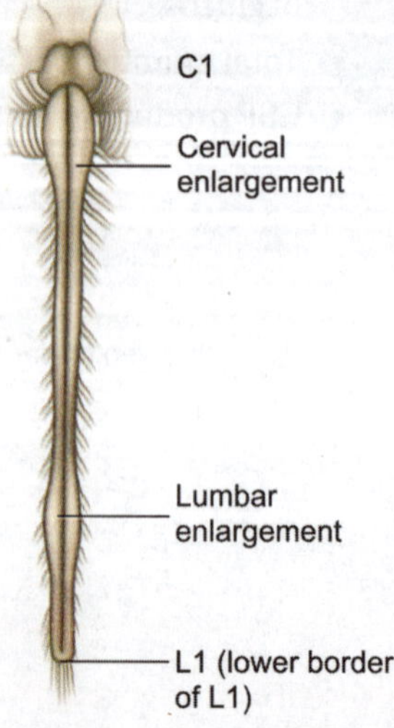

- Cervical enlargement consists of four cervical nerve roots and one thoracic nerve root forming brachial plexus
- Lumbar enlargement consists of four lumbar nerve roots and two sacral nerve roots giving rise to lumbar plexus and sacral plexus respectively
- Distal to lumbar enlargement the spinal cord becomes conical and is known as conus medullaris
- Pia mater condenses into singular filament distal to conus known as filum terminale
- Spinal cord consists of 31 segments namely 8 cervical, 12 thoracic, 5 lumbar, 5 sacral and 1 coccygeal
- In cut section spinal cord can be distinctly divided into H-shaped gray matter (cell bodies) and surrounding white matter (myelinated fibers).

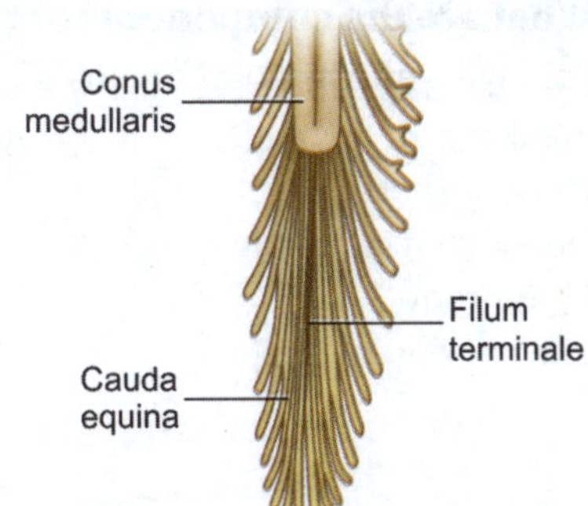

Terminal segment of spinal cord

Q. Depict the transverse section of spinal cord (important cell groups and fiber tract to be shown).

Ans.

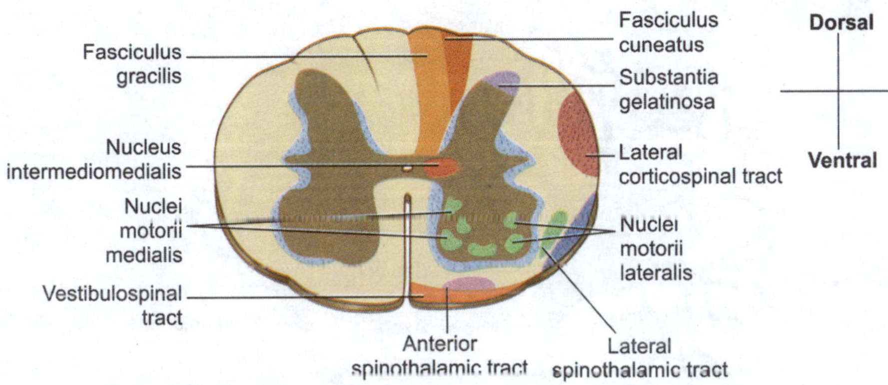

Q. How are the cells of the gray matter of spinal cord classified?

Ans. There are two types of cells:
- *Root cells:* These are present in anterior and lateral horns of spinal cord and gives rise to axons, which leave through ventral root
- *Column cells:* These are neurons whose peripheral processes are within CNS.

Q. At what level does the conus medullaris lie at birth?

Ans. The conus medullaris is at the level of L3 vertebra at birth.

Q. What are the components of reflex arc?

Ans. Following are the components of reflex arc:

- Receptor
- Sensory root
- Dorsal root ganglion
- Motor root
- Effector organ.

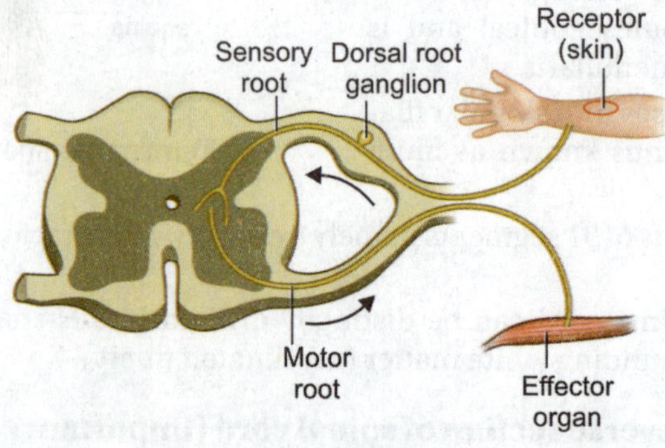

Reflex arc

Q. Draw a neat labeled diagram of a neuron.

Ans.

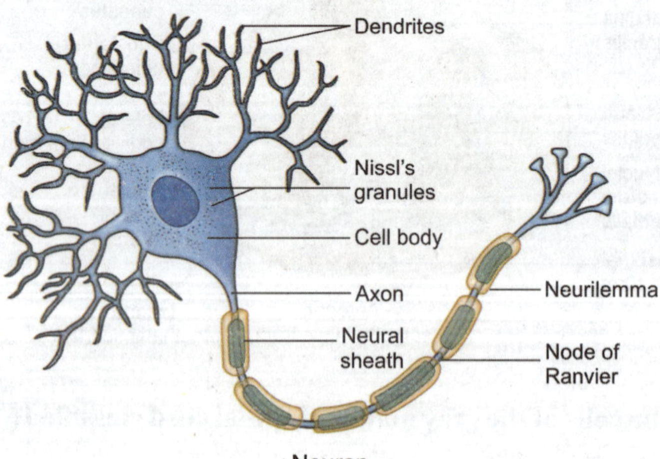

Neuron

Q. What do you understand by nuclei and ganglia?

Ans.

- Collection of cell bodies of neuron within CNS is known as nuclei
- Collection of cell bodies of neuron within PNS is known as ganglia.

Q. What are the major cell types of nervous system?

Ans. There are mainly two cell types of nervous system:
- *Excitable cells:* Neurons
- *Non-excitable cells:* Neuroglia, ependyma, Schwann cells.

Q. How do you classify neuroglial cells?

Ans. Neuroglial cells are broadly classified into:
- *Macroglia:* Astrocytes, oligodendrocytes
- *Microglia:* Phagocytes.

Short Notes: Brain

Key short notes

Key short notes

- White matter of cerebrum
- Superolateral surface and medial surface of cerebral hemisphere
- Components of basal ganglia
- Fourth ventricle
- Cut section of medulla passing through the floor of fourth ventricle
- Features of midbrain
- Fissures and lobules of cerebellum
- Components of diencephalon
- Cut section of medulla at motor (pyramidal) and sensory (medial lemniscus) decussation
- Cut section of lower and upper pons
- Laminar pattern of spinal cord
- Corpus callosum
- Cerebellar peduncles
- Visual pathway
- Auditory pathway

Q. WHITE MATTER OF CEREBRUM

The core of cerebral hemisphere consists of thick myelinated fibers interconnecting subcortical nuclei, this forms the white matter of cerebrum.

The fibers of white matter can be subdivided into three types:

- Projection fibers
- Association fibers
- Commissural fibers.

Projection Fibers

The fibers transmit impulses to and fro from cerebral cortex, and form fan-like bundle of fibers known as corona radiata.

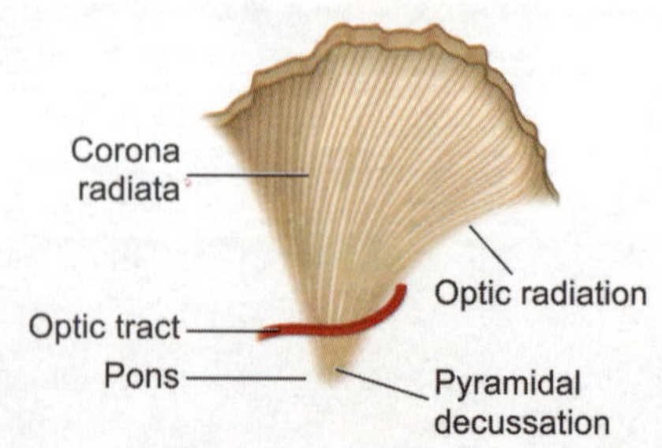

Projection fibers

Association Fibers

The fibers interconnect different cortical areas within the same cerebral hemisphere, e.g. uncinate fasciculus.

Commissural Fibers

The fibers interconnect similar cortical areas between the two cerebral hemispheres, e.g. corpus callosum.

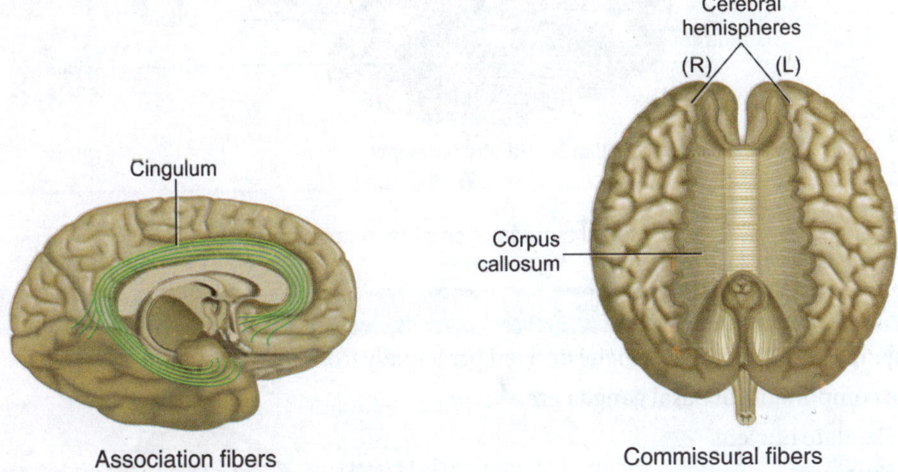

Q. SUPEROLATERAL SURFACE AND MEDIAL SURFACE OF CEREBRAL HEMISPHERE (DIAGRAM ONLY).

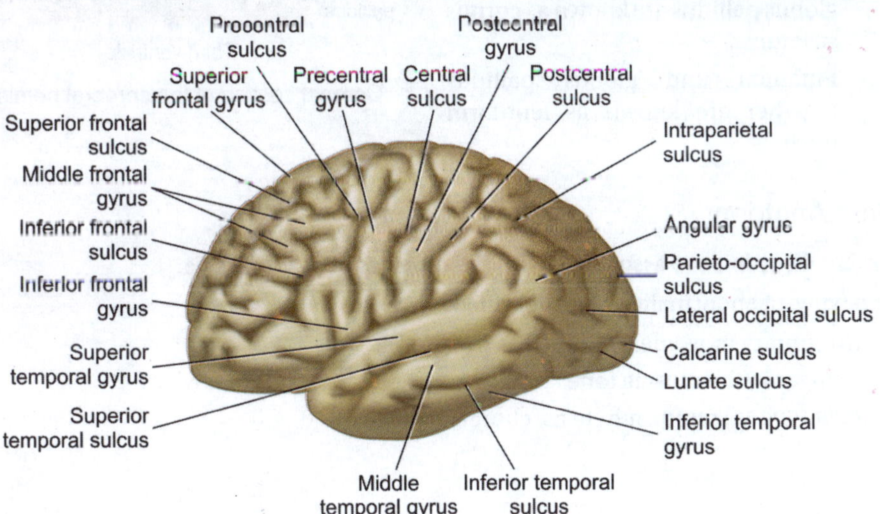

Superolateral surface of cerebral hemisphere

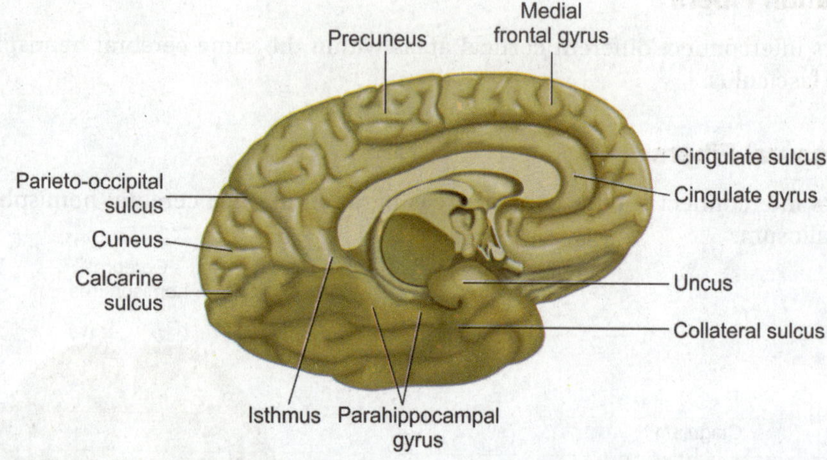

Medial surface of cerebral hemisphere

Q. COMPONENTS OF BASAL GANGLIA

Basal ganglia are subcortical nuclei derived principally from telencephalon.

The components of basal ganglia are:

- Caudate nucleus
- Putamen
- Globus pallidus
- Amygdaloid nuclear complex:
    - Caudate nucleus, putamen and globus pallidus are known as corpus striatum
    - Putamen and globus pallidus together are known as lentiform nucleus.

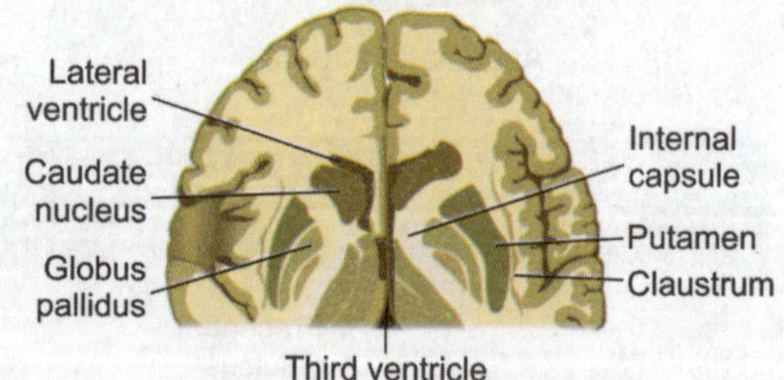

Coronal section of the cerebral hemisphere

Applied Anatomy

Movement disorders are associated with the diseases of basal ganglia.

Two types of abnormalities are identified:

- Involuntary movements known as dyskinesia
- Changes in the muscle tone.

Dyskinesia types: Tremor, athetosis, chorea, ballism.

Q. FOURTH VENTRICLE

Fourth ventricle is a rhomboid-shaped cavity overlying the pons and medulla and hence it can be subdivided into pontine part and medullary part.

Extent

- *Above:* Cerebral aqueduct of midbrain
- *Below:* Central canal of upper cervical spinal cord.

Roof

Superior and inferior medullary veli (like a tent).

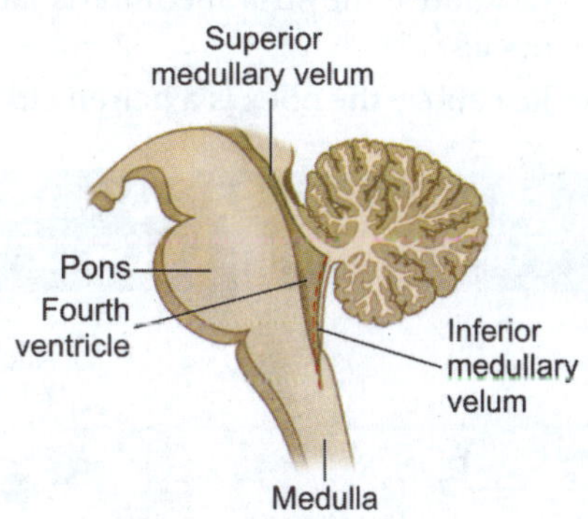

Fourth ventricle location

Apex

Apex extends into the cerebellum where it is known as fastigium.

Recess

Lateral recess: Lies over the surface of inferior cerebellar peduncle and opens into the cerebellomedullary cistern.

Communications

Communicates with the subarachnoid space through foramen of Luschka and foramen of Magendie.

Floor

Features

- Vertically in the center, divided by median sulcus and paramedially divided by sulcus limitans
- Horizontally it is divided by stria medullaris
- Paramedian area has a bulge known as median eminence
- Caudal area of fourth ventricle is known as calamus scriptorius
- The apex of the ventricle is known as obex.

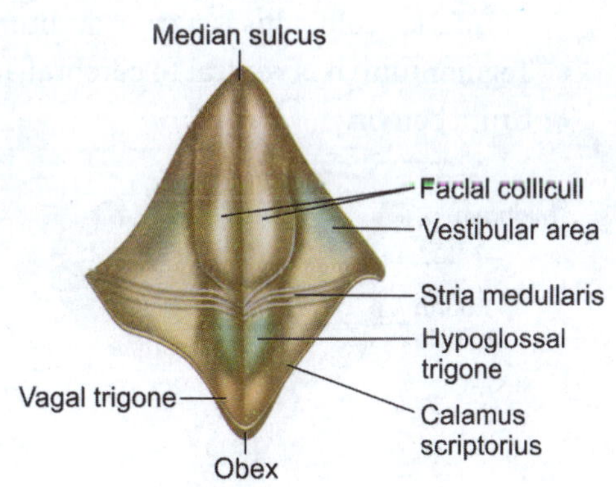

Floor of fourth ventricle

Specific Area

- Just above the stria medullaris paramedially is facial colliculus and hypoglossal trigone is just below it
- Vagal trigone lies paramedially toward the caudal part of fourth ventricle
- Just above the stria medullaris laterally is vestibular area beneath, which is vestibular nuclei
- Just above the obex is a paired circumventricular organ known as area postrema.

Q. DRAW A DIAGRAM OF CUT SECTION OF MEDULLA PASSING THROUGH THE FLOOR OF FOURTH VENTRICLE.

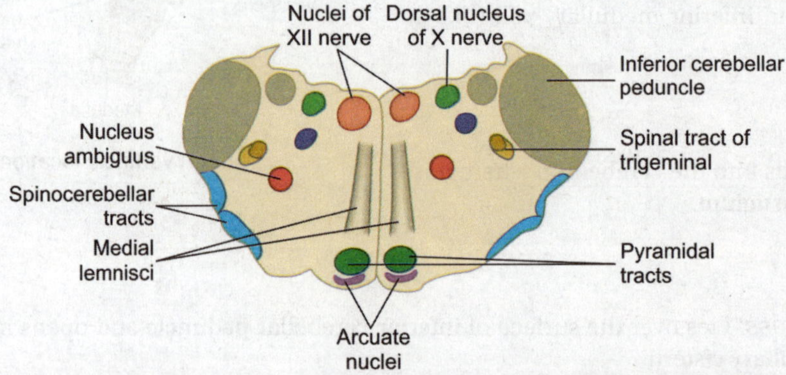

Q. FEATURES OF MIDBRAIN

Midbrain is smallest and least differentiated portion of brainstem. The features of midbrain are as follows:

- Tectum comprises of superior and inferior colliculus:
  - Superior colliculus is part of visual pathway
  - Inferior colliculus is part of auditory pathway.
- Tegmentum: It is ventral to cerebral aqueduct
- Crura cerebri

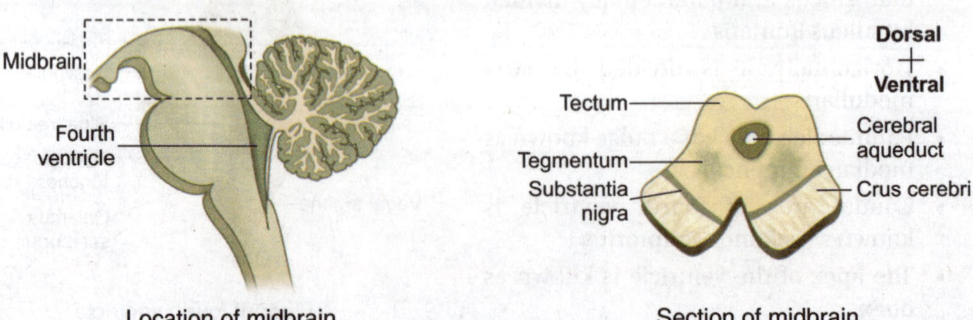

Location of midbrain   Section of midbrain

- Substantia nigra: It is a pigmented area between tegmentum and crura cerebri:
  - The cells of substantia nigra produce dopamine.
- Superior colliculus and an area just above it, is known as pretectum
- Two cranial nerves are related to midbrain namely oculomotor and trochlear
- Superior cerebellar peduncle decussates in caudal midbrain and surrounds a discrete nuclear mass known as red nucleus.

Q. DRAW A NEAT LABELED DIAGRAM SHOWING FISSURES AND LOBULES OF CEREBELLUM.

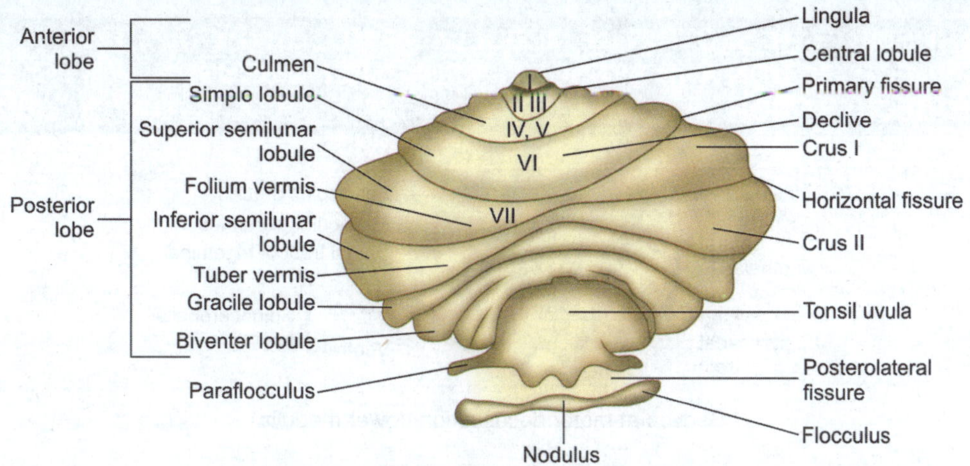

Cerebellum showing lobes and fissures

Q. COMPONENTS OF DIENCEPHALON

The most proximal segment of brainstem is known as diencephalon. It is a paired structure on each side of third ventricle (area between cerebral hemisphere).

It can be subdivided into four parts namely:

- Epithalamus
- Thalamus
- Hypothalamus
- Subthalamic region.

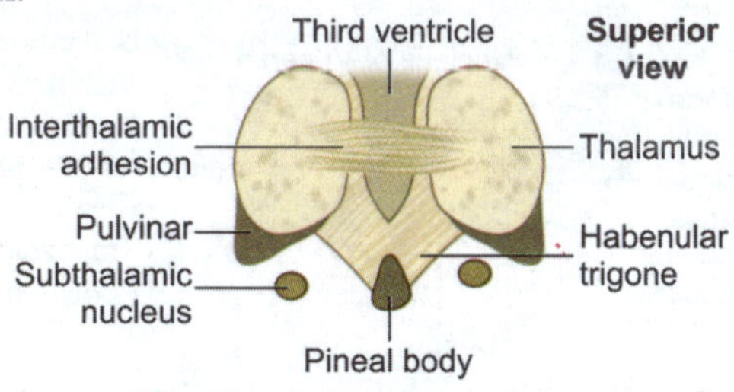

Components of diencephalon

Components of diencephalon

Epithalamus	Thalamus	Hypothalamus	Subthalamic region
Pineal body	Pulvinar (expanded posterior part)	Optic chiasm	Subthalamic nucleus
Habenular nuclei	Medial and lateral geniculate bodies (metathalamus)	Infundibulum	Zona incerta
Striae medullares	Anterior, lateral, medial and ventral nuclear groups	Tuber cinereum	
Tenia thalami		Mammillary bodies	

Q. DEPICT CUT SECTION OF MEDULLA AT MOTOR (PYRAMIDAL) DECUSSATION AND SENSORY (MEDIAL LEMNISCUS) DECUSSATION.

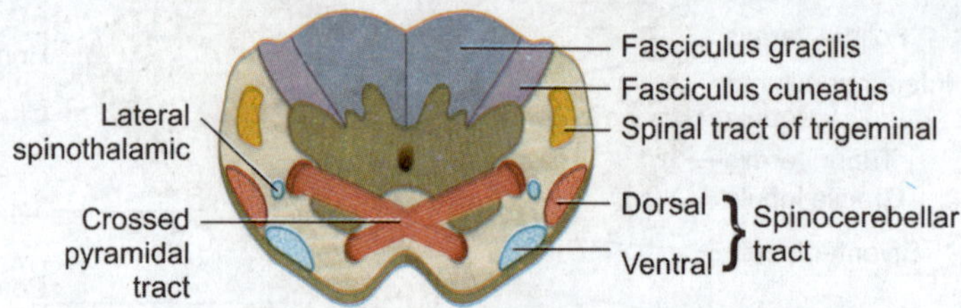

Section at motor decussation (lower medulla)

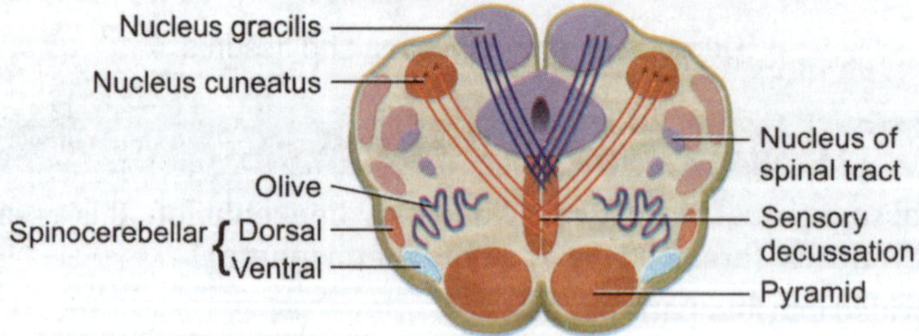

Section at sensory decussation (upper medulla)

Q. DEPICT CUT SECTION OF LOWER AND UPPER PONS.

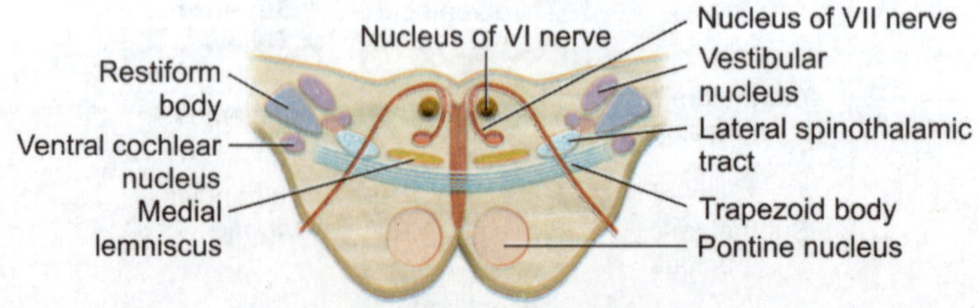

Transverse section at lower pons

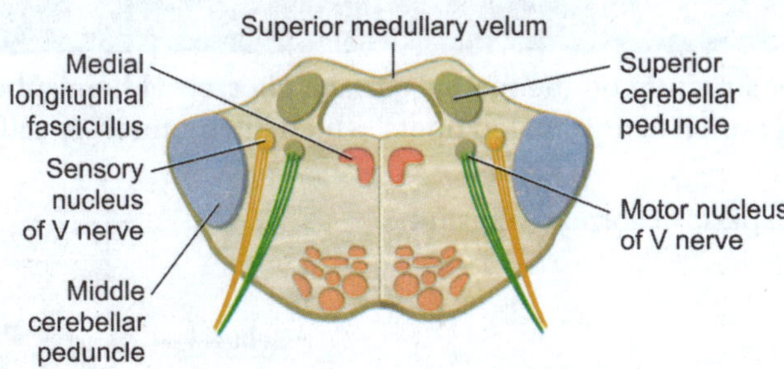

Transverse section at upper pons

Q. LAMINAR PATTERN OF SPINAL CORD

The cells in the gray matter of spinal cord are arranged in the form of layers (like a marble print); this constitutes the laminar pattern of spinal cord.

The layers (laminae) are given in roman numbers. It includes:

1. **Lamina I:** Caps the posterior horn, has posteromarginal nucleus, receives axons from lamina II. Cells in the lamina respond to pain and temperature stimuli, and contribute fibers to contralateral spinothalamic tract.

2. **Lamina II:** Corresponds to substantia gelatinosa, found at all spinal levels, send axons to dorsolateral fasciculus, transmits pain impulses also has opiate receptors.

3. **Lamina III:** Axons of the neurons in this lamina divide number of times to form thick plexus in laminae III and IV, most cells in this laminae are interneurons.

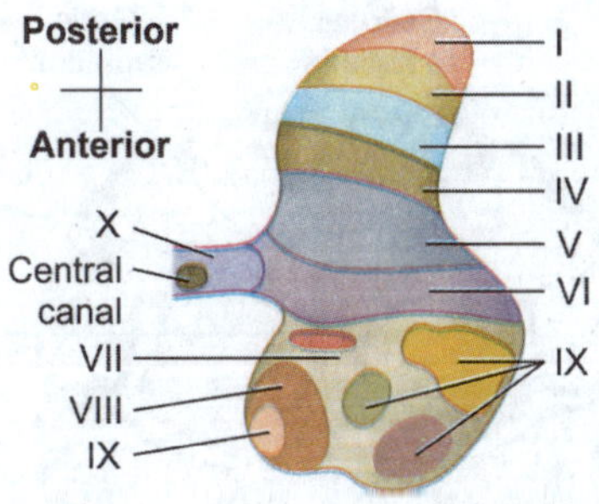

Laminar pattern of spinal cord

4. **Lamina IV:** Contains cells, which respond to light touch.

5. **Lamina V:** Divided into medial and lateral parts (except in thoracic region). Lateral part in cervical region gives rise to reticular process.

6. **Lamina VI:** Present in the region of cord enlargements, divided into medial and lateral parts, group I muscle afferent terminate in medial zone and descending spinal tracts are present in lateral zone.

7. **Lamina VII:** It is also known as zona intermedia, dorsal nucleus of Clarke forms an important cell group in this lamina, gives rise to uncrossed posterior spinocerebellar tract, intermediolateral nucleus gives rise to preganglionic sympathetic fibers.

8. **Lamina VIII:** Most of the descending tracts of spinal cord terminate in the cells of this lamina.

9. **Lamina IX:** Consist of many discrete groups of somatic motor neurons (α and γ) involved in maintaining muscle tone.

10. **Lamina X:** It is a gray matter around the central canal.

Q. CORPUS CALLOSUM

The most prominent structure on the medial surface of cerebral hemisphere is corpus callosum. It comprises of bunch of myelinated fibers, which interconnect specific areas of cerebral hemisphere.

Following are the parts of corpus callosum:

- Rostrum
- Genu
- Body
- Splenium.

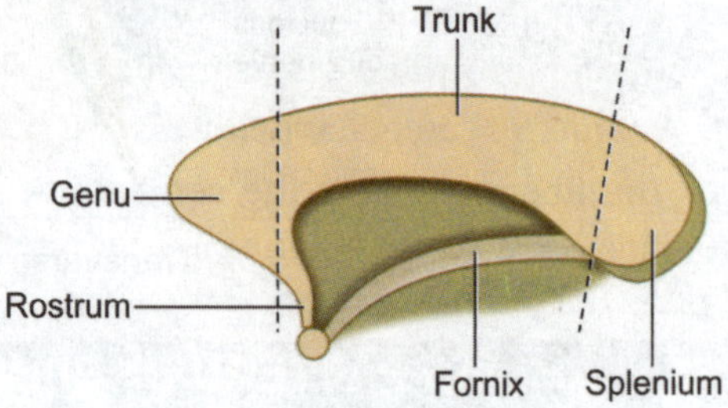

Subdivisions of fibers of corpus callosum:

- Fibers connecting frontal lobes are known as anterior forceps (forceps minor)
- Fibers connecting occipital lobes are known as posterior forceps (forceps major)
- Fibers in splenium lying between lateral wall of posterior horn of lateral ventricle and optic radiation are known as tapetum.

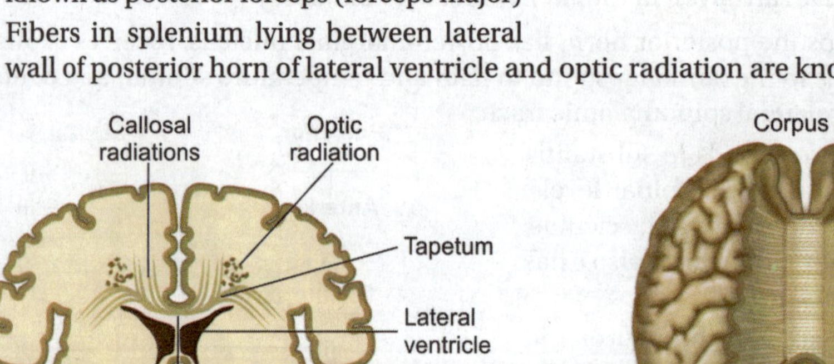

Parts of corpus callosum

Section at splenium of corpus callosum

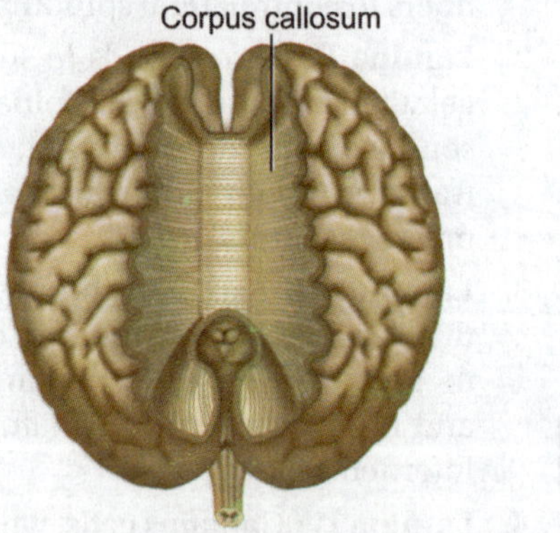

Superior view

Relations of Corpus Callosum

- *Above:* Longitudinal fissure
- *Below:* Lateral ventricle.

Callosal sulcus separates the corpus striatum from cingulate gyrus.

Function

Corpus callosum helps in transferring information learned by one cerebral hemisphere to another, e.g. some experiences in the past memory of certain events.

However, surgical transection of corpus callosum does not show any obvious neurological deficit in experimental animals.

Q. CEREBELLAR PEDUNCLES

The cerebellum is connected to the brainstem by cerebellar peduncles.

There are three cerebellar peduncles:

- Superior cerebellar peduncle
- Middle cerebellar peduncle
- Inferior cerebellar peduncle.

The fibers reaching the cerebellum (afferent system) enter via inferior and middle cerebellar peduncle by and large.

The fibers leaving the cerebellum (efferent system) enter the superior cerebellar peduncle by and large.

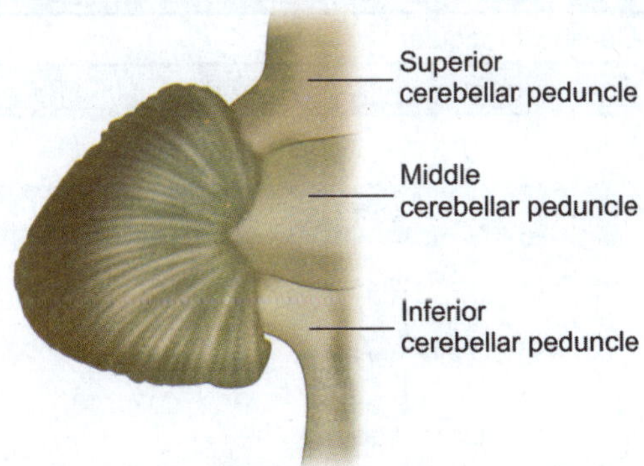

Cerebellar peduncle

Inferior Cerebellar Peduncle

Inferior cerebellar peduncle can be subdivided into two portions:

- Lateral restiform body
- Medial juxtarestiform body.

Afferent fibers	Efferent fibers
Posterior spinocerebellar tract	Cerebello-olivary fibers
Cuneocerebellar tract	Cerebellovestibular fibers
Olivocerebellar tract	Cerebelloreticular fibers
Parolivocerebellar tract	
Reticulocerebellar tract	
Vestibulocerebellar tract	

Middle Cerebellar Peduncle

Middle cerebellar peduncle is the most thick peduncle, which transmits fibers to cerebellum, i.e. pontocerebellar fibers originating from pontine precerebellar nuclei. Pontine precerebellar nuclei receive fibers from ipsilateral cerebral cortex.

Superior Cerebellar Peduncle

Superior cerebellar peduncle comprises of efferent bundle of fibers arising from deep nuclei of cerebellum mostly dentate nucleus. The efferent fibers end in inferior olivary nuclei, reticular formation, red nucleus and thalamus.

Accordingly the fibers are classified as detailed below.

Efferent fibers	Afferent fibers
Cerebello-olivary	Anterior spinocerebellar
Cerebelloreticular	Tectocerebellar
Cerebellorubral	Dentatothalamic

Q. VISUAL PATHWAY (DIAGRAM ONLY)

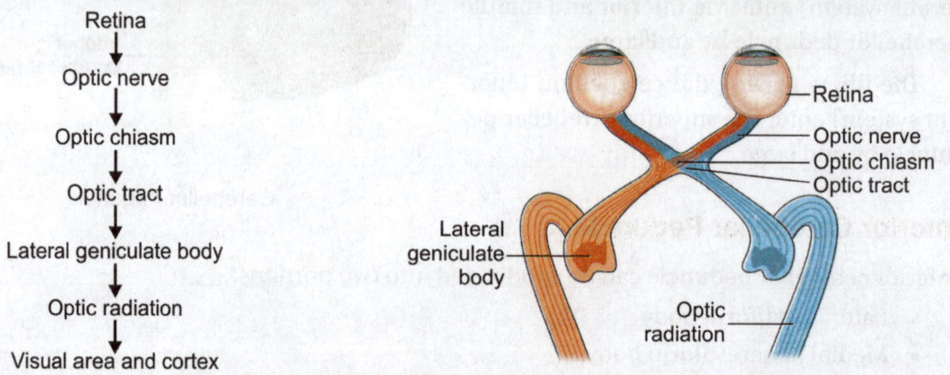

Q. AUDITORY PATHWAY

Auditory receptors (hair cells of organ of Corti in cochlea).

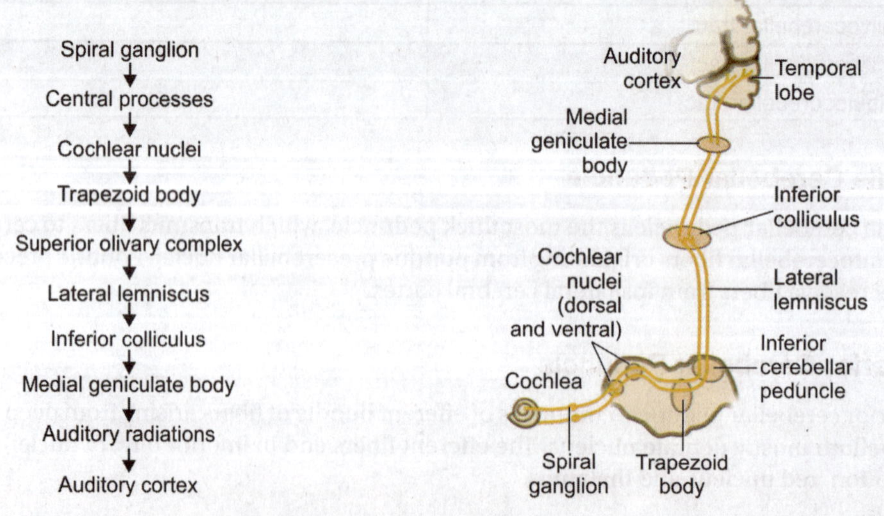

Short Notes: Spinal Cord Tracts

> **Key short notes**
>
> - Tracts of spinal cord
>
> ## ASCENDING SPINAL TRACTS
>
> - Posterior white column
> - Anterior spinothalamic tract
> - Lateral spinothalamic tract
> - Posterior spinocerebellar tract
> - Anterior spinocerebellar tract
>
> ## DESCENDING SPINAL TRACTS
>
> - Corticospinal tract
> - Vestibulospinal tract
> - Medial longitudinal fasciculus

Q. GENERAL FEATURES OF TRACTS OF THE SPINAL CORD.

- Tracts or fasciculi are bundles of nerve fibers having same origin, course and termination (functionally and anatomically having a single link)
- Funiculus is a distinct area in the spinal cord having different tracts
- By and large, long tracts are located peripherally in the white matter and small tracts are close to the gray matter.

Classification

Tracts are classified into:

- Ascending tracts that carry sensory impulses towards the brain by and large
- Descending tracts that carry motor impulses away from the brain.

Ascending tracts	Descending tracts
Posterior white column in spinal cord	Corticospinal (lateral and anterior)
Medial lemniscus in brainstem	Rubrospinal
Anterior spinothalamic	Vestibulospinal
Spinotectal	Reticulospinal
Lateral spinothalamic	Medial longitudinal fasciculus
Posterior spinocerebellar	Autonomic pathways
Anterior spinocerebellar	

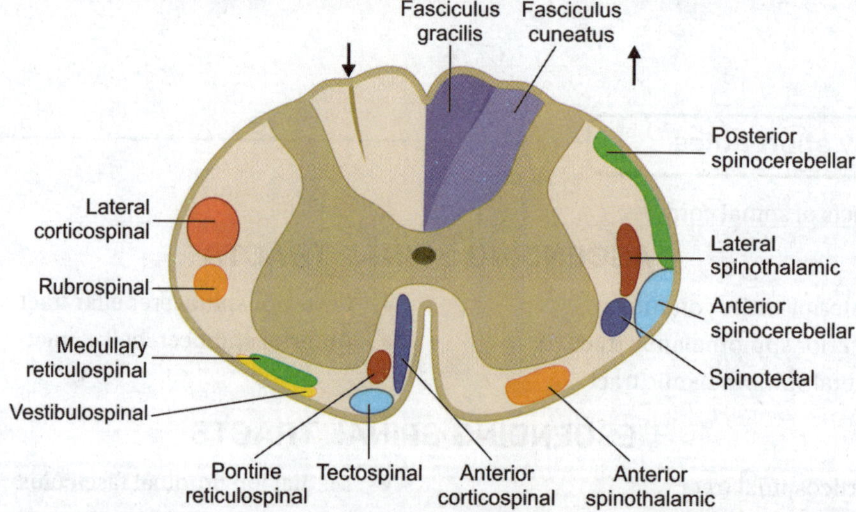

Ascending and descending tracts

▶ ASCENDING TRACTS

Q. POSTERIOR WHITE COLUMN

Functions

Concerned with touch, pressure sensation and proprioception (joint position).

Origin

Dorsal root ganglion (first order neuron) and uncrossed ascending branches of spinal ganglion cells.

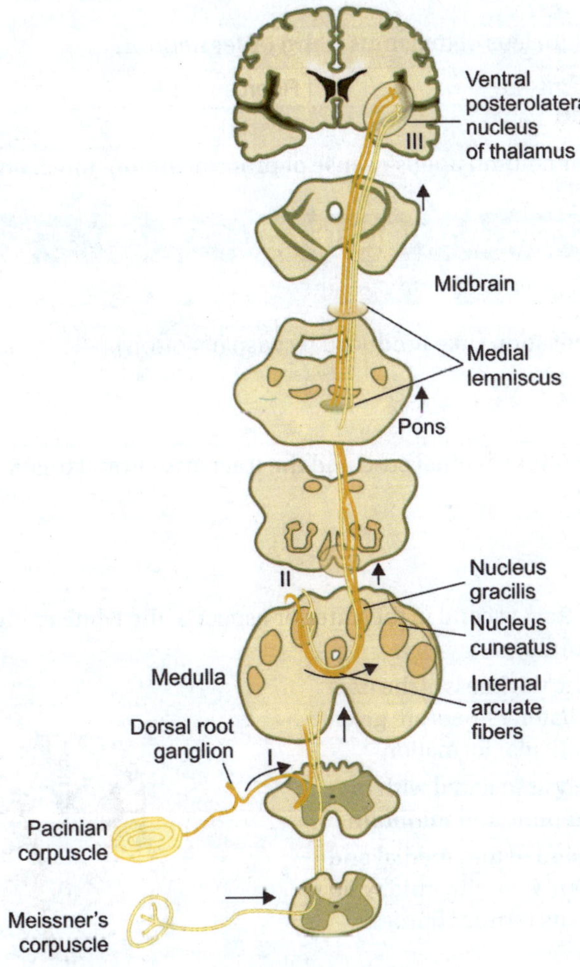

Course

1. Fibers ascend in posterior funiculus medially and dorsally (in thoracic and cervical region, a septum appears within the posterior funiculus dividing it into fasciculus gracilis and fasciculus cuneatus).

2. The fibers synapse at nuclei gracilis and cuneatus (second order neuron).

3. Second order fibers arise from above neurons, which curve anteriorly and medially as internal arcuate fibers.

4. The fibers after crossing the midline, form a bundle known as medial lemniscus. This crossing over occurs at lower medulla.

5. The fibers of medial lemniscus ascend in the brainstem to synapse with ventral posterolateral nucleus of thalamus (third order neuron).

Termination

Ventral posterolateral nucleus of thalamus (third order neuron).

Clinical Importance

Lesions of the posterior column abolish sense of proprioception, touch and pressure.

Q. ANTERIOR SPINOTHALAMIC TRACT

Function

Conveys light touch sensation (like produced by wisp of cotton).

Origin

Cells within the gray matter of spinal cord and the tract arise from laminae I, IV and V contra-laterally.

Course

- The fibers of the tract ascend in the anterior aspect of the white matter of the spinal cord to reach the medulla
- In the medulla, the thickness of the tract reduces since collateral fibers are given to the nuclei in reticular formation
- The tract is closely associated with medial lemniscus in pons and midbrain
- The tract is subdivided into medial and lateral components in the midbrain depending upon its termination.

Termination

1. Medial component terminates into periaqueductal gray matter and the intralaminar thalamic nuclei bilaterally.
2. Lateral component terminates into caudal parts of ventral posterolateral thalamic nuclei.
3. Spinotectal tract is in close association with anterior spinothalamic tract, but terminates in contralateral superior colliculus and periaqueductal gray matter. This tract is concerned with nociceptive sensation.

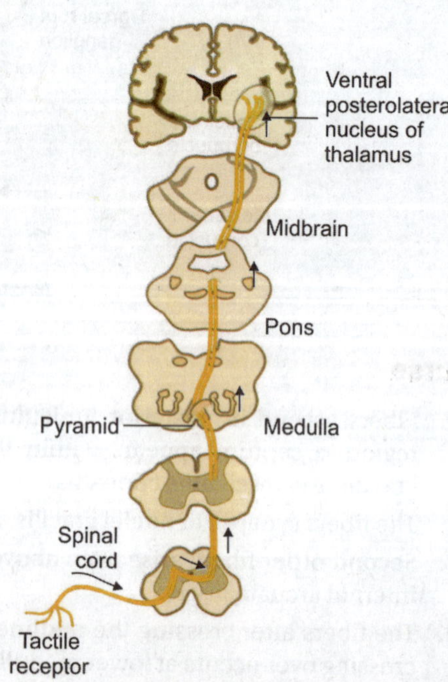

Anterior spinothalamic tract

Clinical Importance

Lesion of this tract does not cause significant changes since the major sensations are carried by posterior column.

Q. LATERAL SPINOTHALAMIC TRACT

Function

Conveys pain and temperature sensation.

Origin

Cells in laminae I, IV and V gives rise to fibers that cross the spinal cord anteriorly and ascend in contralateral lateral funiculus as lateral spinothalamic tract.

Course

- The tract ascends upwards just medial to anterior spinocerebellar tract in spinal cord
- The fibers concerned with temperature sensation are posterior to the fibers concerned with pain
- In the brainstem, collateral fibers are given to the reticular formation
- It terminates in thalamus.

Termination

Ventral posterolateral nucleus of thalamus.

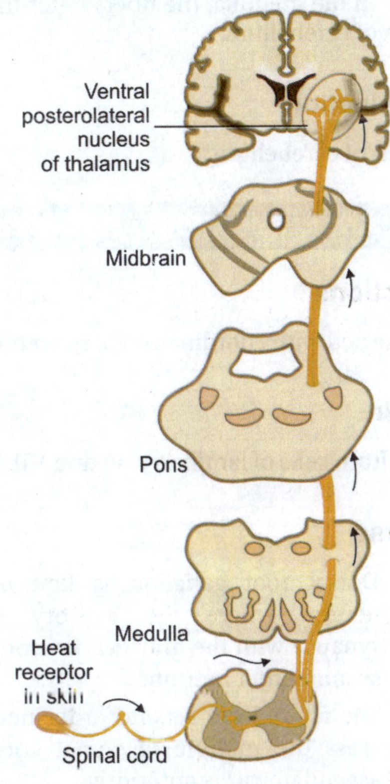

Clinical Importance

Lesion on one side of the lateral spinothalamic tract causes loss of pain and temperature on the opposite side of the body.

Q. POSTERIOR SPINOCEREBELLAR TRACT

Functions

Posterior spinocerebellar tract is involved in fine coordination of posture and movement of individual limb muscles.

Origin

Arises from dorsal nucleus of Clarke (lamina VII).

Course

- Ascends in the posterolateral part of lateral funiculus
- In the medulla, the fibers enter the inferior cerebellar peduncle and end in the vermis of cerebellum.

Termination

Vermis of cerebellum.

Q.   ANTERIOR SPINOCEREBELLAR TRACT

Functions

Concerned with coordination of movement and maintenance of posture of lower limb.

Origin

Arise from cells of laminae V, VI and VII.

Course

1. Dorsal root ganglion is first order neuron where the sensory fiber synapse with the gray cell neuron, i.e. second order neuron.
2. The fibers from second order neuron cross the midline of spinal cord to ascend upwards anteriorly.
3. In the brainstem, at the level of upper pons, the fibers course on the dorsal surface of superior cerebellar peduncle. The tract terminates contralaterally in the anterior cerebellar vermis (lobules I–IV).

Clinical Importance

Lesions of spinocerebellar tract do not cause any significant loss of sensation since the impulses enter the cerebellum and not the cerebrum, which is a conscious brain.

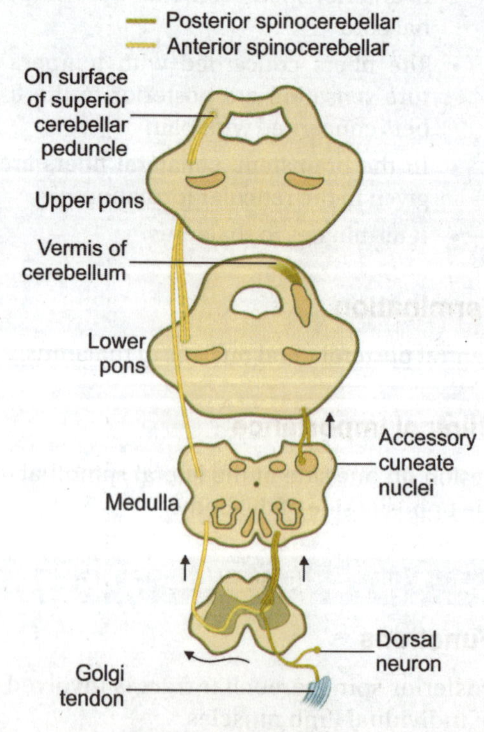

Spinocerebellar tracts

► DESCENDING SPINAL TRACTS

Q. CORTICOSPINAL TRACT

Functions

Concerned with voluntary skilled movements.

Origin

Arises from the cells in the cerebral cortex lamina V (motor area 4, premotor area 6 mainly).

Course

1. The fibers arising from the cerebral cortex converge in corona radiata and descend downwards to enter the posterior limb of internal capsule and form crus cerebri at midbrain level.

2. In the medulla, the fibers form massive pyramids.

3. At the junction of medulla and spinal cord, the tract divides into three separate parts:

   a. 90% of the fibers cross the midline to form lateral corticospinal tract.

   b. 8% forms uncrossed anterior corticospinal tract.

   c. 2% forms uncrossed lateral corticospinal tract.

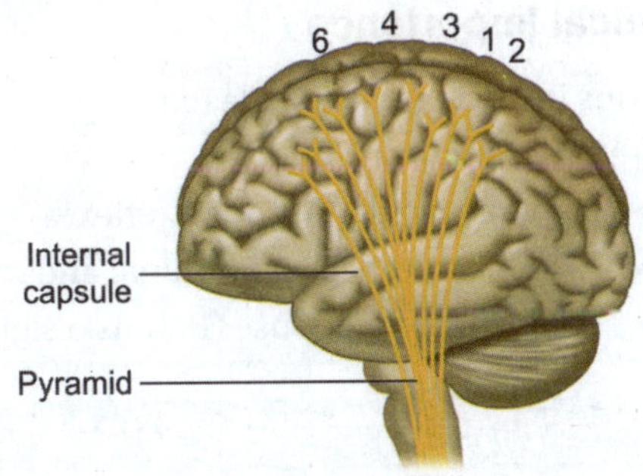

Origin of corticospinal tract

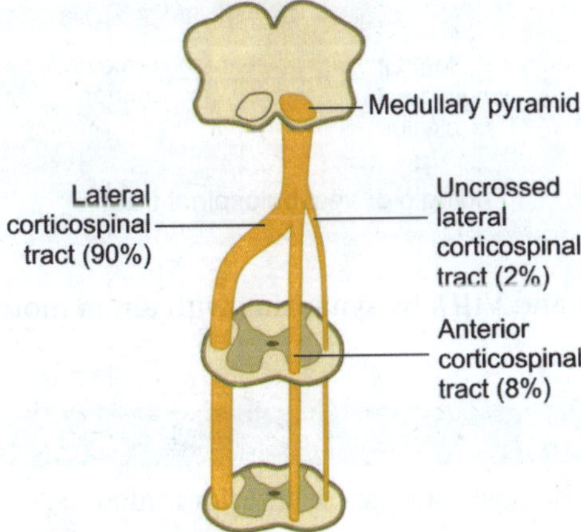

Subdivisions of corticospinal tract

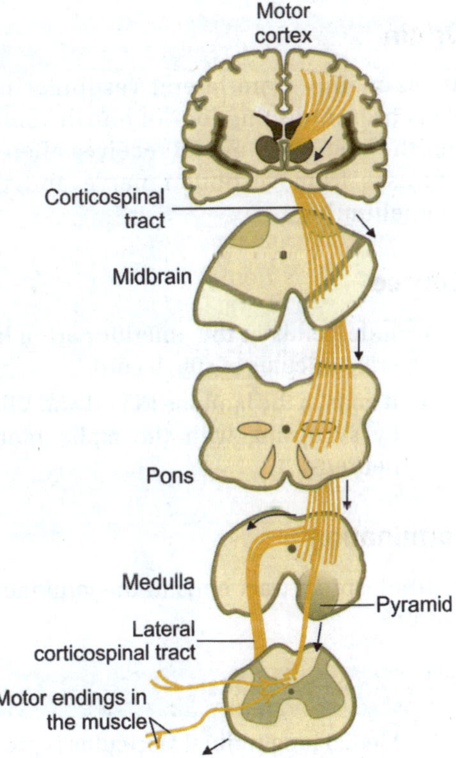

Corticospinal tract

4. The lateral corticospinal tract as it descends along the spinal cord gives fibers to gray matter of laminae IV, V, VI and VII of spinal cord.

Termination

Terminates in the gray matter of laminae IV, V, VI and VII of spinal cord.

Clinical Importance

Lesions involving this tract lead to:

- Loss of muscle tone
- Hyperactive deep tendon reflexes
- Loss of superficial abdominal and cremasteric reflex
- Extensor toe response (Babinski sign).

Q. VESTIBULOSPINAL TRACT

Function

Vestibulospinal tract exerts an excitatory influence on spinal reflex and muscle tone.

Origin

Arises mainly from lateral vestibular nucleus present in the floor of fourth ventricle (the vestibular nuclei receives afferent impulses from vestibular nerve and the cerebellum).

Course

- It descends in the anterior part of lateral funiculus of spinal cord
- It ends in the laminae IX (VII and VIII), by synapsing with the alpha motor neurons.

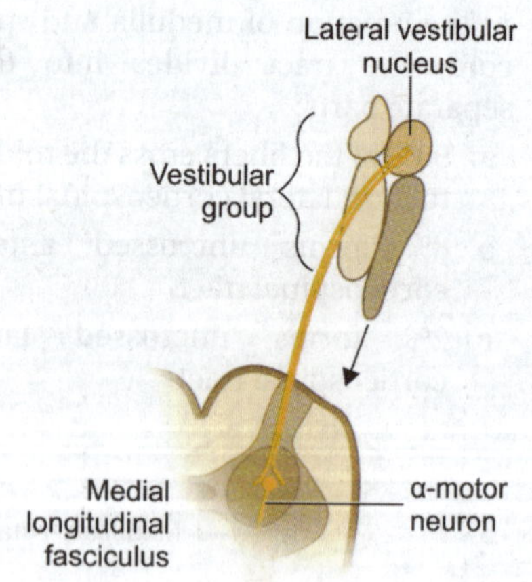

Origin of vestibulospinal tract

Termination

Vestibulospinal tract ends in the laminae IX (VII and VIII), by synapsing with alpha motor neurons.

Q. MEDIAL LONGITUDINAL FASCICULUS

1. Medial longitudinal fasciculus is present in the posterior part of anterior funiculus.
2. It connects the different nuclei in the brainstem.

3. Fibers from superior vestibular nuclei ascend to ipsilateral trochlear nucleus and oculomotor nucleus and also few fibers to contralateral oculomotor nucleus.

4. Fibers arising from medial vestibular nuclei ascend to contralateral abducens nucleus and trochlear and oculomotor nucleus, and few fibers to ipsilateral abducens nucleus.

5. This interconnection between vestibular, abducens, trochlear and oculomotor nucleus forms a composite ascending medial longitudinal fasciculus.

6. The descending medial longitudinal fasciculus begins from the medial vestibular nuclei, and terminate in the laminae VIII and VII of spinal cord.

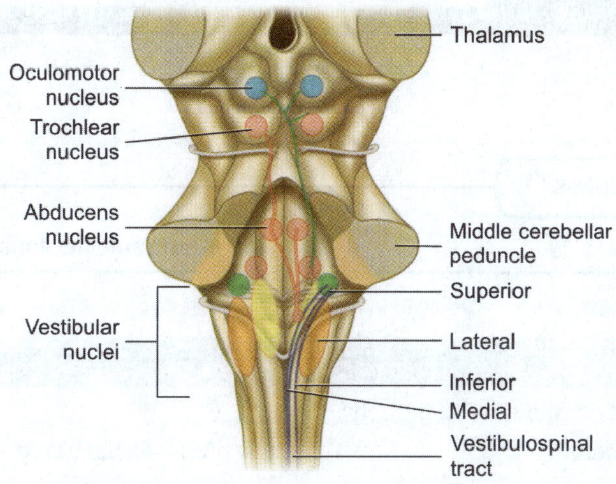

Medial longitudinal fasciculus

Clinical Significance

Medial longitudinal fasciculus play important role in conjugate eye movements. Stimulation of a nerve in the semicircular duct (vestibular component) produces deviations in both eyes by virtue of extraocular muscle action.

Short Notes: Cranial Nerves

Q. CRANIAL NERVES

There are 12 pairs of cranial nerves, namely:

- I—Olfactory nerve
- II—Optic nerve
- III—Oculomotor nerve
- IV—Trochlear nerve
- V—Trigeminal nerve
- VI—Abducens nerve
- VII—Facial nerve
- VIII—Vestibulocochlear nerve
- IX—Glossopharyngeal nerve
- X—Vagus nerve
- XI—Spinal accessory nerve
- XII—Hypoglossal nerve.

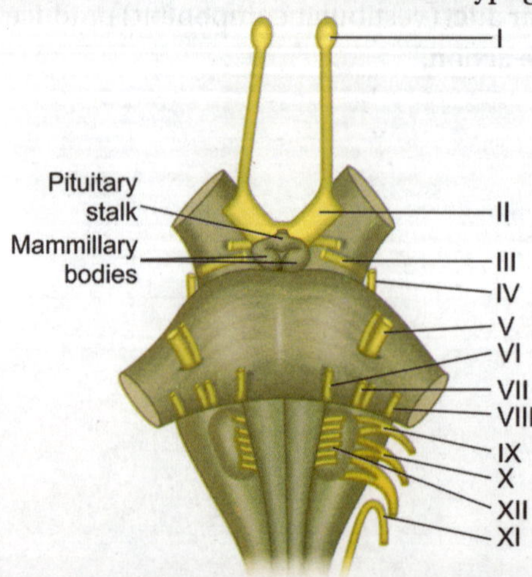

Inferior surface of brain showing cranial nerves

General Features

As the topic implies, we will be dealing with the functions of the cranial nerves:

- Each nerve may have a specific or general function and afferent (sensory) or efferent (motor) fibers
- A nerve supplying specific group of muscle, e.g. facial muscles, which are derived from branchial arch, will have a branchial efferent (special efferent) component
- A nerve supplying a gland will produce secretion by contraction of myoepithelial cell, which is considered to have general efferent component
- Glands are considered as general viscera, and tongue and branchial muscles are considered as special viscera

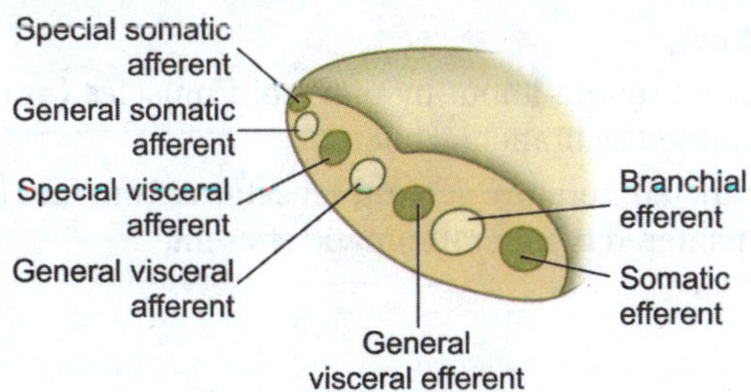

Cranial nerve fibers

- Skin, eye, pinna, nose are organs on the exterior and fibers ending on from them are considered as somatic afferent
- Fibers going to the muscles or glands are known as efferent fibers.

Functional Components of Cranial Nerve

Olfactory Nerve (I)

- *Function:* Smell
- *Component:* It carries smell (special sense) from exterior, so functionally the fibers are named as special somatic afferent.

Optic Nerve (II)

- *Function:* Vision
- *Component:* It conveys the sight (special sense) of objects in the external environment to brain. So functionally the fibers are named as special somatic afferent.

Oculomotor Nerve (III)

- *Function:* Bring about movements in extraocular muscles (special muscles)
- *Component:* Eye is on exterior aspect, so considered somatic; and fiber is going to the muscle. So the component of the nerve is considered as somatic efferent.

- *Function:* Constriction of pupil
- *Component:* It is due to contraction of pupillary muscles and hence the functional component is considered as general visceral efferent.

Trochlear Nerve (IV)

- *Function:* Bring about movements in extraocular muscles (special muscles)
- *Component:* Eye is on exterior aspect, so considered somatic; and fiber is going to the muscle. So the component of the nerve is considered as somatic efferent.

Trigeminal Nerve (V)

- *Functions:* As follows:
  - Movement of jaw brought about by pterygoid muscles (branchial muscles); so the component is named as branchial efferent
  - Carry touch, pain, temperature general sensations from face (exterior) and hence the component considered is general somatic afferent.

Abducens Nerve (VI)

- *Function:* Bring about movements in extraocular muscles (special muscles)
- *Component:* Eye is on exterior aspect, so considered somatic; and fiber is going to the muscle. So the component of the nerve is considered as somatic efferent.

Facial Nerve (VII)

- *Functions:* As follows:
  - Supply fibers to facial muscles (branchial), so the component is named as branchial efferent
  - Carry special taste sensation from tongue (viscera), so the component is named as special visceral afferent
  - Supply fibers to salivary glands (viscera) like submandibular and produce secretion (general saliva), so the component is named as general visceral efferent.

Vestibular Cochlear Nerve (VIII)

- *Function:* Hearing (special sense)
- *Component:* Ear is on the exterior and carries special hearing sense, hence the component is named as special somatic afferent.

Glossopharyngeal Nerve (IX)

- *Functions:* As follows:
  - Brings about movement in special (branchial) muscles of larynx, hence the component is named as branchial efferent

- Supplies fibers to parotid (viscera) gland and produces secretion of saliva (general fluid) and hence the component is named as general visceral efferent
- Carries special taste sensation from posterior one third of tongue (viscera) and hence the component is named as special visceral afferent.

Vagus Nerve (X) and Cranial Part of XI Nerve

- *Functions:* As follows:
  - Brings about movements in special (branchial) muscles of palate, pharynx and larynx, hence the component is named as branchial efferent
  - Produces general secretions in the bronchi and gut, hence the component is named as general visceral efferent
  - Carries general sensations from abdominal viscera, so the component is named as general visceral afferent
  - Carries special taste sensation from epiglottis (viscera) and hence the component is named as special visceral afferent.

Spinal Part of Spinal Accessory (XI)

- *Function:* Supplies fibers to special (branchial) muscles, i.e. sternocleidomastoid and trapezius, and hence the component is named as branchial efferent.

Hypoglossal Nerve (XII)

- *Function:* Brings about movements of tongue by supplying fibers to tongue muscles. Tongue is considered on exterior aspect, so the component is named as somatic efferent.

Q. AUTONOMIC NERVOUS SYSTEM

- Autonomic nervous system comprises of sympathetic and parasympathetic components, which are under the control of centers in the brainstem, hypothalamus and cerebral cortex
- Each component has efferent and afferent fibers
- All efferent fibers synapse on its way with a ganglion
- All afferent fibers have their cell bodies in cranial and dorsal spinal nerve
- Preganglionic fibers are medullated
- Postganglionic fibers are nonmedullated
- Afferent sensory fibers from blood vessels viscera traverse via both pre- and post-ganglionic fibers.

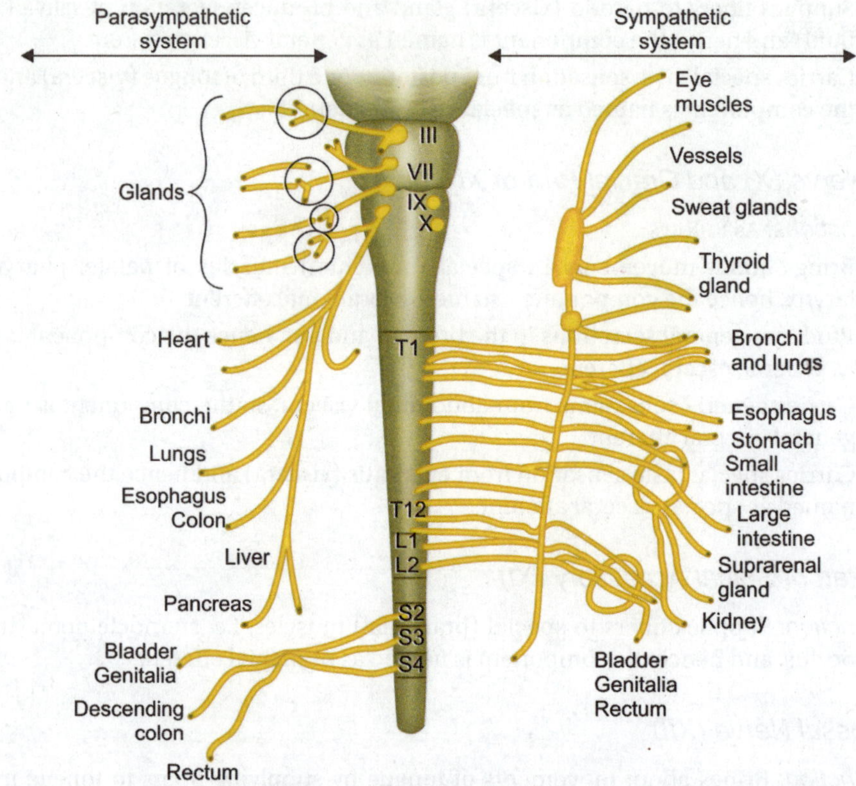

Autonomic nervous system

Features	Sympathetic system	Parasympathetic system
Preganglionic fibers arise from	Axons of lateral column of gray matter	III, VII, IX, X cranial nerve nuclei Gray matter of S2, S3, S4
Origin	Thoracolumbar outflow	Craniosacral outflow
Preganglionic fibers length	Short	Long
Postganglionic synapse	Many	Few
Effect	Widespread	Limited
Ganglia	Away from the structure to be innervated	Close to the structure to be innervated

Neurotransmitters:
    In preganglionic
    In postganglionic
	Acetylcholine
	Noradrenaline (except sweat glands, it Is acetylcholine)
		Acetylcholine
		Acetylcholine

Spinal cord segments giving origin	All thoracic, L1, L2	III, VII, IX, X cranial nerve nuclei and S2, S3, S4
Distribution of fibers	Vasoconstrictors To arterioles, sweat glands, skin	Mainly visceral

Long Questions

Q. DESCRIBE INTERNAL CAPSULE IN DETAIL (PARTS, ASCENDING AND DESCENDING FIBERS, BLOOD SUPPLY, APPLIED ANATOMY).

Internal capsule is a bundle of fibers stacked between the basal nuclei components. It has both ascending and descending fibers interconnecting the cortex to brainstem, spinal cord. Since it is a closely packed area, damage to even a small region will cause involvement of many fibers leading to extensive signs and symptoms.

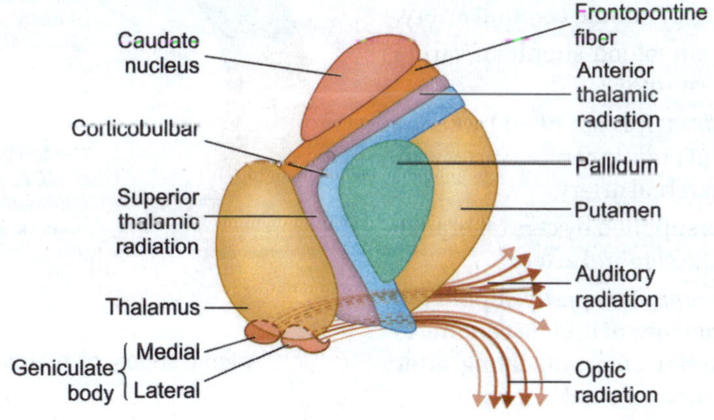

Horizontal section of internal capsule

Parts

In horizontal section, it can be subdivided into following parts:

- Anterior limb
- Genu
- Posterior limb
- Retrolentiform part
- Sublentiform part.

Composition of Each Part

1. **Anterior limb:** It lies between caudate nucleus and lentiform nucleus. It contains anterior thalamic radiation and frontopontine fibers.
2. **Genu:** The anterior and the posterior limb meet at an angle known as genu. It contains corticobulbar and corticoreticular fibers.
3. **Posterior limb:** It lies between lentiform nucleus and thalamus. It contains superior thalamic radiation, corticopontine fibers, corticofugal fibers and corticospinal fibers.
4. **Retrolentiform part:** It is a part behind the lentiform nucleus. It contains posterior thalamic radiation including optic radiation and other fibers included are parietopontine and occipitopontine fibers.
5. **Sublentiform part:** It is a part below the lentiform nucleus. It contains inferior thalamic peduncle, auditory radiation and other fibers included are parietopontine and temporopontine.

Blood Supply

Arterial Supply

The chief source of arterial blood is lenticulostriate branches of middle cerebral artery.

Following is the blood supply of various parts of internal capsule:

- *Anterior limb:* It is supplied by central branches of middle cerebral artery and anterior cerebral artery
- *Genu:* It is supplied by central branches of middle cerebral artery
- *Posterior limb:* It is partly supplied by central branches of middle cerebral artery, posterior communicating artery and anterior choroidal artery.

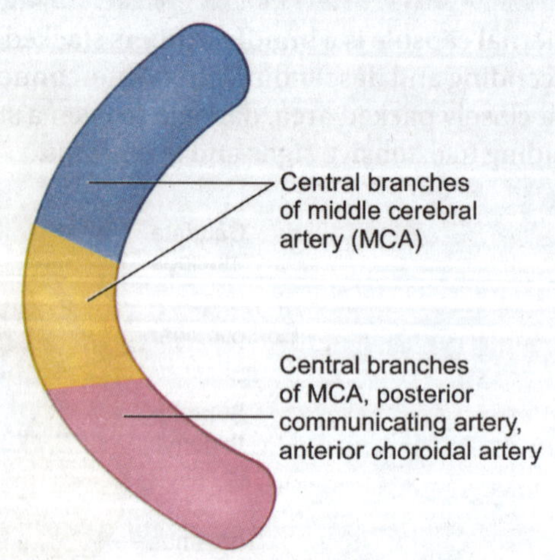

Arterial supply of internal capsule

Venous Drainage

Striate branches of cerebral veins drain into various cranial venous sinuses.

Applied Anatomy

Thrombosis or hemorrhage of middle cerebral artery or anterior choroidal artery lead to the lesions of internal capsule, i.e.:

- Vascular injury in the posterior limb of internal capsule results in the contralateral hemianesthesia
- Lesion in the genu leads to contralateral hemiplegia
- Vascular lesion in the retro- or sub-lentiform part causes hemianesthesia, hemianopsia and hemihypacusis.

Q. DISCUSS VENTRICLES TO BRAIN IN DETAIL WITH ITS CLINICAL SIGNIFICANCE.

Cavities within the forebrain, midbrain and hindbrain form ventricular system of the brain. These cavities communicate with each other and then the subarachnoid space and permit circulation of cerebrospinal fluid (CSF).

The choroid plexus within the ventricular system, produces the CSF.

Following are the divisions of ventricles:

- *Lateral ventricle:* Cavity in cerebral hemisphere
- *Third ventricle:* Cavity in diencephalon
- *Cerebral aqueduct:* It is a passage connecting third ventricle to fourth ventricle
- *Fourth ventricle:* Cavity within the medulla.

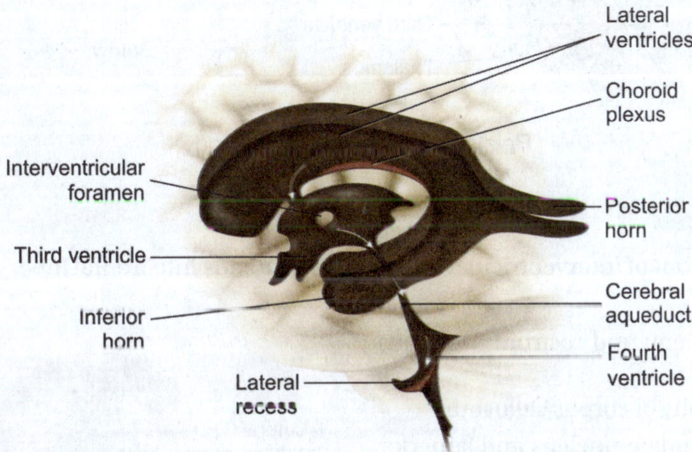

Ventricles of brain (arrow shows flow of CSF)

Communications

- The lateral ventricles communicate with third ventricle through interventricular foramen (foramen of Monro)
- The third ventricle communicates with fourth ventricle through the cerebral aqueduct

- The fourth ventricle communicates with subarachnoid space through foramen of Magendie and foramen of Luschka.

Lateral Ventricle: Cavity in Cerebral Hemisphere

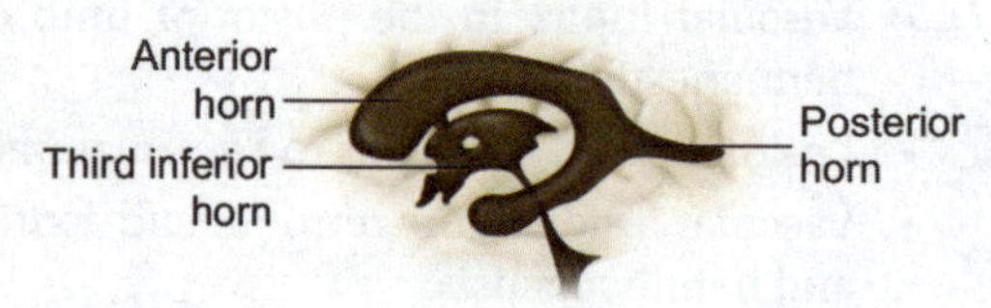

Lateral ventricle has following parts: A central part and three horns—anterior, posterior and inferior.

Central Part

Central part is related to corpus callosum. It extends from interventricular foramen to splenium of corpus callosum.

Relations
- *Above:* Corpus callosum
- *Below:* Caudate nucleus and thalamus
- *Medially:* Septum pellucidum.

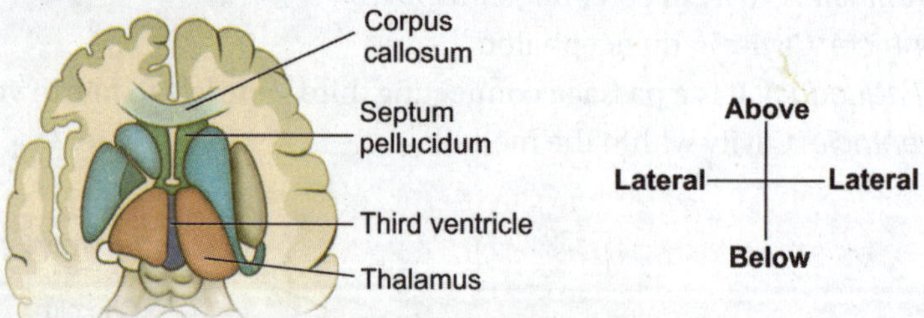

Relations of lateral ventricle body

Anterior Horn

The part lies in front of interventricular foramen and extends into frontal lobe.

Relations
- *In front:* Genu and rostrum of corpus callosum
- *Above:* Body of corpus callosum
- *Below:* Caudate nucleus and superior surface of rostrum of corpus callosum.

Posterior Horn

The part lies behind the splenium of corpus callosum and extends into occipital lobe.

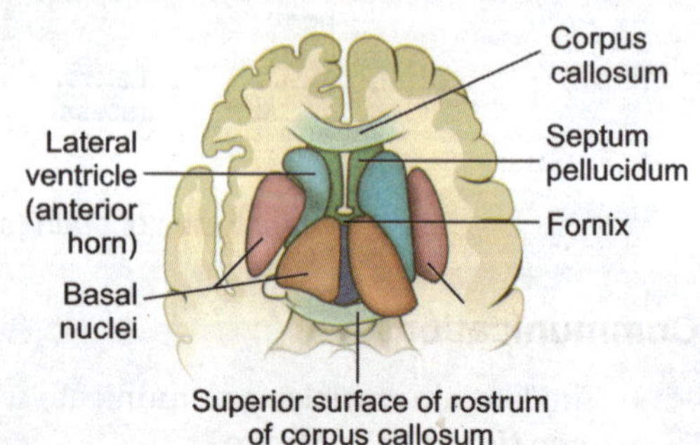

Relations

- *Above and laterally:* Tapetum and optic radiation
- *Below and medially:* Forceps major (fibers of corpus callosum)

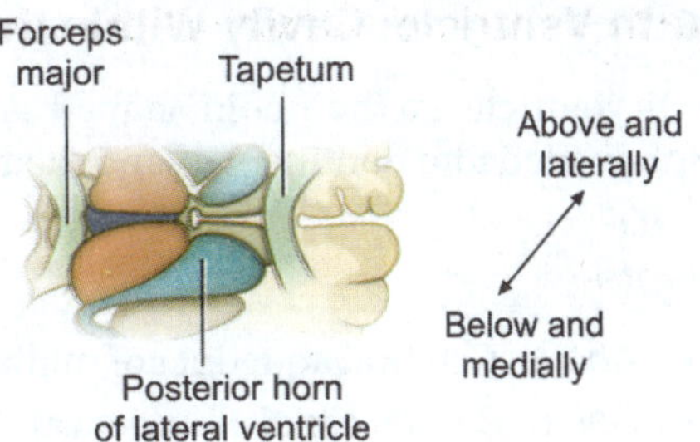

Inferior Horn

Inferior horn is the largest horn of lateral ventricle extending into the temporal lobe.

Relations

- *Above and laterally:* Tapetum and caudate nucleus
- *Below and medially:* Collateral sulcus and hippocampus.

Third Ventricle

Cavity of diencephalon has extensions namely suprapineal, pineal, infundibular and optic. The cavity lies between thalami on either side.

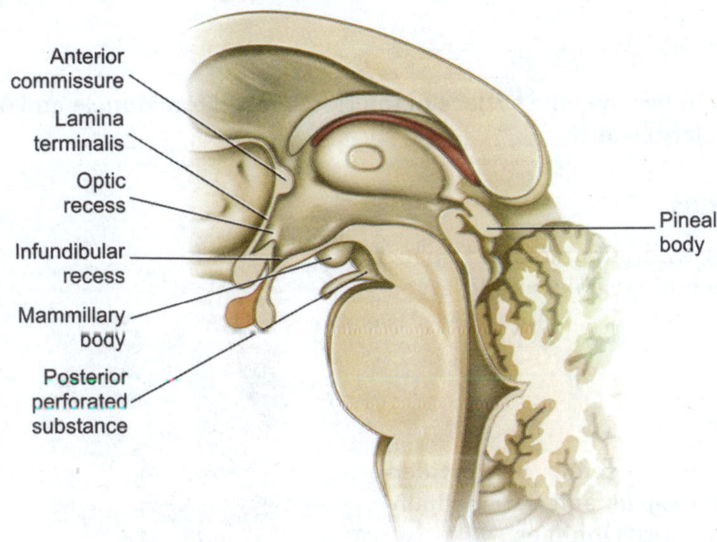

Boundaries of III ventricle

Relations

- *In front:* Lamina terminalis
- *Behind:* Pineal body, posterior commissure, cerebral aqueduct
- *Above:* Choroid plexus
- *Below:* Optic chiasm, tuber cinereum, pituitary stalk, mammillary bodies, posterior perforated substance and tegmentum of midbrain
- *On either side:* Thalamus.

Fourth Ventricle: Cavity Within the Medulla

Fourth ventricle is a rhomboid-shaped cavity overlying the pons and medulla and hence it can be subdivided into pontine part and medullary part.

Extent

- *Above:* Cerebral aqueduct of midbrain
- *Below:* Central canal of upper cervical spinal cord.

Roof

Superior and inferior medullary vela (like a tent).

Apex

Apex extends into the cerebellum, where it is known as fastigium.

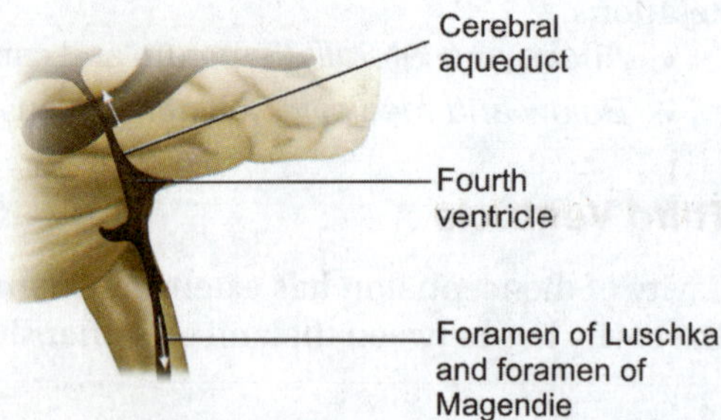

Recess

Lateral recess: It lies over the surface of inferior cerebellar peduncle and opens into the cerebellomedullary cistern.

Communications

Communicates with subarachnoid space through foramen of Luschka and foramen of Magendie.

Floor

Features

- Vertically in the center, it is divided by median sulcus and paramedially divided by sulcus limitans
- Horizontally, it is divided by stria medullaris
- Paramedian area has a bulge known as median eminence
- Caudal area of fourth ventricle is known as calamus scriptorius
- The apex of the ventricle is known as obex.

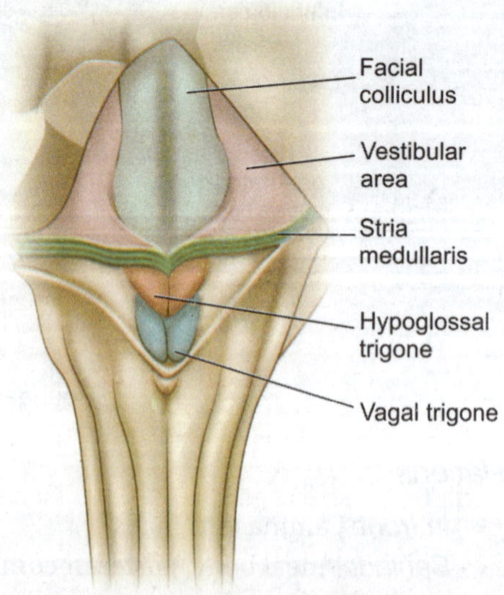

Floor of fourth ventricle

Specific area

- Just above the stria medullaris, paramedially is facial colliculus and hypoglossal trigone is just below it
- Vagal trigone lies paramedially toward the caudal part of fourth ventricle
- Just above the stria medullaris, laterally is vestibular area beneath, which is vestibular nuclei
- Just above the obex is a paired circumventricular organ known as area postrema.

Clinical Importance

In case of blockage of communicating passages of ventricular system or excessive production of CSF, due to brain tumors will lead to dilatation of ventricles giving rise to hydrocephalus.

Q. DISCUSS THE BLOOD SUPPLY OF BRAIN AND SPINAL CORD.

Brain is the most active system of the body with an average blood supply of 50 mL/100 g of brain tissue per minute. Compromise of the blood supply to the brain even for 5 minutes can cause neurological deficit. Thus, the blood supply of brain and spinal cord assumes great clinical significance.

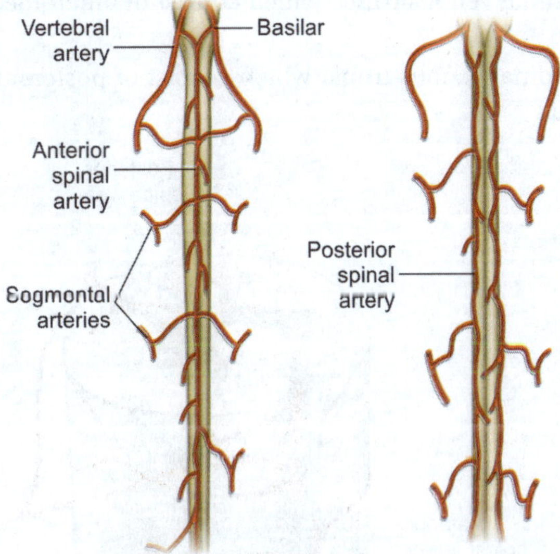

Arterial Supply of Spinal Cord

The spinal cord receives blood from following sources:

- Branches of vertebral arteries
- Branches of segmental arteries.

Descending Branches of Vertebral Arteries

Posterior spinal artery: These are paired arteries on posterior surface of spinal cord and form plexiform channels or may be so small in size, hardly visible.

Anterior spinal artery: Paired anterior spinal arteries soon unite after its origin from vertebral arteries and form a single midline vessel, which lies on the anterior median fissure of the spinal cord. They anastomose with radicular arteries.

Branches of Segmental Arteries

Radicular arteries: These arteries traverse the intervertebral foramina and divide into anterior and posterior radicular arteries. A prominent anterior radicular artery in lumbar region is known as artery of Adamkiewicz.

Spinal arteries and radicular arteries through their small branches, i.e. sulcal branches, form a rich network of arteries all around the spinal cord.

Venous Drainage of Spinal Cord

The venous blood of the spinal cord is drained mainly by two venous trunks namely:

- Anterior longitudinal venous trunk, which consist of anteromedian and anterolateral spinal veins
- Posterior longitudinal venous trunk, which consist of posteromedial vein and paired posterolateral vein.

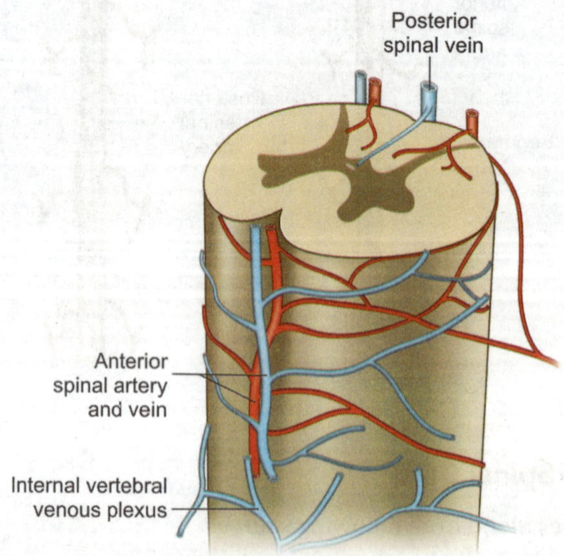

Blood supply of spinal cord

Communications of Venous Channels

The internal vertebral venous plexus lies between dura mater and vertebral periosteum. At the level of intervertebral space the plexus is connected to thoracic, abdominal and intercostal veins and also with the external vertebral venous plexus. The blood can flow in both directions since there are no valves. When there is rise in intra-abdominal pressure or block in jugular veins the blood may flow in the internal vertebral venous system. This communication within the venous channels may cause spread of tumor.

Arterial Supply of the Brain

The brain is supplied by the branches of internal carotid artery and vertebral artery. Following are the branches of internal carotid artery.

Internal Carotid Artery

- Anterior cerebral
- Middle cerebral
- Ophthalmic
- Posterior communicating
- Anterior choroidal.

Vertebral Artery

Vertebral artery arises from the first part of subclavian artery and runs along the anterolateral surface of medulla, and unites to form basilar artery at the lower border of pons.

Intracranial branches of vertebral and basilar artery supply the brainstem, cerebellum, posterior parts of diencephalon and occipital, and temporal lobes of the brain. Labyrinthine, a branch of basilar artery, supplies the inner ear.

An anastomotic arterial circle is formed by branches of internal carotid artery and basilar artery. This arterial circle is known as circle of Willis.

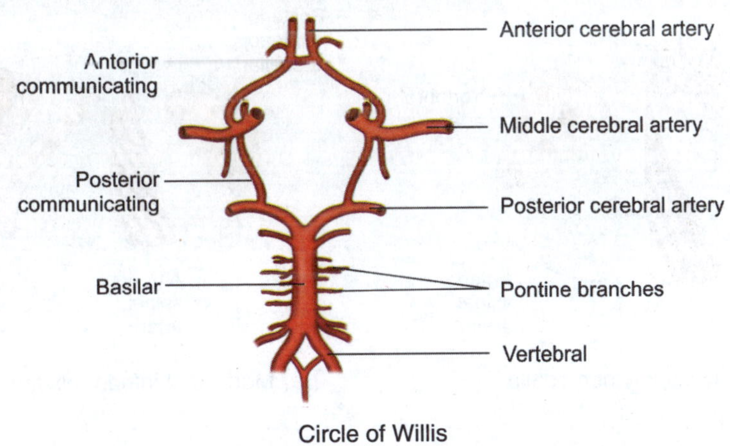

Circle of Willis

Regional Arterial Supply

1. Cortical branches of anterior, middle and posterior cerebral arteries supply the cerebral hemisphere.

2. The anterior choroidal artery supplies the choroidal plexus, hippocampal formation, portions of globus pallidus, posterior limb of internal capsule and retrolenticular portion of internal capsule. Small branches also supply portions of basal ganglia and ventrolateral part of thalamus.

3. The posterior choroidal artery supplies the choroid plexus in lateral ventricle mainly.

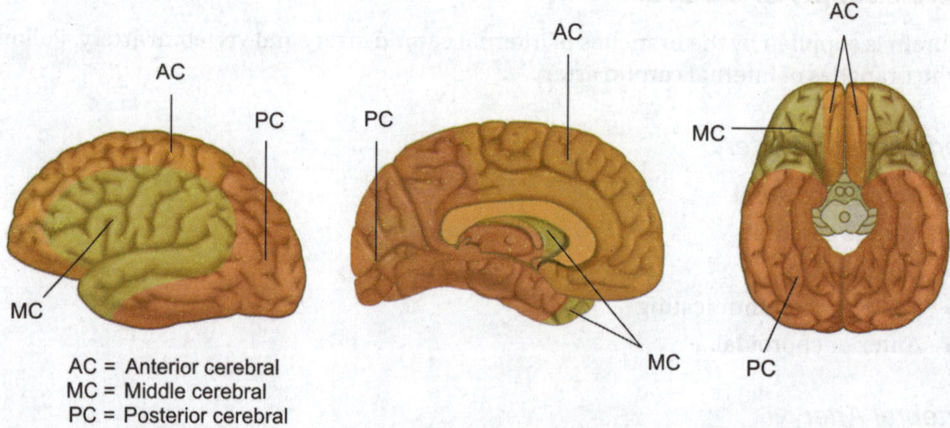

4. The corpus striatum, internal capsule (anterior and posterior limb) receives arterial blood mainly from lateral striate branches of middle cerebral artery.

5. Thalamus receives blood mainly from posterior cerebral artery.

6. Pons and medulla receive arterial blood from spinal arteries, cerebellar arteries, and branches of vertebral and basilar arteries.

7. The cerebellum is supplied by superior, anterior and posterior inferior cerebellar arteries.

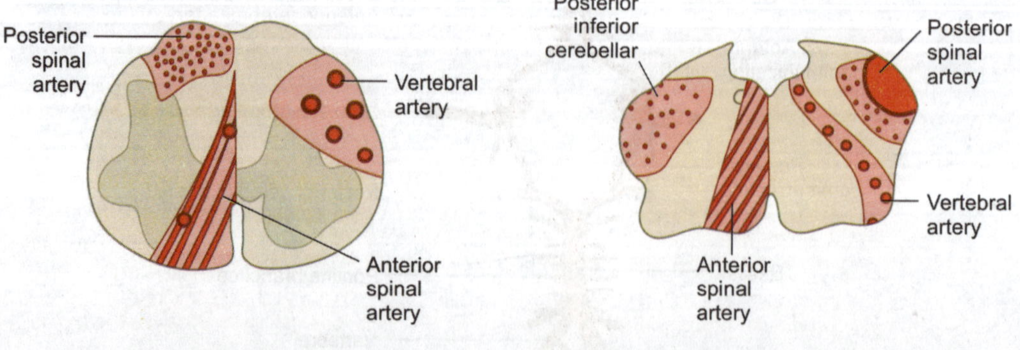

Arterial supply of medulla   Medulla at inferior olivary nucleus

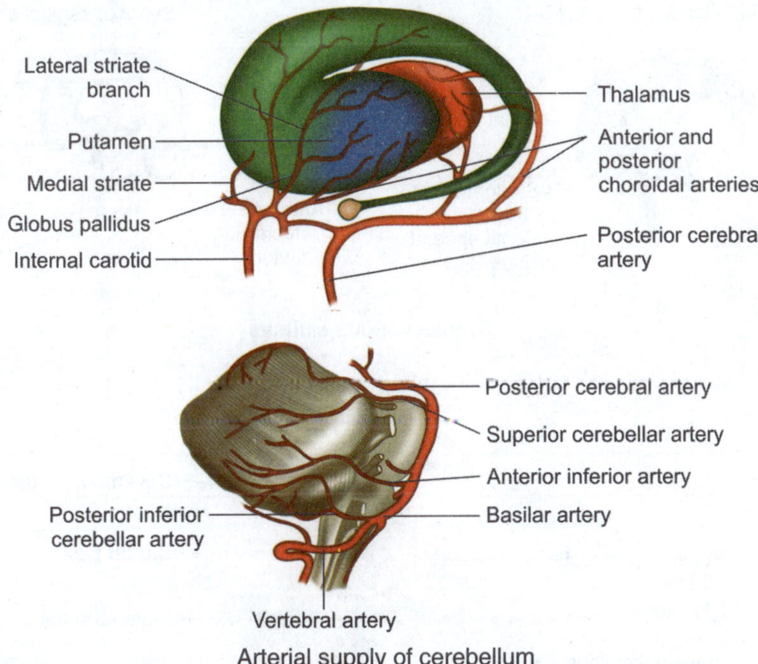

Arterial supply of cerebellum

Venous Drainage

The venous blood of brain is mainly drained by cerebral veins and dural venous sinuses.

Cerebral Vein

- The cerebral veins can be classified into superficial and deep groups
- Superficial cerebral veins drain the cortex and the subcortical white matter and end in various cranial sinuses.

Tributaries

Superficial cerebral vein	Deep cerebral vein
Superior cerebral	Internal cerebral
Inferior cerebral	Basal (Rosenthal)
Superficial middle cerebral	Great cerebral (Galen)

Dural Venous Sinuses

The dural venous sinuses lie between periosteal and meningeal layers of dura, and are very tough in nature and have no valves.

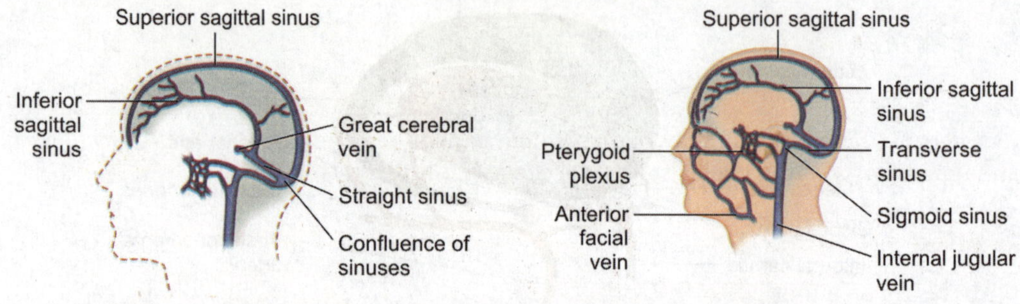

Cranial venous sinuses

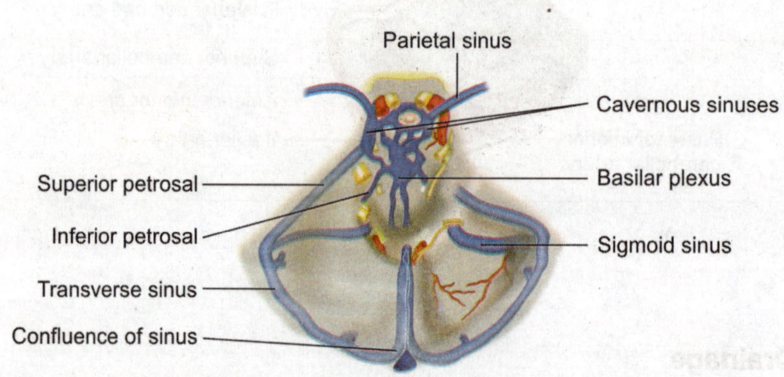

Dural venous sinuses

Following are the dural sinuses:
- Superior and inferior sagittal sinus
- Transverse sinus
- Cavernous sinus
- Sigmoid sinus.

Clinical Importance

- Sudden occlusion of posterior inferior cerebellar artery gives rise to lateral medullary syndrome
- In this syndrome, there is loss of pain and temperature on the same side of the face and opposite side of the body, dysphagia and Horner's syndrome
- Thrombosis of lenticulostriate branch of middle cerebral artery gives rise to hemiplegia
- Sudden rupture of pontine artery can be fatal.

Q. DISCUSS THALAMUS UNDER FOLLOWING HEADINGS: LOCATION, GROSS FEATURES, RELATIONS, CONNECTIONS AND APPLIED ANATOMY.

Thalamus is a large mass of gray matter, which constitutes one of the subdivisions of diencephalon and is a sensory relay station for the ascending tracts.

Location

Thalamus lies on either side of third ventricle and is disposed obliquely with the axis running backward and laterally.

Gross Features

- *Shape:* Oval (like an egg)
- *Surfaces:* Medial, superior, lateral and inferior
- *Ends:* Anterior end, posterior end.

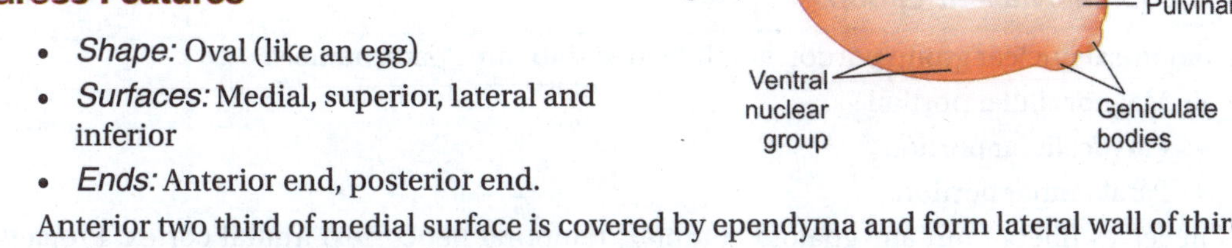

Anterior two third of medial surface is covered by ependyma and form lateral wall of third ventricle above hypothalamic sulcus.

Posterior end of thalamus is wide and is known as pulvinar and overhangs the midbrain.

The superior surface tapers anteriorly in a rounded tubercle just posterior to interventricular foramen.

Posterior part of inferior surface of thalamus has two swellings namely medial and lateral geniculate bodies (metathalamus).

Important Relations

- *Medially:* Third ventricle, habenular triangle
- *Laterally:* Stria terminalis, internal capsule.

Subdivisions

Major thalamic nuclei can be classified into specific relay nuclei and association nuclei. Specific relay nuclei receive definite ascending pathways and project to definite cerebral areas. Association nuclei of thalamus project to associated areas of cerebrum. Following are the nuclear groups of thalamus and their main connections.

Anterior Nuclear Group

- Anteroventral (AV)
- Accessory nuclei
- Anterodorsal (AD)
- Anteromedial (AM).

Receives fibers from mammillothalamic tract, fornix projects fibers to cingulate gyrus via anterior limb of internal capsule.

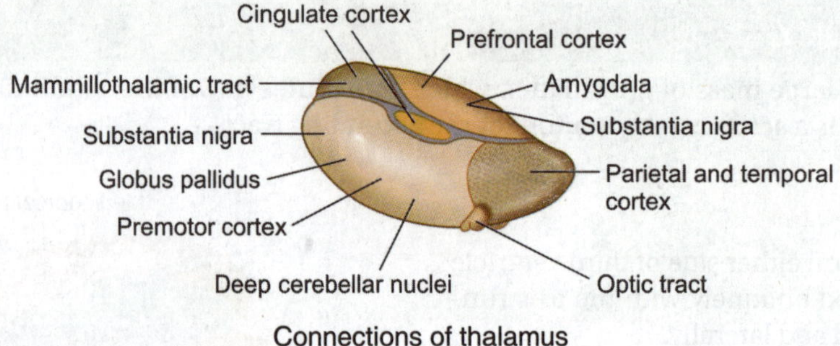

Connections of thalamus

Mediodorsal Nuclear Group

Mediodorsal nuclear group portion is subdivided into three parts namely:

- Magnocellular portion
- Parvocellular portion
- Paralaminar portion.

Receives fibers from amygdaloid complex, temporal neocortex, frontal cortex. Projects fibers to frontal cortex and coordinates somatic and visceral activities.

Lateral Nuclear Group

Lateral nuclear group lies on the dorsomedial surface of the thalamus caudal to anterior nuclear group. It consist of three nuclear masses—lateral dorsal nucleus, lateral posterior nucleus and pulvinar. It is reciprocally connected to temporal cortex.

Ventral Nuclear Group

Ventral nuclear group is subdivided into three nuclei namely:

- Ventral anterior
- Ventral lateral
- Ventral posterior.

The ventral posterior is further subdivided into ventral posterolateral and ventral postero-medial nuclei. It receive impulses from substantia nigra, globus pallidus, contralateral deep cerebellar nuclei, medial lemniscus and spinothalamic tract; project fibers to premotor cortex and sensory cortex.

There are other less distinct nuclei groups like midline nuclei and intralaminar nuclei group. Thalamic reticular nucleus is a neuronal shell, which surrounds lateral, superior and anteroinferior aspect of dorsal thalamus.

Applied Anatomy

Neurosurgically, thalamotomy may control rigidity and tremors in diseases of corpus striatum.

Multiple Choice Questions (MCQs)

1. Weight of the adult brain is approximately ___________
    a. 1,500 g
    b. 500 g
    c. 1,500 mg
    d. 500 mg

   Answer: a

2. Following constitute hind brain ___________
    a. Diencephalon + Metencephalon
    b. Mesencephalon + Metencephalon
    c. Metencephalon + Myelencephalon
    d. Diencephalon + Myelencephalon

   Answer: c

3. Leptomeninges means ___________
    a. Dura + Pia
    b. Pia + Arachnoid
    c. Dura + Arachnoid
    d. Dura + Pia + Arachnoid

   Answer: b

4. Dura chiefly receives blood from ___________ artery.
    a. Middle meningeal
    b. Ophthalmic
    c. Ethmoidal
    d. All of the above

   Answer: a

5. What is the approximate quantity of CSF?
    a. 1 L
    b. 500 mL
    c. 150 mL
    d. 5 mL

   Answer: c

6. Match the following spinal cord segments:

Column A	Column B
1. Cervical	a. 12
2. Thoracic	b. 1

3. Lumbar

c. 5

4. Coccygeal

d. 8

Answer: 1-d, 2-a, 3-c, 4-b

7. The spinal cord ends at ______________ level in adults.

a. L1

c. L3

b. L2

d. L4

Answer: a

8. The spinal cord ends at ______________ level at birth.

a. L1

c. L3

b. L2

d. L4

Answer: c

9. Lentiform nucleus is a combination of following nuclei ______________

a. Caudate nucleus + Putamen

b. Putamen + Globus pallidus

c. Caudate nucleus + Globus pallidus

d. Caudate nucleus + Putamen + Globus pallidus

Answer: b

10. The least differentiated segment of brainstem is ______________

a. Pons

c. Midbrain

b. Medulla

d. All of the above

Answer: c

11. Following cranial nerves are related to midbrain:

a. I, II

c. IV, V

b. III, IV

d. V, VI

Answer: b

12. Following are the areas noted in the floor of fourth ventricle except ______________

a. Facial colliculus

c. Hypoglossal trigone

b. Vestibular area

d. Oculomotor area

Answer: d

13. Which lamina surrounds the central canal?

a. Lamina I

c. Lamina X

b. Lamina IV

d. Lamina VIII

Answer: c

14. The lamina, which forms many discrete groups in the anterior horn of the gray matter of spinal cord is ______________

a. Lamina IX

c. Lamina III

b. Lamina VII

d. Lamina V

Answer: a

15. Zona intermedia is __________
    a. Lamina I
    b. Lamina VII
    c. Lamina IX
    d. Lamina VIII

    Answer: b

16. The tract, which carries crude touch and pressure is __________
    a. Posterior white column
    b. Anterior spinothalamic tract
    c. Lateral spinothalamic tract
    d. Posterior spinocerebellar tract

    Answer: a

17. The tract, which carries light touch sensation is __________
    a. Posterior white column
    b. Anterior spinothalamic tract
    c. Lateral spinothalamic tract
    d. Posterior spinocerebellar tract

    Answer: b

18. The tract, which conveys pain and temperature is __________
    a. Posterior white column
    b. Anterior spinothalamic tract
    c. Lateral spinothalamic tract
    d. Posterior spinocerebellar tract

    Answer: c

19. The sensory relay station in the brain is __________
    a. Epithalamus
    b. Hypothalamus
    c. Metathalamus
    d. Thalamus

    Answer: d

20. Following are the ascending crossed tracts except __________
    a. Lateral spinothalamic
    b. Medial lemniscus
    c. Anterior spinocerebellar
    d. Posterior spinocerebellar

    Answer: d

21. Following are the uncrossed descending fibers except __________
    a. Lateral corticospinal
    b. Anterior corticospinal
    c. Uncrossed lateral corticospinal
    d. Vestibulospinal

    Answer: a

22. Medial longitudinal fasciculus connect following nucleus except __________
    a. Oculomotor
    b. Trochlear
    c. Abducens
    d. Facial

    Answer: d

23. Carotid siphon is referred to __________ parts of internal carotid artery.
    a. Cervical + Cerebral portion
    b. Intrapetrosal + Intracavernous
    c. Intracavernous + Cerebral portion
    d. Intrapetrosal + Cervical

    Answer: c

24. The lateral medullary syndrome is produced by __________
    a. Anteroinferior cerebellar artery
    b. Posteroinferior cerebellar artery
    c. Middle cerebral artery
    d. Basilar artery

    Answer: b

25. Pulvinar is a portion of ________________
    a. Hypothalamus
    b. Epithalamus
    c. Thalamus
    d. Internal capsule

    Answer: c

26. Fornix is an efferent system of ________________
    a. Hypothalamus
    b. Epithalamus
    c. Thalamus
    d. Hippocampus

    Answer: d

27. Following is a part of metathalamus ________________
    a. Habenular trigone
    b. Pineal body
    c. Medial geniculate body
    d. Thalamus

    Answer: c

28. Restiform body is ________________
    a. Superior cerebellar peduncle
    b. Inferior cerebellar peduncle
    c. Middle cerebellar peduncle
    d. All of the above

    Answer: b

Glossary

Fornix: It is a main efferent system of hippocampus, which includes projection and commissural fibers. The fibers are axons of cells in subicular cortex and pyramidal cells of hippocampus. The fibers from fornix end in mammillary body and from the mammillary body, the fibers go to anterior nuclei of thalamus.

Hypothalamus: It is a part of diencephalon, which lies ventral to hypothalamic sulcus and extends from optic chiasm to mammillary bodies. It is divided into medial and lateral nuclear groups by fornix. It grossly comprises of infundibulum, tuber cinereum and mammillary bodies. Functionally related to visceral, endocrine, metabolic activities and temperature regulation, sleep and emotional behavior.

Habenular nuclei: Part of epithalamus, which consist of medial and lateral nuclei, receive fibers from stria medullaris and gives rise to fasciculus retroflexus; it is a site of convergence of limbic pathway, which conveys impulses to midbrain.

Limbus of the cerebrum: The hippocampus, dentate gyrus, indusium griseum, septum pellucidum and fornix form the limbus of the cerebrum. It forms a part of rhinencephalon (literally means smell brain).

Olivary complex: It has two subdivisions namely, superior and inferior:

1. Superior olivary complex: It comprises of several nuclei, located in lateral position in reticular formation, medial to it is trapezoid body. It is involved in auditory sound source localization and are main relay stations of cochlear nuclei.
2. Inferior olivary complex: It is the most striking feature in medulla comprising of three parts—principal nuclei, medial accessory nuclei and dorsal accessory nuclei. These nuclei have short dendrites and the axons of the cells cross the median raphe to enter the inferior cerebellar peduncle. These fibers end as climbing fibers in cerebellar cortex, which cause excitatory action upon Purkinje cells.

Precerebellar nuclei: The nuclei in the brainstem, which project to cerebellum are collectively known as precerebellar nuclei.

Pyramid: On the anterior surface of medulla, there are two pyramids separated by anterior median fissure. The pyramids are bundles of nerve fibers originating from precentral gyrus and descend downward through crura and the pons to form the pyramid in medulla.

Restiform body: It is equivalent to inferior cerebellar peduncle.

Red nucleus: It is an ovoid mass, dorsomedial to substantia nigra of midbrain, appear pink in fresh specimens due to ferric pigment in the neurons. Its function in human beings is uncertain.

Reticular formation: It lies dorsal and lateral to red nucleus, and fibers of superior cerebellar peduncle traverse this nucleus and referred as locomotor center (walking movements elicited).

Stria terminalis: It is a well-defined amygdaloid nuclear complex. Fibers of stria terminalis arch along medial border of caudate nucleus to end in nuclei of stria terminalis. Amygdaloid complex stimulation causes fear confusion and amnesia.

Stria medullaris of diencephalon: It is a bundle of fibers arising from septal nuclei, lateral preoptic region and anterior thalamic nuclei.

Septal area: The subcallosal region and paraterminal gyrus constitute septal area. Beneath this area lie septal nuclei. The septal nuclei receive afferent from hippocampus via fornix and efferent fibers project via stria medullaris to medial habenular nucleus, medial forebrain bundle to lateral hypothalamus and fornix to hippocampus.

Syndrome of Benedikt: Ipsilateral III nerve paresis and contralateral involuntary motor movements like tremor, ataxia is known as syndrome of Benedikt. It occurs in the lesions of midbrain tegmentum.

Stria medullaris of fourth ventricle: Arcuate nucleus is an inferior extension of pontine nuclei; fibers arising from arcuate nucleus pass posteriorly through midline of medulla and run across the floor of fourth ventricle forming the striae medullares of fourth ventricle.

Trapezoid body: Mostly regarded as auditory relay station, but the axons of trapezoid body may enter medial longitudinal fasciculus connecting V, VII, III, IV, VI nuclei. Thus, coordinating stapedial reflex, action of tensor tympanic and extraocular muscle.

Tectum of midbrain: It is the roof of midbrain (dorsal to cerebral aqueduct) bearing two dorsal swellings namely, superior colliculus and inferior colliculus, detailed as follows:

1. Superior colliculi: It is a laminated structure having alternate gray and white matter. Superficial layers receive fibers from retina and visual cortex, and are involved in detection of movements in visual field. The deep layers receive fibers from auditory system, motor cortex, reticular formation. Efferent fibers of deep layers are concerned with head and eye movements.

2. Inferior colliculi: It is an ovoid cellular mass in caudal tectum concerned with transmitting signals from lateral lemniscus to medial geniculate body involved in auditory pathway.

Weber's syndrome: Lesions affecting III nerve and corticospinal fibers in midbrain cause ipsilateral III nerve paralysis and contralateral hemiplegia. This is known as Weber's syndrome (superior alternating hemiplegia).

SECTION - VII

EMBRYOLOGY

General Embryology

Contd...

Contd...

▪ Follicular phase	▪ Primitive gut formation
▪ Occurence of ovulation	▪ Embryonic disk
▪ Rhythm method	▪ Implantation of blastocyst
▪ Hormones influencing ovulation	▪ Decidual reaction
▪ Oral contraceptive pills	▪ Parts of decidua
▪ Blastocyst formation	▪ Types of villi
▪ Zona pellucida	▪ Placental barrier
▪ Primary yolk sac formation	▪ Functions of placenta
▪ Extraembryonic mesoderm and celom	▪ Upper and lower uterine segments
▪ Chorion formation	▪ Site of placenta implantation
▪ Amnion	▪ Placenta previa
▪ Primitive streak	▪ Ectopic pregnancy
▪ Gastrulation	▪ Anomalies of placenta
▪ Critical period	▪ Normal disposition of embryo in uterine cavity
▪ Fertilization morula	
▪ Formation of notochord	▪ Membrane
▪ Division intraembryonic mesoderm	▪ Fate of somites
▪ Fate of intraembryonic mesoderm	▪ Mesenchyme and its derivatives
▪ Septum transversum	▪ What is the fate of occipital myotomes

Q. What do you understand by embryology?

Ans. Embryology can also be described as developmental anatomy. Embryology is the study of the formation and development of the embryo from the time of its inception till birth.

Q. What is an embryo?

Ans. From the time of inception to first 2 months is known as embryo.

Q. What is a fetus?

Ans. From 3rd month onwards till birth is known as fetus.

Q. What are gametes?

Ans. The sex organs, i.e. testes and ovaries produce highly specialized cells known as gametes. Male gamete is spermatozoa and female gamete is ova.

Q. What is fertilization?

Ans. Fusion of male and female gamete is known as fertilization.

Q. Where does fertilization take place?

Ans. Fertilization occurs in the ampulla of uterine tube.

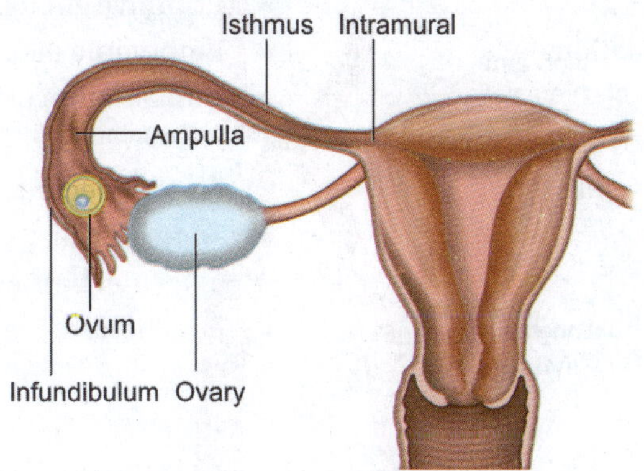

Parts of fallopian tube

Q. Why does fertilization take place in ampulla?

Ans. Fertilization takes place in ampulla for following reasons:
- Ampulla is the widest portion of uterine tube
- Close to ovary and is easy to pick up ova.

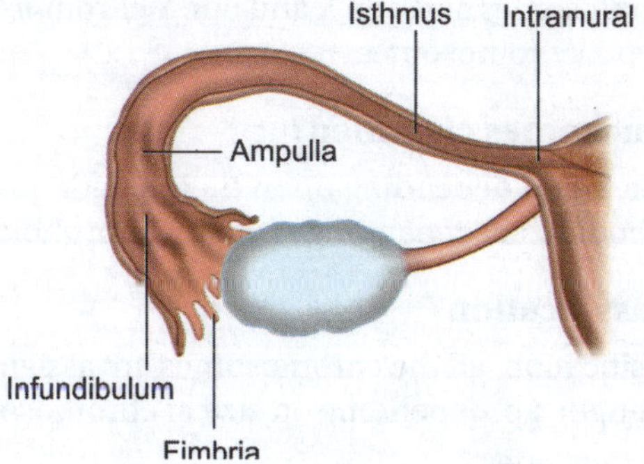

Fallopian tube showing ampulla

Q. How many chromosomes are there in each human cell?

Ans. The number of chromosomes in each human cell is 46. This is a diploid number.

Q. How many chromosomes are there in the gametes?

Ans. The gametes, i.e. spermatozoa and ova have 23 number of chromosomes. It is a haploid number.

Q. How are the chromosomes classified in each cell?

Ans. The 46 chromosomes in each cell can be divided into 44 autosomes and two sex chromosomes.

Q. Draw a neat labeled diagram of typical chromosome.

Ans.

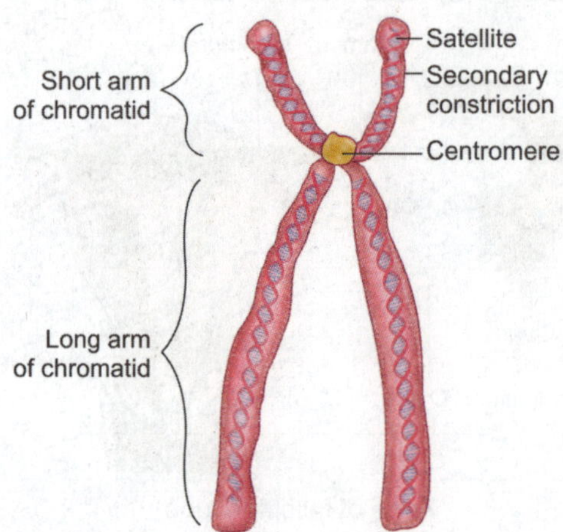

Q. What are sex chromosomes?

Ans. Sex chromosomes are of two types: X and Y.

Q. How are the chromosomes classified in man and woman?

Ans. In man, there are 44 autosomes and one X and one Y chromosome. In woman, there are 44 autosomes and two X chromosomes.

Q. How are the chromosomes classified?

Ans. Chromosomes are classified depending upon their length, position of centromere and presence of satellite bodies, i.e. depending upon the morphology.

Q. What is Denver classification?

Ans. In this system of classification, all the chromosomes are assigned groups from A to G, in order of decreasing length, i.e. depending on size of chromosome:

1. Group A—1, 2, 3 chromosomes.
2. Group B—4, 6 chromosomes.
3. Group C—6, 7, 8, 9, 10, 11, 12, X chromosomes.
4. Group D—13, 14, 15 chromosomes.
5. Group E—16, 17, 18 chromosomes.
6. Group F—19, 20 chromosomes.
7. Group G—1, 22, Y chromosomes.

Q. Classify X chromosome.

Ans. X chromosome is a member of group C, it is a submetacentric chromosome.

Q. Classify Y chromosome.

Ans. Y chromosome is a member of group G and is an acrocentric chromosome.

Q. How do you classify chromosomes depending upon the position of centromere?

Ans.

1. Telocentric—centromere is at one end.

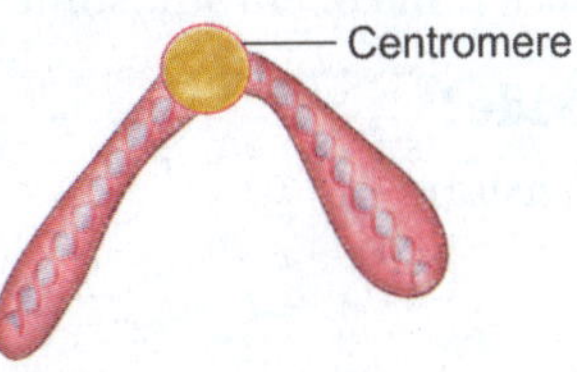

2. Acrocentric—centromere is near one end.

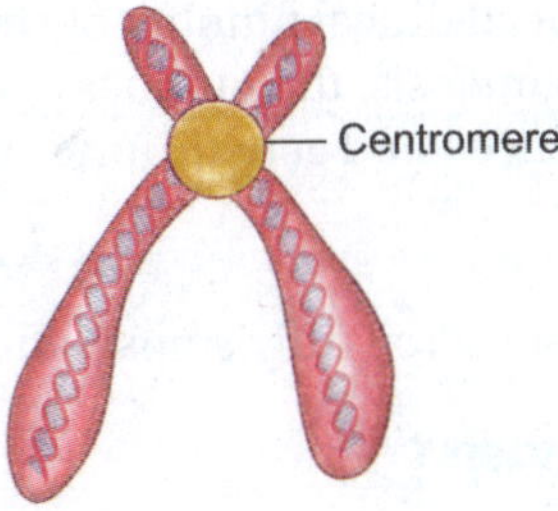

3. Submetacentric—centromere is submedian.

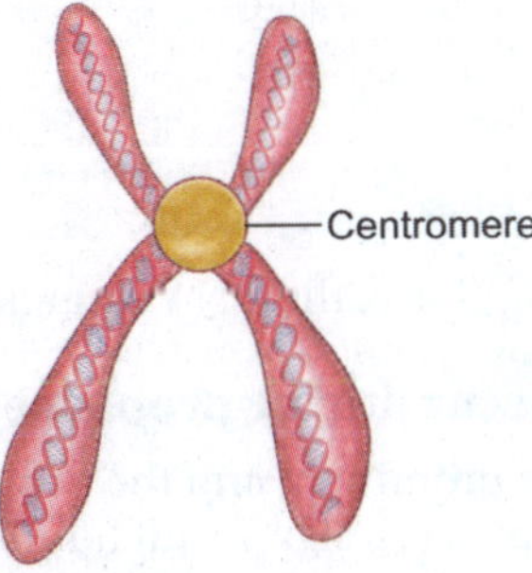

4. Metacentric—centromere is in the center.

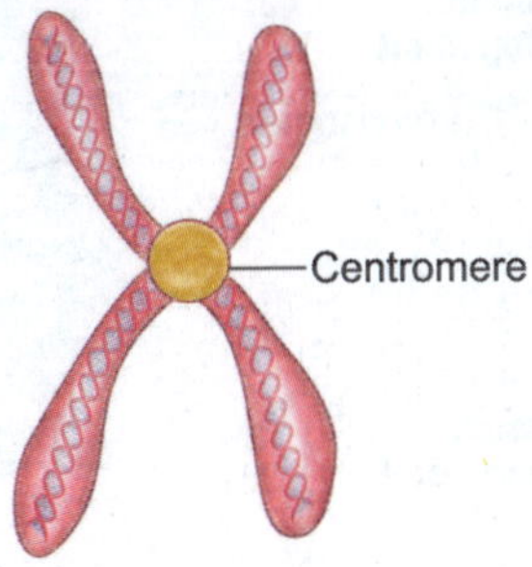

Q. What is the significance of chromosomes?

Ans. Chromosomes are made up of predominantly nucleic acid called deoxyribonucleic acid (DNA). It carries the information necessary for the formation of numerous tissues and organs of the body, and for their orderly assembly and function. This information is imprinted on genes, i.e. structural units of chromosomes.

Q. In what ways the cells divide?

Ans. There are two types of cell divisions:

1. Mitosis.
2. Meiosis.

Q. What is the main difference between mitosis and meiosis?

Ans. In mitosis, daughter cells have identical number of chromosomes and genetic information as that of the mother. In meiosis, the number of chromosomes in daughter cells is reduced to half that of mother cell and genetic information is not identical.

Q. What is interphase?

Ans. The period between the two successive divisions is interphase.

Q. What are the stages of mitosis?

Ans. Following are the stages of mitosis:

1. Prophase.
2. Metaphase.
3. Anaphase.
4. Telophase.

Q. What happens in interphase?

Ans. During specific period of interphase, the DNA content of chromosome is duplicated.

Q. What important events occur during prophase?

Ans. Chromosomes become more prominent and the two centrioles move to opposite poles in early prophase. In late prophase, a significant number of microtubules develop giving rise to spindle formation.

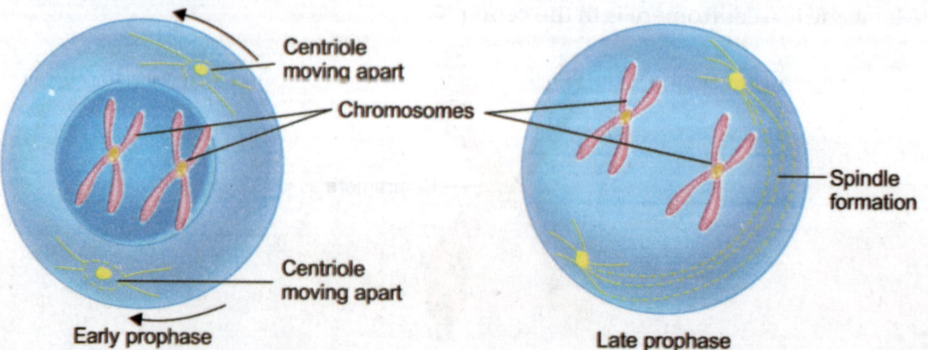

Q. What happens in metaphase?

Ans. Chromosomes occupy a central position in between the centrioles and get attached to the microtubule of the spindle.

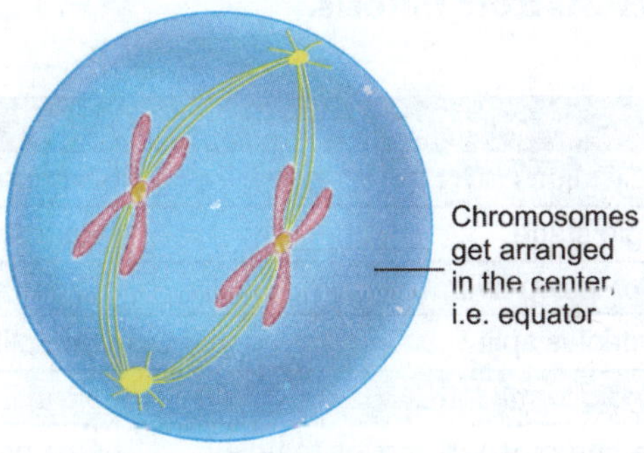

Metaphase

Q. What events occur in anaphase?

Ans. The centromere of each chromosome splits longitudinally to give rise to independent chromosomes.

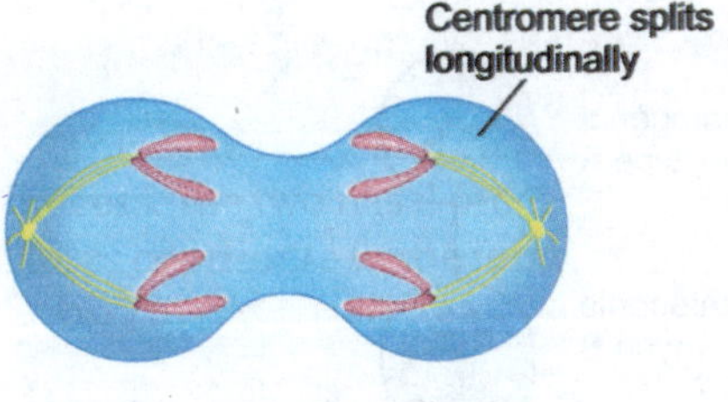

Anaphase

Q. How is the telophase marked by?

Ans. During telophase, nuclear membrane appears and two daughter cells are formed, cytoplasm also divides.

Q. What are the stages of prophase in first meiotic division?

Ans. Following are the stages of prophase in first meiotic division:

1. Leptotene.
2. Zygotene.
3. Pachytene.
4. Diplotene.

Q. In what stage of prophase 'crossing over' takes place?

Ans. In pachytene stage of prophase, crossing over takes place.

Q. How does the anaphase of meiosis differ from mitosis?

Ans. There is no splitting of centromere in meiosis during anaphase.

Q. How does the interphase of meiosis differ from mitosis?

Ans. There is no duplication of DNA during the interphase of meiosis.

Q. Differentiate meiosis from mitosis.

Ans.

Stages	Mitosis	Meiosis
Interphase	Duplication of DNA	No duplication of DNA
Prophase	Single stage	Four stages
Prophase I	No crossing over	Crossing over takes place
Anaphase	Centrioles split	No splitting of centrioles
Metaphase	Spindle formation	No spindle formation
Anaphase	One chromosome moves to pole	One pair moves to pole

Q. To what does second meiotic division resemble?

Ans. Second meiotic division resembles mitosis.

Q. Enumerate spermatogenesis.

Ans.

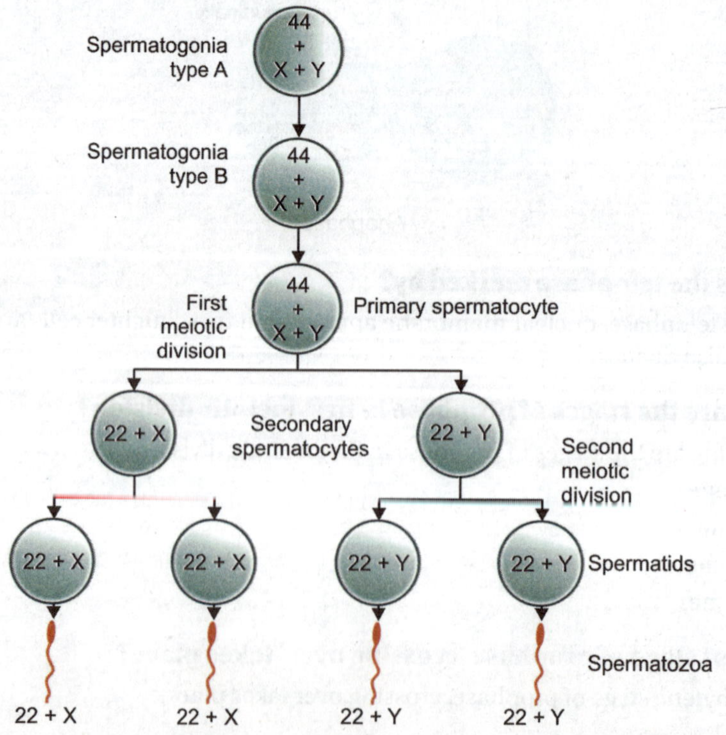

Q. What is spermiogenesis?

Ans. The process of transformation of spermatid to spermatozoa is known as spermiogenesis.

Q. Enumerate stages in oogenesis.

Ans.

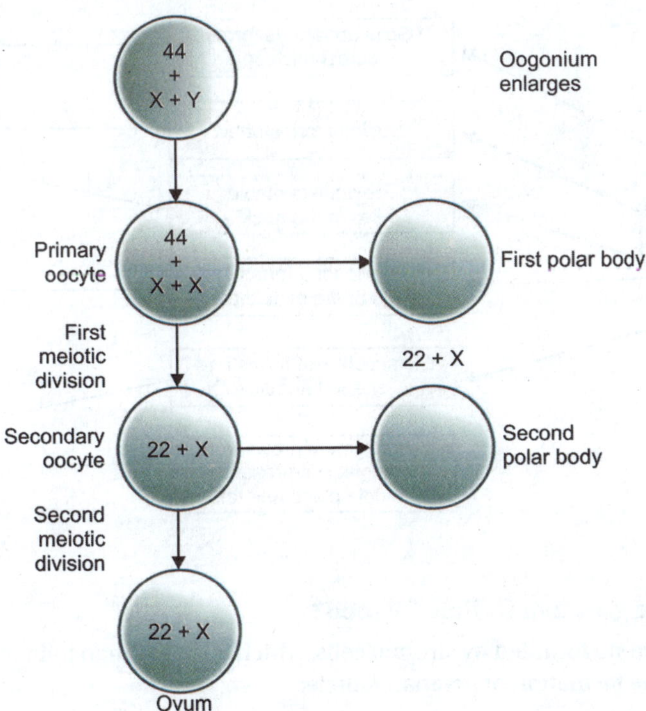

Q. How is the sex of offspring decided?

Ans. Sex of the offspring is determined by which type of sperm unites with ovum. Sperm could be either 22X or 22Y, while ovum is only 22X.

Q. What are the parts of spermatozoa?

Ans. A spermatozoa has a head, neck, middle piece and tail.

Q. What is capacitation?

Ans. Spermatozoa acquire the ability to fertilize ovum only after they have been in the female genital tract. This final stage of maturation is called capacitation.

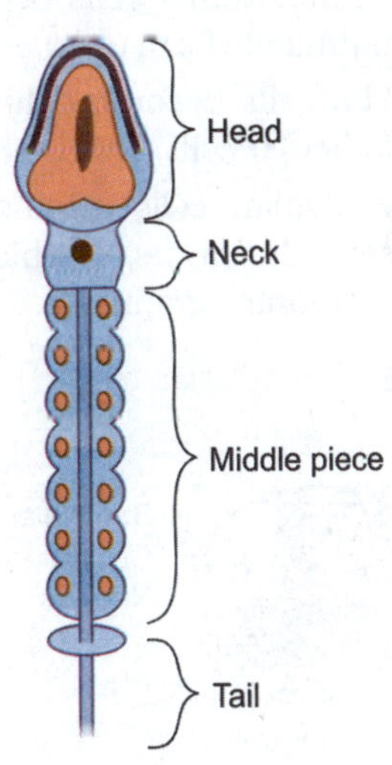

Spermatozoa pouts

Q. What is spermiogenesis?

Ans.   The process by which a spermatid becomes spermatozoa is called spermiogenesis.

Q. How are the parts of spermatozoa derived?

Ans.

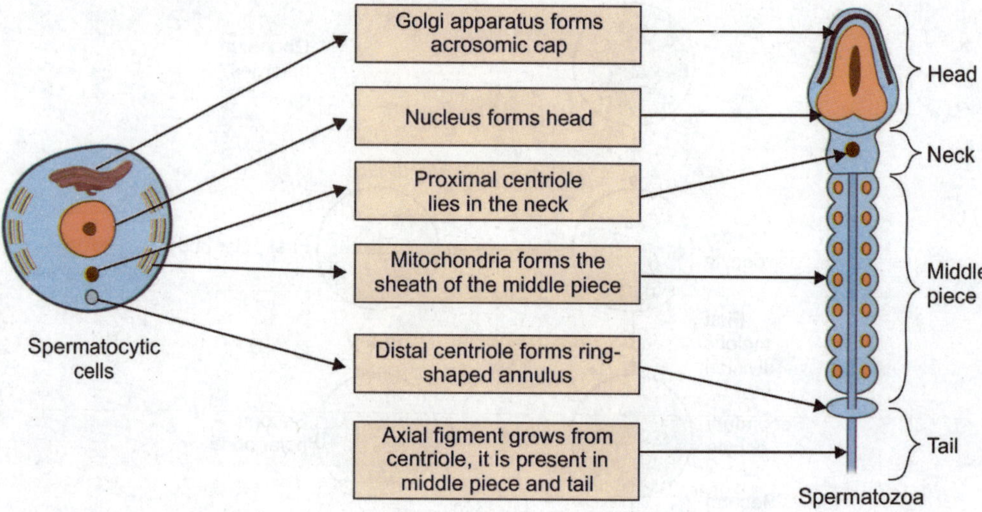

Q. How is the graafian follicle formed?

Ans.   Oogonia are surrounded by stromal cells, which form graafian follicle. Following are the stages in the formation of graafian follicle:

1. Some stromal cells become flattened and surround an oocyte. These flattened cells ultimately form ovarian follicle and therefore called follicular cells.

2. Flat cells become columnar and a homogenous layer appears between oocyte and follicular cells. This is known as zona pellucida.

3. Follicular cells proliferate to form several layers, which constitute membrana granulosa.

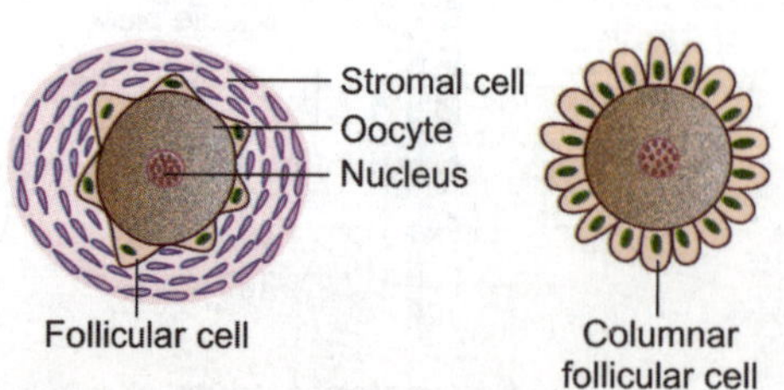

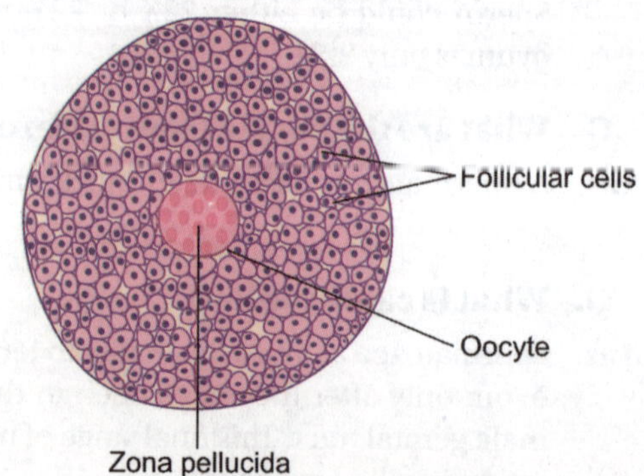

4. A cavity appears within membrana granulosa, which gradually increase in size. Oocyte lies eccentrically surrounded by granulosa cells, i.e. cumulus oophorus. The cells which attach it to the wall is discus proligerus.

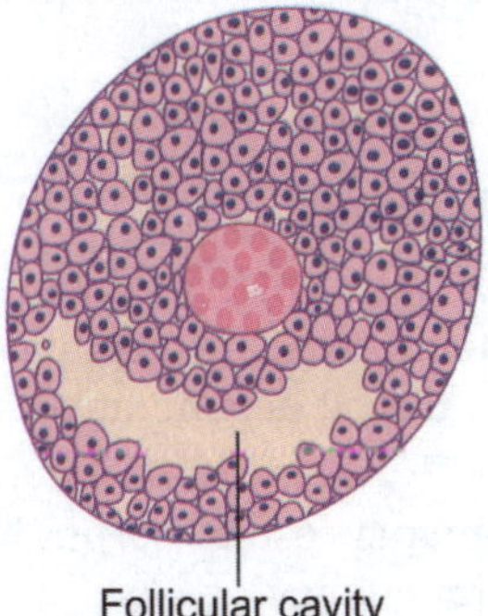

Formation of graafian follicle

5. Stromal cells surrounding the membrana granulosa become condensed to form theca interna, while the surrounding fibrous tissue forms theca externa.

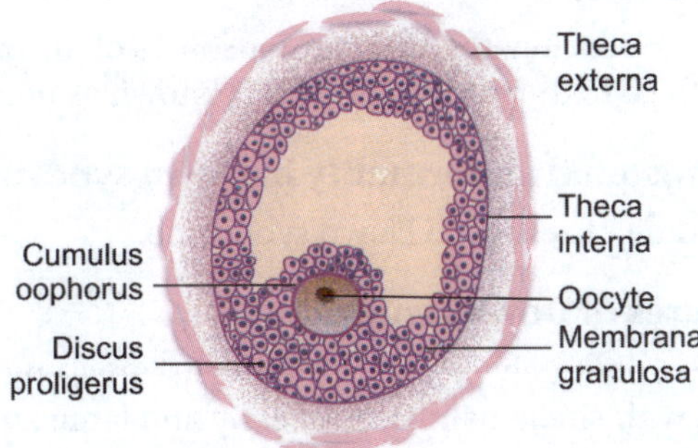

Graafian follicle

Q. What is the stage of ovum? When it is shed from the ovary?

Ans. Ovum is in the secondary oocyte stage, which is undergoing division to shed off second polar body.

Q. Depict the structure of ovum at the time of ovulation.

Ans.

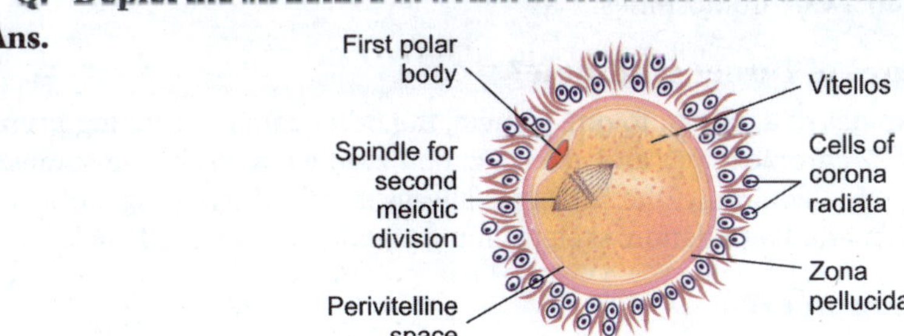

Structure of ovum

Q. How long does the ovum take to reach the uterus?

Ans. Ovum takes 3–4 days to reach the uterus.

Q. What is corpus luteum?

Ans. Ovarian follicle after ovulation is corpus luteum.

Q. What is the fate of corpus luteum?

Ans. Fate of corpus luteum depends upon whether the ovum is fertilized or not. If the ovum is not fertilized, the corpus luteum persists for 14 days. It is known as corpus luteum of menstruation. At the end of 14 days it degenerates and forms a fibrous mass known as corpus albicans.

If ovum is fertilized and pregnancy results, corpus luteum persists for 3–4 months and is known as corpus luteum of pregnancy.

Q. What is the importance of corpus luteum?

Ans. Corpus luteum secretes hormone progesterone, which maintains pregnancy.

Q. What is nondisjunction?

Ans. During the first meiotic division, the two chromosomes of the pair instead of separating at anaphase may both go to the same pole. This is known as nondisjunction.

Q. What is the chromosomal abnormality in Down syndrome?

Ans. Trisomy of chromosome 21 results in Down syndrome.

Q. What are the features of Down syndrome?

Ans. Child has a broad face, obliquely placed palpebral fissures, epicanthus, furrowed lower lip and broad hands with single palmar crease. By and large are mentally retarded and have heart defects.

Q. What are the features associated with extra X or Y chromosome?

Ans. The presence of extra X or Y chromosome can give rise to syndromes associated with abnormal genital development, mental retardation and abnormal growth.

Q. Who are superfemales?

Ans. These are patients with XXX chromosomes.

Q. What are the features of Turner syndrome?

Ans. When both chromosomes of a pair go to one gamete, the other gamete resulting from the division has only 22 chromosomes and at fertilization zygote has 45 chromosomes. This is monosomy. In this syndrome, the subject is always female. There is agenesis of ovary associated with mental retardation, skeletal abnormalities and webbed neck.

Q. What are isochromosomes?

Ans. During cell division, centriole splits transversely to give rise to isochromosomes.

Q. What are the phases of menstrual cycle?

Ans. Menstrual cycle is divided into following phases:

1. Postmenstrual.
2. Proliferative.
3. Secretory.
4. Menstrual.

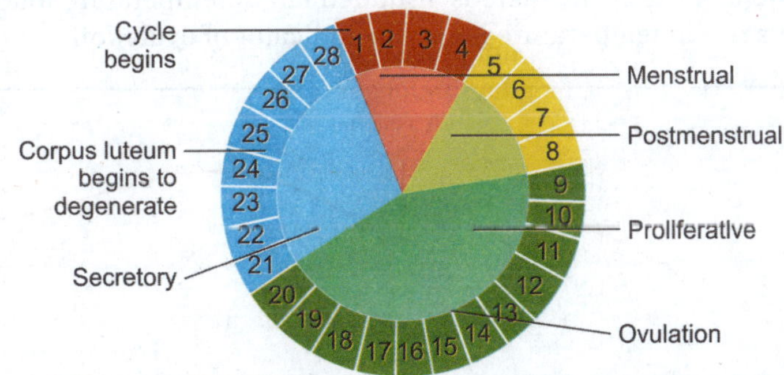

Phases of menstrual cycle

It is also divided in other ways:

1. Follicular phase.
2. Luteal phase.

Q. Which hormone influences the luteal phase?

Ans. Progesterone hormone influences the luteal phase.

Q. Which hormone influences the follicular phase?

Ans. Estrogen hormone influences the follicular phase.

Q. Depict the changes in the epithelium of uterine glands during a menstrual cycle.

Ans.

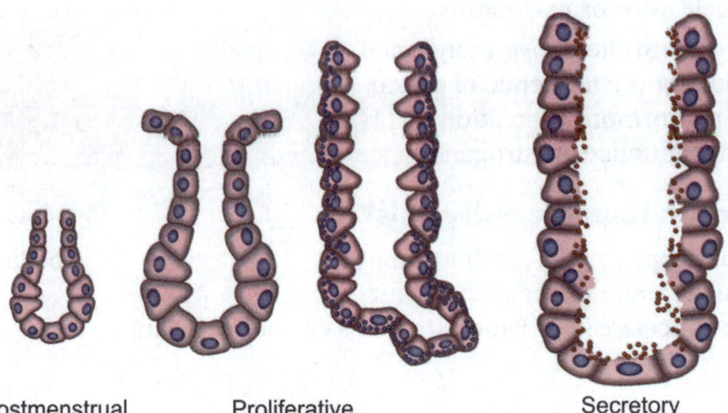

Q. What layers of endometrium are shed off during menstruation?

Ans. Stratum compactum and stratum spongiosum are shed off during menstruation.

Q. When does ovulation occur? How does one detect ovulation?

Ans. In a 28 days cycle, ovulation takes place at about middle of the cycle. The period between ovulation and next menstrual cycle is fixed, i.e. 14 days.

At about middle of the cycle, there is a sudden fall in temperature followed by a rise in temperature. This rise in temperature is a crude indicator of ovulation.

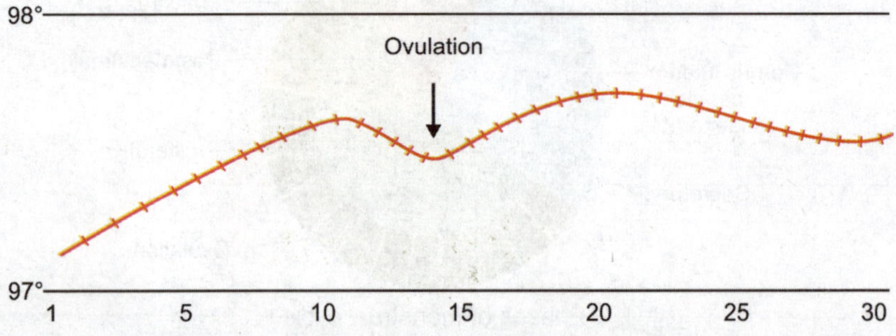

Q. What is rhythm method of family planning?

Ans. After ovulation, ovum remains viable for maximum 2 days. Spermatozoa introduced into vagina die within 4 days. Therefore, fertilization occurs only if intercourse takes place during a period between 4 days before ovulation to 2 days after ovulation. The remaining days have been regarded as safe period. This forms the basis of rhythm method of family planning.

Q. What hormones influence the ovulation and menstruation?

Ans. Follicular stimulating hormone (FSH)—stimulates formation of follicle. Luteinizing hormone (LH)—converts follicle into corpus luteum.

Secretions of both the above mentioned hormones are under the influence of gonadotropin-releasing hormone. Secretion of LH is also under the influence of estrogens.

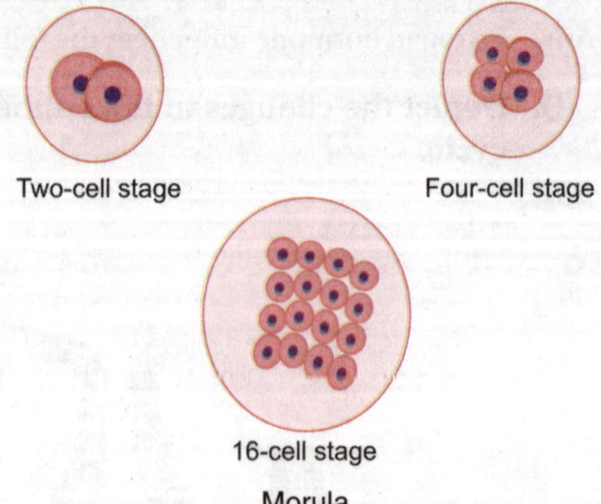

Q. What are oral contraceptive pills?

Ans. Oral contraceptive pills are hormonal pills, which contain progestin as norethisterone acetate (1 μg) and estrogen as estradiol (50 μg).

Q. Describe the formation of blastocyst.

Ans.

1. After fertilization, the two-cell stage undergoes further divisions to give rise to 16-cell stage known as morula.

2. A section of morula shows inner cell mass covered by outer layer of cells known as trophoblast.

3. Fluid appears between trophoblast and inner cell mass. As the fluid accumulates, the cells of the trophoblast become flattened.

4. The inner cell mass gets attached to the inner side of the trophoblast. This is known as the blastocyst.

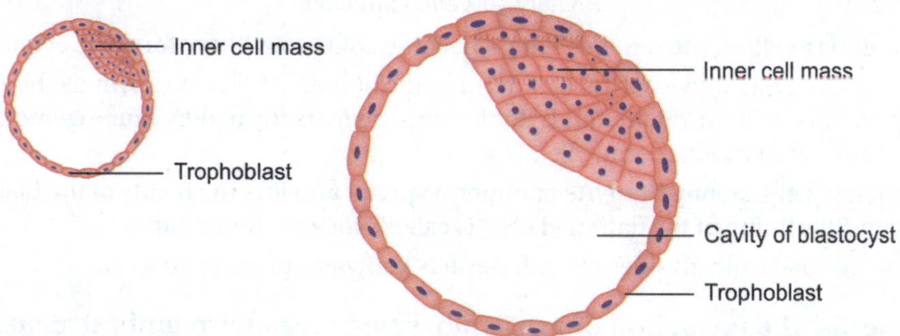

Blastocyst formation

Q. What is the function of the zona pellucida?

Ans. Trophoblast has the property of being able to stick to uterine epithelium and eat up other cells. They can invade and burrow into tissues. Zona pellucida prevents abnormal implantation of blastocyst.

Q. Discuss the formation of primary yolk sac.

Ans.

1. Few cells of the inner cell mass of blastocyst get converted into flattened cells that lie against the free surface. This forms the endoderm.

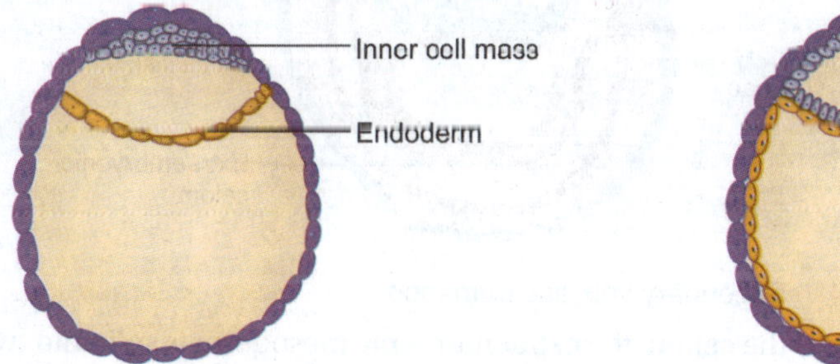

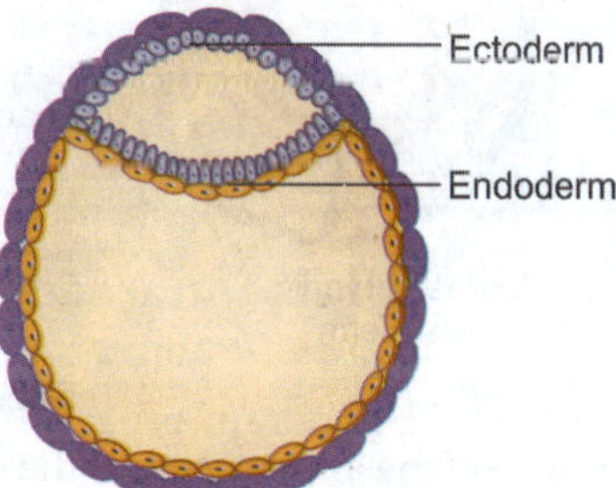

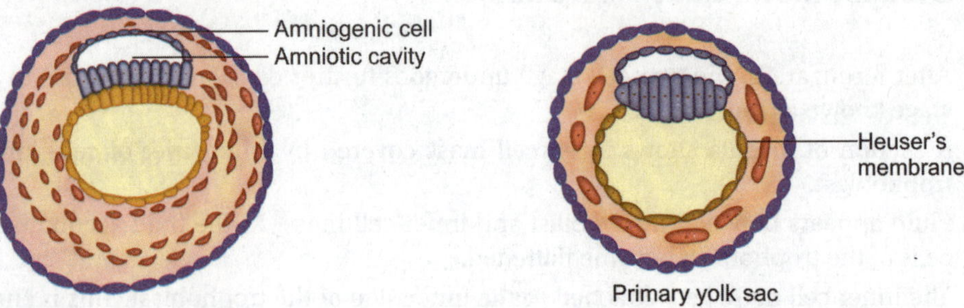

Primary yolk sac formation

2. Remaining cells of the inner cell mass become columnar. These form the ectoderm.

3. A space appears between the ectoderm and trophoblast this is known as the amniotic cavity, filled with amniotic fluid. Roof of this cavity is formed by amniogenic cells and floor is formed by ectoderm.

4. Flattened cells arising from the endoderm spread and line the inside of the blastocystic cavity. This lining of the flattened cells is called Heuser's membrane.

5. A cavity lined from all sides by endoderm is known as primary yolk sac.

Q. Describe the formation of extraembryonic mesoderm and extraembryonic celom.

Ans. The trophoblastic cells lining the primary yolk sac gives rise to the extraembryonic mesoderm. These cells come to lie between the endoderm and trophoblast below, and amniogenic cells and trophoblast above.

Small cavities appear in the extraembryonic mesoderm, which coalesce to form a large cavity, i.e. extraembryonic celom.

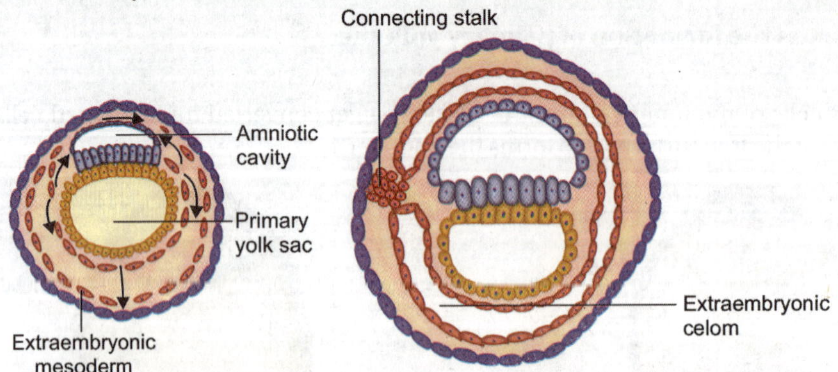

Secondary yolk sac formation

Because of the appearance of the celom, the extraembryonic mesoderm is split into two layers. The part lining the outside of the amniotic cavity is parietal extraembryonic mesoderm. The part lining the yolk sac is visceral extraembryonic mesoderm. The extraembryonic celom does not extend beyond the amniotic cavity and this region of unsplit extraembryonic mesoderm forms connecting stalk. The yolk sac becomes smaller and now known as secondary yolk sac.

Q. How is the chorion formed?

Ans. The chorion is formed by the combination of parietal extraembryonic mesoderm and overlying trophoblast.

Q. What is amnion?

Ans. The amnion is constituted by amniogenic cells forming the wall of amniotic cavity.

Q. How does one decide about the head end or tail end of the embryo?

Ans. When the embryo is made of bilaminar disk, made up of ectoderm and endoderm one cannot make out, which is the head end or tail end.

Soon a circular area develops near the margin of the embryonic disk, the cubical cells become columnar. This area is known as prochordal plate. It determines the central axis of the embryo.

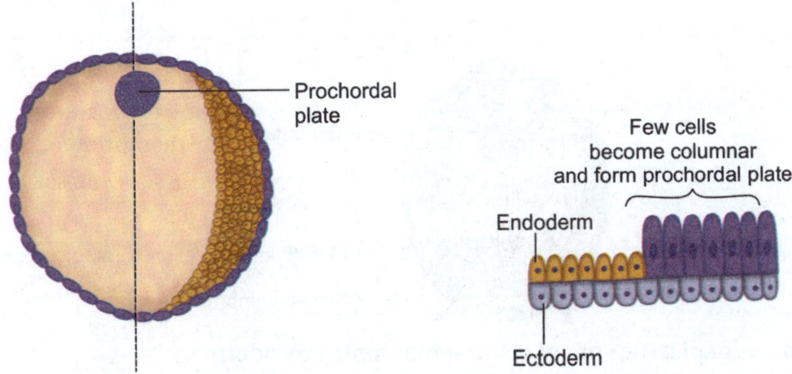

Axis of embryonic disk formation of prochordal plate

Q. What is primitive streak? What is its importance?

Ans.

1. Some of the ectodermal cells toward the tail end of the embryonic disk proliferate (increase in number). This elevation is known as the primitive streak.

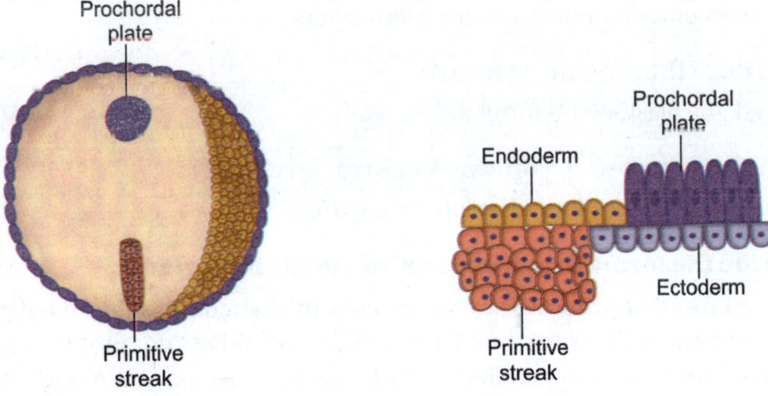

2. The cells of the primitive streak proliferate and grow in between the ectoderm and endoderm. These cells form the intraembryonic mesoderm.

3. With the formation of the primitive streak, the third germinal layer is formed. This marks the process of gastrulation.

Q. What is gastrulation?

Ans. The process of formation of primitive streak and of intraembryonic mesoderm is referred to as gastrulation.

Q. In which two areas the intraembryonic mesoderm does not split?

Ans. The intraembryonic mesoderm does not spread in the region of prochordal plate, which forms the buccopharyngeal membrane.

It also does not spread in an area caudal to primitive streak. This region forms the cloacal membrane.

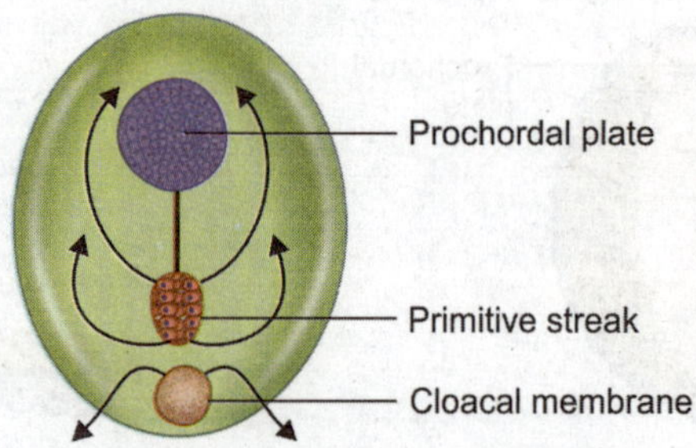

Here, arrows depict the spread of intraembryonic mesoderm.

Q. Which is the critical period of development?

Ans. Critical period of development is considered for 3–8 weeks since this period is characterized by organogenesis and any environmental insult in the form of drugs, radiation, infections, etc. can lead to development of congenital anomalies.

Q. After how many days of fertilization morula is formed?

Ans. Embryo becomes morula 3 days after fertilization.

Q. When does the blastocyst form?

Ans. On day 4, the blastocyst is formed.

Q. When does intraembryonic mesoderm develops?

Ans. Intraembryonic mesoderm develops by day 16.

Q. Describe the formation of notochord and its importance.

Ans. The cranial end of primitive streak becomes thickened. This thickened part is called primitive knot or Hensen's node. Cells in the primitive knot proliferate grow cranially in midline between ectoderm and endoderm reaching up to the caudal margin of prochordal plate. These cells form a solid rod called notochord.

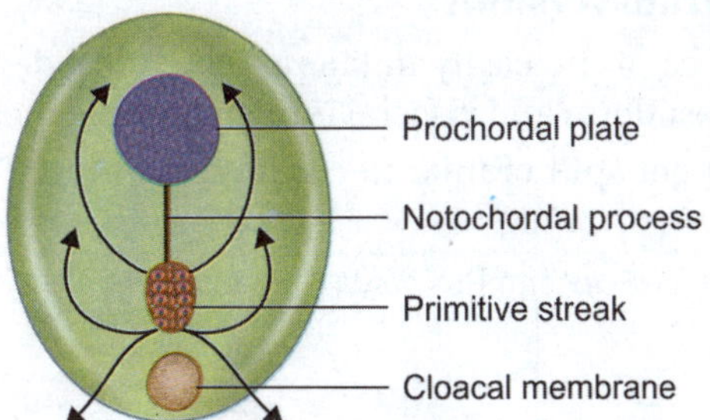

Formation of notochord

Notochord remains in the center position later to be occupied by the vertebral column. Most of the notochord disappears, but parts of it remain in the region of each intervertebral disk as nucleus pulposus.

Q. At which sites in an embryo the ectoderm and the endoderm are in close contact? Or at which sites the intraembryonic mesoderm does not reach?

Ans. The intraembryonic mesoderm does not develop in the following regions:

1. Prochordal plate.
2. Cloacal membrane.
3. In the midline caudal to prochordal plate.

Q. How is the intraembryonic mesoderm divided?

Ans. The intraembryonic is subdivided into:

1. Para-axial mesoderm.
2. Lateral plate mesoderm.
3. Intermediate mesoderm.

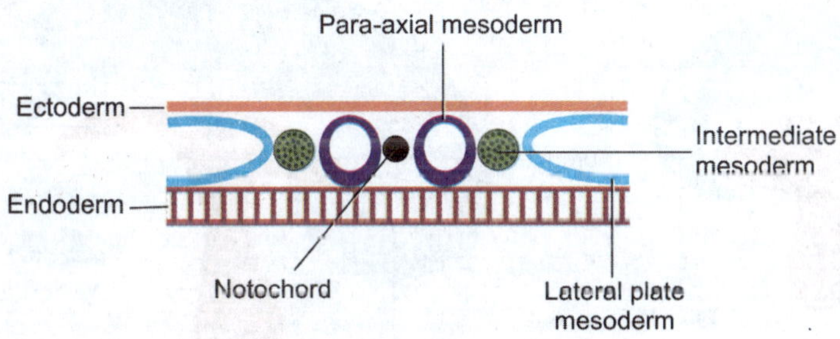

Intraembryonic mesoderm

Q. What is the fate of intraembryonic mesoderm?

Ans.

1. Para-axial mesoderm gives rise to somites.
2. Intermediate mesoderm gives rise to nephrogenic cord.
3. A cavity develops in the lateral plate mesoderm, which gives rise to pericardial, pleural and peritoneal cavities.

Q. What is septum transversum?

Ans. With the appearance of the cavity in lateral plate mesoderm it gets split into parietal intraembryonic mesoderm and visceral intraembryonic mesoderm.

However, it does not get split cranial to cardiogenic area. This unsplit area forms the septum transversum.

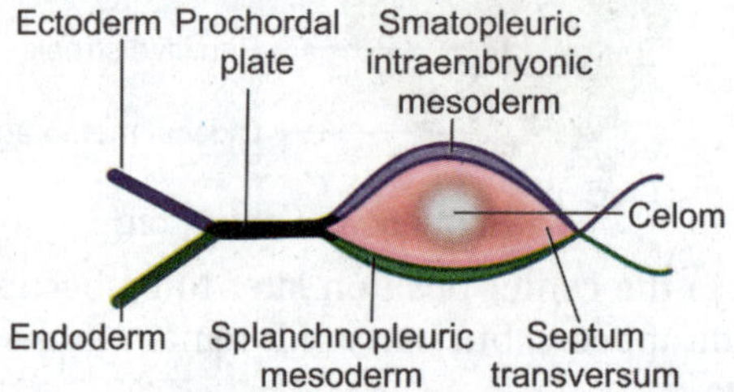

Septum transversum

Q. Draw neat labeled diagrams to depict folds of embryonic disk and formation of primitive gut.

Ans.

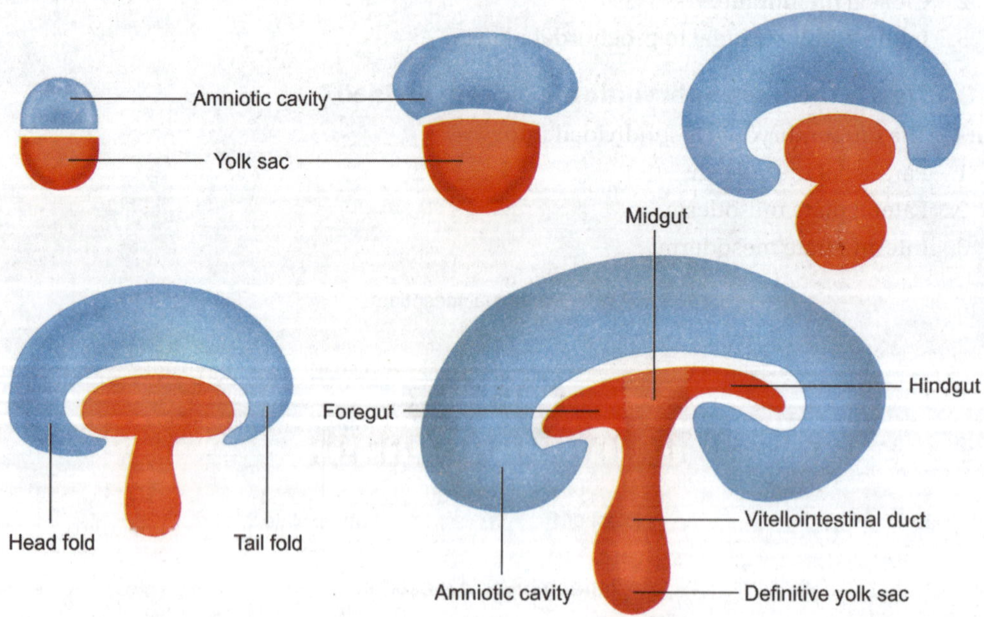

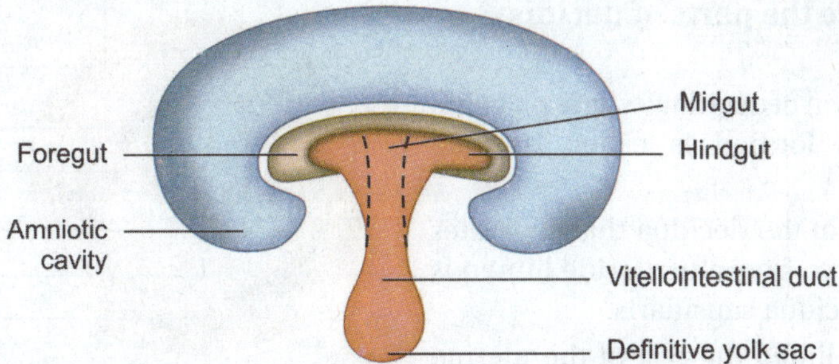

Q. Draw neat labeled diagrams to show embryonic disk before and after formation of head and tail end.

Ans.

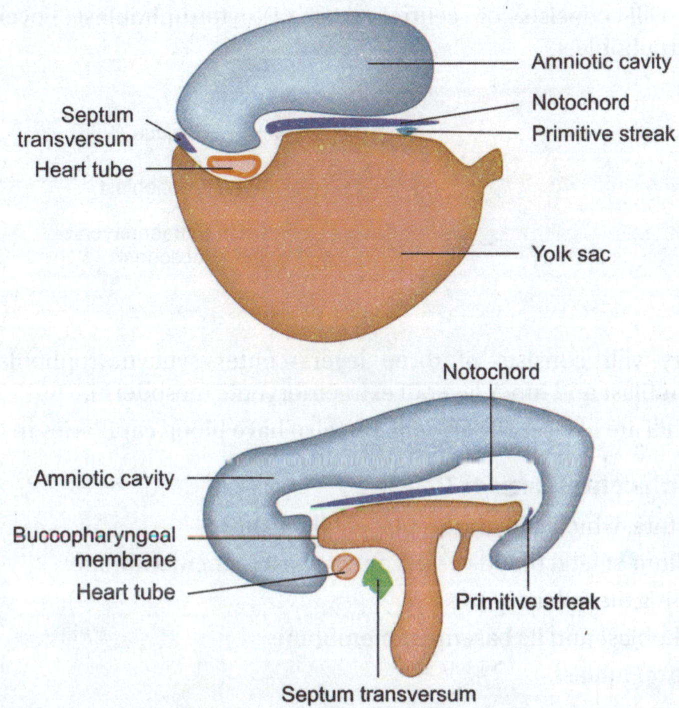

Q. When does the implantation of blastocyst occur?

Ans. Implantation begins after 6 days of fertilization. Blastocyst goes deeper and deeper into uterine mucosa till it lies within the thickness of the endometrium. This is called interstitial implantation.

Q. What is decidual reaction?

Ans. After implantation, the uterine endometrium is known as decidua. The stromal cells of the endometrium enlarge, become vacuolated, store glycogen and lipids. This change in stromal cells is called decidual reaction.

Q. What are the parts of decidua?

Ans.

1. The portion of decidua, where placenta is to be formed is called decidua basalis.

2. The part of the decidua that separates the embryo from the uterine lumen is called decidua capsularis.

3. The part lining the rest of the uterine cavity is decidua parietalis.

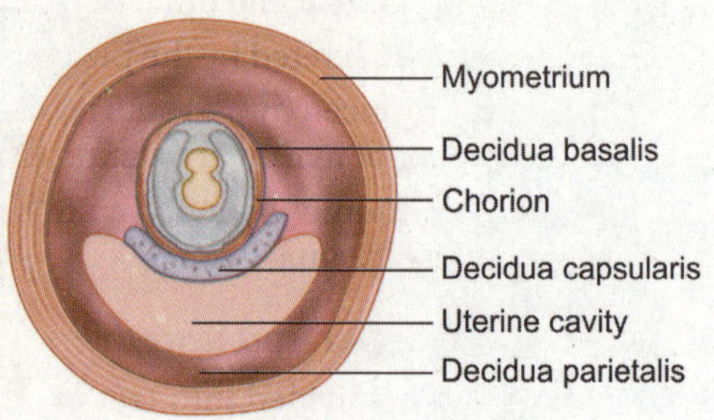

Parts of decidua

Q. What are the different types of villi?

Ans. There are three types of villi:

1. Primary villi consists of central core of cytotrophoblast covered by layer of syncytiotrophoblast.

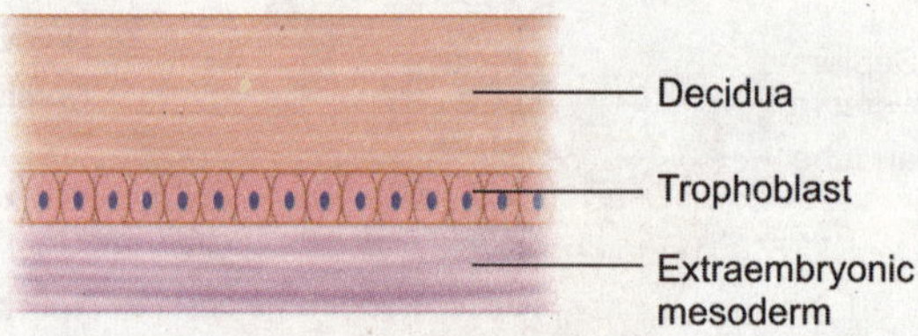

Types of villi

2. Secondary villi consists of three layers—outer syncytiotrophoblast, intermediate cytotrophoblast and inner layer of extraembryonic mesoderm.

3. Tertiary villi are like secondary villi, but also have blood capillaries in the mesoderm.

Q. What is placental barrier?

Ans. The structure, which constitutes placental barrier:

1. Endothelium of fetal blood vessels and its basement membrane.

2. Surrounding mesoderm.

3. Cytotrophoblast and its basement membrane.

4. Syncytiotrophoblast.

Q. What are the functions of placenta?

Ans.

1. Placenta helps in transport of oxygen, water, electrolytes and nutrition from maternal blood to fetal blood.

2. It provides excretion of carbon dioxide, urea and other waste products produced by fetus.

3. Maternal antibodies reach fetus through the blood and give immunity to fetus.

4. It prevents bacteria and other harmful substances reaching the fetus.
5. Progesterone secreted by the placenta is essential for the maintenance of pregnancy.
6. Estrogen produced by placenta reach maternal blood and promotes uterine growth and development of mammary gland.
7. Human chorionic gonadotropin and somatomammotropin are other hormones secreted by placenta.

Q. What are upper and lower uterine segments?

Ans. Uterus can be divided into two parts. An upper part, consisting of the fundus and the greater part of the body is known as upper uterine segment. The lower part of the body and cervix is known as lower uterine segment.

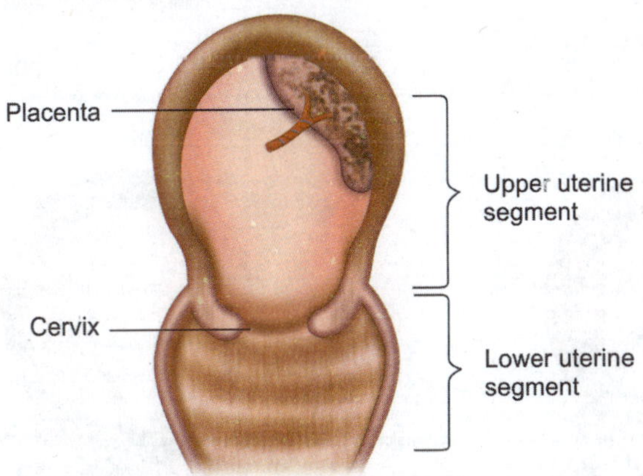

Upper and lower uterine segments

Q. What is the normal site of implantation of placenta?

Ans. The placenta is normally attached to the upper uterine segment only.

Q. What is placenta previa? What are its various degrees?

Ans. The attachment of placenta may partially or completely extend into lower uterine segment. This condition is known as placenta previa.

Various degrees of placenta previa are as follows:

1. First degree—the attachment of placenta extends into the lower uterine segment, but does not reach internal os.
2. Second degree—the margin of the placenta reaches the internal os, but does not cover it.
3. Third degree—the edge of the placenta covers the internal os, but when the os dilates during childbirth, the placenta no longer occludes it.
4. Fourth degree—the placenta completely covers the internal os even after it is dilated.

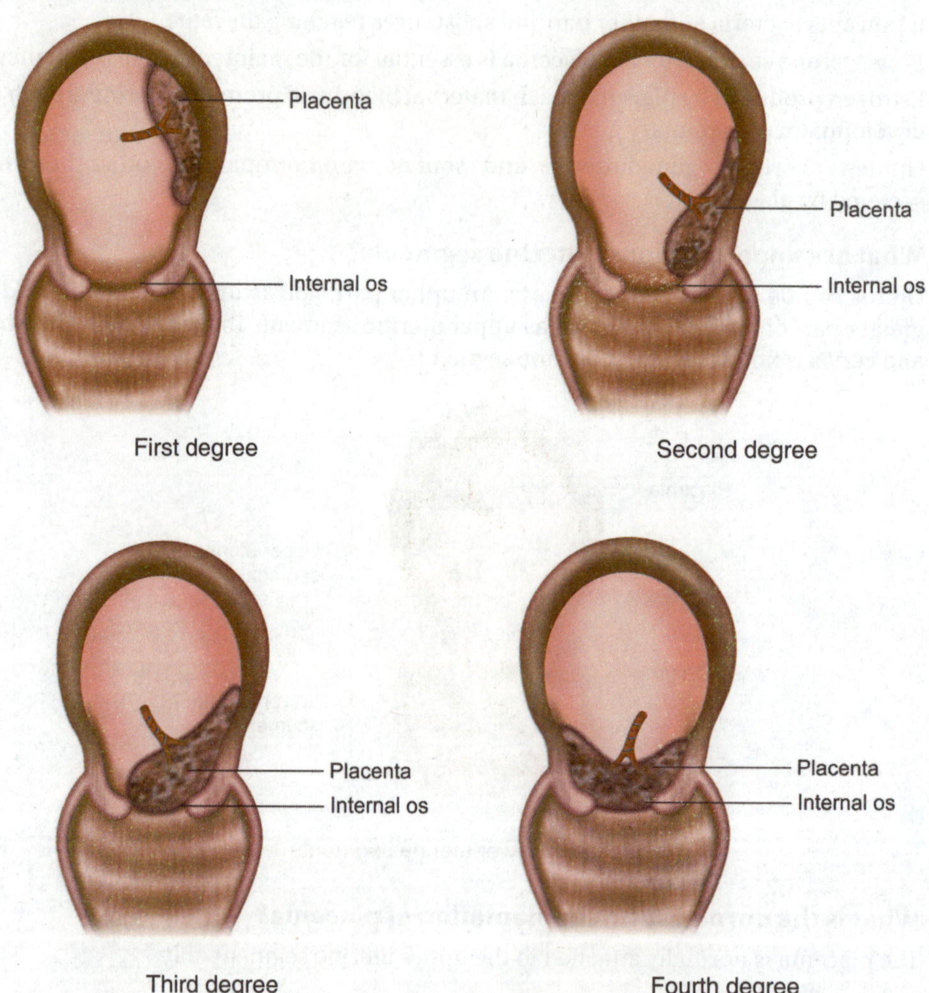

Types of placenta previa

Q. What are the sites of ectopic pregnancy?

Ans. When the fertilized ovum gets implanted at any site outside the uterus, is called ectopic pregnancy. Following are the sites of ectopic pregnancy:

1. Tubal pregnancy—the blastocyst gets implanted in the uterine tube. Such a pregnancy cannot go on to full term, may result into rupture of the tube. After the rupture, the blastocyst may acquire a secondary implantation in the abdominal cavity giving rise to abdominal pregnancy.

2. Interstitial tubal implantation—the blastocyst gets implanted in the intramural part of the uterine tube.

3. Implantation in the ovary—fertilization and implantation may occur in the ovary.

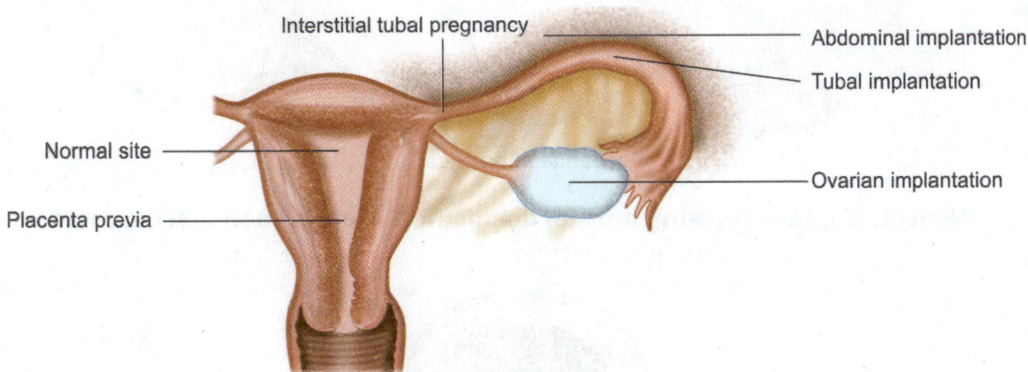

Sites of ectopic pregnancy

Q. Draw neat labeled diagrams of anomalies of placenta.

Ans. Variations in the attachment of umbilical cord to placenta are shown in figures below.

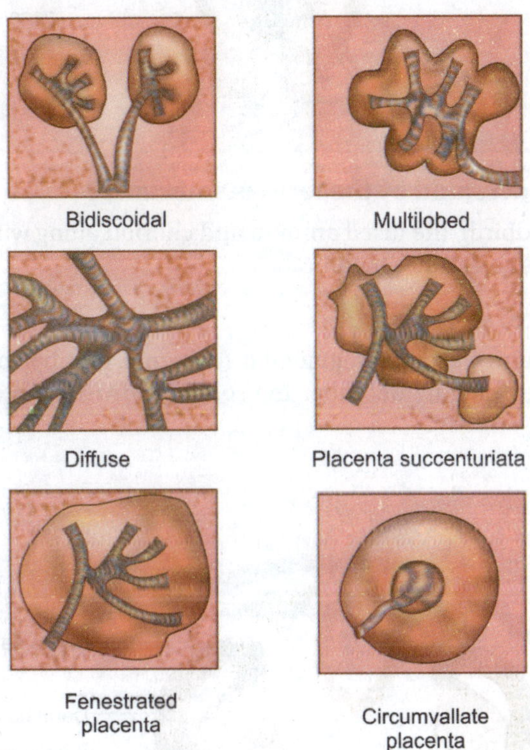

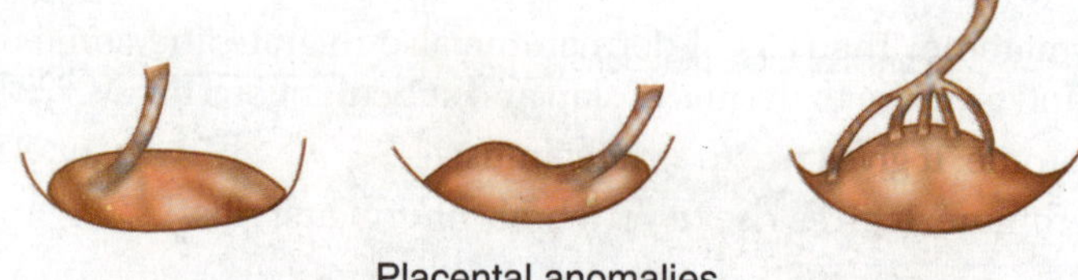

Placental anomalies

Q. Depict a diagram showing normal disposition of embryo in uterine cavity.

Ans.

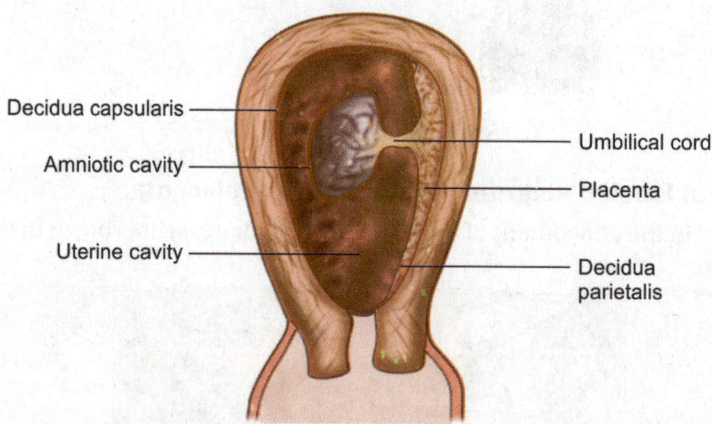

Q. What do you understand by the term membranes?

Ans. At the time of childbirth, the fused amnion and chorion along with the greatly thinned decidua capsularis constitutes membranes.

Q. Discuss the fate of somites.

Ans. Para-axial mesoderm becomes segmented to form a number of somites that lie on either side of developing neural tube. The somite is divisible into three parts namely:

- Dermatome
- Myotome
- Sclerotome.

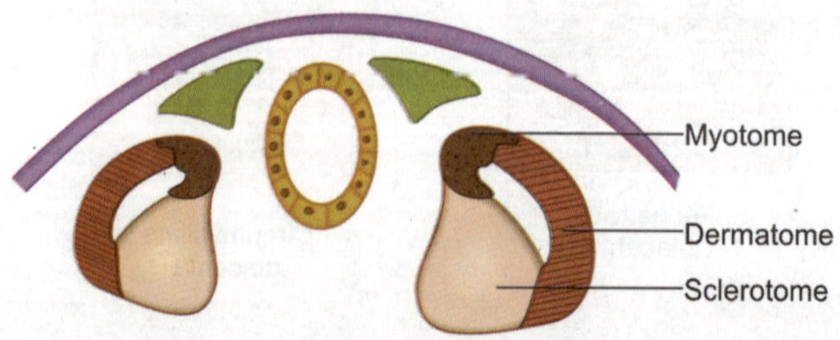

Fate of somites

1. Fate of dermatome: The cells of dermatome also migrate and come to lie beneath the ectoderm and give rise to dermis of skin and subcutaneous tissue.
2. Fate of myotome: It gives rise to striated muscle.
3. Fate of sclerotome: It gives rise to vertebral column and ribs.

Q. What is mesenchyme? What are the derivatives of mesenchyme?

Ans. Cells of mesoderm, which gives rise to loose connective tissue are known as mesenchymal cells. Following are the derivatives of mesenchyme (as shown in the figure).

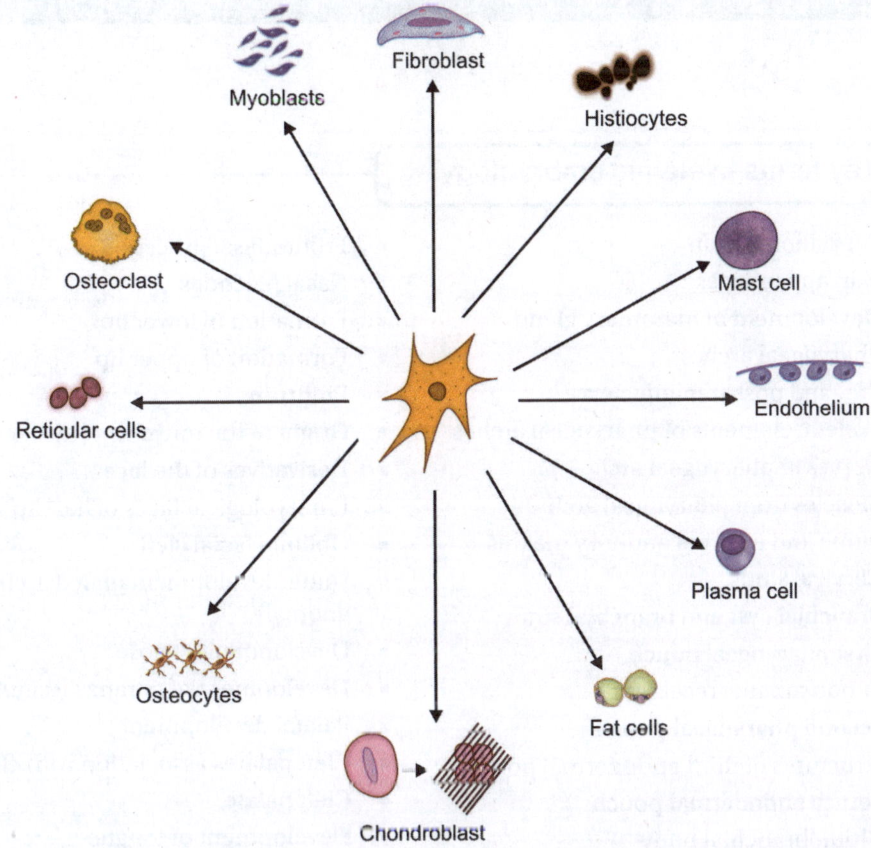

Derivatives of mesenchyme

Q. What is the fate of occipital myotomes?

Ans. Occipital myotomes give rise to muscles of the tongue.

Systemic Embryology

Key terms systemic embryology

- Formation of skin
- Skin appendages
- Development of mammary gland
- Pharyngeal arches
- Pre- and post-trematic nerve
- Skeletal elements of pharyngeal arches
- Nerves of pharyngeal arch
- Muscles from pharyngeal arch
- Pinna and external auditory meatus
- Cervical sinus
- Branchial cyst and branchial sinus
- First pharyngeal pouch
- Tubotympanic recess
- Second pharyngeal pouch
- Structures of third endodermal pouch
- Fourth endodermal pouch
- Ultimobranchial body
- Pharyngeal pouches
- Parathyroid glands
- Thyroid gland
- Anomalies of thyroid gland
- Path of thyroglossal duct
- Formation of face
- Frontonasal process
- Nasal placodes
- Formation of lower lip
- Formation of upper lip
- Philtrum
- Origin of the muscles of the face
- Derivatives of the face
- Embryological basis of harelip
- Oblique facial cleft
- Underdevelopment of first arch anomaly
- Development of nose
- Development of paranasal sinuses
- Palatal development
- Cleft palates association with cleft lips
- Cleft palate
- Development of tongue
- Tongue innervations
- Origin of muscles of tongue
- Development of palatine tonsils
- Parts of the primitive gut
- Arteries of primitive gut
- Rotation of midgut loop

Contd...

Contd...

- Foregut
- Subdivisions of cloaca
- Midgut
- Hindgut
- Cecum
- Developmental anomalies of the gut
- Development of liver
- Gall bladder
- Development of pancreas
- Development of spleen
- Classification of anomalies
- Respiratory diverticulum
- Cavities of the body
- Development of diaphragm
- Innervation of diaphragm
- Development of heart
- Parts of heart tube
- Veins drain into sinus venosus
- Arterial and venous ends of heart tube
- Openings in the right atrium
- Heart tube
- Derivatives of pericardium
- Sinus venosus
- Interatrial septum
- Septum primum and septum secundum
- Right atrium
- Left atrium
- Subdivisions and fate of bulbus cordis
- Remnant of first arch
- Interventricular septum
- Tetralogy of Fallot
- Genesis of arteries
- Recurrent laryngeal nerve
- Axis artery of upper and lower limb
- Superior vena cava
- Inferior vena cava
- Features of fetal circulation
- Components of fetal circulation
- Fetal circulation at birth
- Formation of urogenital system
- Nephrogenic cord
- Components of urethra
- Subdivisions of cloaca
- Subdivisions of urogenital sinus
- Distinct sources of kidney
- Anomalies of kidney
- Development of ureter
- Development of urinary bladder
- Paramesonephric ducts in females
- Anomalies of uterus
- Paramesonephric ducts in males
- Male homologue of uterus
- Development of external genitalia
- Descent of testis
- Formation of neural tube
- Subdivisions of neural tube
- Neural tube in adult
- Neural tube fold
- Cavities of brain subdivisions
- Neural crest cells
- Derivatives of neural crest cells
- Development of pituitary gland
- Layers of neural tube
- Components of eyeball
- Formation of optic vesicle
- Lens vesicle
- Otic vesicle
- Middle ear
- External auditory canal
- Formation of pinna
- Ectoderm
- Endoderm
- Mesoderm

Q. What components take part in the formation of skin?

Ans. Skin is derived from three diverse components:
1. Epidermis is derived from surface ectoderm.
2. Melanoblasts of the epidermis are derived from the neural crest.
3. Dermis is formed by condensation and differentiation of mesenchyme underlying the surface ectoderm. This mesenchyme is a derivative of dermatome of somites.

Q. What are skin appendages? How do they develop?

Ans. Following are the skin appendages:
1. Nails.
2. Hair.
3. Sebaceous glands.
4. Sweat glands.

All the above structures develop from the ectoderm.

Q. Discuss the development of mammary gland. Add a note on its anomalies.

Ans. The ectoderm becomes thickened along a line from axilla to inguinal region. This is known as milk line or mammary ridge or line.

In the region, where the mammary gland is to form a thickened mass of epidermal cells is seen projecting into the dermis. From this thickened mass, 16–20 solid outgrowths arise. Eventually these thickened outgrowths get canalized. The secretory elements are formed by the proliferation of the terminal parts of the outgrowths. The proximal part forms the lactiferous duct.

The ducts open into a pit. However due to growth of underlying mesoderm, the pit is pushed outside and forms the nipple.

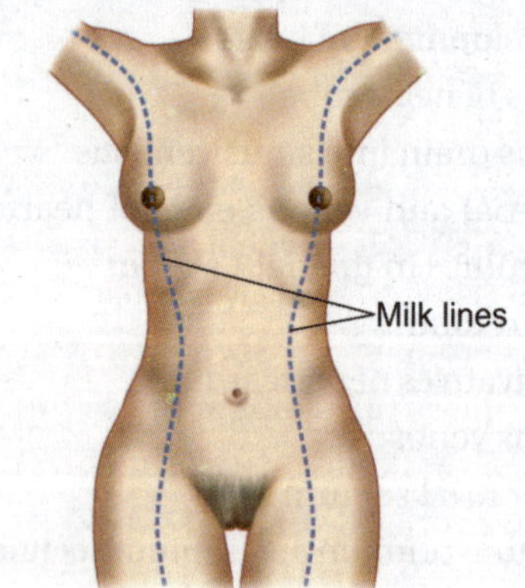

Development of mammary gland

Anomalies

1. Amastia—gland is absent on one or both sides.
2. Athelia—nipple is absent.
3. Polythelia and polymastia—supernumerary nipples may be present along the milk line.
4. Accessory breasts may be found outside the milk line, like in the neck, cheeks, femoral triangle and vulva.
5. Inverted/Crater nipple—failure of development of nipple.
6. Gland may be abnormally small (micromastia) or abnormally large (macromastia).

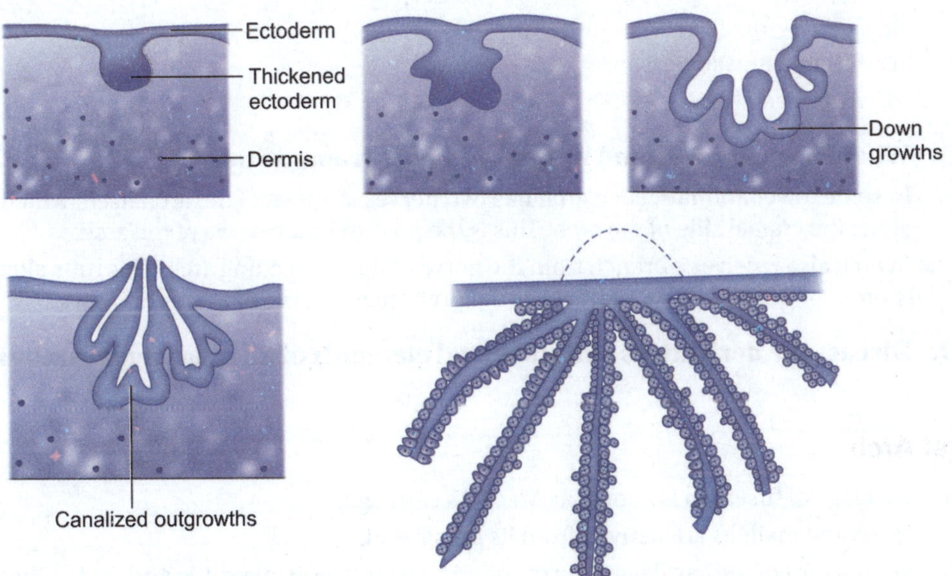

Canalized outgrowths

Q. What are pharyngeal arches?

Ans. A series of mesodermal thickenings appear in the cranial most portion of the foregut. These are known as the pharyngeal arches or branchial arches.

Structure of pharyngeal arch is as follows:

1. Each pharyngeal arch has a endodermal lining, which dips outward to form endodermal pouch (there are six pharyngeal arches, arch five disappears).

2. Ectoderm also dips at the same place to form ectodermal cleft.

3. In between the ectoderm and endoderm is the mesoderm. The mesoderm gives rise to the following structures:

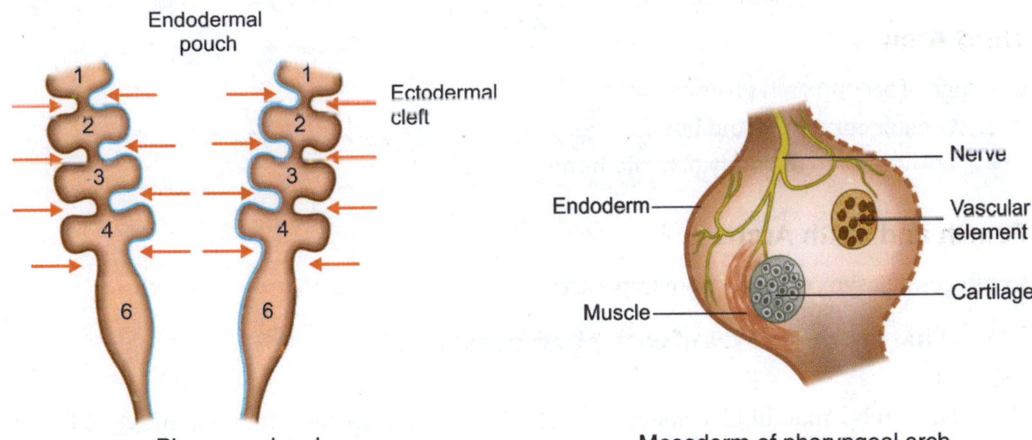

Pharyngeal arches   Mesoderm of pharyngeal arch

   a. Cartilage.
   b. Nerve.
   c. Striated muscle.
   d. Arterial arch.

Q. What do you understand by pre- and post-trematic nerve?

Ans. In some lower animals, each arch has two nerves. A nerve of the arch itself, which runs along the cranial side of the arch. This is the post-trematic nerve of the arch.

Each arch also receives a branch from the nerve of the succeeding arch. This runs along the caudal border of the arch. This is known as the pretrematic nerve of the arch.

Q. Discuss the derivatives of the skeletal elements of all pharyngeal arches.

Ans.

First Arch

1. Cartilage of first arch is known as Meckel's cartilage.
2. Incus and malleus are derived from its dorsal end.
3. Ventral part of the cartilage is surrounded by developing mandible and is absorbed.
4. The part of perichondrium from middle ear to mandible forms the anterior ligament of malleus and sphenomandibular ligament.

Second Arch

Cartilage of second arch gives rise to:
1. Stapes.
2. Styloid process.
3. Stylohyoid ligament.
4. Smaller cornu of hyoid bone.
5. Superior part of the body of hyoid bone.

Third Arch

Cartilage of second arch gives rise to:
1. Greater cornu of hyoid bone.
2. Lower part of the body of hyoid bone.

Fourth and Sixth Arches

Cartilages of larynx develop from these arches.

Q. What are the nerves of each pharyngeal arch?

Ans.

1. First arch—mandibular nerve (mandibular nerve is the post-trematic nerve of the first arch, while the chorda tympani nerve is the pretrematic nerve of the first arch).

2. Second arch—facial nerve.
3. Third arch—glossopharyngeal nerve.
4. Fourth arch—superior laryngeal nerve.
5. Sixth arch—recurrent laryngeal nerve.

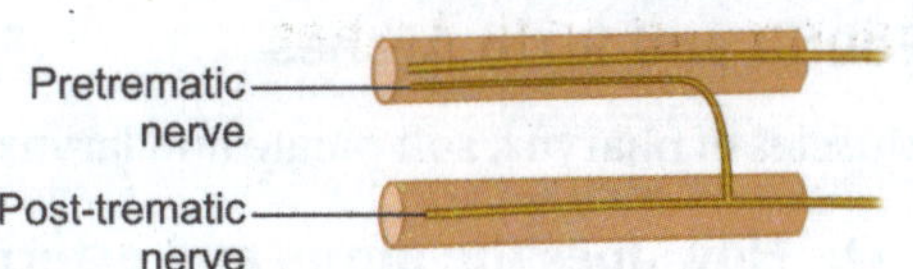

Q. What are the muscles developing from each arch?

Ans.

First Arch

Tensor tympani, tensor palati, medial and lateral pterygoids, masseter, temporalis, mylohyoid and anterior belly of digastric.

Second Arch

Stapedius, stylohyoid, posterior belly of digastric, muscles of the face, auricular muscles, occipitofrontalis and platysma.

Third Arch

Stylopharyngeus.

Derivatives of the skeletal elements of pharyngeal arches

Fourth and Sixth Arches

Muscles of pharynx, soft palate and larynx.

Q. How does the pinna and external auditory meatus develop?

Ans.

1. The dorsal part of the first cleft develops into the epithelial lining of external auditory meatus.
2. The pinna is formed from the series of swellings that arise around the first and the second arch, where they adjoin the first cleft.
3. Swellings around the mandibular arch form the tragus, while rest of the auricle develops from the hyoid arch.

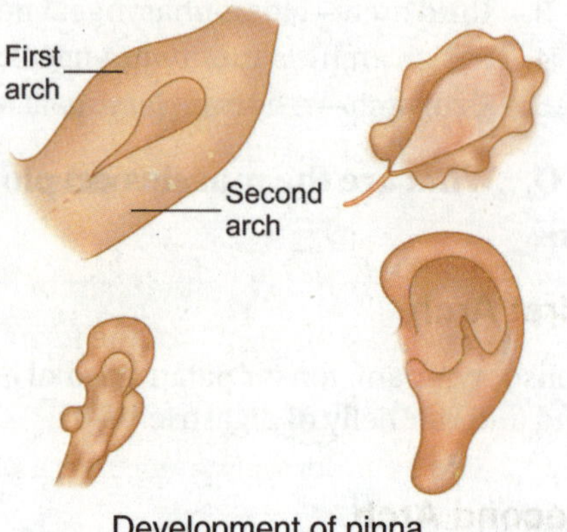

Development of pinna

Q. What is cervical sinus?

Ans. The second arch grows much faster than the succeeding arches and overhangs them. The space between the overhanging second arch and third, fourth and sixth arches is called the cervical sinus.

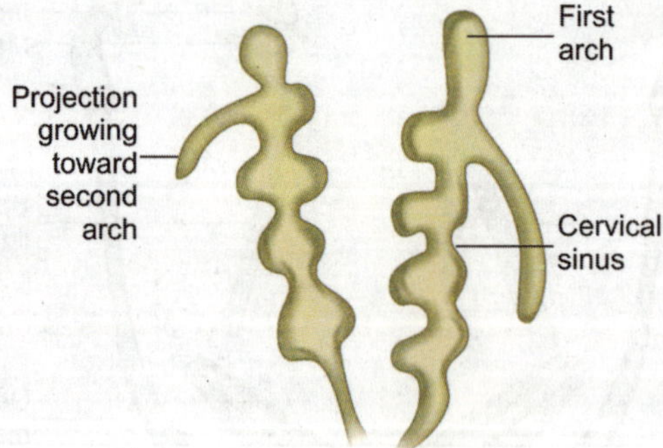

Cervical sinus

Q. What is the embryological basis of branchial cyst and branchial sinus?

Ans. Normally, the cavity of cervical sinus gets obliterated. Sometimes part of the cavity may persist and gives rise to swellings that lie in the neck along the anterior border of sterno-cleidomastoid, these are branchial cysts. If such a cyst opens on the surface, it becomes branchial sinus.

Q. What is the fate of first pharyngeal pouch?

Ans.

1. Ventral part of first pharyngeal pouch gets obliterated due to formation of tongue.
2. Dorsal part of first pouch and a part of second pouch form a diverticulum toward developing ear. This diverticulum is called tubotympanic recess.

Q. What is the fate of the tubotympanic recess?

Ans.

1. Proximal part of tubotympanic recess gives rise to auditory tube.
2. Distal part of tubotympanic recess gives rise to middle ear cavity.

Q. Discuss the fate of second pharyngeal pouch.

Ans.

1. Epithelium of the ventral part of this pouch contributes to the formation of tonsil.
2. Dorsal part takes part in the formation of the tubotympanic recess.

Q. Third endodermal pouch gives rise to which structures?

Ans. Third endodermal pouch gives rise to inferior parathyroid glands and thymus.

Q. What is the fate of fourth endodermal pouch?

Ans. Fourth endodermal pouch gives rise to superior parathyroid glands and may contribute to thyroid gland.

Q. What is the fate of ultimobranchial body?

Ans. Ultimobranchial body gives rise to parafollicular cells of thyroid gland.

Q. Draw a diagram to show the fate of pharyngeal pouches.

Ans.

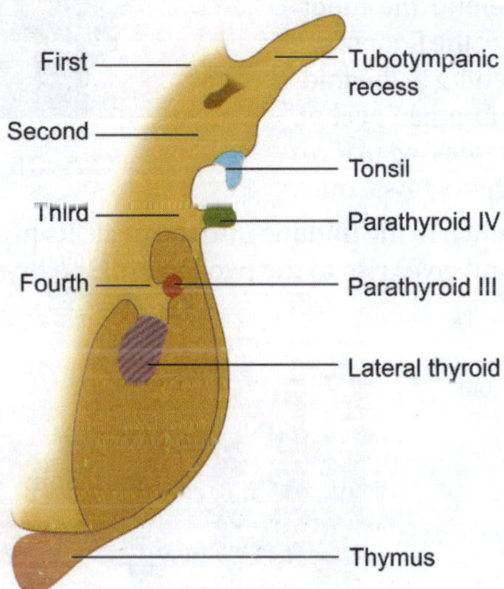

Q. Discuss the development of parathyroid glands.

Ans.

1. Endoderm of third pharyngeal pouch gives rise to inferior parathyroid gland (parathyroid IV).

2. Endoderm of fourth pharyngeal pouch gives rise to superior parathyroid gland (parathyroid III).

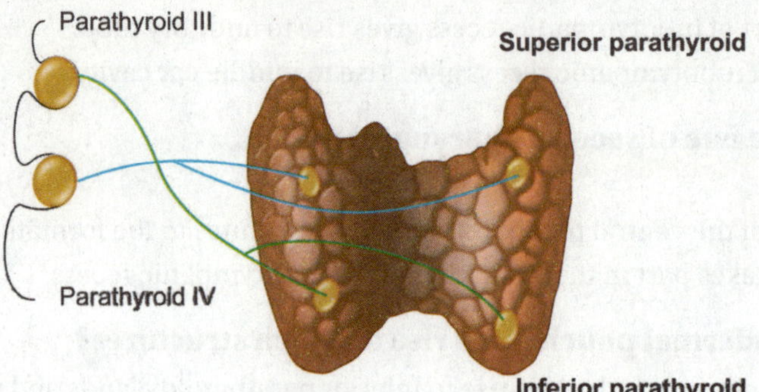

Parathyroid gland

Third pouch also gives rise to thymus; this organ is closely related to parathyroid III. When the thymus descends towards the thorax parathyroid III is carried caudally along with it.

Q. Discuss the development of thyroid gland.

Ans. Thyroid gland appears as a structure in the midline in between the two mandibular arches known as tuberculum impar. Immediately behind the tuberculum, the epithelium of the floor of the pharynx shows a thickening in the midline. This is the site of foramen cecum. This region soon gets depressed to form a diverticulum called thyroglossal duct.

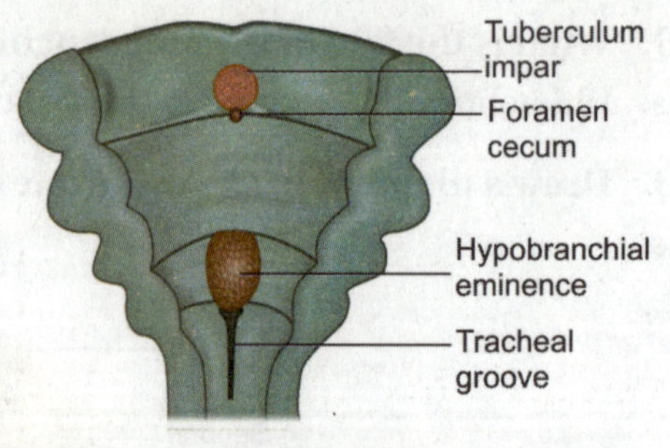

Thyroid gland

The diverticulum grows down in the midline into the neck. Its tip soon bifurcates. Proliferation of the cells of this bifid end gives rise to the two lobes of the thyroid gland.

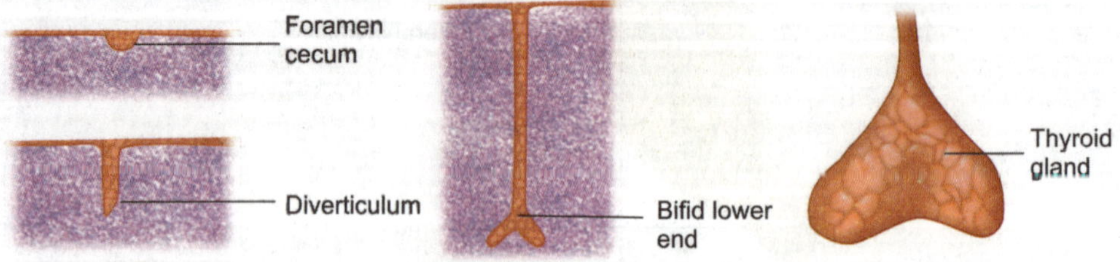

Development of thyroid gland

Q. Discuss the anomalies of thyroid gland.

Ans. Anomalies of thyroid gland can be classified under following headings.

Anomalies of the Shape

1. The pyramidal lobe may arise from isthmus or from one of the lobes.
2. The isthmus may be absent.
3. One of the lobes may be small.

Anomalies of the Position

1. Lingual thyroid—the thyroid tissue may be under the mucosa of the tongue.
2. Suprahyoid thyroid—the gland may lie in the midline of the neck.
3. Infrahyoid thyroid.
4. Intrathoracic.

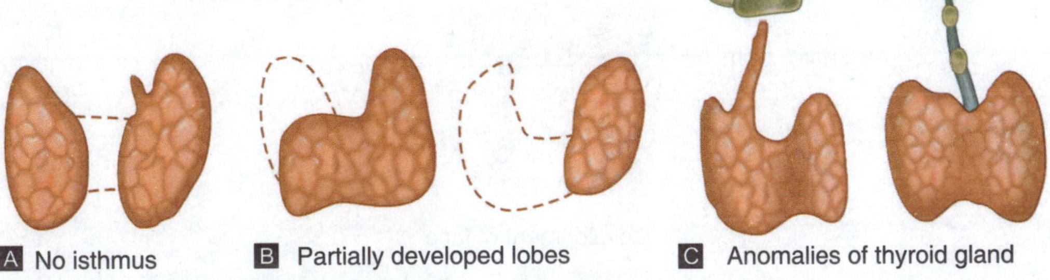

Ectopic Thyroid Tissue

Small masses of thyroid tissue have been observed in the larynx, trachea, esophagus, pons, pleura, pericardium and ovaries.

Remnants of thyroglossal duct may be in the form of thyroglossal cysts or thyroglossal fistula.

Q. Trace the path of thyroglossal duct (diagram only).

Ans.

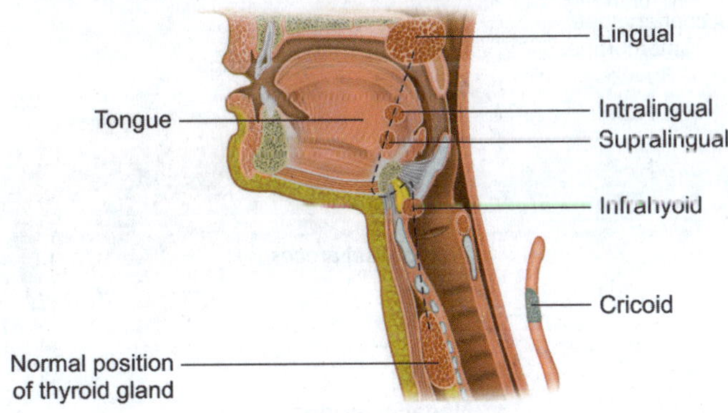

Path of thyroglossal duct

Q. What embryological structures take part in the formation of face?

Ans. The face is derived from following embryological structures:

1. Frontonasal process.
2. First pharyngeal or mandibular arch.

Q. What is frontonasal process?

Ans. Mesoderm over the developing forebrain proliferates and forms a downward projection that overlaps the upper part of the stomodeum. This forms the frontonasal process.

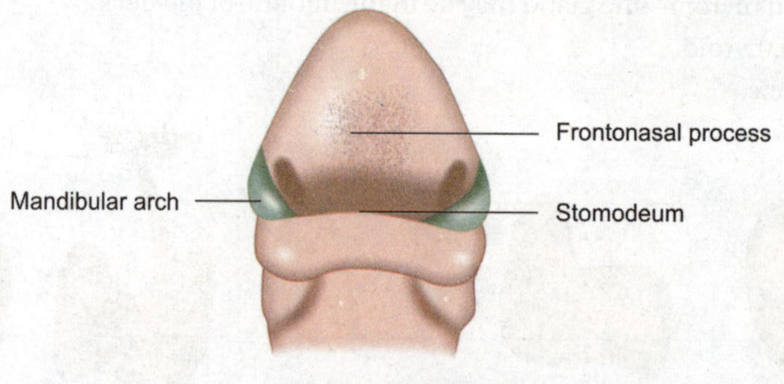

Development of face

Q. What are nasal placodes?

Ans. The ectoderm over the frontonasal process shows bilateral localized thickenings. These are called nasal placodes. The nasal placodes soon sink to form nasal pits. The edges of nasal pits are raised above the surface, the medial raised edge is called medial nasal process and lateral edge is called lateral nasal process.

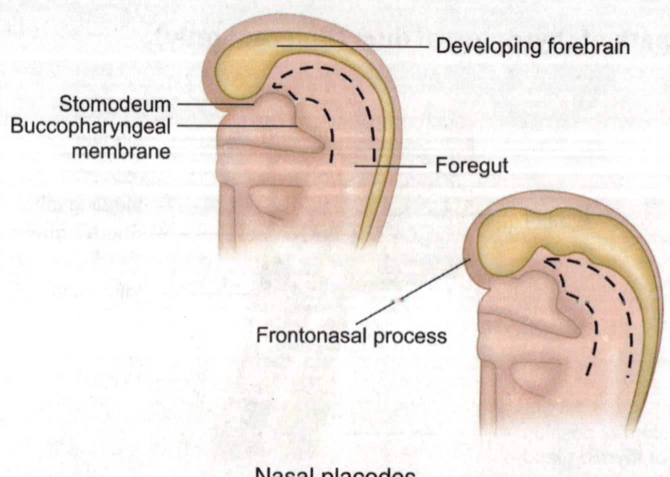

Nasal placodes

Q. Describe the formation of lower lip.

Ans. Mandibular process of the two sides grows toward each other and fuses in the midline to form the lower lip. The mouth develops from the stomodeum.

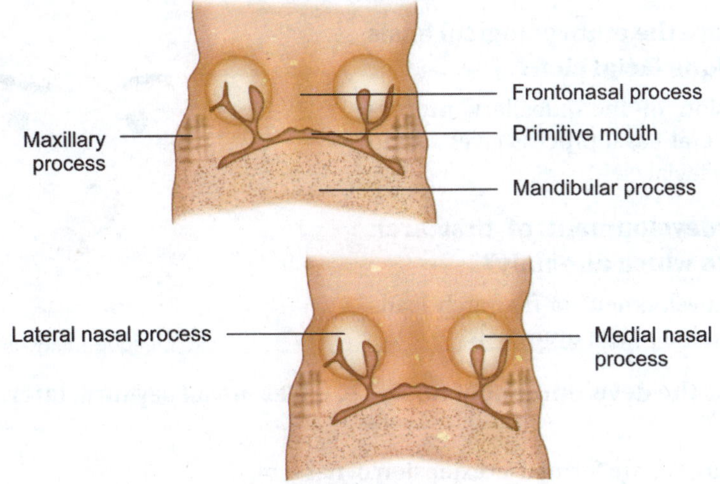

Formation of lower lip

Q. Discuss the formation of upper lip.

Ans. Each maxillary process grows medially and fuses with the lateral nasal process, and then the medial nasal process. The two nasal processes also fuse with each other. All the above mentioned structures contribute to the formation of upper lip.

Q. What structures form the philtrum?

Ans. Frontonasal process forms the philtrum.

Q. What is the origin of the muscles of the face?

Ans. Muscles of the face are derived from second branchial arch and are therefore supplied by the facial nerve.

Q. Depict derivatives of the face in the form of a diagram.

Ans.

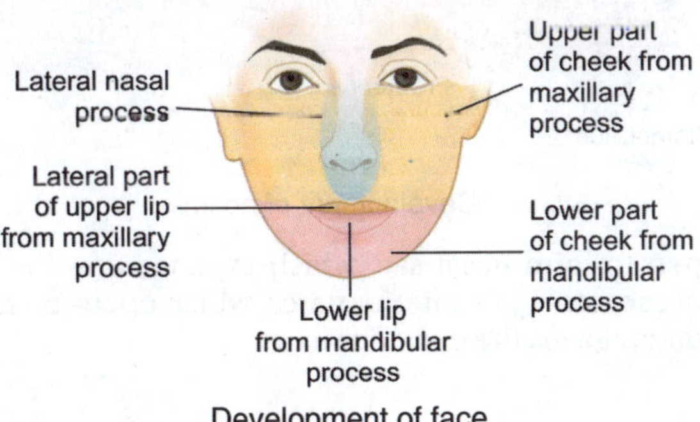

Development of face

Q. Discuss the embryological basis of harelip, i.e. cleft lip.

Ans. Nonfusion of the maxillary process with medial nasal process gives rise to the defects of upper lip.

Q. What are the embryological basis of oblique facial cleft?

Ans. Nonfusion of the maxillary process with lateral nasal process gives rise to oblique facial cleft.

Q. Underdevelopment of first arch leads to which anomaly?

Ans. Underdevelopment of first arch leads to mandibulofacial dysostosis.

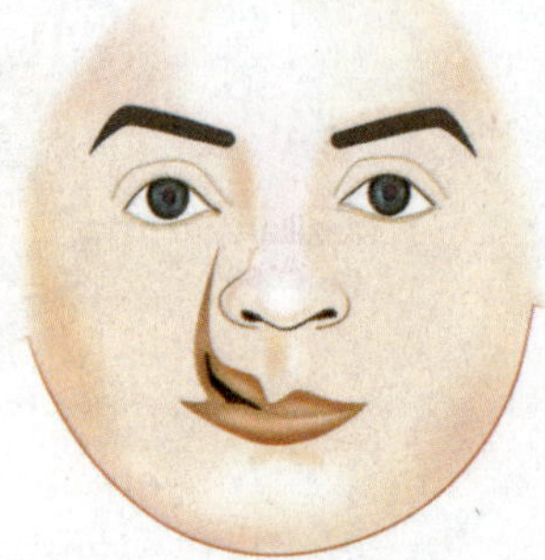

Oblique facial cleft

Q. Discuss the development of nose, i.e. nares, nasal septum, lateral nasal wall.

Ans.

1. Nasal cavities are formed as extension of nasal pits.

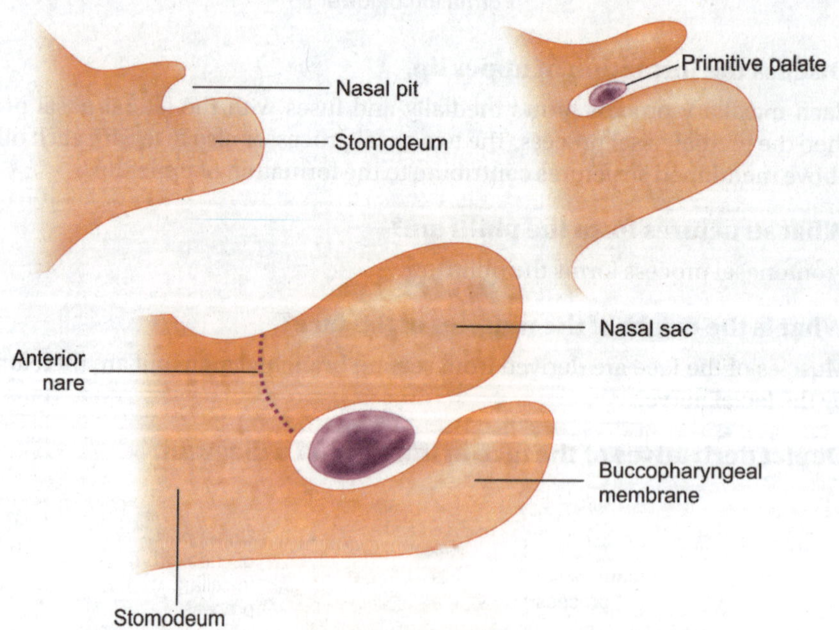

Development of nose

2. Nasal pits deepen to form nasal sac, which expands dorsally and caudally. Anterior opening of nasal sac forms the anterior nares, which opens on the face. Dorsal opening into the stomodeum forms the posterior nares.

3. The nasal sacs are separated from each other by frontonasal process. With the enlargement of nasal sacs the frontonasal process diminishes in size to form the nasal septum.

4. Lateral wall of the nose is derived from lateral nasal process.

Q. How do the paranasal sinuses develop?

Ans. The paranasal sinuses appear as a diverticuli from nasal cavities. The diverticuli grow within the facial bones after which they are named. Maxillary and sphenoidal sinuses begin to develop before birth and are rudimentary at birth. Frontal and ethmoidal sinuses begin to develop after birth.

Q. Discuss the embryological basis of palatal development.

Ans. Three components contribute to the development of palate:

1. Primitive palate, which develops from the frontonasal process.

2. Palatal process, which is an outgrowth of maxillary process.

3. Medial edge of palatal process fuse with lower edge of nasal septum.

   Mesoderm in the palate undergoes intramembranous ossification to form the hard palate. This ossification fails to extend backwards; this unossified part forms the soft palate.

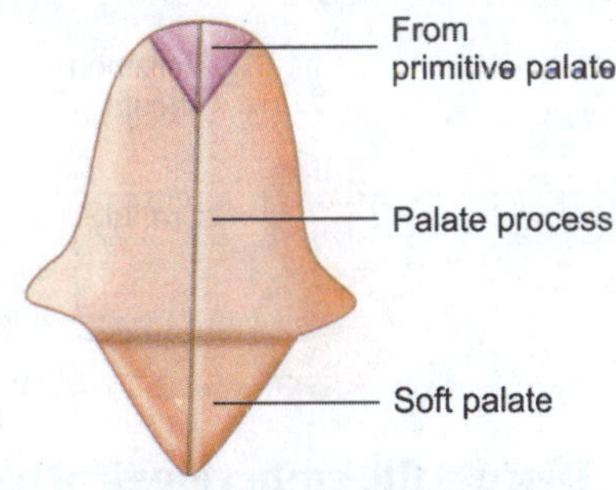

Development of palate

Q. Why are cleft palates associated with cleft lips?

Ans. Both upper lip and palate develop from fusion of maxillary process with frontonasal process.

Q. What is the embryological basis of cleft palate?

Ans. Defective fusion of various components of palate, i.e. premaxilla and palatal process.

Q. Discuss the development of tongue.

Ans. Development of tongue can be discussed under following headings:

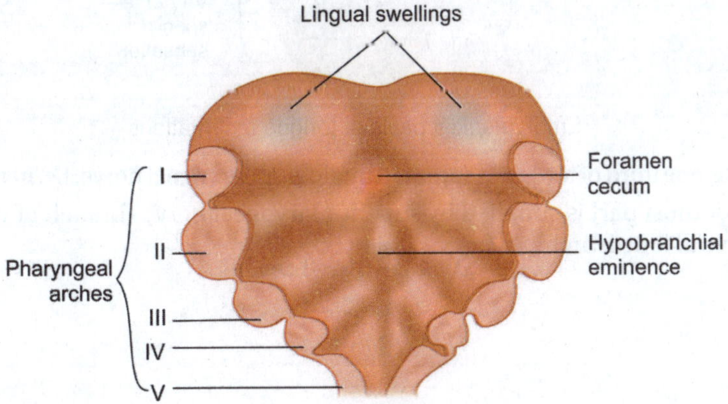

1. Development of anterior two third of tongue develops from:
   a. Lingual swellings.
   b. Tuberculum impar.
   c. Cranial part of hypobranchial eminence.
2. Development of posterior one third of tongue. The third pharyngeal arch grows over the second and thus contributes to the development of posterior one third of tongue.

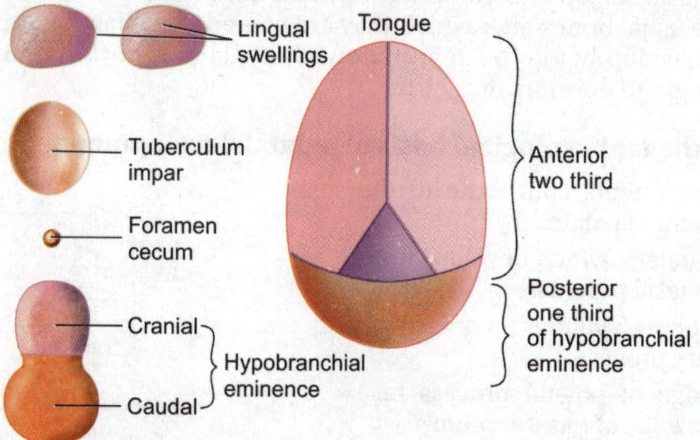

Q. Discuss the embryological basis of tongue innervations.

Ans.

1. Anterior two third of tongue is supplied by lingual branch of mandibular nerve, which is the post-trematic nerve of first arch and by the chorda tympani, which is the pretrematic nerve of this arch.

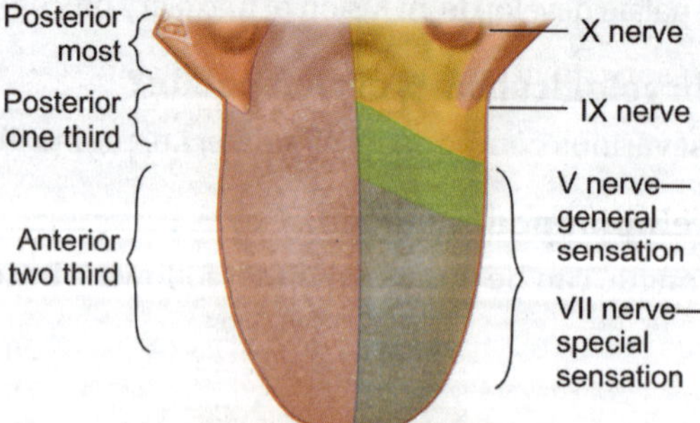

Embryological basis of tongue innervations

2. Posterior one third of tongue is supplied by glossopharyngeal nerve, i.e. nerve of third arch.
3. Posterior most part is supplied by superior laryngeal nerve (branch of vagus), which is the nerve of fourth arch.

Q. Discuss the origin of muscles of tongue.

Ans. Musculature of tongue is derived from occipital myotomes. Occipital myotomes are supplied by hypoglossal nerve thus the muscles of the tongue.

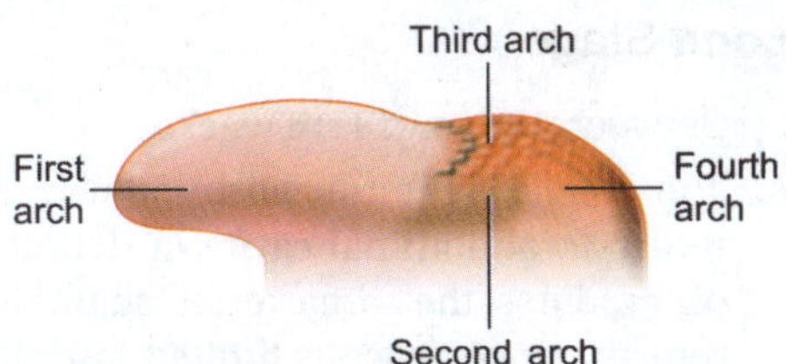

Q. In relation to which pouch palatine tonsils develop?

Ans. Palatine tonsils develop in relation to second pharyngeal pouch.

Q. Draw a diagram showing parts of the primitive gut.

Ans.

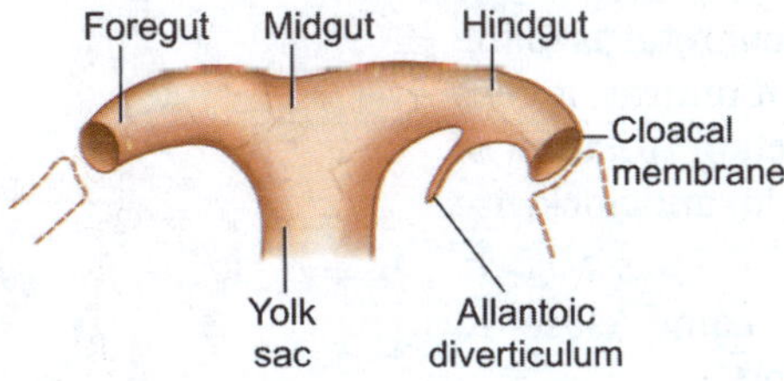

Q. What are the arteries of primitive gut?

Ans.

1. The artery of abdominal part of foregut is celiac artery.
2. The artery of midgut is superior mesenteric artery.
3. The artery of hindgut is inferior mesenteric artery.

Q. Discuss rotation of midgut loop.

Ans. Rotation of midgut loop can be studied in three stages

First Stage

1. Between 5th and 10th weeks in umbilical cord.
2. Development of liver, forces the portion of midgut proximal to superior mesenteric artery, downwards and to the right.
3. Thus the postarterial segment goes upwards and to the left.
4. Viewed from ventral side, the loop undergoes anticlockwise rotation by 90°, so that it lies in horizontal plane.
5. The prearterial segment now undergoes great increase in length to form coils of jejunum.

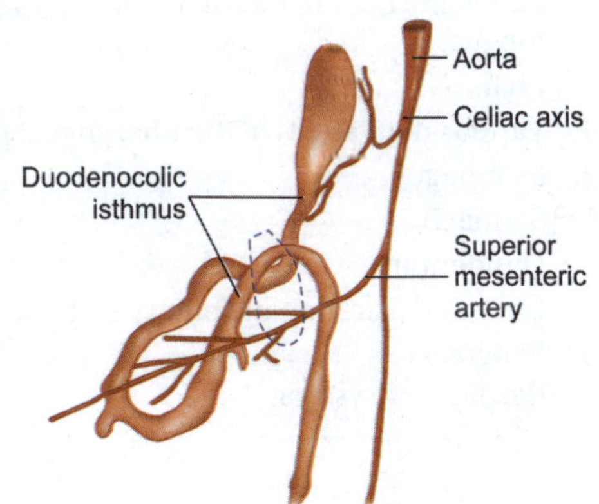

Second Stage

1. Between 10th and 11th weeks.
2. The coils of jejunum and ileum now return to abdominal cavity in definite order. First the prearterial segment returns, since space is limited in right side, further coils of intestine enter left side of abdominal cavity. As they do so the midgut loop undergoes a further anticlockwise rotation. As a result, the coils of jejunum and ileum pass behind the superior mesenteric artery. Finally the postarterial segment returns to the abdominal cavity. As it returns, it goes in anticlockwise direction (rotation of the gut takes place in anticlockwise direction).
3. Eventually the coils come close to adult intestinal position.

Third Stage

1. From 11th week to shortly after birth.
2. Cecum lies in right iliac fossa.
3. Mesentery of cecum, ascending colon, hepatic flexure and hindgut get obliterated.

Q. What are the derivatives of foregut?

Ans. Derivatives of foregut are as follows:

1. Part of the floor of mouth including the tongue.
2. Pharynx.
3. Various derivatives of the pharyngeal pouches and the thyroid.
4. Esophagus.
5. Stomach.
6. Duodenum.
7. Liver and extrahepatic biliary system.
8. Pancreas.
9. Respiratory system.

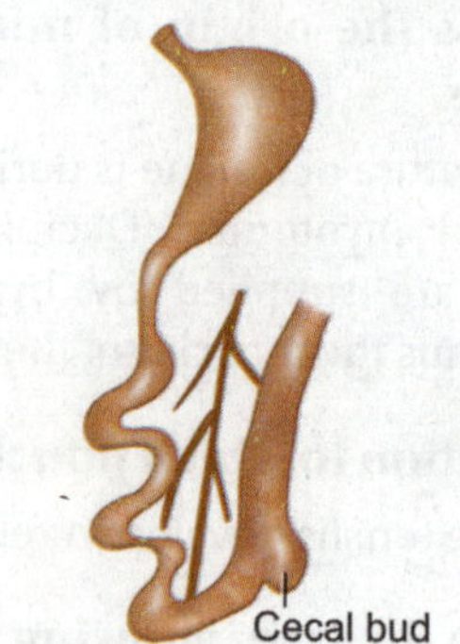

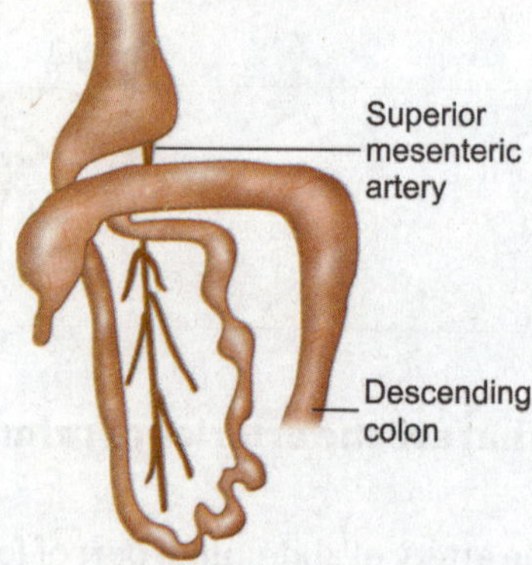

Rotation of midgut

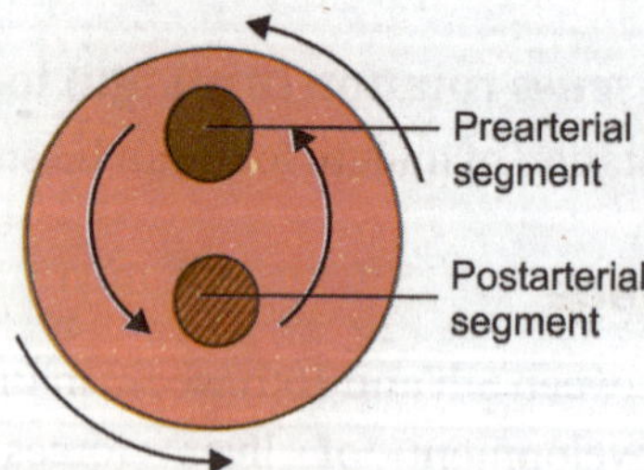

Q. What are the subdivisions of cloaca?

Ans. With the formation of urorectal septum, cloaca divides into primitive urogenital and rectum (dorsally).

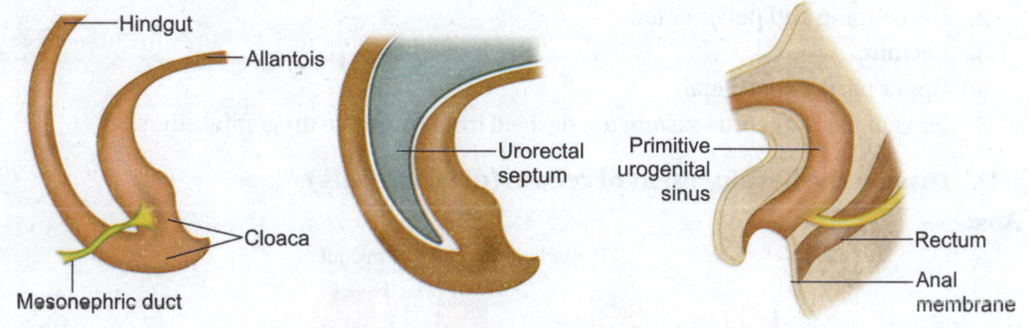

Subdivisions of cloaca

Q. Draw a diagram showing derivatives of primitive gut.

Ans.

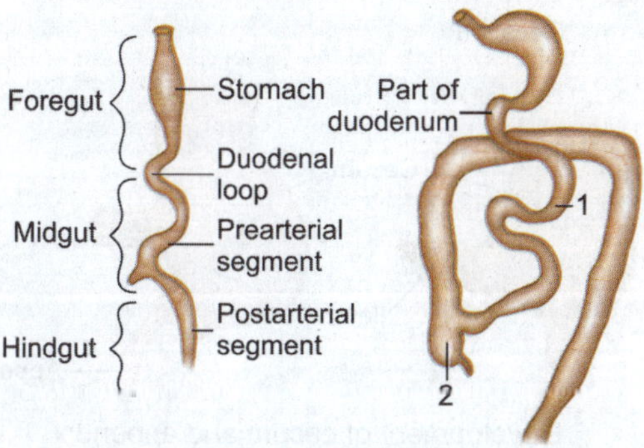

1. Duodenum below entry of bile duct, jejunum and most of ileum from prearterial segment of midgut.

2. Terminal ileum, cecum, ascending colon, right two third of transverse colon from postarterial segment of midgut.

Q. What are the derivatives of midgut?

Ans. Following are the derivatives of midgut:

1. Duodenum.
2. Jejunum.
3. Ileum.
4. Cecum and appendix.
5. Ascending colon.
6. Right two third of transverse colon.

Q. **What are the derivatives of hindgut?**

Ans. Following are the derivatives of hindgut:
1. Left one third of transverse colon.
2. Descending and pelvic colon.
3. Rectum.
4. Upper part of anal canal.
5. Parts of the urogenital system are derived from primitive urogenital sinus.

Q. **Discuss the development of cecum (diagram only).**

Ans.

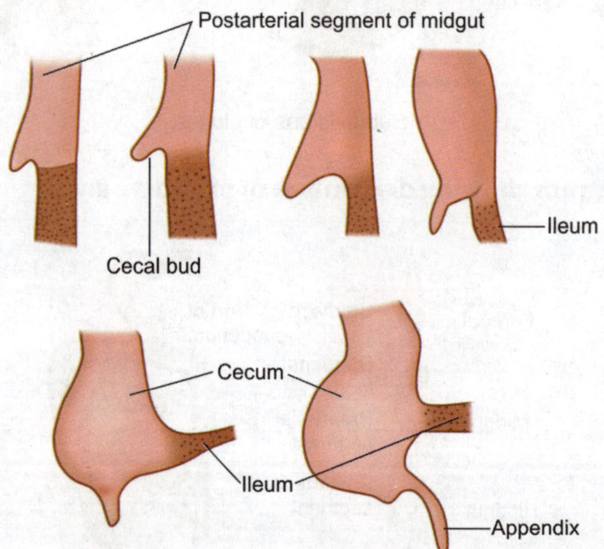

Development of cecum and appendix

Ans. Cecal bud is a diverticulum that arises from the postarterial segment of midgut loop. The cecum and appendix are formed by enlargement of this bud.

Q. **Discuss the developmental anomalies of the gut.**

Ans.

Congenital Obstruction

1. Atresia—continuity of the lumen is interfered.
2. Stenosis—narrowing of the lumen.
3. Abnormal thickening of the muscular wall is seen at the pyloric end of the stomach.
4. External pressure by abnormal peritoneal bands.

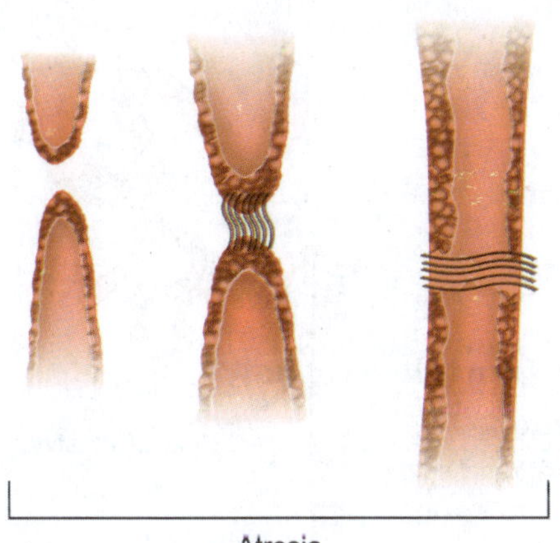
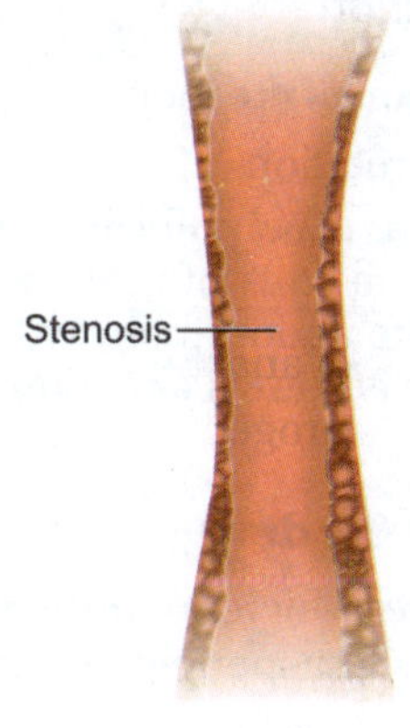

Anomalies of gut

Abnormal Communications

Tracheoesophageal fistula.

Duplication

Various lengths of intestine may get duplicated.

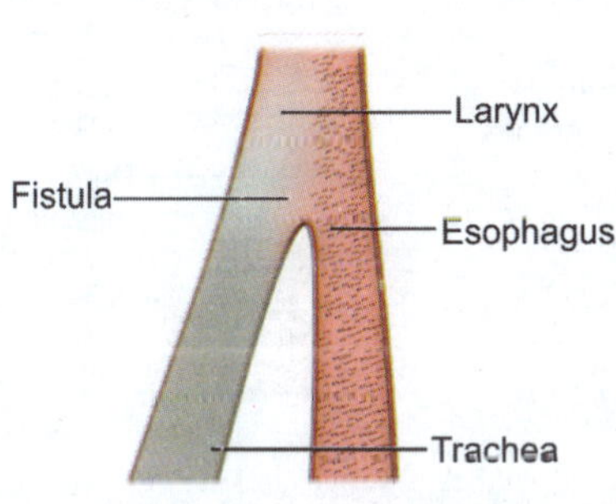

Tracheoesophageal fistula

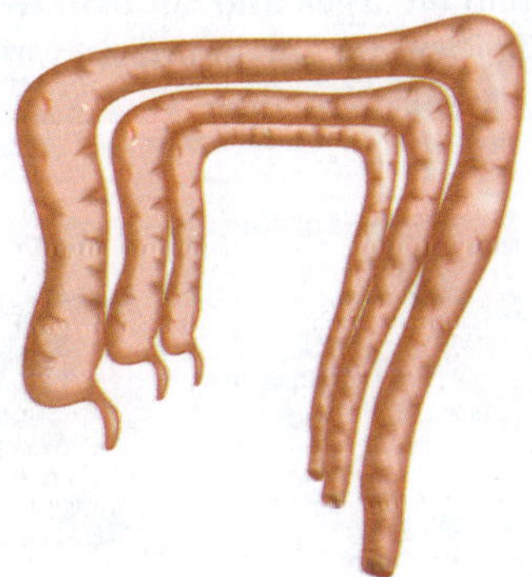

Intestinal duplication

Diverticuli

Persistence of vitellointestinal duct may give rise to the presence of diverticulum attached to the terminal part of ileum. This is called Meckel's diverticulum.

Errors of Rotation

- Nonrotation of the loop
- Reversed rotation
- Nonreturn of umbilical hernia, i.e. wherein the coils of intestine remain outside the abdominal cavity. Such a condition is known as exomphalos.

Errors of Fixation

Parts of intestine, which are normally retroperitoneal may get suspended by mesentery.

Situs Inversus

There is a lateral inversion of all the abdominal organs (e.g. liver is on the left side, heart on right side).

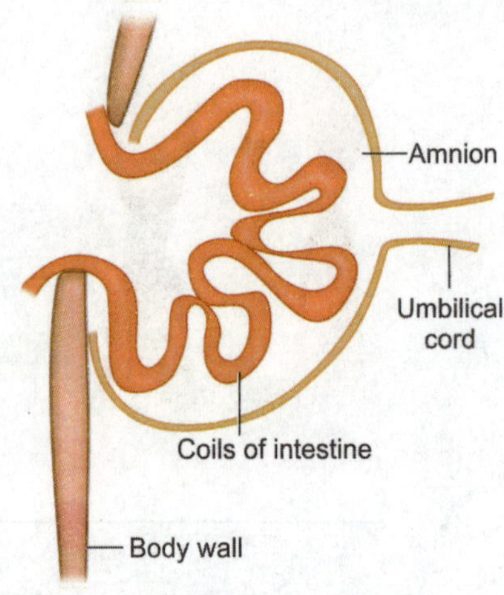

Exomphalos

Q. Discuss the development of liver.

Ans. Liver develops from an endodermal bud that arises from the ventral aspect of the gut at the point of junction between foregut and midgut. This bud grows into ventral mesogastrium and passes through it into the septum transversum.

This bud enlarges and soon shows a division into larger cranial part called pars hepatica and smaller caudal portion pars cystica. Pars hepatica divides into right and left parts, which forms the lobes of the liver.

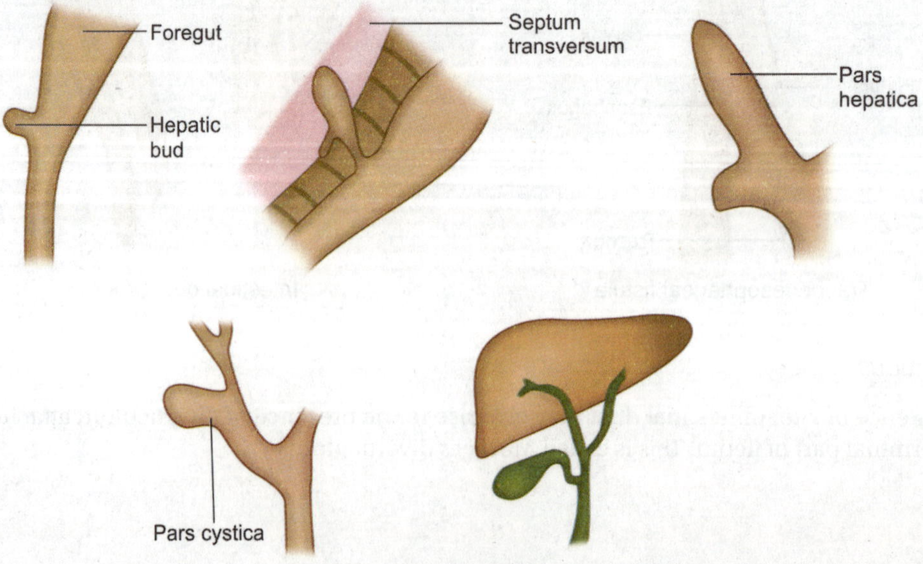

Development of liver

Q. Which embryonic structure gives rise to gallbladder?

Ans. Pars cystica gives rise to gallbladder.

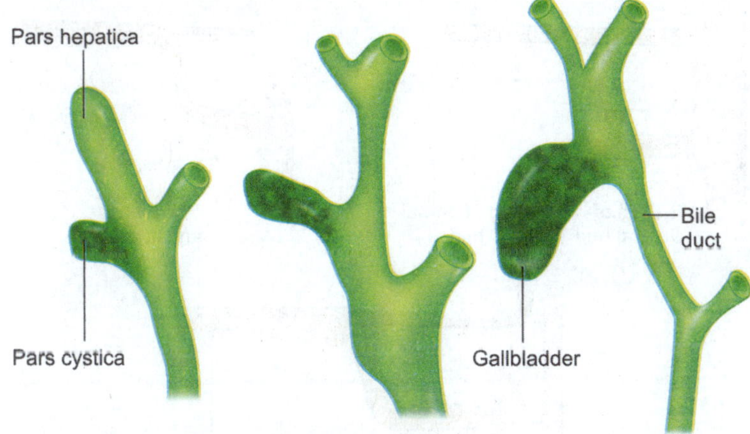

Development of gallbladder

Q. How does the pancreas develop?

Ans. Pancreas develops by two buds originating from the endoderm lining of the duodenum:

- Dorsal pancreatic bud is in the dorsal mesentery
- Ventral pancreatic bud is close to the bile duct.

When the duodenum rotates to the right and becomes C-shaped, the ventral pancreatic bud moves dorsally, and comes to lie immediately below and behind the dorsal bud.

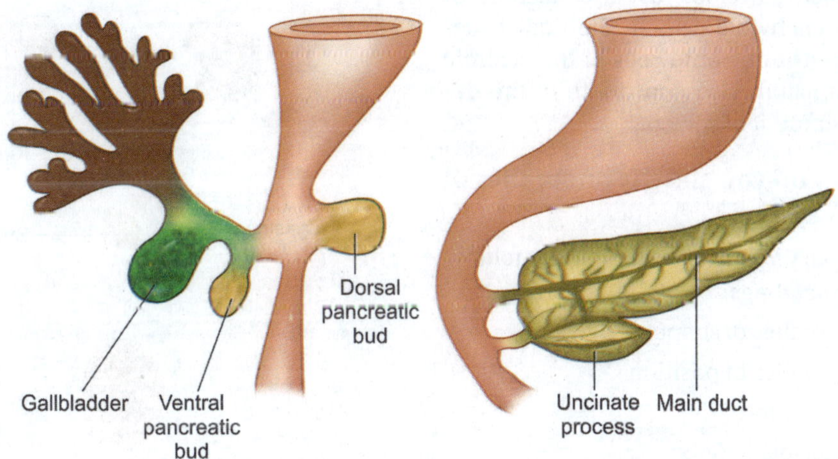

Development of pancreas

Ventral bud forms the lower part of the head and the uncinate process. Dorsal bud forms the upper part of the head, body and tail.

Duct System of Pancreas

The ducts of dorsal and ventral bud anastomose with each other.

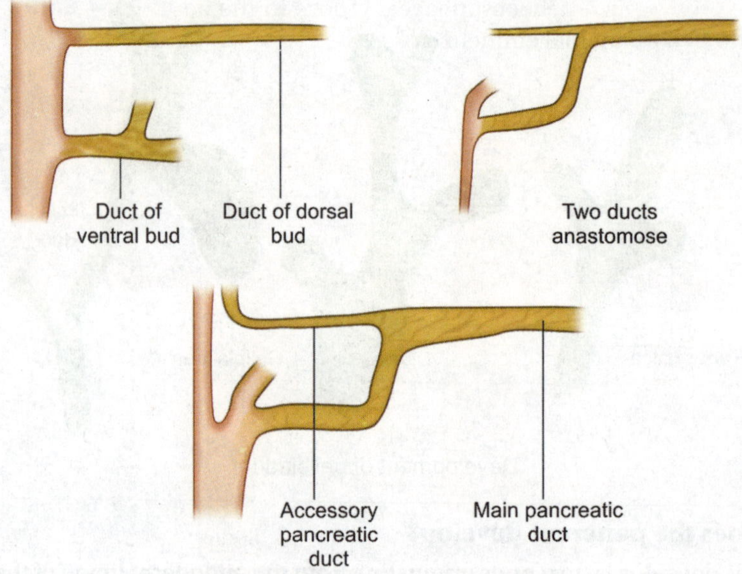

Duct system of pancreas

Part of dorsal duct proximal to anastomosis forms accessory pancreatic duct. Main pancreatic duct is a combination of ventral duct and dorsal duct distal to the anastomosis.

Q. How does the spleen develop?

Ans. Spleen develops as a collection of mesenchymal cells in the dorsal mesogastrium. Some cells of the celomic epithelium also contribute in the development of spleen.

Q. How do you classify anomalies of any system?

Ans. Anomalies are classified under following headings:

- Anomalies of shape
- Anomalies of position
- Duplication
- Abnormal length
- Abnormal termination
- Nondevelopment of duct, i.e. atresia
- Accessory tissue at ectopic sites.

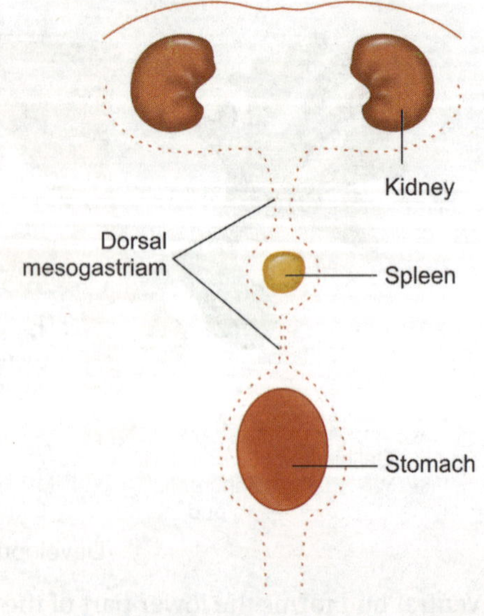

Spleen development

Q. How does the respiratory diverticulum develop? What is its fate?

Ans. The diverticulum, which is destined to form respiratory system is initially spotted as midline groove, i.e. tracheoesophageal groove in the floor of developing pharynx just caudal to hypobranchial eminence.

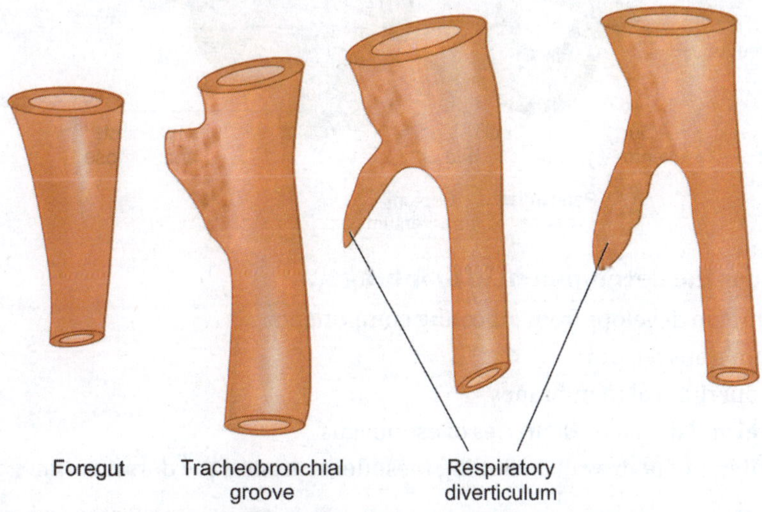

Respiratory diverticulum formation

This groove is flanked by sixth pharyngeal arches. The free caudal end of the diverticulum becomes bifid giving rise to lung bud.

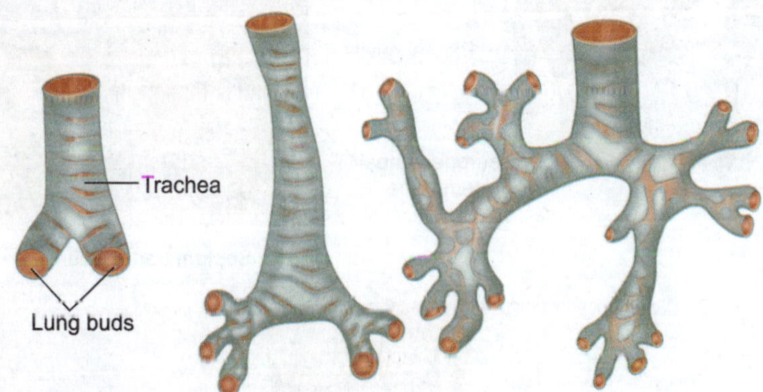

Respiratory diverticulum gives rise to larynx, trachea, bronchi and lung parenchyma. The connective tissue, cartilage and muscle in relation to the organs of respiratory system are derived from splanchnopleuric mesoderm.

Q. Cavities of the body develop from which structure?

Ans. The pericardial, pleural and peritoneal cavities are derivatives of the intraembryonic celom.

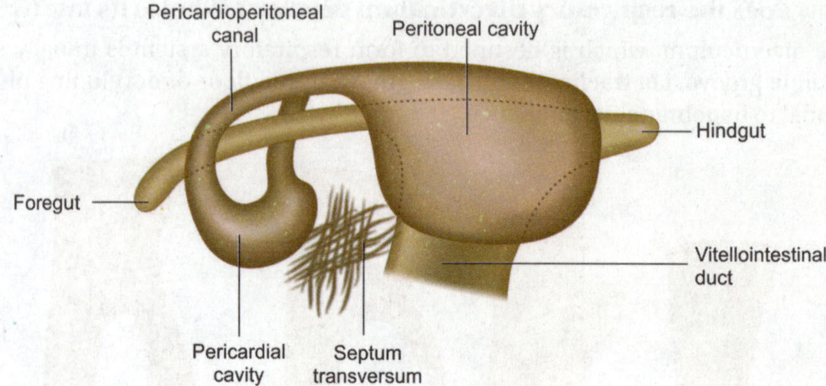

Q. Discuss the development of diaphragm.

Ans. Diaphragm develops from following components:

- Septum transversum
- Pleuroperitoneal membranes
- Ventral and dorsal mesenteries of esophagus
- Mesoderm of body wall, including mesoderm around the dorsal aorta.

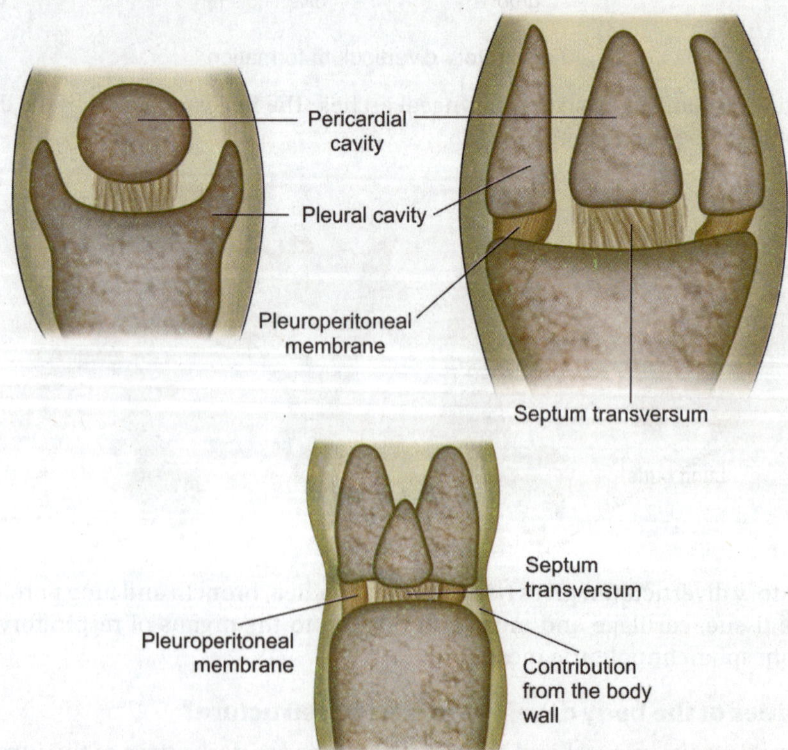

Development of diaphragm

Q. **Give the embryological basis of the innervation of diaphragm.**

Ans. Diaphragm is supplied by C3, C4, C5 and intercostal nerve. Innervation by C3, C4 and C5 implies the migration of diaphragm to caudal direction. Intercostal nerve innervations depict the contribution of body wall.

Q. **From which embryological structure does the heart develop?**

Ans. The heart develops from angioblastic tissue that arises from this splanchnopleuric mesoderm, i.e. from the cardiogenic area.

Q. **Depict the parts of heart tube.**

Ans.

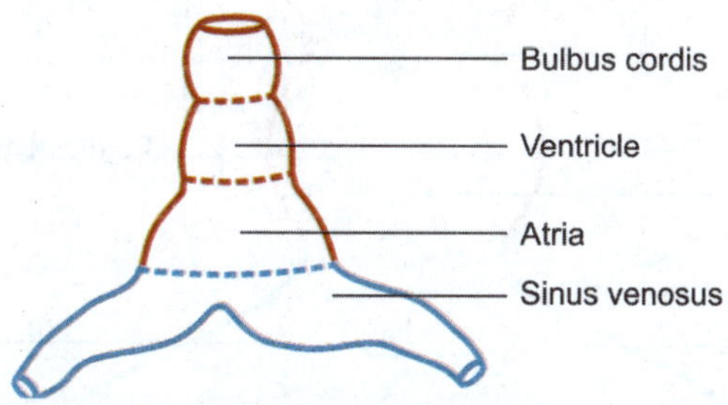

Q. **Which veins drain into sinus venosus?**

Ans. Common cardinal vein, umbilical vein and vitelline vein drains into sinus venosus.

Q. **Which is the arterial end and venous end of the heart tube?**

Ans. Bulbus cordis represents the arterial end of the heart tube, while sinus venosus represents the venous end of the heart tube.

Q. **Discuss the embryological basis of the openings in the right atrium.**

Ans.

1. The body and right horn of sinus venosus are absorbed into common atrial chamber and form part of right atrium.
2. Thus the common cardinal vein, which forms the terminal part of superior vena cava and right vitelline vein forms the terminal part of inferior vena cava, which opens into right atrium.
3. The left horn of the sinus venosus forms part of the coronary sinus, which opens into right atrium.

Q. **What are the derivatives of pericardium?**

Ans. Visceral layer of pericardium is derived from splanchnopleuric mesoderm. The parietal layer is derived from somatopleuric mesoderm.

Q. Depict the fate of heart tube.

Ans.

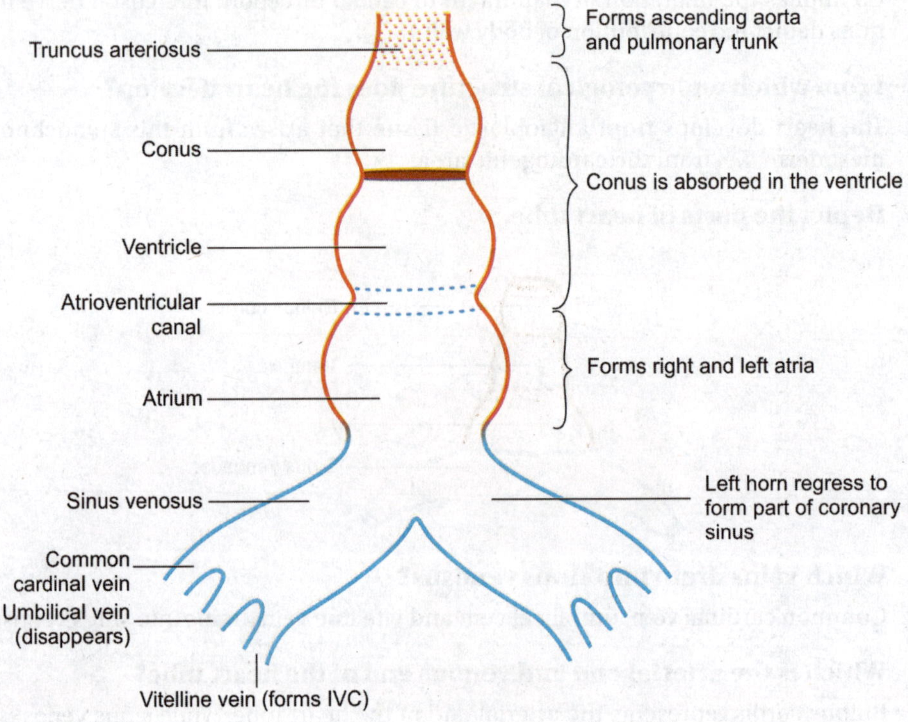

Q. Discuss the fate of sinus venosus (diagram only).

Ans.

1.

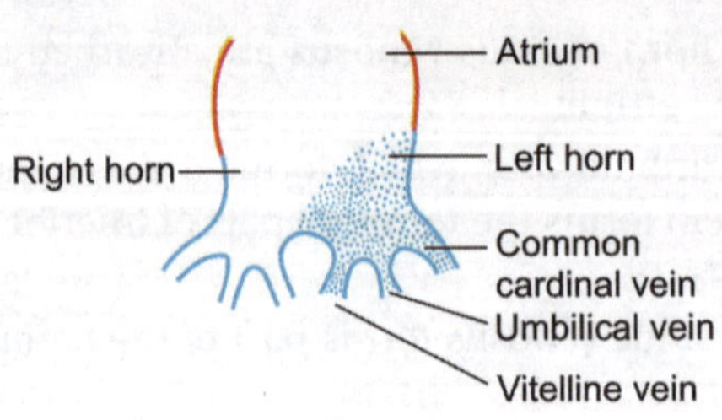

2.

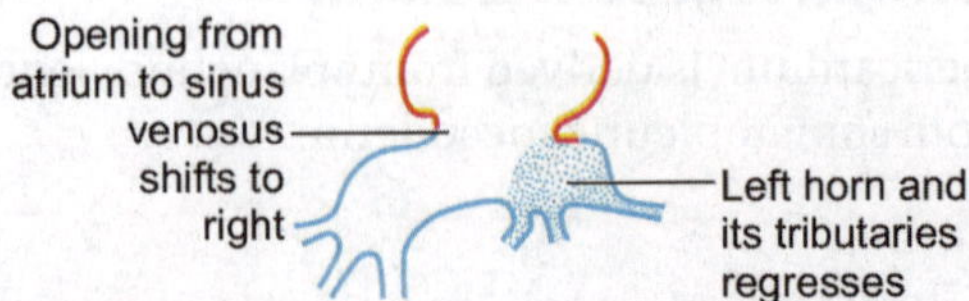

3.

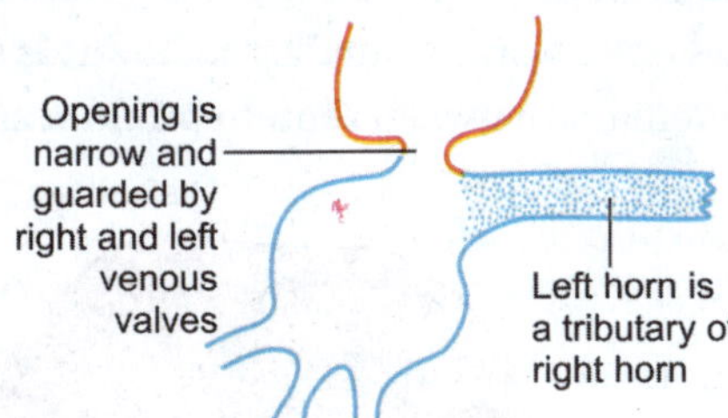

Q. Discuss the formation of interatrial septum.

Ans.

1. A septum arises from the roof of the atrial chamber, a little to the left of the opening of sinus venosus. This is septum primum.

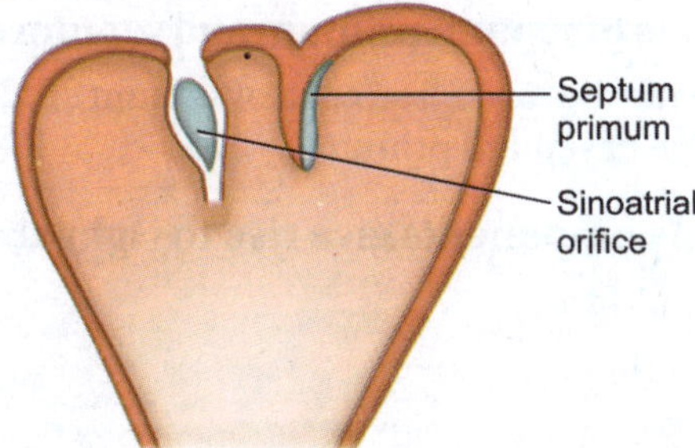

2. The septum primum grows downwards towards atrioventricular cushions.

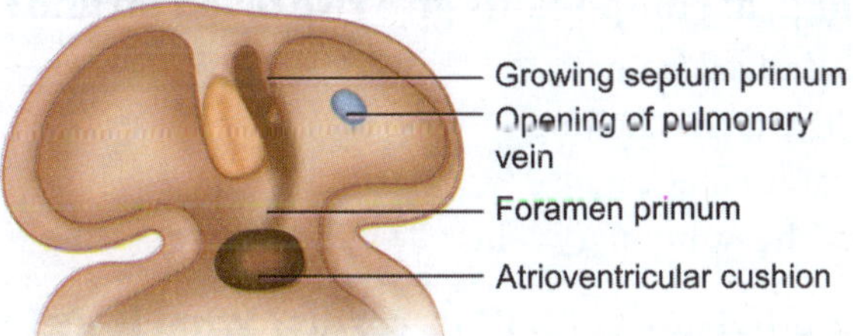

3. A second septum arises from the roof of atrial chamber, i.e. to the right of septum primum.

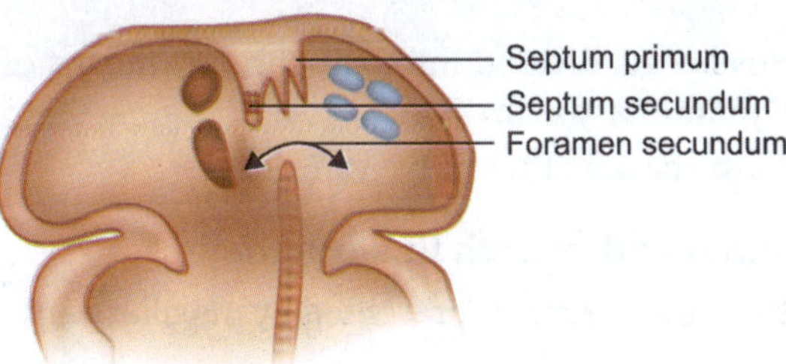

4. As septum gets detached from the roof, it gives rise to foramen secundum.

5. Septum secundum grows downwards from the roof towards septum primum.

6. An oblique valvular gap remains between septum primum and secundum.

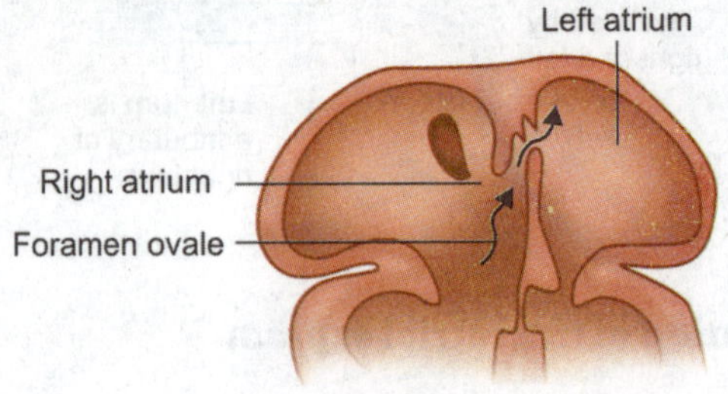

Pressure changes in the atrial chamber closes the foramen ovale.

Q. What are the remnants of septum primum and septum secundum in adult life?

Ans. Annulus ovalis represents the lower free edge of septum secundum. Fossa ovalis represents the lower free edge of septum primum.

Q. What embryological components give rise to right atrium?

Ans. The right atrium develops from:
- Right half of primitive atrium
- Sinus venosus
- Right half of atrioventricular canal.

Q. What embryological components give rise to left atrium?

Ans. The left atrium is derived from:
- Left half of primitive atrial chamber
- Left half of atrioventricular canal
- Absorbed parts of the pulmonary veins.

Q. What are the subdivisions of bulbus cordis? What is their fate?

Ans.
- Bulbus cordis is divisible into proximal part the conus and the distal part called the truncus arteriosus
- The truncus arteriosus gets divided into two parts by means of spiral septum into ascending aorta and pulmonary trunk
- Conus merges with the cavity of primitive ventricle.

Q. What is the remnant of first arch in adult life?

Ans. In adult life, the first arch artery is represented by maxillary artery.

Q. What are the components of interventricular septum?

Ans. Following are the components of interventricular septum:

- Bulbar septum
- Atrioventricular cushions
- Proliferation of tissue from bulboventricular cavity.

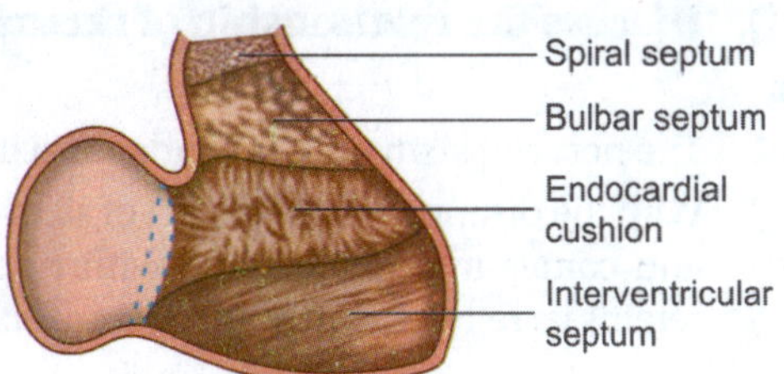

Interventricular septum

Q. Depict the components of tetralogy of Fallot.

Ans.

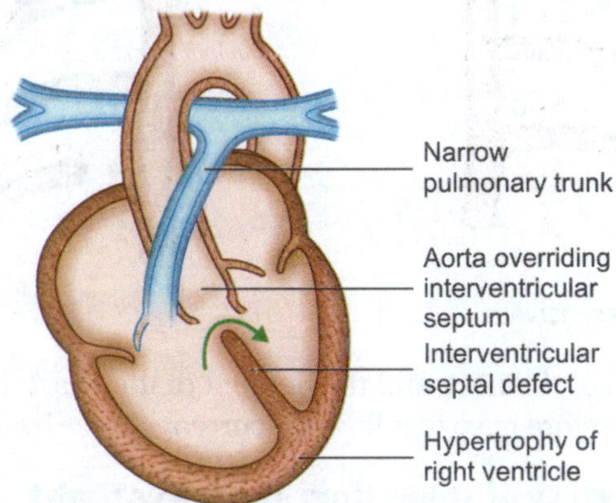

Tetralogy of Fallot components

Q. Give the genesis of following arteries:

- **Ascending aorta and pulmonary trunk**
- **Arch of aorta**
- **Descending aorta**
- **Subclavian artery right and left**
- **External carotid artery.**

Ans.

1. Ascending aorta and pulmonary trunk are formed from truncus arteriosus.
2. Ventral part of aortic sac, left horn and left fourth arch form arch of aorta.
3. Left dorsal aorta below the attachment of fourth arch artery with fused median vessel form descending aorta:

   a. Right fourth arch artery and seventh cervical intersegmental artery form right subclavian artery.

   b. Left subclavian artery is derived from seventh intersegmental artery.

   c. External carotid artery arises as a bud from third arch artery.

Q. Discuss the relationship of recurrent laryngeal nerve on right and left side.

Ans.

1. The nerve of sixth arch is caudal to sixth arch artery on both sides initially.

2. With the disappearance of part of sixth arch artery on right side the nerve moves cranially and comes into relationship with right fourth arch artery (subclavian). On left side, it retains its relationship to that part of sixth arch, which forms ductus arteriosus.

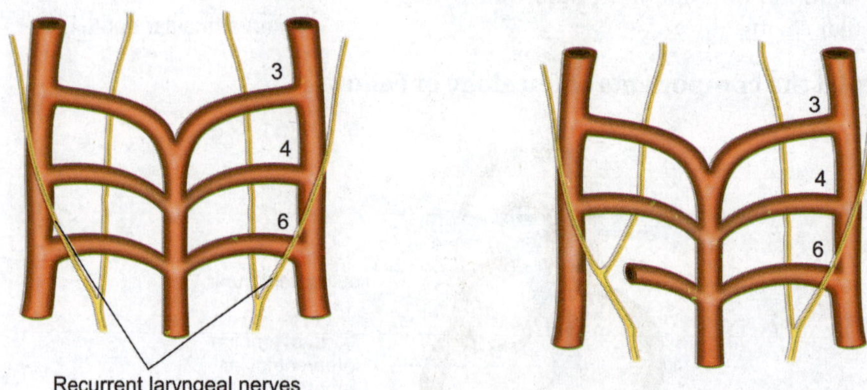

3. With the elongation of the neck and the descent of the heart these nerves are dragged downwards and therefore have to follow a recurrent course back to larynx.

Q. What is the axis artery of upper limb and lower limb?

Ans. Axis artery of the upper limb is formed by the seventh intersegmental artery. Axis artery of lower limb is derived from fifth lumbar intersegmental artery.

Q. How is portal vein formed?

Ans. Portal vein develops from following embryological components:

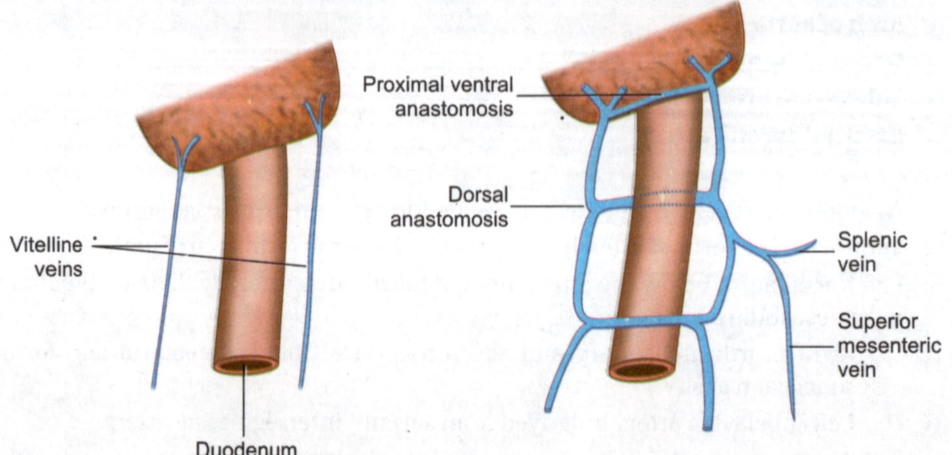

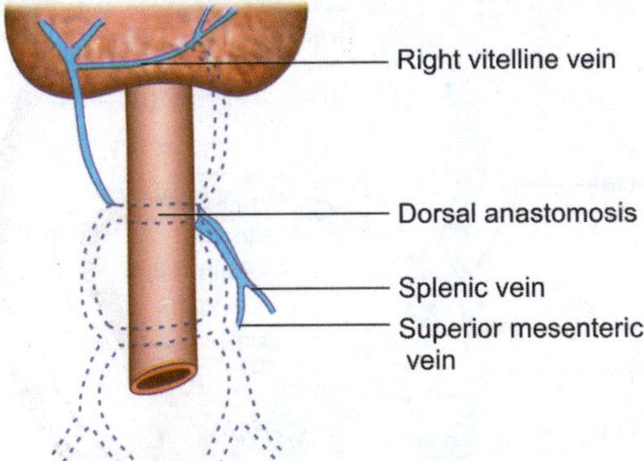

Portal vein formation

- Left vitelline vein between the entry of superior mesenteric and splenic veins and the dorsal anastomosis
- Dorsal anastomosis itself
- Right vitelline vein between the dorsal anastomosis and the cranial ventral anastomosis.

Q. How is superior vena cava formed?

Ans. Superior vena cava is derived from:

- Right anterior cardinal vein caudal to the transverse anastomosis
- Right common cardinal vein.

Q. What are the components of inferior vena cava?

Ans. Following components give rise to inferior vena cava, i.e.:

- Subcardinal veins
- Supracardinal veins
- Subcardinal-hepatocardiac anastomosis
- Hepatocardiac channel
- Supracardinal-subcardinal anastomosis.

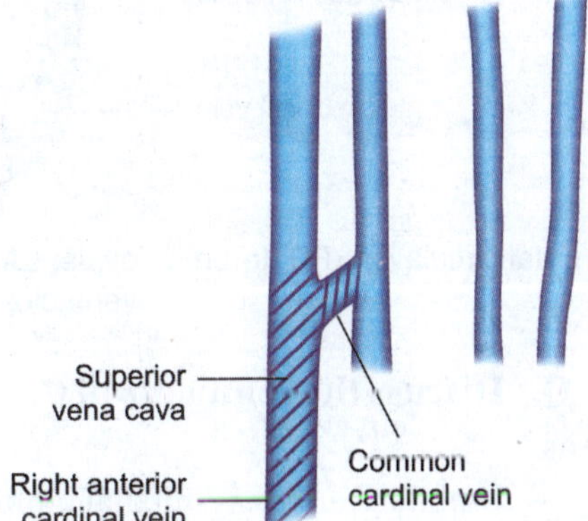

Formation of superior vena cava

Q. Discuss the features of fetal circulation.

Ans.

1. The source of oxygenated blood is placenta.
2. Oxygenated blood from placenta passes through ductus venosus to inferior vena cava.
3. Most of the oxygenated blood from right atrium passes through foramen ovale into left atrium. Rest goes from right atrium into right ventricle.
4. Most of the blood from right ventricle is directed into ductus arteriosus and thence into the aorta.

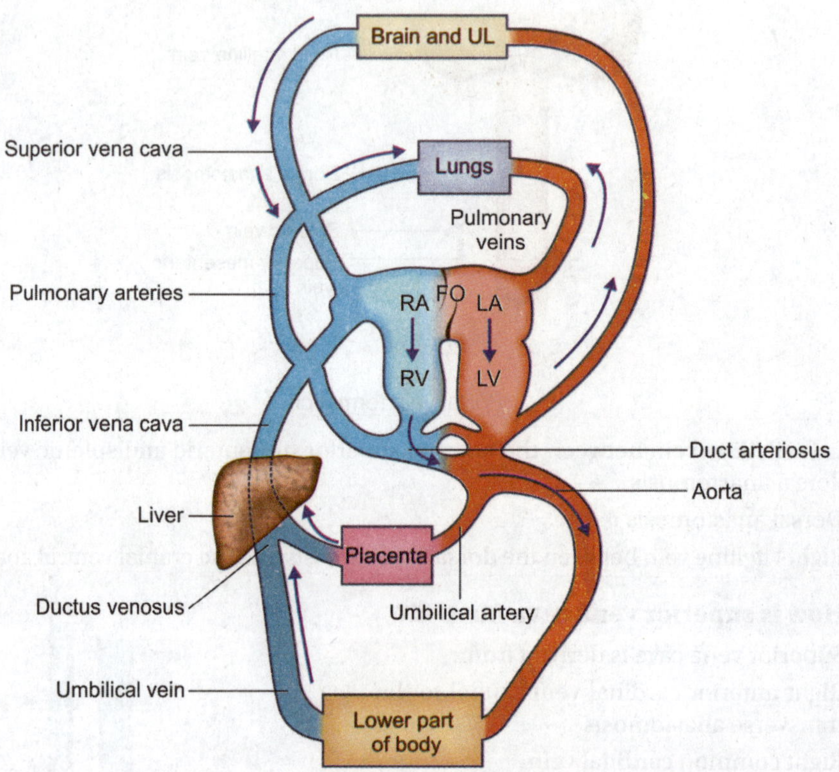

Fetal circulation (FO, foramen ovale; LA, left atrium; LV, left ventricles; RA, right atrium; RV, right ventricle; SVC, superior vena cava)

Q. Discuss the remnants of the components of fetal circulation.

Ans.

- Umbilical arteries—medial umbilical ligament
- Left umbilical vein—ligamentum teres of liver
- Ductus venosus—ligamentum venosum
- Ductus arteriosus—ligamentum arteriosum.

Q. What are the changes in fetal circulation at birth?

Ans.

1. The muscle in the wall of umbilical arteries immediately contracts after birth. This prevents loss of fetal blood into the placenta.
2. Lumen of umbilical vein and ductus venosus is also occluded, but this takes few minutes after birth.
3. Ductus arteriosus is occluded.
4. Pulmonary vessels increase in size and proportionately a much larger volume of blood reaches left atrium from lungs.

Q. Which embryological structure plays role in the formation of urogenital system?

Ans. The intermediate mesoderm plays an important role in the development of urogenital system.

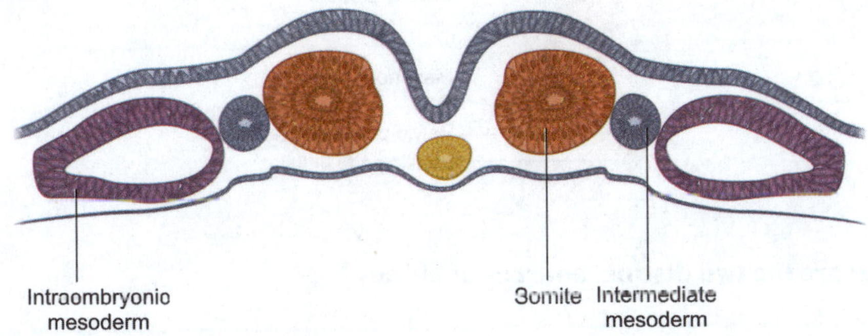

Q. What is nephrogenic cord?

Ans. Intermediate mesoderm forms a bulge on the posterior abdominal wall lateral to the attachment of dorsal mesentery of the gut. This is the nephrogenic cord. It extends from cervical region to sacral region.

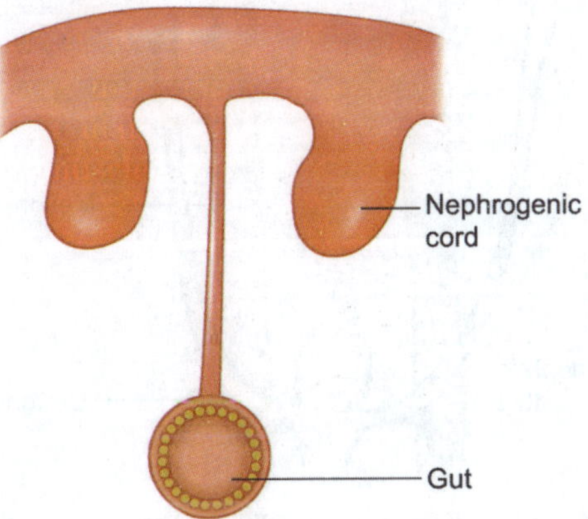

Q. What components give rise to urethra?

Ans. Definitive urogenital sinus and caudal part of vesicourethral canal give rise to urethra.

Q. What are the subdivisions of cloaca?

Ans. Cloaca is subdivided into:
- Primitive urogenital sinus
- Rectum.

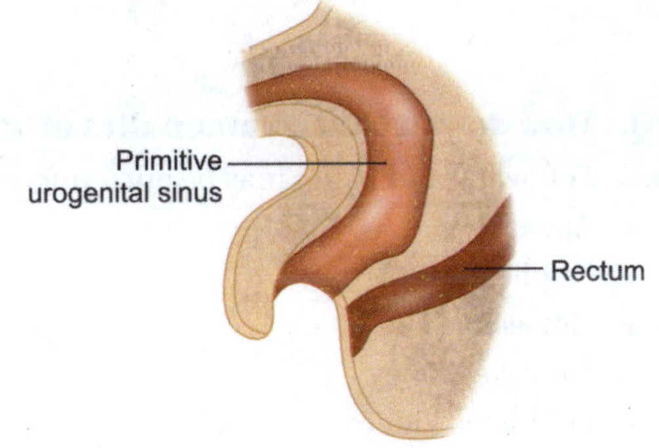

Primitive urogenital sinus

Q. Depict the subdivisions of urogenital sinus.

Ans.

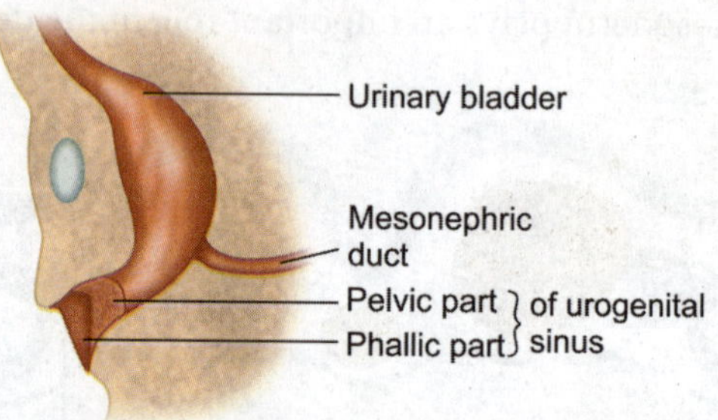

Q. What are the two distinct sources of kidney?

Ans.

- The excretory tubules are derived from the lowest part of nephrogenic cord of cells of which form the metanephric blastema
- The collecting part of the kidney is derived from a diverticulum called ureteric bud.

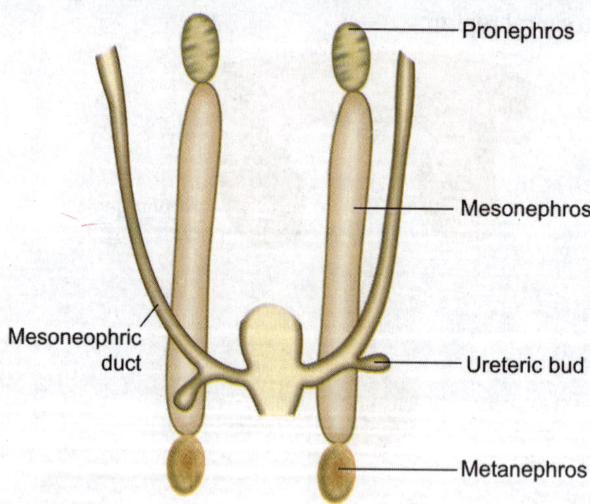

Q. How do you classify anomalies of kidney?

Ans. Following anomalies may be encountered:

- Agenesis
- Duplication
- Horseshoe kidney
- Pancake kidney
- Lobulated kidney.

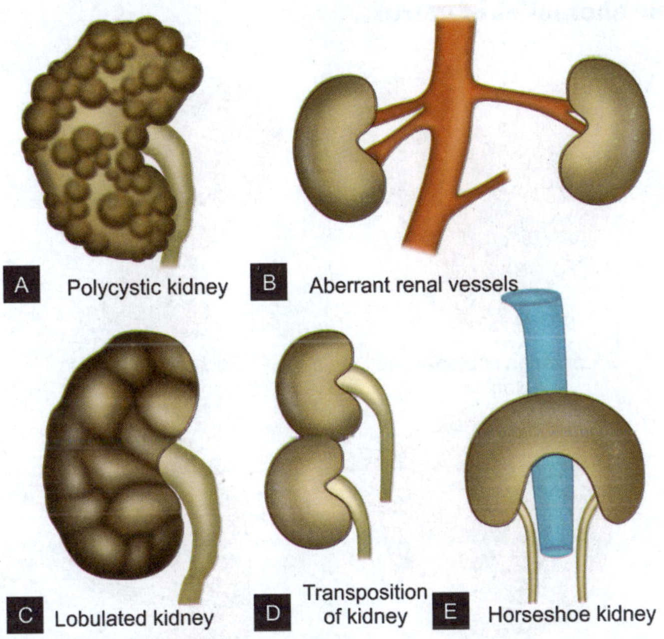

Anomalies of kidney

Q. How does the ureter develop?

Ans. Ureter is derived from the part of ureteric bud that lies between the pelvis of the kidney and the vesicourethral canal.

Q. Discuss the development of urinary bladder.

Ans.
- The epithelium of urinary bladder develops from the cranial part of vesicourethral canal
- Epithelium of trigone of the bladder is derived from the absorbed mesonephric duct
- Muscular and serous walls are derived from splanchnopleuric mesoderm.

Q. What is the fate of paramesonephric ducts in females?

Ans. In the females, paramesonephric duct gives origin to uterine tubes, uterus and part of vagina.

Q. What is the fate of paramesonephric ducts in males?

Ans.
- Paramesonephric duct remains rudimentary in males
- Cranial end of each duct persists as a small rounded body attached to the testis—appendix of testis
- Uterovaginal canal remnant is prostatic utricle.

Q. Depict the anomalies of uterus.

Ans.

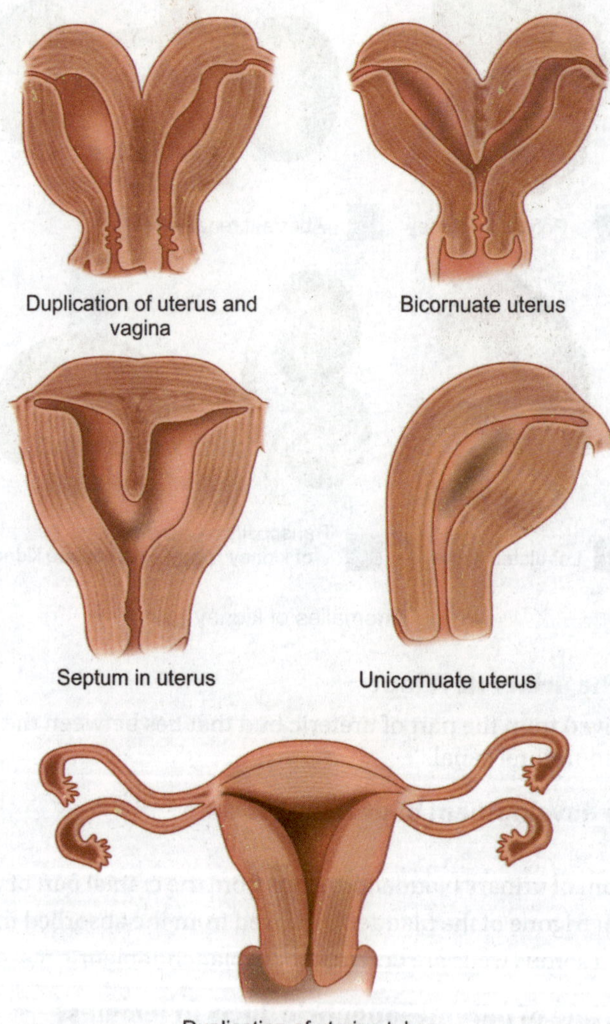

Anomalies of uterus

Q. What is the male homologue of uterus?

Ans. Prostatic utricle is the male homologue of uterus.

Q. Discuss the development of external genitalia.

Ans. In females:
- Genital tubercle forms clitoris
- Genital swellings form labia majora
- Primitive urethral folds form labia minora.

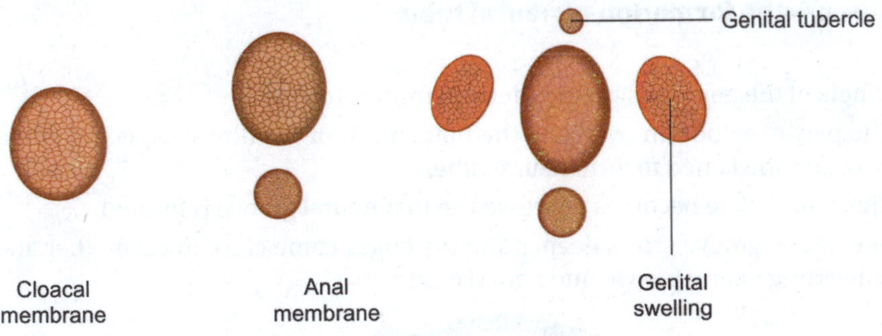

In males:

- Genital tubercle forms penis
- Genital swellings form scrotal sac
- Urethral folds form penile urethra.

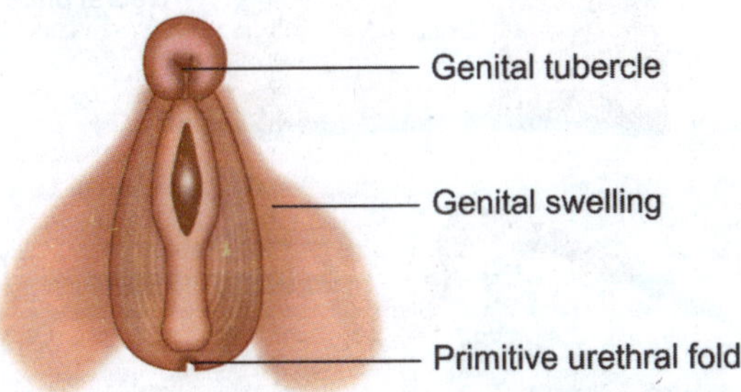

Q. Discuss the descent of testis.

Ans.

- The testis develops in relation to the lumbar region of the posterior abdominal wall
- During fetal life, they gradually descend to the scrotum
- They reach the iliac fossa during the third month
- They lie at the site of deep inguinal ring up to 7th month of intrauterine life
- They pass through the inguinal canal during the 7th month
- They reach the scrotum during 8th month.

Factors affecting descent of testis:

- Differential growth of the body wall
- Formation of inguinal bursa
- Shortening of gubernaculums
- Processus vaginalis is a diverticulum of peritoneal cavity, which grows towards scrotum
- The descent of testis is greatly influenced by hormones
- Appendix of epididymis represents the remnant of mesonephric duct
- Appendix of testis is the remnant of paramesonephric duct.

Q. Discuss the formation of neural tube.

Ans.

1. Whole of the nervous system is derived from ectoderm.
2. The part of ectoderm overlying the notochord on the dorsal aspect of embryonic disk becomes thickened to form neural tube.
3. The neural plate becomes depressed so that neural groove is formed.
4. The neural groove grows deeper and the edges come close to each other and fuse thus converting neural groove into neural tube.

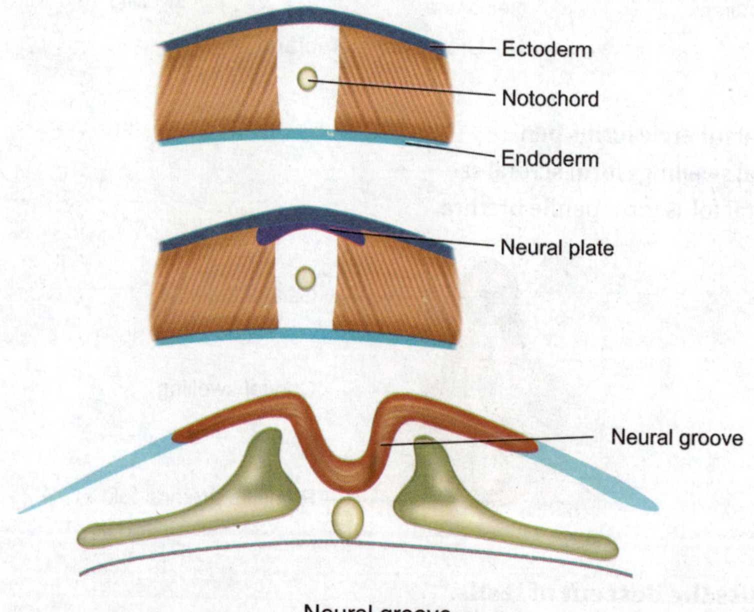

Q. What are the subdivisions of neural tube?

Ans. Neural tube is broadly divided into three parts:

1. Prosencephalon.
2. Mesencephalon.
3. Rhombencephalon.

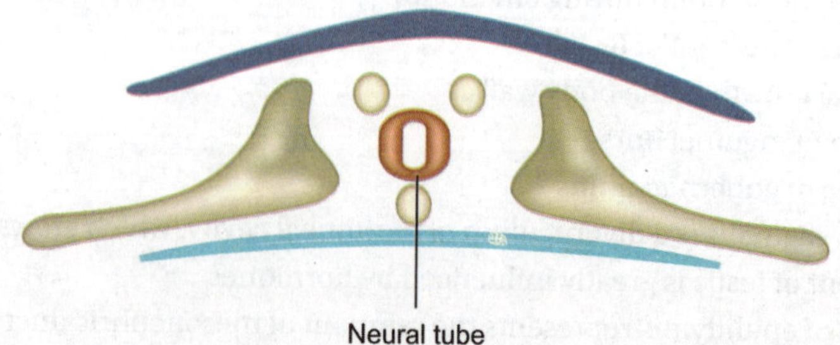

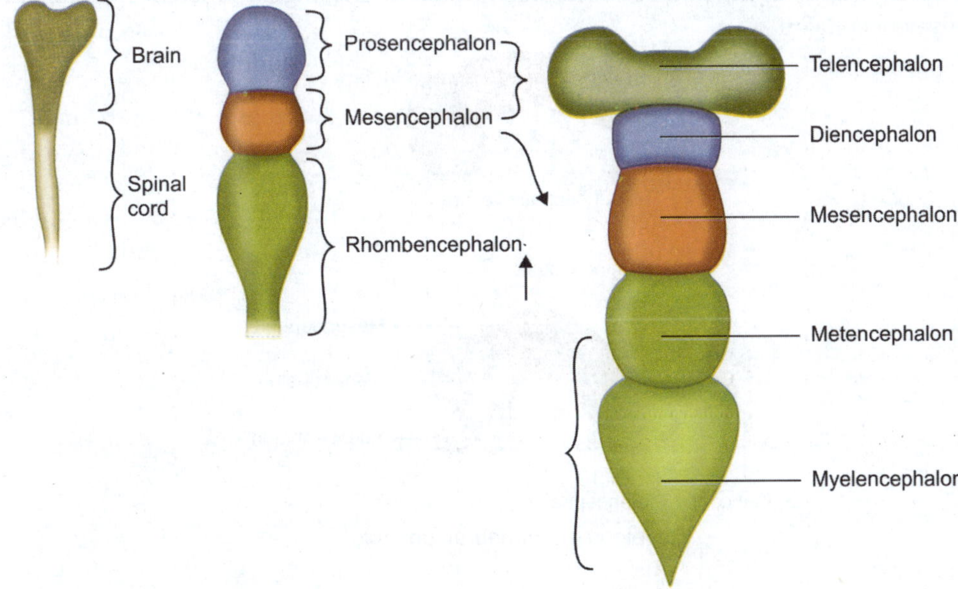

Q. What is the fate of neural tube in adult?

Ans.

- Telencephalon—cerebral cortex, corpus striatum
- Diencephalon—thalamus, hypothalamus, optic stalk, pars nervosa of hypophysis
- Mesencephalon—midbrain
- Metencephalon—pons, cerebellum
- Mylencephalon—medulla oblongata.

Q. How does the neural tube fold?

Ans. Neural tube folds by the development of several flexures such as:

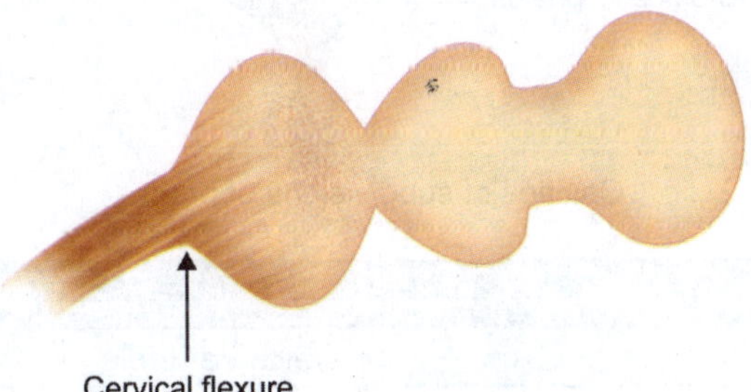

1. Cervical flexure between rhombencephalon and spinal cord.
2. Mesencephalic flexure in the region of midbrain.

3. Pontine flexure at the middle of rhombencephalon dividing into metencephalon and myelencephalon.

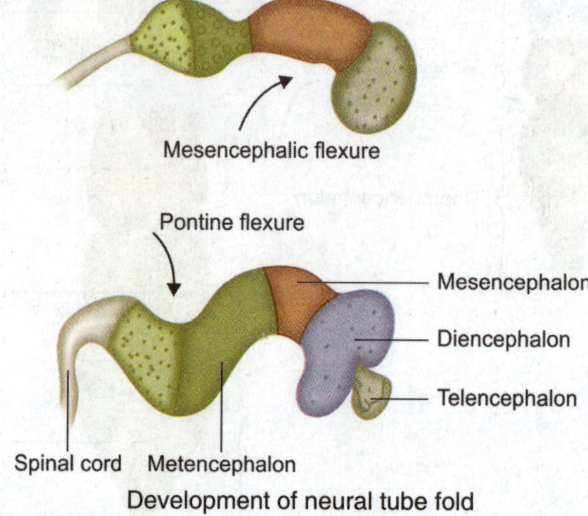

Development of neural tube fold

Q. What are the cavities of subdivisions of brain?

Ans.   The cavities of subdivisions of brain are explained in the table given below.

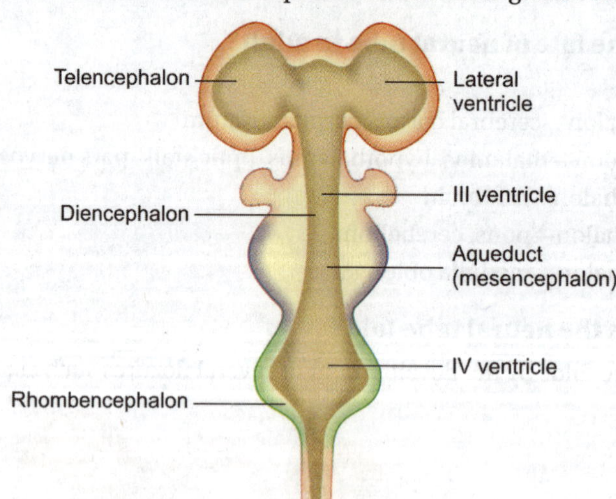

Cavities of subdivisions of brain

Subdivision of brain	Cavity
Telencephalon	Lateral ventricle
Diencephalon	Third ventricle
Mesencephalon	Aqueduct
Rhombencephalon	Fourth ventricle

Q.   What are neural crest cells?

Ans.   At the time when the neural plate is being formed, some cells at the junction between the neural plate and rest of the ectoderm becomes specialized to form the primordium of neural crest.

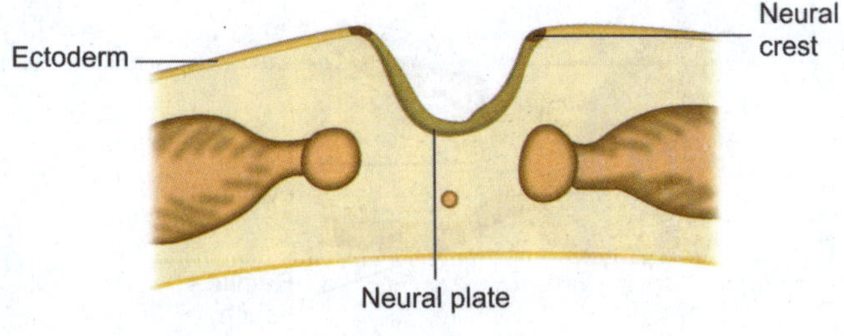

Neural crest cells

Q.   What are the derivatives of neural crest cells?

Ans.   Following are the derivatives of neural crest cells:

- Neurons of the spinal posterior nerve root ganglia
- Neurons of the sensory ganglia of V, VII, VIII, IX and X cranial nerves
- Neurons of sympathetic ganglia
- Schwann cells
- Some cells of adrenal medulla
- Chromaffin cells, pigment cells
- Pia- and arachnoid-mater
- Mesenchyme of dental papillae.

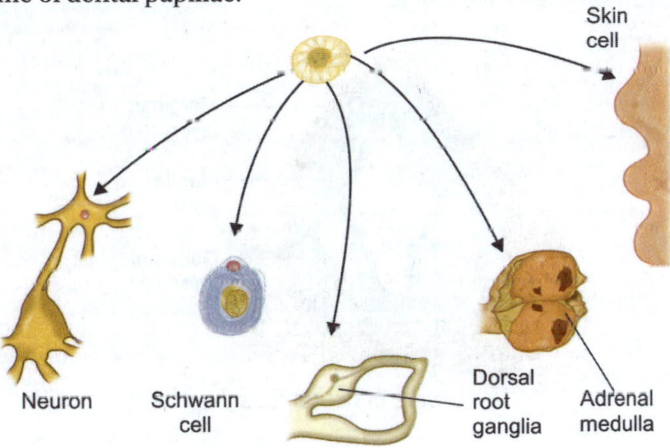

Neural crest cell derivatives

Q. How does pituitary gland develop?

Ans.

1. The anterior and the intermediate part of the organ develops from ectodermal diverticulum that grows upwards from the roof of stomodeum, i.e. Rathke's pouch.

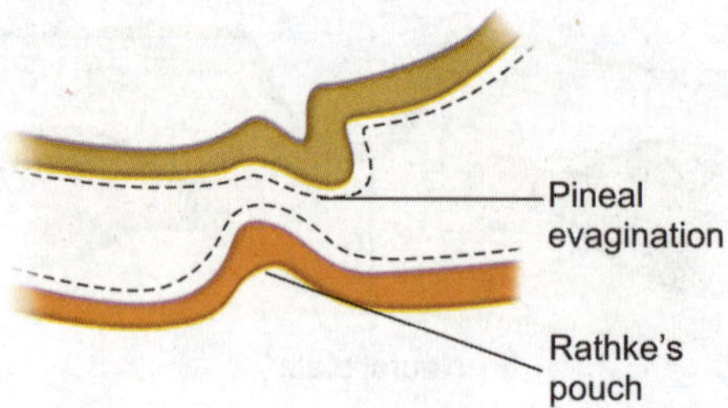

2. Posterior lobe is formed as downgrowth of infundibulum from the floor of third ventricle.

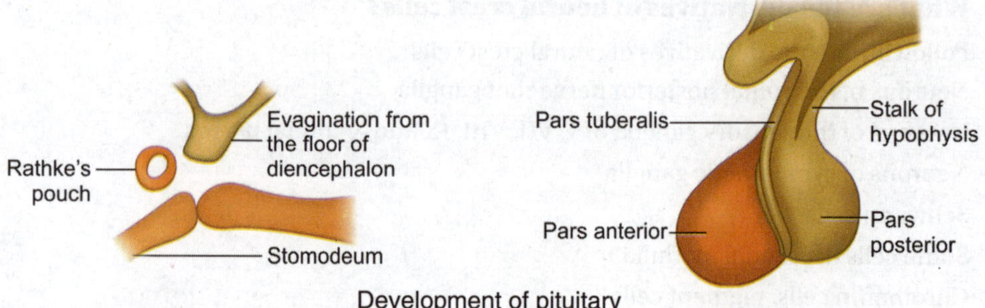

Development of pituitary

Q. Depict the layers of neural tube.

Ans.

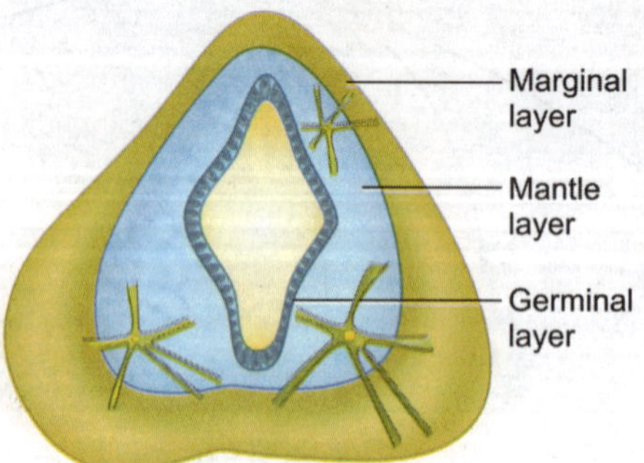

Layers of neural tube

Q. What embryological components give rise to eyeball?

Ans. The various components are derived from following primordia:
- Outgrowth from prosencephalon called optic vesicle
- Specialized area of surface ectoderm gives rise to lens
- Mesoderm covering optic vesicle.

Q. Depict the formation of optic vesicle.

Ans.

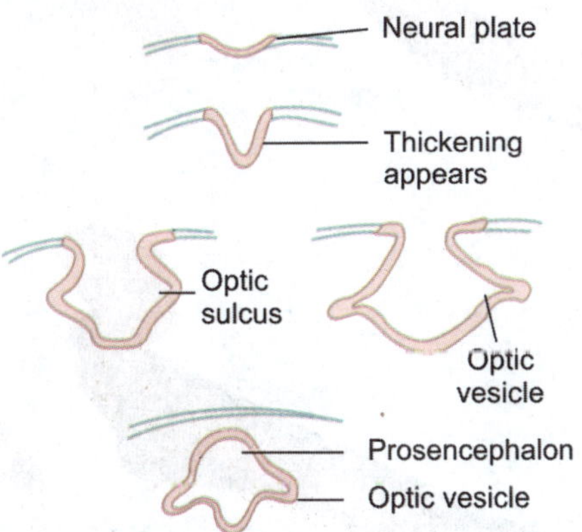

Q. How does the lens vesicle form?

Ans.

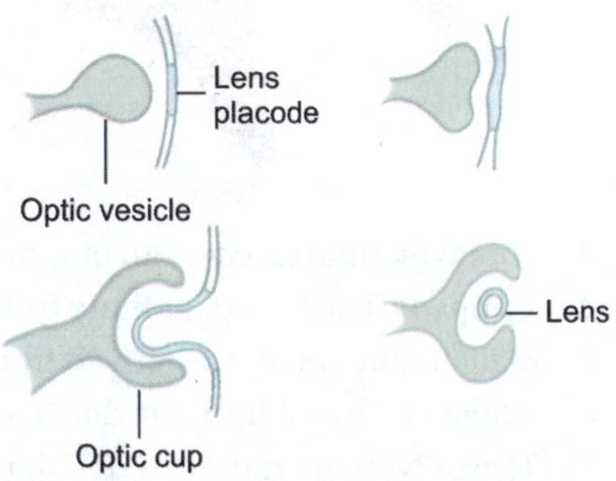

- Optic vesicle grows laterally and comes to lie into relation with surface ectoderm
- An area of this surface ectoderm over-lying optic vesicle becomes thickened to form lens placode.

Q. How does otic vesicle develop? What is its fate?

Ans.

- Part of surface ectoderm overlying the developing hindbrain gets thickened
- This area of thickening is called otic placode
- Otic placode soon gets depressed to form otic pit
- Otic vesicle by differential growth gives rise to membranous labyrinth.

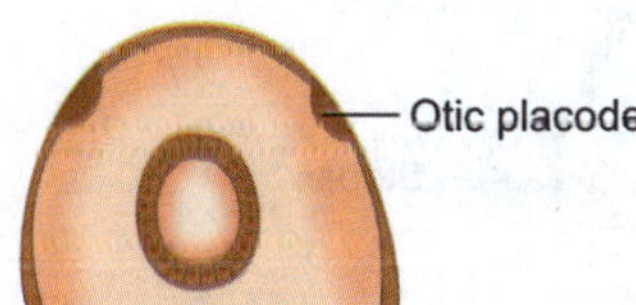

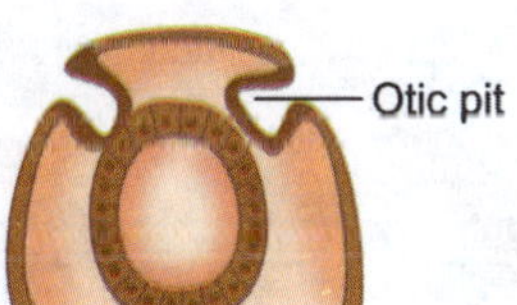

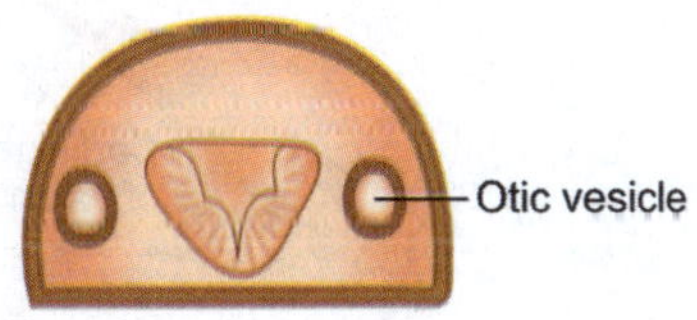

Q. Discuss the middle ear development.

Ans.

1. Epithelial lining of middle ear and of the pharyngotympanic tube is derived from tubotympanic recess.
2. Mastoid antrum is a dorsal extension of tympanic cavity.

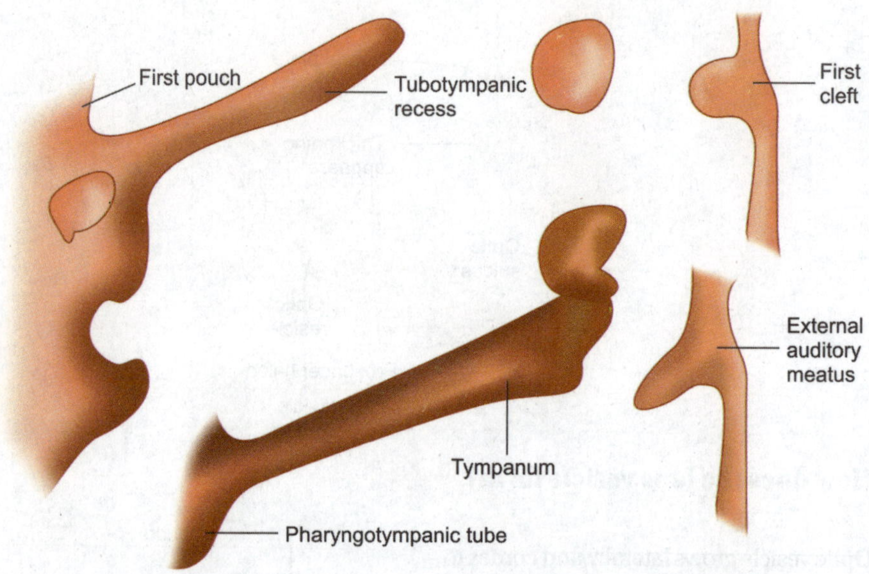

3. Tubotympanic recess is an outgrowth of first pharyngeal pouch.
4. Tympanic cavity and auditory tube develop from tubotympanic recess.
5. Malleus and incus are derived from the dorsal end of Meckel's cartilage.
6. Stapes is derived from the dorsal end of the cartilage of the second pharyngeal pouch.
7. Tensor tympani muscle is derived from the mesoderm of the first pharyngeal pouch.
8. Stapedius muscle from second pharyngeal pouch.

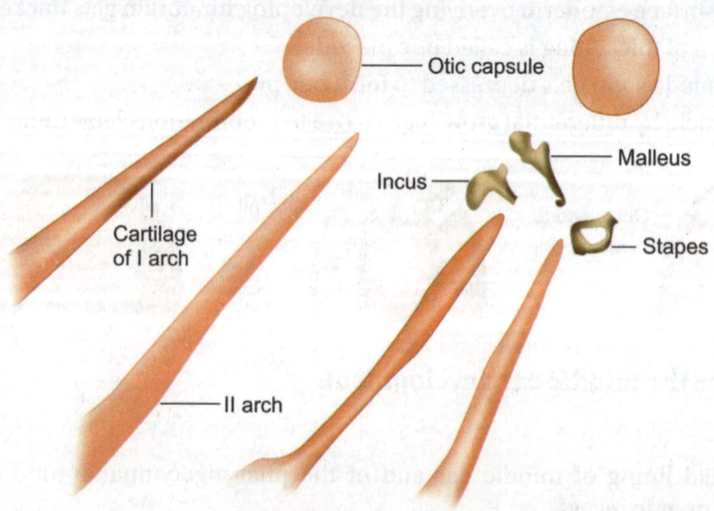

Development of middle ear

Q. How does the external auditory canal develop?

Ans. External auditory canal develops from the dorsal part of first ectodermal cleft.

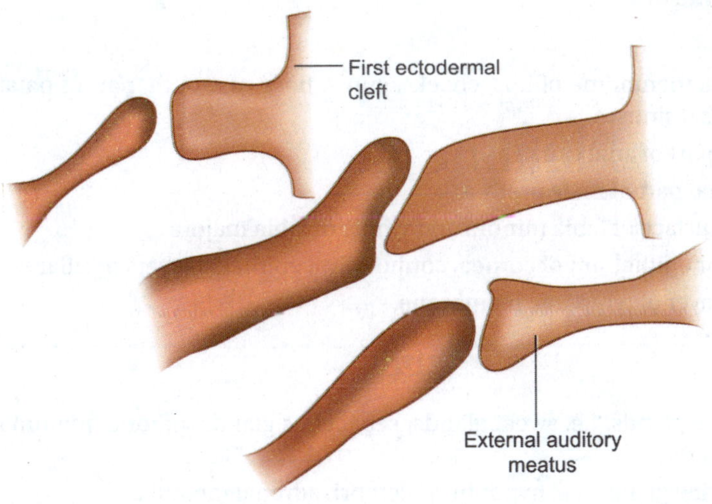

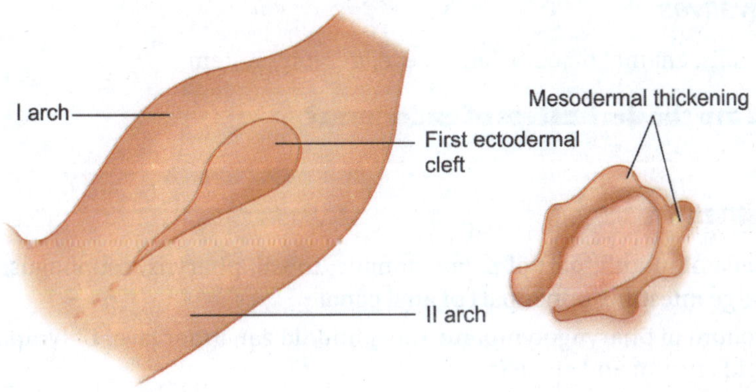

Q. How is pinna formed?

Ans. Pinna is formed from a series of meso-dermal thickenings that appear on the mandibular and hyoid arches around the opening of the dorsal part of the first ectodermal cleft.

Tympanic membrane is formed by the contribution of tubotympanic recess and outer epithelial layer.

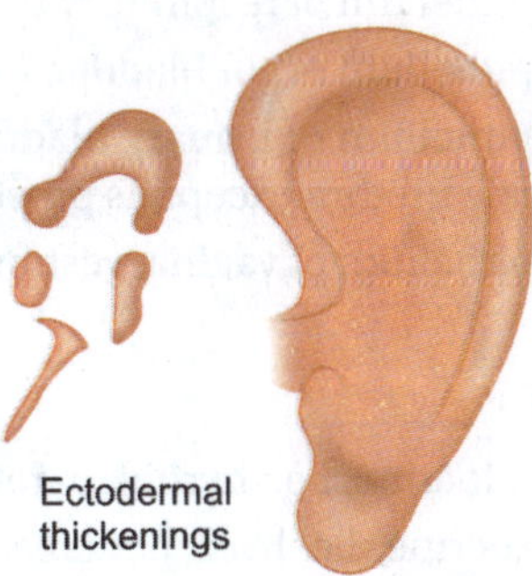

Development of pinna

Q. What are the derivatives of ectoderm?

Ans.

Lining Epithelia

- Skin
- Mucous membrane of lips, cheeks, gums, floor of mouth, part of palate, nasal cavities paranasal sinuses
- Lower part of anal canal
- Terminal part of male urethra
- Outer surface of labia minora and whole of labia majora
- Anterior epithelium of cornea, conjunctiva, epithelial layers of ciliary body and iris
- Outer layer of tympanic membrane.

Glands

- Exocrine glands, i.e. sweat glands, sebaceous glands, parotid, mammary glands, lacrimal glands
- Endocrine glands, i.e. hypophysis cerebri, adrenal medulla.

Other Derivatives

- Hair, nails, enamel of teeth, lens of eye, nervous system.

Q. What are the derivatives of endoderm?

Ans.

Lining Epithelia

- Epithelia of mouth, part of palate, tongue, tonsil, pharynx, esophagus, stomach, small and large intestine, upper part of anal canal
- Epithelium of pharyngotympanic tube, middle ear, inner layer of tympanic membrane, mastoid antrum and air cells
- Epithelium of respiratory tract
- Epithelium of gallbladder, extrahepatic duct system, pancreatic duct
- Epithelium of urinary bladder except trigone, female urethra except its posterior wall, male urethra except its prostatic posterior part and penile urethra
- Epithelium of vagina, vestibule and inner surface of labia minora.

Glands

- Endocrine, i.e. thyroid, parathyroid, thymus, islets of Langerhans
- Exocrine, i.e. liver, pancreas, glands of gastrointestinal tract (GIT) and greater part of prostate.

Q. What are the derivatives of mesoderm?

Ans.

1. All connective tissue including loose areolar tissue, superficial and deep fascia, ligaments, tendons, aponeuroses, dermis of skin.
2. Adipose tissue, reticular tissue, cartilage and bone.
3. Dentine of teeth.
4. All the muscles—smooth, striated, cardiac.
5. Heart, blood vessels, lymphatics, blood vessels.
6. Kidneys, ureters, trigone of bladder, posterior wall of part of female and male urethra.
7. Ovary, uterus, uterine tube.
8. Testis, epididymis, vas deferens, seminal vesicle, ejaculatory ducts.
9. Lining mesothelium of pleura, pericardia, peritoneal cavities.
10. Lining epithelium of bursae and joints.

Chapter 35

Multiple Choice Questions (MCQs)

1. Embryo is from the time of inception till first _____________ month(s).
   a. 1
   b. 2
   c. 3
   d. 4

   Answer: b

2. From _____________ month till birth is called fetus.
   a. 1st
   b. 2nd
   c. 3rd
   d. 4th

   Answer: c

3. Fertilization occurs in _____________ part of the fallopian tube.
   a. Intramural
   b. Isthmus
   c. Ampulla
   d. Infundibulum

   Answer: c

4. X chromosome is a member of _____________ group (Denver classification).
   a. A
   b. B
   c. C
   d. D

   Answer: c

5. Y chromosome is a member of _____________ group.
   a. E
   b. F
   c. G
   d. E

   Answer: c

6. DNA content of chromosome is duplicated during _____________ phase.
   a. Prophase
   b. Interphase
   c. Metaphase
   d. Anaphase

   Answer: b

7. Spindle formation occurs during _____________ of cell division.
   a. Prophase
   b. Metaphase
   c. Anaphase
   d. Telophase

   Answer: a

8. 'Crossing over' takes place during what stage of prophase?
    a. Leptotene
    b. Zygotene
    c. Pachytene
    d. Diplotene

Answer: c

9. At the time of ovulation, the stage of ovary is ___________
    a. Primary oocyte
    b. Secondary oocyte
    c. Oogonium
    d. None of the above

Answer: b

10. How many days it takes for the ovum to reach the uterus?
    a. 1–2 days
    b. 2–3 days
    c. 3–4 days
    d. Within 24 hours

Answer: c

11. If the ovum is not fertilized, the corpus luteum persists for ___________ days.
    a. 10
    b. 12
    c. 14
    d. 16

Answer: c

12. Corpus luteum secretes ___________ hormone.
    a. Estrogen
    b. Luteinizing hormone
    c. Progesterone
    d. Follicle-stimulating hormone

Answer: c

13. Superfemales have ___________ number of chromosomes.
    a. XX
    b. XXY
    c. XO
    d. XXX

Answer: d

14. In isochromosomes, the centriole splits ___________
    a. Longitudinally
    b. Transversely
    c. Obliquely
    d. Diagonally

Answer: b

15. Hormone influencing luteal phase is ___________
    a. Estrogen
    b. Progesterone
    c. LH
    d. FSH

Answer: b

16. Hormone influencing follicular phase is ___________
    a. Estrogen
    b. Progesterone
    c. LH
    d. FSH

Answer: a

17. Ovum remains viable for ___________ number of days.
    a. 1
    b. 2
    c. 3
    d. 4

Answer: b

18. Spermatozoa introduced into vagina die within ___________ days.
    - a. 2
    - b. 3
    - c. 4
    - d. 5

    Answer: c

19. Chorion is formed by the union of ___________
    - a. Visceral extraembryonic mesoderm with trophoblast
    - b. Parietal extraembryonic mesoderm and trophoblast
    - c. Parietal extraembryonic mesoderm with amnion
    - d. Visceral with parietal extraembryonic mesoderm

    Answer: b

20. Morula is ___________ cell stage.
    - a. 10th
    - b. 12th
    - c. 14th
    - d. 16th

    Answer: d

21. ___________ decides the axis of embryonic disk.
    - a. Primitive streak
    - b. Chorion
    - c. Prochordal plate
    - d. Amnion

    Answer: c

22. Prochordal plate is the modification of ___________ cells of embryonic disk.
    - a. Ectoderm
    - b. Mesoderm
    - c. Endoderm
    - d. None

    Answer: c

23. Primitive streak is the proliferation of ___________ cells toward tail end of disk.
    - a. Ectoderm
    - b. Mesoderm
    - c. Endoderm
    - d. All

    Answer: a

24. What gives rise to intraembryonic mesoderm?
    - a. Prochordal plate
    - b. Primitive streak
    - c. Trophoblast
    - d. Extraembryonic mesoderm

    Answer: b

25. Gastrulation is the formation of ___________
    - a. Prochordal plate and primitive streak
    - b. Prochordal plate and extraembryonic mesoderm
    - c. Primitive streak and intraembryonic mesoderm
    - d. Primitive streak and extraembryonic mesoderm

    Answer: c

26. Morula formation occurs after ___________ days of embryo formation.
    - a. 1
    - b. 2
    - c. 3
    - d. 4

    Answer: c

27. Blastocyst formation occurs in ____________ days after embryo formation.
    a. 2
    b. 4
    c. 5
    d. 6

Answer: b

28. Intraembryonic mesoderm develops by the day ____________
    a. 8
    b. 10
    c. 14
    d. 16

Answer: d

29. Hensen's node is the thickened part of ____________
    a. Cranial end of primitive streak
    b. Caudal end of primitive streak
    c. Cranial end of prochordal plate
    d. Caudal end of prochordal plate

Answer: a

30. Para-axial mesoderm gives rise to ____________
    a. Nervous system
    b. Body cavities
    c. Somites
    d. Vertebral column

Answer: c

31. Pleural, pericardial and peritoneal cavities develop from ____________
    a. Para-axial mesoderm
    b. Lateral plate mesoderm
    c. Intermediate mesoderm
    d. Extraembryonic celom

Answer: b

32. Intermediate mesoderm gives rise to ____________
    a. Cardiogenic area
    b. Peritoneal cavities
    c. Nephrogenic area
    d. Genitalia

Answer: c

33. Normally, placenta is implanted in ____________
    a. Upper uterine segment
    b. Lower uterine segment
    c. Both (a and b)
    d. Partially in upper segment

Answer: a

34. Muscles of tongue develop from ____________
    a. Mesoderm of 1st branchial arch
    b. Occipital myotomes
    c. Sclerotome
    d. Dermatome

Answer: b

35. Meckel's cartilage is the cartilage of ____________ pharyngeal arch.
    a. 1st
    b. 2nd
    c. 3rd
    d. 4th

Answer: a

36. Which of the following pharyngeal arch disappears during embryological development?
    a. 2nd
    b. 3rd
    c. 4th
    d. 5th

Answer: d

37. Stapes develops from ___________ pharyngeal arch.
    a. 1st
    b. 2nd
    c. 3rd
    d. 4th

Answer: b

38. Hyoid bone develops from ___________ pharyngeal arch.
    a. 1st
    b. 2nd
    c. 3rd
    d. 4th

Answer: c

39. Cartilages of larynx develop from ___________ pharyngeal arches.
    a. 1st and 2nd
    b. 2nd and 3rd
    c. 3rd and 4th
    d. 4th and 6th

Answer: d

40. Pretrematic nerve of 1st pharyngeal arch is ___________
    a. Chorda tympani
    b. Mandibular
    c. XI
    d. X

Answer: a

41. Post-trematic nerve of 1st arch is ___________
    a. Chorda tympani
    b. Mandibular
    c. Facial
    d. Glossopharyngeal

Answer: b

42. Third pharyngeal arch nerve is ___________
    a. V
    b. VII
    c. X
    d. IX

Answer: d

43. Muscles of mastication develop from ___________ pharyngeal arch.
    a. 1st
    b. 2nd
    c. 3rd
    d. 4th

Answer: a

44. Anterior belly of digastric develops from ___________ pharyngeal arch.
    a. 1st
    b. 2nd
    c. 3rd
    d. 4th

Answer: a

45. Posterior belly of digastric develops from ___________ pharyngeal arch.
    a. 1st
    b. 2nd
    c. 3rd
    d. 4th

Answer: b

46. Auditory tube develops from ___________
    a. Proximal part of tubotympanic recess
    b. Distal part of tubotympanic recess
    c. Second pharyngeal pouch
    d. Ventral part of first pharyngeal pouch

Answer: a

47. Tubotympanic recess is formed by contribution of following two structures __________
    a. Ventral and dorsal part of 1st pouch
    b. Dorsal part of 1st pouch and 2nd pouch
    c. Dorsal and ventral part of 2nd pouch
    d. Tympanic cavity

Answer: b

48. Third endodermal pouch gives rise to __________
    a. Superior parathyroid
    b. Thyroid
    c. Inferior parathyroid
    d. Thymus

Answer: c

49. Fourth endodermal pouch gives rise to __________
    a. Superior parathyroid
    b. Thyroid
    c. Inferior parathyroid
    d. Thymus

Answer: a

50. Ultimobranchial body gives rise to __________
    a. Follicular cells of thyroid
    b. Parafollicular cells of thyroid
    c. Stromal cells of thyroid
    d. Myoepithelial cells of thyroid

Answer: b

51. Face develops from __________
    a. Frontonasal process and 1st arch
    b. 1st and 2nd arch
    c. Frontonasal process only
    d. 1st pharyngeal arch only

Answer: a

52. Lower lip develops from __________
    a. Maxillary process
    b. Mandibular process
    c. Nasal process
    d. All of the above

Answer: b

53. All contributes to the formation of upper lip except __________
    a. Maxillary process
    b. Lateral nasal process
    c. Medial nasal process
    d. Mandibular process

Answer: d

54. Philtrum develops from __________
    a. Mandibular process
    b. Medial nasal process
    c. Frontonasal process
    d. Lateral nasal process

Answer: c

55. Muscles of the face develop from __________ branchial arch.
    a. 1st
    b. 2nd
    c. 3rd
    d. 4th

Answer: b

56. Harelip is due to nonfusion of ____________
    a. Maxillary process with medial nasal process
    b. Mandibular process with medial nasal process
    c. Maxillary process with lateral nasal process
    d. Medial and lateral nasal process

    Answer: a

57. Oblique facial cleft is due to nonfusion of ____________
    a. Mandibular process with lateral nasal process
    b. Maxillary process with the medial nasal process
    c. Maxillary process with lateral nasal process
    d. Mandibular process with medial nasal process

    Answer: c

58. Lateral wall of nose is derived from ____________
    a. Frontonasal process
    b. Medial nasal process
    c. Lateral nasal process
    d. Maxillary process

    Answer: c

59. The paranasal sinus absent at birth is ____________
    a. Frontal
    b. Maxillary
    c. Sphenoid
    d. All

    Answer: a

60. The paranasal sinus absent at birth is ____________
    a. Ethmoid
    b. Maxillary
    c. Sphenoid
    d. All

    Answer: a

61. Sinuses rudimentary at birth are ____________
    a. Frontal and sphenoidal
    b. Frontal and ethmoidal
    c. Maxillary and sphenoidal
    d. Maxillary and ethmoidal

    Answer: c

62. Palatine tonsils develop in relation to ____________ pharyngeal pouch.
    a. 1st
    b. 2nd
    c. 3rd
    d. 4th

    Answer: b

63. Artery of foregut is ____________
    a. Celiac
    b. Superior mesenteric
    c. Gastric
    d. Duodenal

    Answer: a

64. Artery of midgut is ____________
    a. Inferior mesenteric
    b. Celiac
    c. Superior mesenteric
    d. Duodenal

    Answer: c

65. Artery of hindgut is _______________
    a. Inferior mesenteric
    b. Celiac
    c. Superior mesenteric
    d. Duodenal

    Answer: a

66. Rotation of midgut loop occurs between _______________
    a. 3rd and 8th week
    b. 5th and 10th week
    c. 4th and 6th week
    d. 2nd and 6th week

    Answer: b

67. Spleen develops in _______________
    a. Dorsal mesogastrium
    b. Ventral mesogastrium
    c. Midgut
    d. Foregut

    Answer: a

68. Arterial end of the heart tube is _______________
    a. Bulbus cordis
    b. Sinus venosus
    c. Ventricle
    d. Atria

    Answer: a

69. Annulus ovalis is the remnant of _______________
    a. Septum primum
    b. Septum secundum
    c. Foramen ovalis
    d. Foramen primum

    Answer: b

70. First arch artery remnant in adult life is _______________
    a. Facial artery
    b. Superior thyroid artery
    c. Maxillary artery
    d. Superficial temporal artery

    Answer: c

71. External carotid artery is a bud from _______________ arch artery.
    a. 1st
    b. 2nd
    c. 3rd
    d. 4th

    Answer: c

72. Axis artery of upper limb is _______________
    a. 1st intersegmental
    b. 4th intersegmental
    c. 7th intersegmental
    d. None

    Answer: c

73. Axis artery of lower limb is _______________
    a. 1st lumbar intersegmental
    b. 2nd lumbar intersegmental
    c. 4th lumbar intersegmental
    d. 5th lumbar intersegmental

    Answer: d

74. Ligamentum teres is the remnant of _______________
    a. Umbilical artery
    b. Right umbilical vein
    c. Left umbilical vein
    d. Ductus venosus

    Answer: c

75. A 2 months pregnant woman happens to get exposed to radiation; there is a risk of development of anomalies to the baby due to ______________

    a. Radiation is dangerous

    b. Exposure to radiation falls in period of organogenesis

    c. Genetic predisposition

    d. All the above

Answer: b

Section - VIII

HISTOLOGY

Histology

Key terms in histology

- Cell structure
- Simple squamous epithelium
- Simple cuboidal epithelium
- Simple columnar epithelium
- Pseudostratified columnar epithelium
- Transitional epithelium
- Stratified squamous epithelium
- Loose areolar tissue
- Adipose tissue
- Hyaline cartilage
- Elastic cartilage
- Fibrocartilage
- Compact bone
- Cancellous bone
- Skeletal muscle
- Smooth muscle
- Cardiac muscle
- Peripheral nerve
- Sensory ganglion
- Elastic artery
- Muscular artery
- Vein
- Lymph node
- Spleen
- Thymus
- Palatine tonsil
- Skin
- Tongue
- Circumvallate papilla
- Serous salivary gland
- Mixed salivary gland
- Mucous salivary gland
- Esophagus
- Cardiac end of stomach
- Body of the stomach
- Pyloric end of stomach
- Jejunum
- Duodenum
- Ileum
- Large intestine
- Vermiform appendix
- Liver
- Gallbladder
- Trachea

Contd...

Contd...

▪ Lung	▪ Uterus in secretory phase
▪ Kidney	▪ Vagina
▪ Ureter	▪ Mammary gland
▪ Urinary bladder	▪ Pituitary gland
▪ Testis	▪ Thyroid gland
▪ Epididymis	▪ Parathyroid gland
▪ Ductus deferens	▪ Suprarenal gland
▪ Seminal vesicle	▪ Cornea
▪ Prostate	▪ Wall of eyeball
▪ Penis (low magnification)	▪ Cochlea
▪ Ovary	▪ Spinal cord (special stain)
▪ Uterine tube	▪ Cerebellum
▪ Uterus in proliferative stage	▪ Cerebral cortex

Q. Cell structure

Ans. Cell is bounded by cell membrane (plasma membrane):

- Within the cell membrane is protoplasm
- Protoplasm consists of central nucleus and surrounding cytoplasm
- Nucleus is covered by nuclear membrane
- Many structures are present within the cytoplasm, which are referred as organelle.

Organelles	Functions
Endoplasmic reticulum (ER) (smooth, rough)	Rough ER—protein synthesis; smooth ER–metabolic processes, e.g. carbohydrate metabolism
Ribosomes (free in cytoplasm)	Protein synthesis
Mitochondria	ATP, GTP are produced, exhibit important part in Krebs cycle
Golgi complex	Protein-carbohydrate complexes are formed
Phagosomes	Engulf bacteria by phagocytosis
Pinocytic vesicle	Fluid taken in by pinocytosis
Exocytic vesicle	Cell products expelled out by exocytosis
Storage vesicle	Stores lipid, carbohydrate
Lysosomes	Contain enzymes, which destroy unwanted material in the cell
Microtubule	Provide stability to cell, facilitate transport within the cell, form mitotic spindle in dividing cell
Centriole	Crucial role in formation of cilia, flagella, mitotic spindles

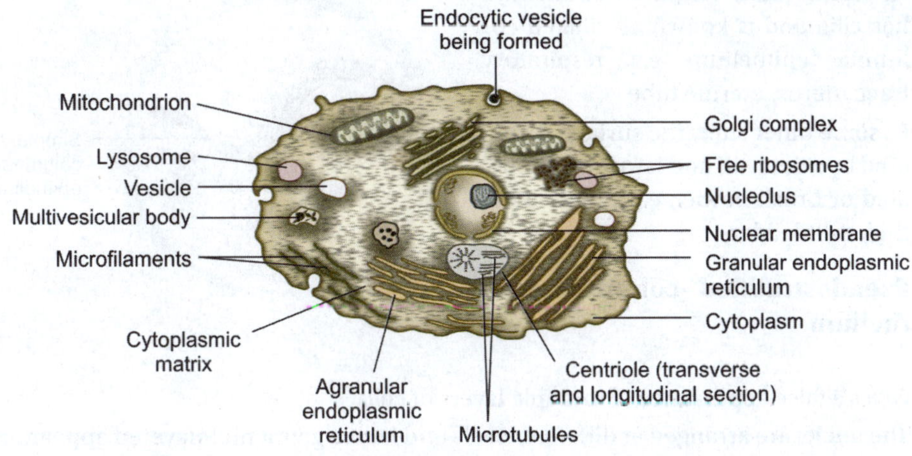

Structure of a cell

Q. Simple squamous epithelium

Ans.

- Single layer of flattened cells
- Very thin cell membrane; hence the nuclei bulge on the surface
- Lines the alveoli of lungs, free surface of serous pericardium, pleura peritoneum
- Lines the interior of heart (endocardium), blood vessels and lymphatics (endothelium).

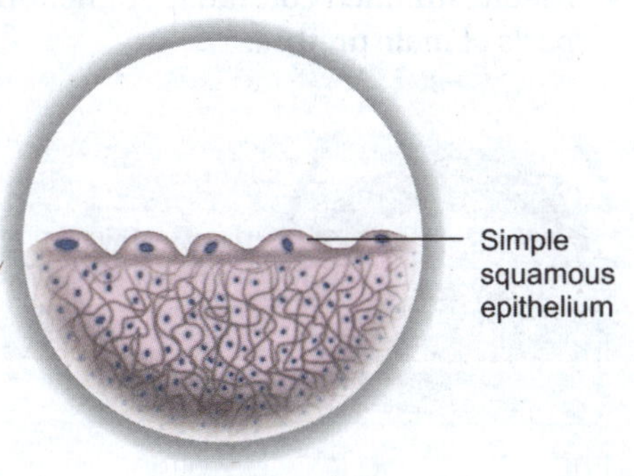

Q. Simple cuboidal epithelium

Ans.

- Single layer of cube-like cells (length and breadth equal)
- By and large, lines the glands
- Typical cuboidal epithelium is seen in thyroid gland, surface of ovary
- Cuboidal epithelium with brush border is seen in proximal convoluted tubule of kidney.

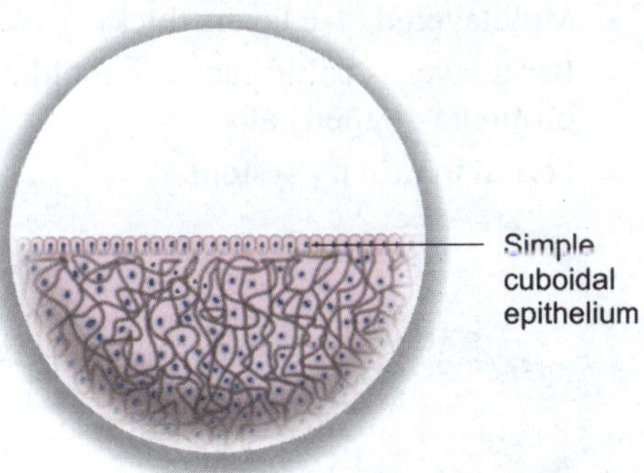

Q. Simple columnar epithelium

Ans.

- Single layer of tall cells (height > width)
- Nuclei oval vertically lie near the base of the cell

- At certain sites, columnar epithelium has cilia and is known as ciliated columnar epithelium, e.g. respiratory tract, uterus, uterine tube
- In some other sites, the surface is covered by microvilli and is known as striated or brush border, e.g. small intestine, gallbladder.

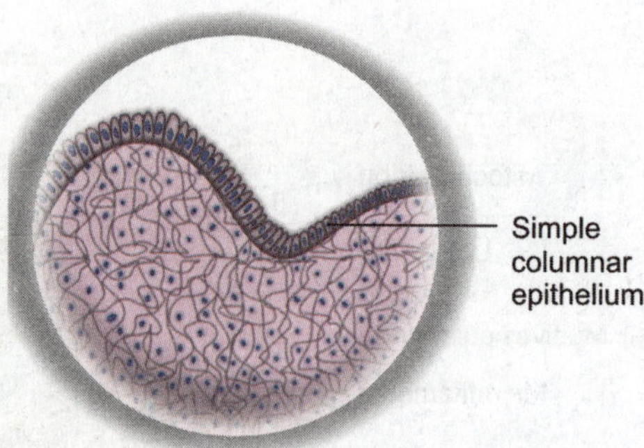

Q. Pseudostratified columnar epithelium

Ans.

- Gives a false appearance of multiple layers of cells
- The nuclei are arranged at different levels and hence gets a multilayered appearance
- At certain sites, may have cilia and is known as ciliated pseudostratified columnar epithelium, e.g. trachea and bronchi
- Pseudostratified columnar epithelium present in auditory tube partly, ductus deferens, parts of male urethra.

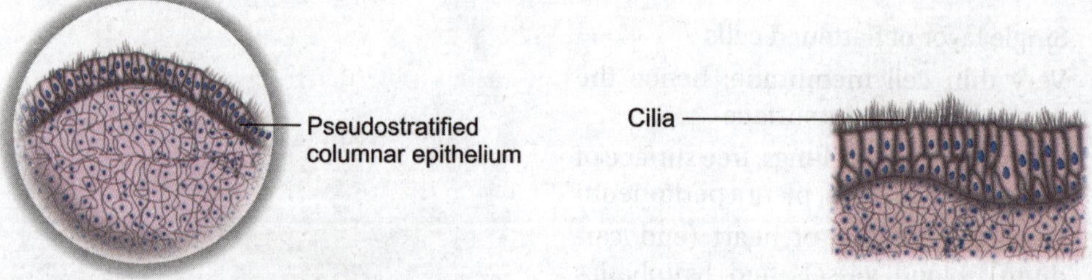

Q. Transitional epithelium

Ans.

- Multilayered (4–6 layers thick)
- Basal layer is columnar or cuboidal, middle layer is pear shaped, upper layer is large umbrella-shaped cells
- Found in urinary system.

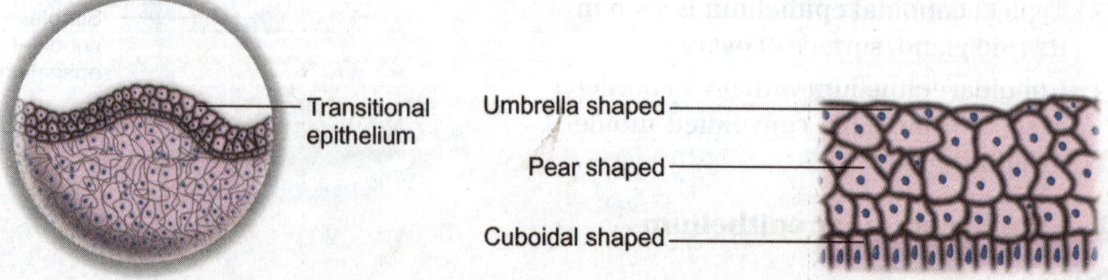

Q. Stratified squamous epithelium

Ans.

- Multilayered epithelium
- Basal layer is columnar, middle layer polyhedral, while superficial layer is made up of flat cells
- Nuclei are oval in basal layer, round in middle layer, transversely elongated in superficial layer, e.g. epidermis of skin
- Following layers are identified in the epidermis of skin:
    - Basal layer, stratum spinosum, stratum granulosum, stratum lucidum, stratum corneum.

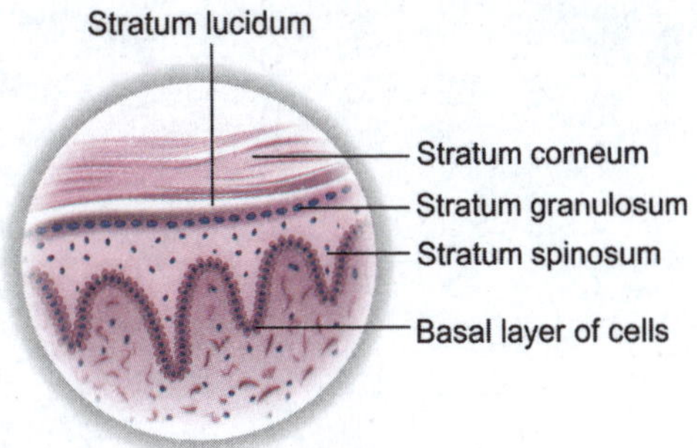

Mnemonic	Layers
"*Bombay*	**Basal**
Shall	**Spinosum**
Give	**Granulosum**
Lot of	**Lucidum**
Coins"	**Corneum**

- Thick skin has prominent stratum corneum
- Stratum lucidum is present only in thick skin
- Majority of the body is covered by thin hairy skin
- Thick hairless skin is present on the palms of the hand and sole of the feet.

Q. Loose areolar tissue

Ans.

- Bundle of collagen fibers are seen and have a wavy course
- Dark branching elastic fibers visible
- Connective tissue cells are mostly fibroblasts
- Elastic fibers need special stains for visualization, e.g. omentum.

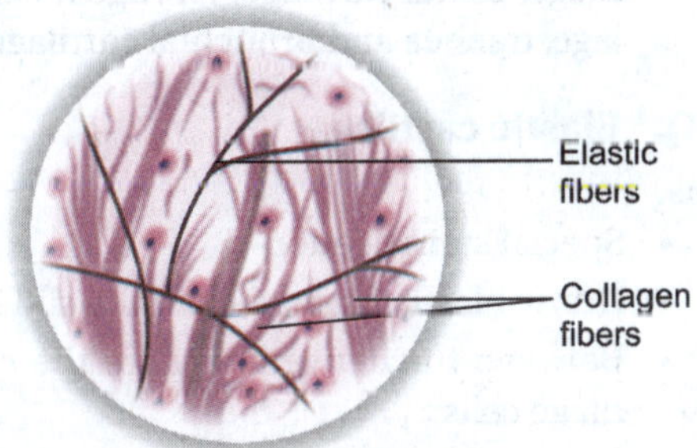

Loose areolar tissue

Q. Adipose tissue

Ans.

- Made up of fat cells
- The cells appear vacant, since the fat gets dissolved during the preparation of section
- Cytoplasm reduced to thin rim and nucleus lies at a periphery, e.g. omentum.

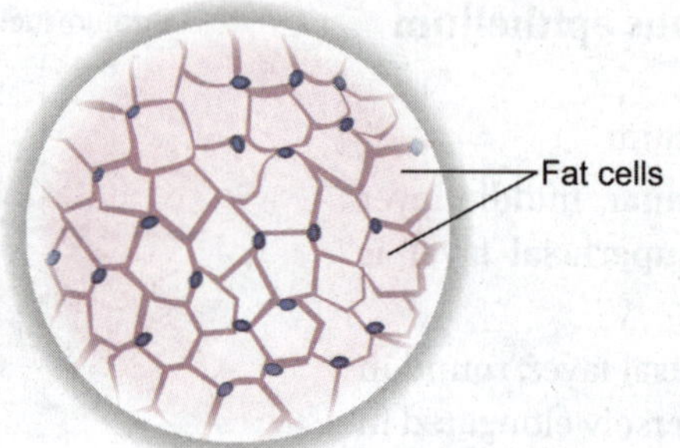

Adipose tissue

Q. Hyaline cartilage

Ans.

- On the surface of cartilage, the cells are flat and in continuation with the overlying connective tissue forming perichondrium
- Within the perichondrium, is a homogenous matrix (glass like)
- The matrix is packed with collagen fibers
- The Groups of cartilage cells that are present within the matrix known as chondrocytes
- Groups of cells due to mitosis are known as cell nests, e.g. articular cartilage, costal cartilage, laryngeal cartilage, trachea and bronchial cartilage.

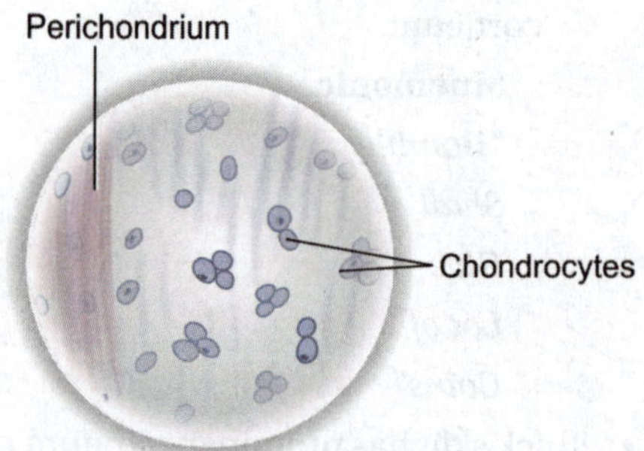

Hyaline cartilage

Q. Elastic cartilage

Ans.

- Special stain needed
- Dense elastic fibers seen in the slide
- Between the dense fibers are the cartilage cells
- Perichondrium is visible at upper end, e.g. pinna, lateral part of external acoustic meatus, medial part of auditory tube epiglottis.

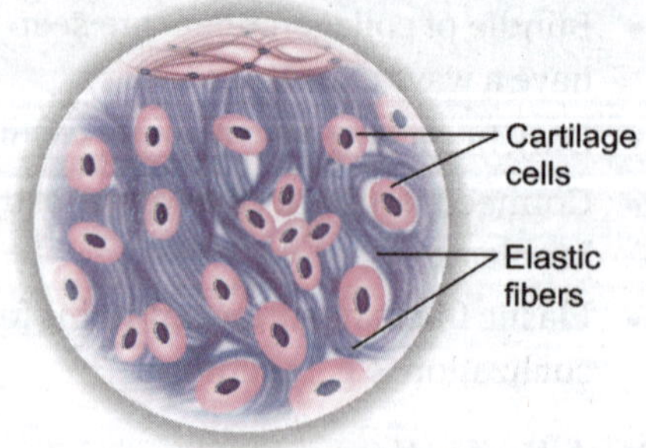

Elastic cartilage

Q. Fibrocartilage

Ans.

- Section contains typical cartilage cell groups surrounded by capsule
- Dense collagen bundles are present within the matrix
- Has no perichondrium, e.g.:
  - Secondary cartilaginous joints, pubic symphysis, intervertebral disk, manubriosternal joints
  - Synovial joints of membrane bones like clavicle, mandible are covered by fibrocartilage.

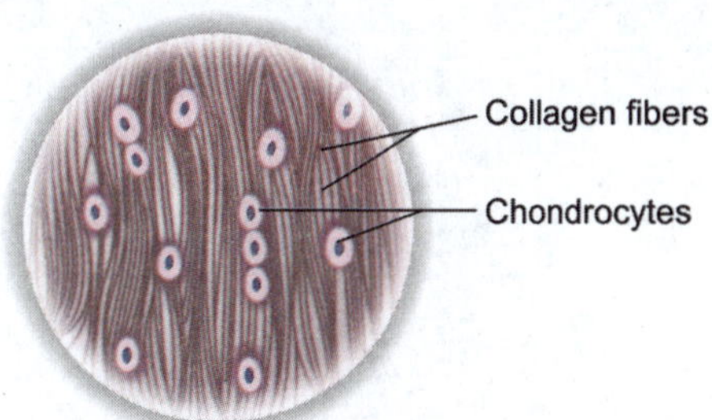

Fibrocartilage

Q. Compact bone

Ans.

- Made up of haversian system, i.e. ring like osteons
- In the center has a canal known as haversian canal
- Around the canal are layers of lamellae of bone
- Within the lamellae are small spaces, lacunae filled with osteocytes
- Canaliculi radiate from lacunae.

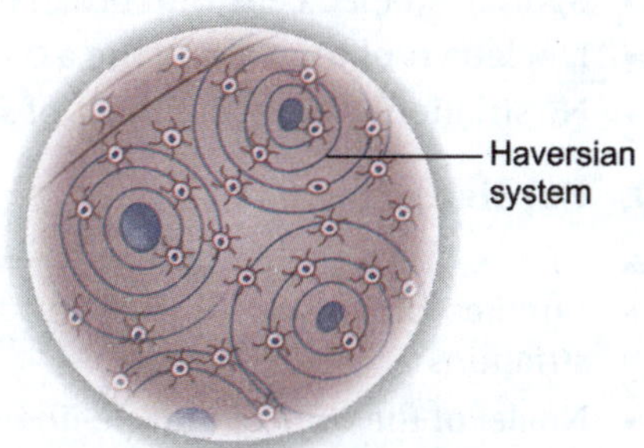

Compact bone

Q. Cancellous bone

Ans.

- Incomplete bony trabeculae are seen
- Within the trabeculae are osteocytes
- The spaces within the trabeculae are filled by bone marrow in which fat cells are present
- Blood-forming elements are present within the bone forming space.

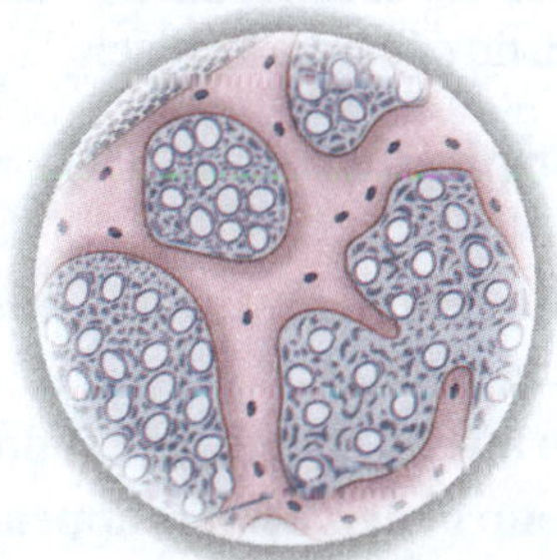

Cancellous bone

Q. Skeletal muscle (LS)

Ans.

- Vertical bundle of the muscle fibers are identified
- Cross striations are visible on the muscle fibers
- Peripherally located nuclei.

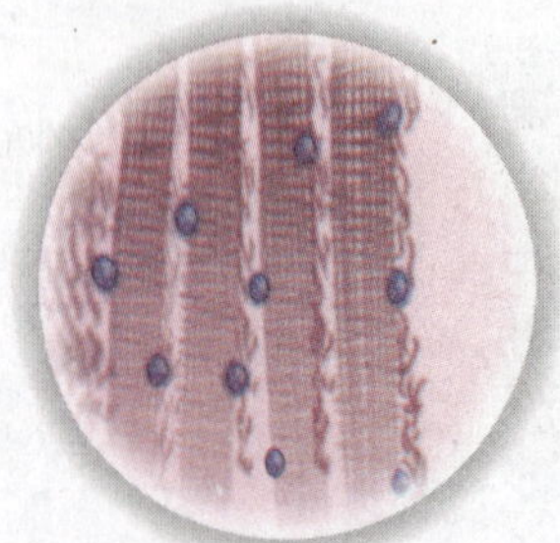

Skeletal muscle

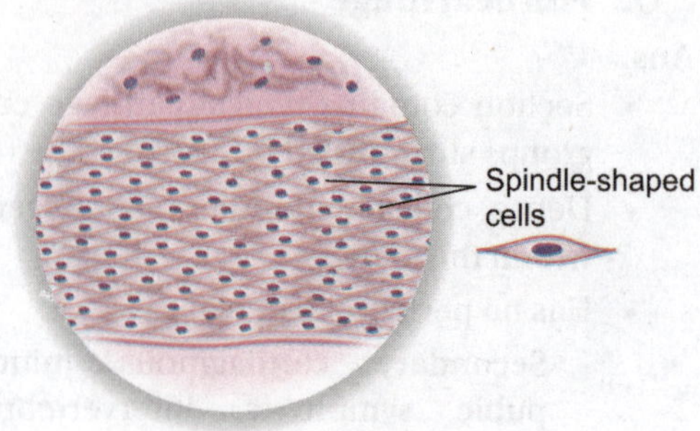

Smooth muscle

Q. Smooth muscle (LS)

Ans.

- Spindle-shaped cells with broad central part and tapering ends
- Nucleus is oblong along the axis of the cell
- No striations visible, e.g. walls of stomach, intestine.

Q. Cardiac muscle (LS)

Ans.

- Bundles of muscle fibers show faint striations
- Nuclei of the cells of muscle fibers are centrally located
- The muscle fibers branch an anastomose with each other
- Presence of intercalated disk is characteristic of cardiac muscle.

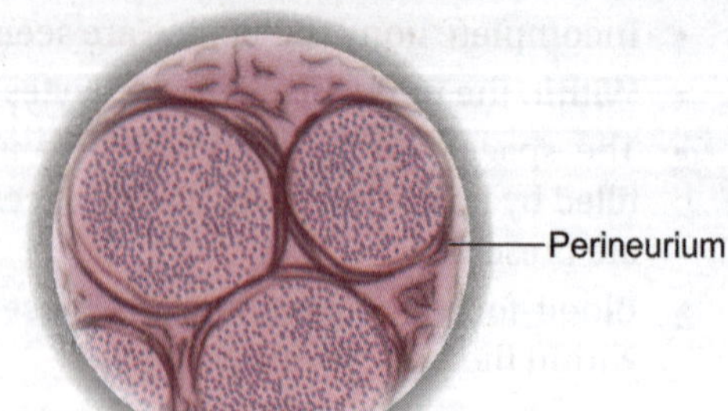

Cardiac muscle

Q. Peripheral nerve (TS)

Ans.

- The nerve tissue fixation needs special stain, osmic acid
- The myelin sheaths are stained black
- Group of nerve fibers appear as collection of empty black rings
- The bundle of nerve fibers is covered by connective tissue known as perineurium.

Peripheral nerve

Q. Sensory ganglion

Ans.

- Groups of neurons can be identified
- Each neuron has vesicular nucleus with prominent nucleoli
- Neuron is surrounded by satellite cells
- Collection of nerve fibers can be identified between groups of neurons.

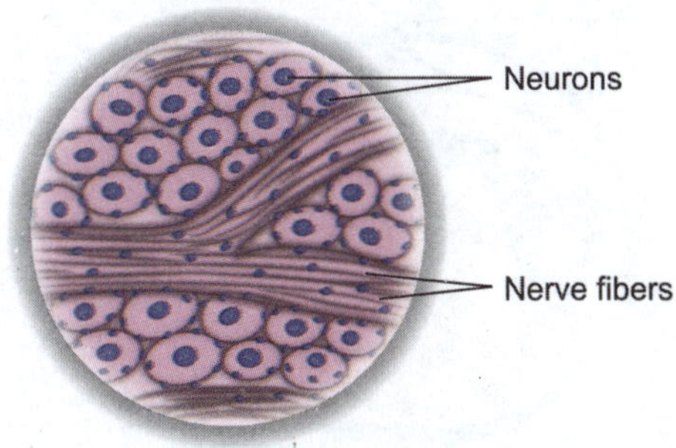

Sensory ganglion

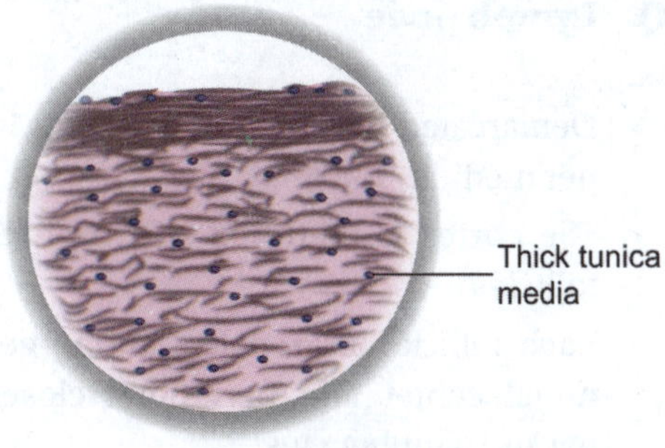

Elastic artery

Q. **Elastic artery**

Ans.

- Tunica media is very thick
- It is made up of fenestrated concentric elastic membranes
- In between the membranes there is connective tissue and few smooth muscle cells
- Internal elastic lamina is not distinct
- Tunica adventitia is thin, e.g. aorta, large arteries supplying head, neck and limbs.

Q. **Muscular artery**

Ans.

- The internal elastic membrane is very distinct
- Clear separation of tunica media and tunica intima can be appreciated
- Tunica media is made up of smooth muscle cells
- Tunica adventitia is made up of collagen and elastic fibers, e.g. all other arteries in the body except aorta, the large arteries supplying head, neck and limbs.

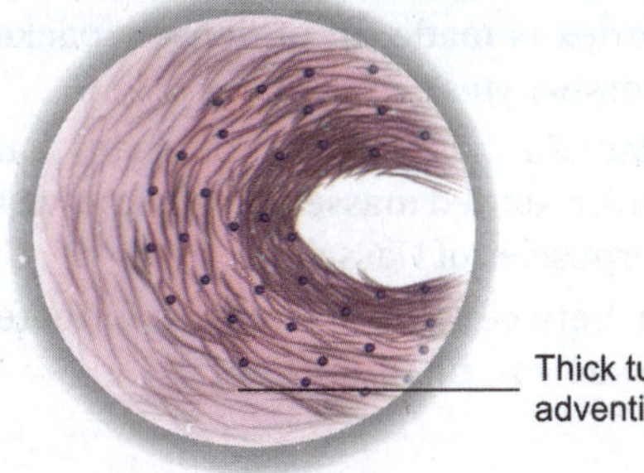

Muscular artery

Q. **Vein**

Ans.

- Vein has a collapsed wall and a large lumen within
- Tunica intima, media and adventitia cannot be separately identified and merge with each other
- Tunica adventitia is very thick
- Tunica media is thin and contain few muscle fibers.

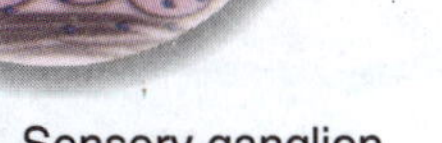

Vein

Q. Lymph node

Ans.

- Demarcated into outer cortex and inner medulla
- The cortex is made up of lymphatic follicles
- Each follicle has a pale staining germinal center and peripheral closely packed lymphocytes
- Lymphocytes are present within the follicles
- Medulla consists of blood vessels and collection of lymphocytes in the form of cords.

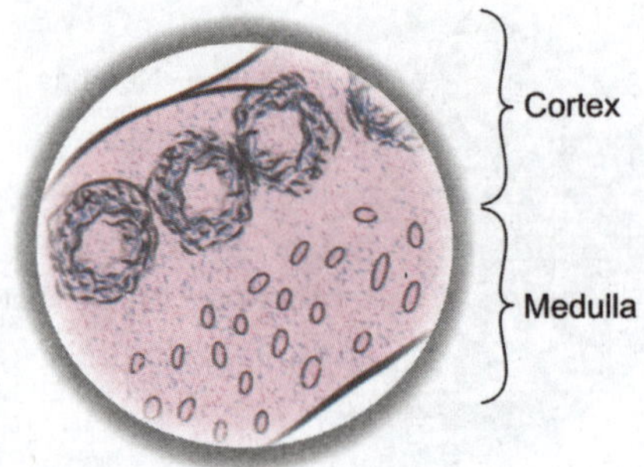

Lymph node

Q. Spleen

Ans.

- Parenchyma of spleen is divisible into red pulp and white pulp
- Red pulp comprises of numerous sinusoids and few lymphocytes
- White pulp is a dense collection of lymphocytes in the form of cords
- Capsule can be identified
- Incomplete septae or trabeculae can be identified within the parenchyma.

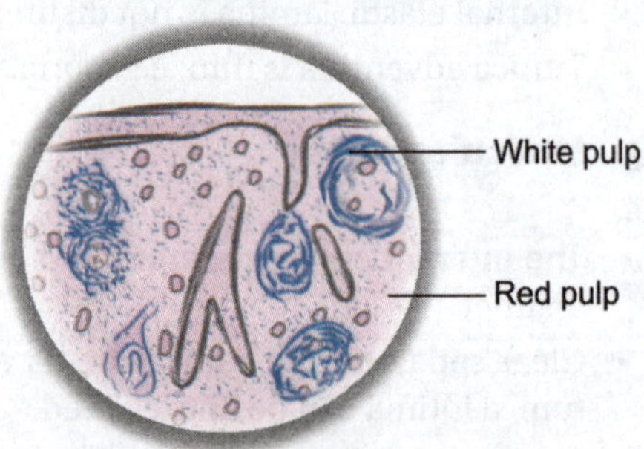

Spleen

Q. Thymus

Ans.

- Distinct lobules can be identified
- Each lobule has an outer cortex and inner medulla
- Cortex is made up of densely packed lymphocytes
- Medulla has few lymphocytes and pink rounded masses of cells known as corpuscles of Hassall
- In between the lobules, connected tissue can be identified.

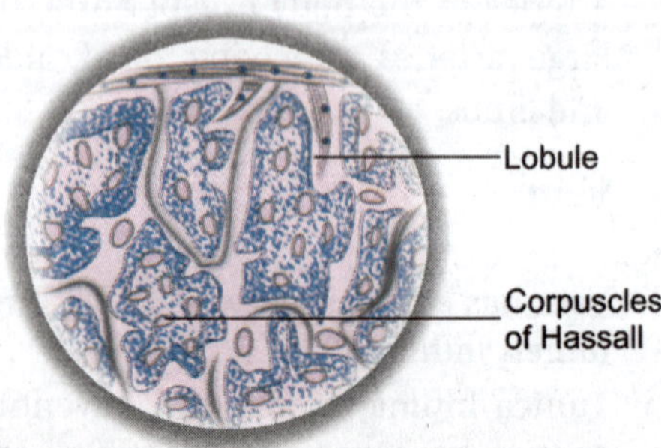

Thymus

Q. Palatine tonsil

Ans.

- It is the only lymphatic tissue covered by stratified squamous epithelium
- Epithelium dips at certain places and these sites are known as crypts
- Beneath the epithelium, there are lymphatic follicles, which have densely packed lymphocyte in the periphery and diffuse lymphocytes in the center.

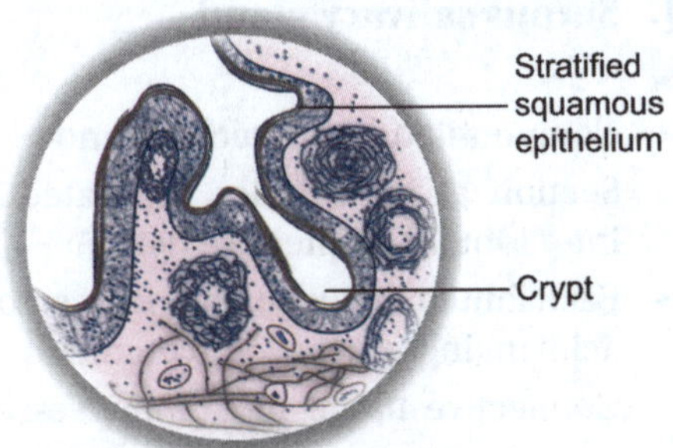

Palatine tonsil

Q. Skin

Ans.

- Comprises of epidermis and dermis
- Hair follicle with arrector pili muscle visible
- Sebaceous gland present near the hair follicle
- The parts of sweat gland can be appreciated.

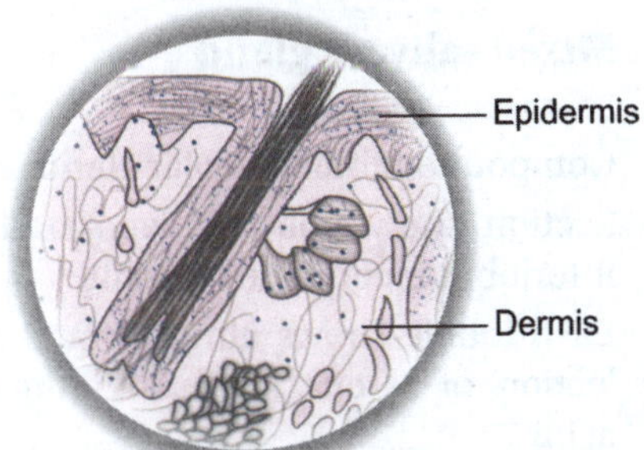

Skin

Q. Tongue

Ans.

- Section of tongue shows group of skeletal muscle fibers in various directions
- Collection of serous and mucous glands are present in between the muscle fibers
- Surface is covered by stratified squamous epithelium
- Papillae are seen on the dorsum, each papilla has connective tissue covered by stratified squamous epithelium.

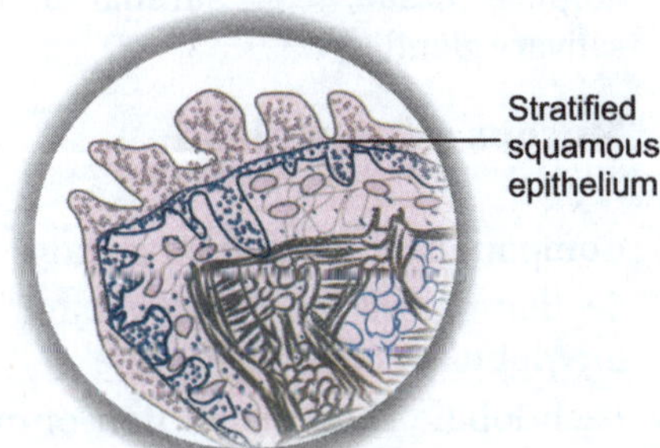

Tongue

Q. Circumvallate papilla

Ans.

- It is the largest papilla of the tongue
- Top of the papilla is broad and covered by stratified squamous epithelium
- It has a lateral wall that forms a deep groove
- The lateral wall has taste buds
- Core of the papilla shows serous glands and muscle fibers.

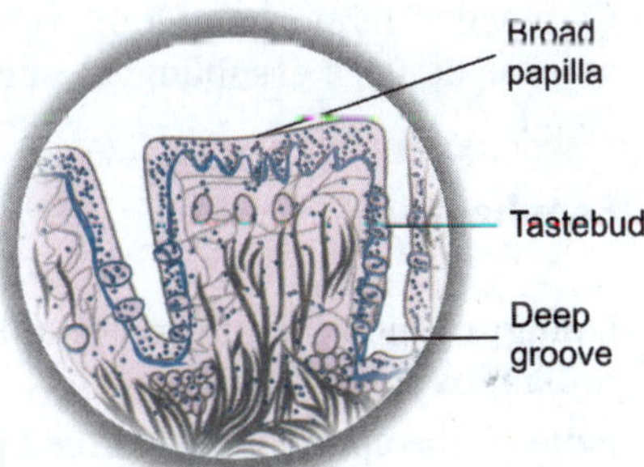

Circumvallate papilla

Q. **Serous salivary gland**

Ans.

- Compound tubuloalveolar gland
- Section shows lobules separated by inter lobular connective tissue
- Each lobule shows collection of serous acini mainly and few mucous acini
- Connective tissue has blood vessels, adipose tissue, e.g. parotid salivary gland.

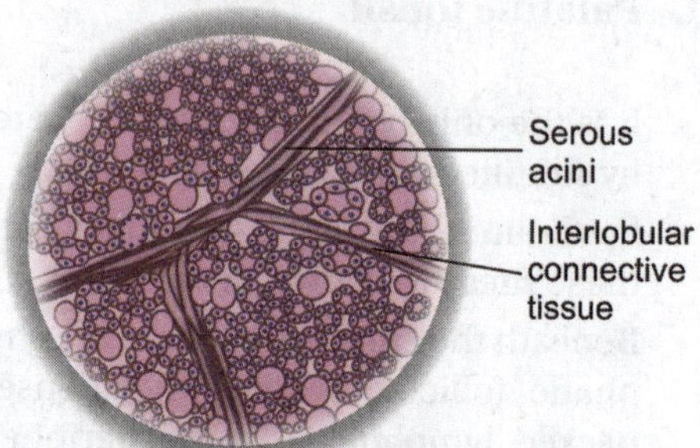

Serous salivary gland

Q. **Mixed salivary gland**

Ans.

- Compound tubuloalveolar gland
- Section shows lobules separated by interlobular connective tissue
- Each lobule shows almost equal collection of serous acini and mucous acini
- Connective tissue has blood vessels, adipose tissue, e.g. submandibular salivary gland.

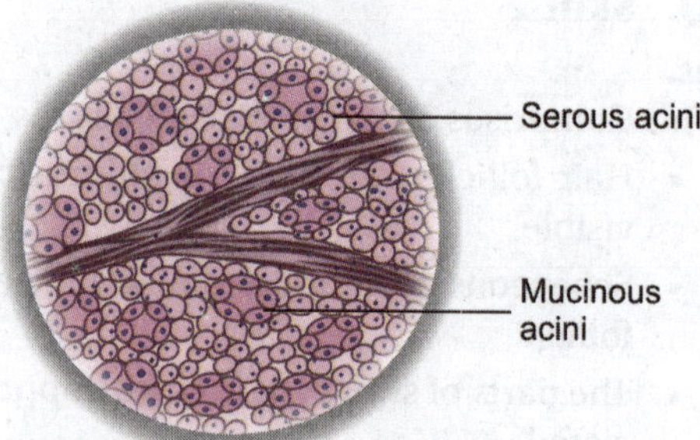

Mixed salivary gland

Q. **Mucous salivary gland**

Ans.

- Compound tubuloalveolar gland
- Section shows lobules separated by interlobular connective tissue
- Each lobule shows collection of only mucous acini; occasionally a serous demilune may be seen
- Connective tissue has blood vessels, adipose tissue, e.g. sublingual salivary gland.

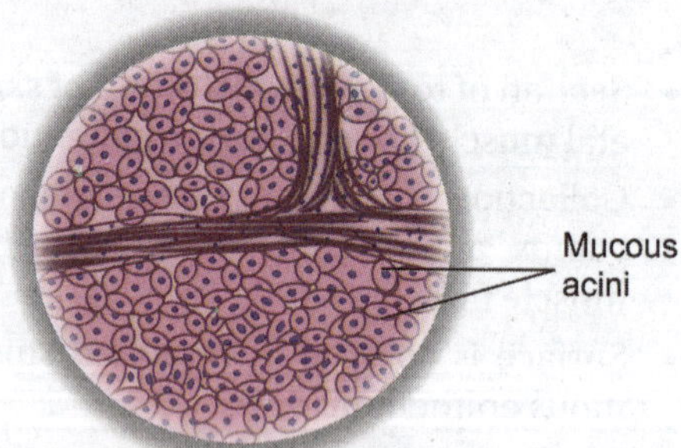

Mucous salivary gland

Q. **Esophagus**

Ans.

- Lining of non-keratinized stratified squamous epithelium seen
- Beneath the epithelium is lamina propria, a connective tissue layer
- Cut muscle fibers are seen below the lamina propria

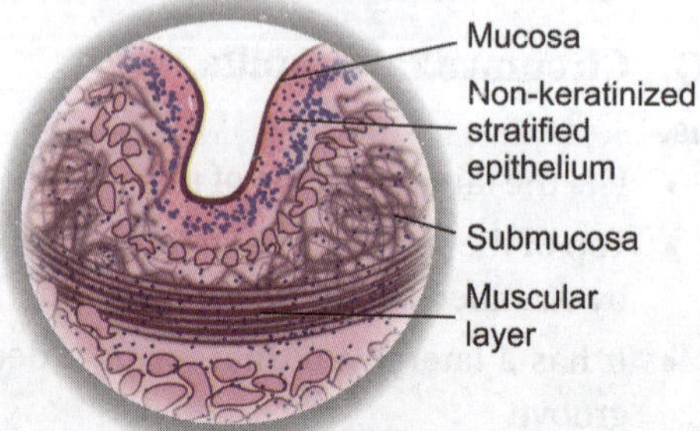

Esophagus

- Thick submucosal layer comprising of mucous glands, lymphoid tissue, plasma cells, macrophages
- Muscular layer consists of inner circular and outer longitudinal muscles.

Q. Cardiac end of stomach

Ans.

- The mucosa is thin in this area and gastric pits are shallow
- Junction of stratified squamous epithelium of esophagus and columnar epithelium of stomach is seen
- Cardiac glands are simple tubular or compound tubuloalveolar packed within the mucosa
- Other layers seen are muscularis mucosa, submucosa, circular muscle layer and longitudinal muscle layer.

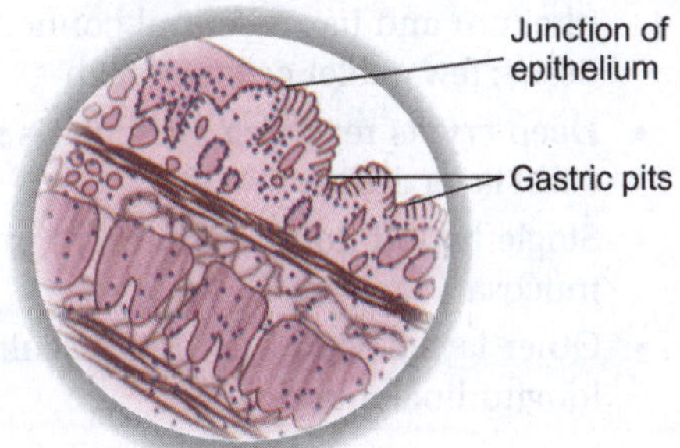

Cardiac end of stomach

Q. Body of the stomach

Ans.

- Mucosal lining is of the columnar epithelium
- Relatively deep gastric pit
- Numerous gastric glands are visible in the mucosa, viz. chief cells (peptic cells), parietal cells (oxyntic cells)
- Near the neck of the gastric glands are mucous neck cells, while at the base are endocrine cells and some undifferentiated cells
- Other layers seen are muscularis mucosa, submucosa, circular muscle layer and longitudinal muscle layer.

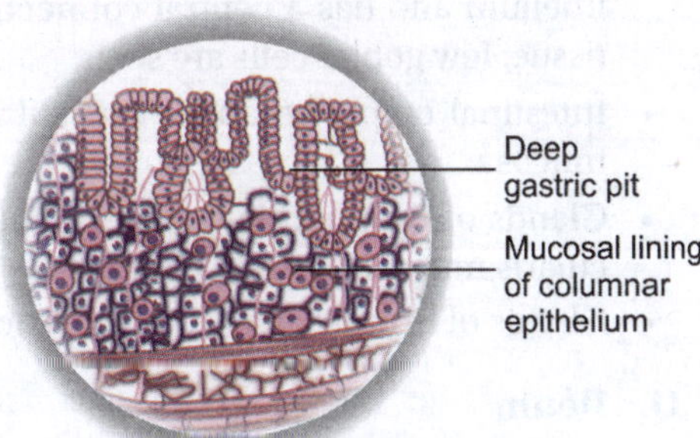

Body of the stomach

Q. Pyloric end of stomach

Ans.

- Gastric pits are deep and occupy two third of the mucosa
- Pyloric glands are seen in the deeper part of mucosa
- Other layers seen are muscularis mucosa, submucosa, circular muscle layer and longitudinal muscle layer.

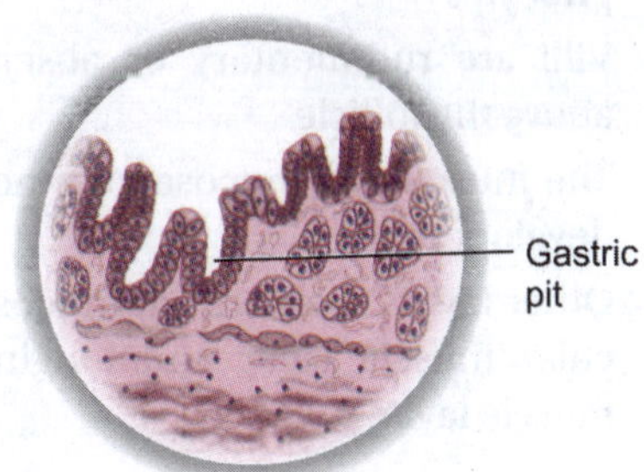

Pyloric end of stomach

Q. Jejunum

Ans.

- Mucosa shows numerous finger-like projections known as villi
- Each villus is covered by columnar epithelium and has a central connective tissue; few goblet cells are seen
- Deep crypts reaching muscularis mucosal layer are seen
- Single lymph nodule is present in the mucosa
- Other layers seen are the muscularis mucosa, submucosa, circular muscle layer and longitudinal muscle layer.

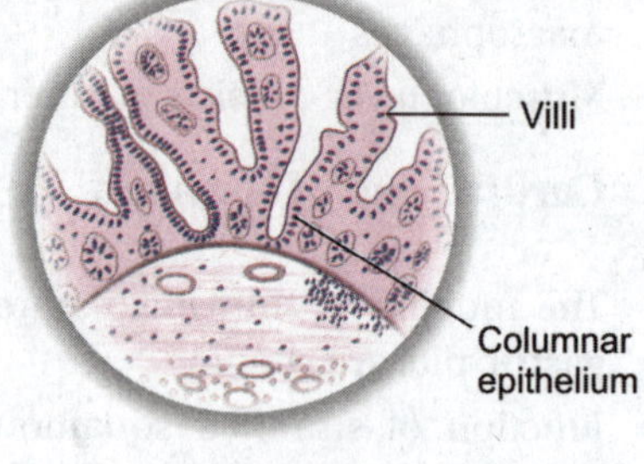

Jejunum

Q. Duodenum

Ans.

- Mucosa shows numerous finger-like projections known as villi
- Each villus is covered by columnar epithelium and has a central connective tissue; few goblet cells are seen
- Intestinal crypts lie above muscularis mucosa
- Glands of Brunner lie below the muscularis mucosa
- Glands of Brunner pack the submucosa and is distinguishing feature of duodenum.

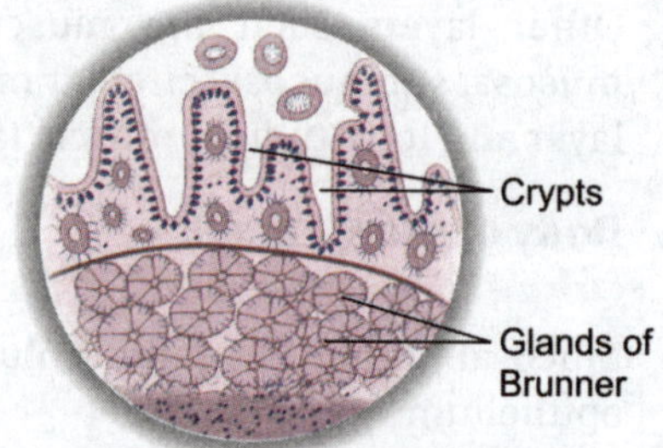

Duodenum

Q. Ileum

Ans.

- Presence of lymphatic follicles (Peyer's patch) is the distinguishing feature
- The lamina propria is filled with lymphocytes
- Villi are rudimentary or absent just above the follicle
- The muscularis mucosae are not well developed
- Other layers seen are submucosa, circular muscle layer and longitudinal muscle layer.

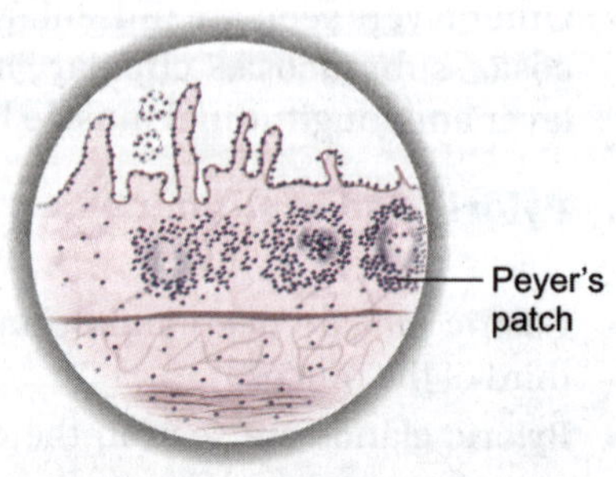

Ileum

Q. Large intestine

Ans.

- Mucosal surface and the crypts are lined by columnar cells amongst which are numerous goblet cells
- Villi are absent
- Paneth cells absent
- Lymphatic nodule is seen in lamina propria
- Longitudinal muscle coat is in the form of three bands called teniae coli
- Other layers seen are muscularis mucosa, submucosa and circular muscle layer.

Q. Vermiform appendix

Ans.

- Mucosa is poorly developed
- Lamina propria filled with lymphocytes and numerous lymphatic nodules
- Other layers seen are muscularis mucosa, submucosa, circular muscle layer and longitudinal muscle layer.

Q. Liver

Ans.

- Section is made up of hexagonal hepatic lobules
- Each lobule has a central vein from which radial sinusoids are visible
- Lobules are separated by connective tissue
- Within connective tissue is portal triad, which comprises of branch of portal vein, hepatic artery and interlobular bile duct.

Q. Gallbladder

Ans.

- The mucosa is lined by tall columnar epithelium
- Goblet cells are absent

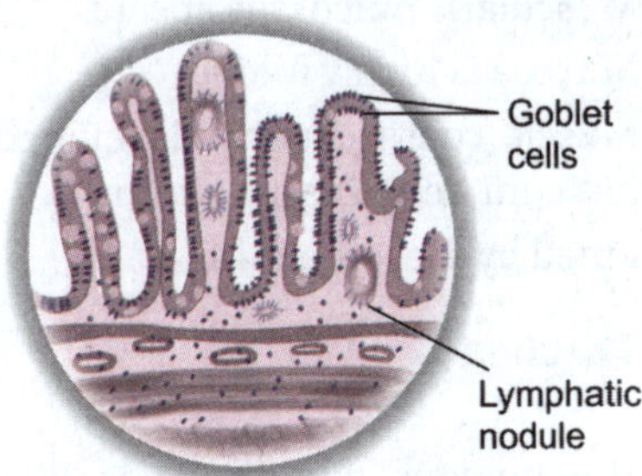

Large intestine

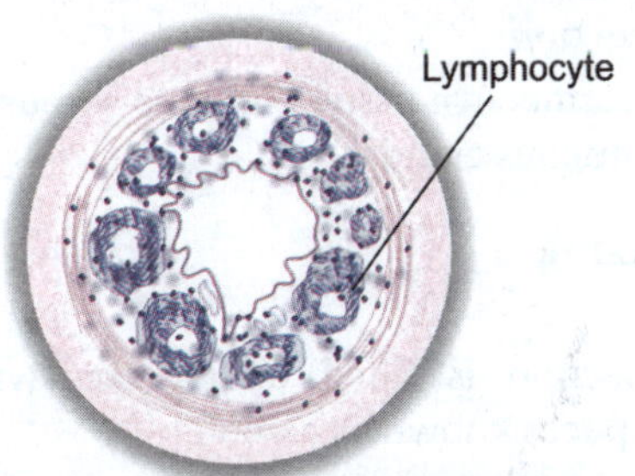

Vermiform appendix

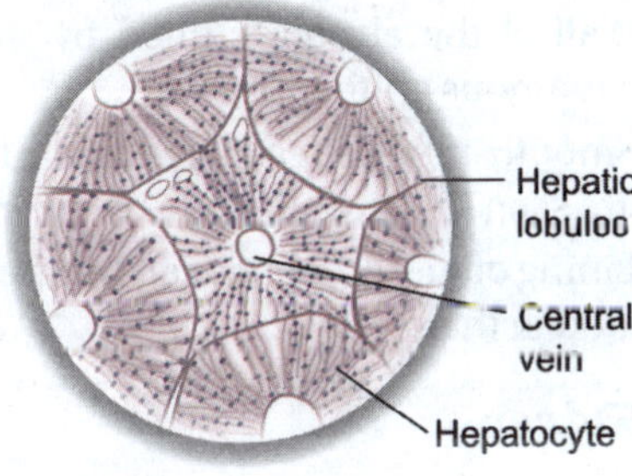

Liver

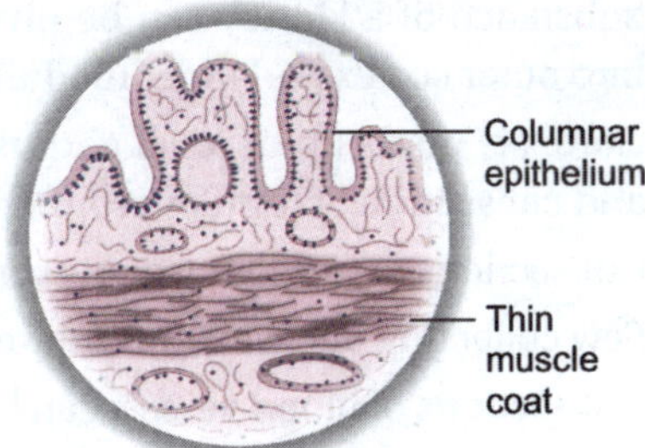

Gallbladder

- Muscularis mucosa is absent
- Mucosa is highly folded
- Muscle coat is poorly developed and has connective tissue within
- Lined by mesothelium.

Q. Trachea

Ans.

- The mucous membrane is lined by pseudostratified ciliated columnar epithelium
- Hyaline cartilage structure seen in the section
- Connective tissue contains serous and mucous glands.

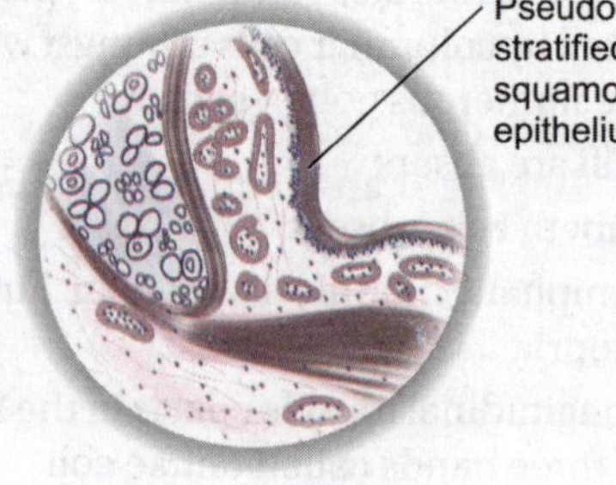

Trachea

Q. Lung

Ans.

- Section is filled up by thin-walled spaces known as alveoli
- Alveoli filled up with air
- Cut section of bronchi can be seen in the slide
- Wall of the alveoli is lined by simple squamous epithelium
- Smooth muscle, cartilage and glands are seen in the wall of the bronchus
- Lining of mesothelium can be appreciated in the section.

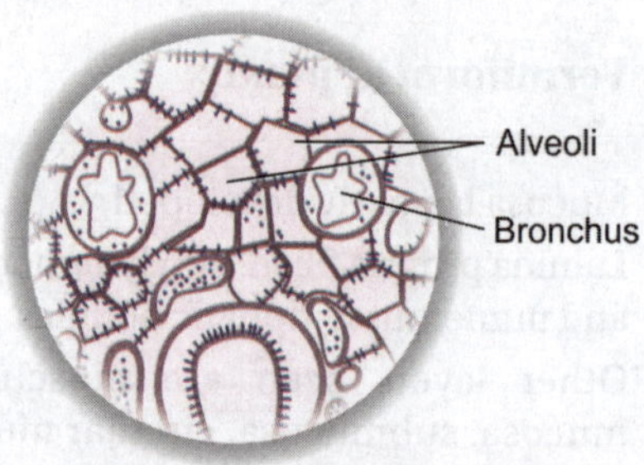

Lung

Q. Kidney

Ans.

- Covered by a capsule
- Substance of a kidney can be divided into outer cortex and inner medulla
- Cortex is made up of renal corpuscles and cut section of tubules around it
- Cut sections of collecting ducts running vertically can be seen in medulla
- Few collecting duct sections may extend into the cortex known as medullary ray
- Cut sections of blood vessels can be seen in the cortex.

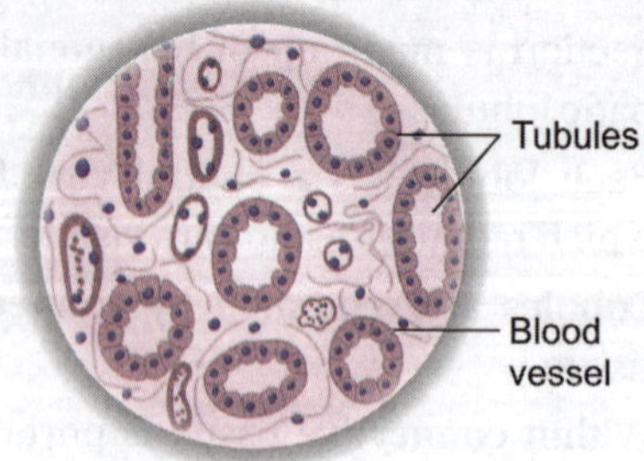

Kidney

Q. Ureter

Ans.

- Slide shows star-shaped lumen
- Mucous membrane is lined by transitional epithelium
- Muscle coat comprises of inner longitudinal layer and outer circular layer
- Muscle layer is covered by connective tissue layer in which fat cells and blood vessels are seen.

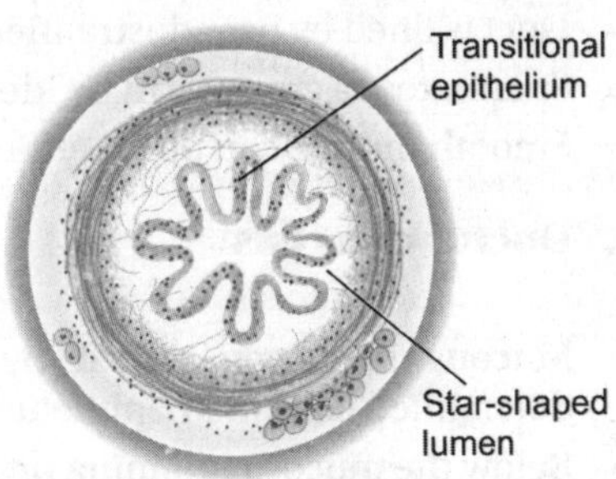

Ureter

Q. Urinary bladder

Ans.

- Mucous membrane is lined by transitional epithelium
- Subepithelial connective tissue layer is present
- Very thick muscular layer is present
- No clear demarcation can be appreciated between longitudinal and circular muscle
- By and large, circular muscle fibers are seen in between outer and inner longitudinal layer.

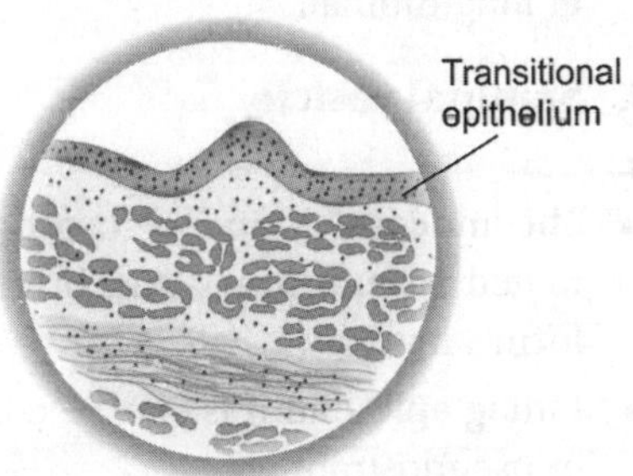

Urinary bladder

Q. Testis

Ans.

- Outer fibrous layer, tunica albuginea can be appreciated
- Cut section of seminiferous tubules are seen
- Several layers of cells (different stages of spermatogenesis) can be appreciated within the tubules
- In between the tubules, there is connective tissue with blood vessels and groups of interstitial cells.

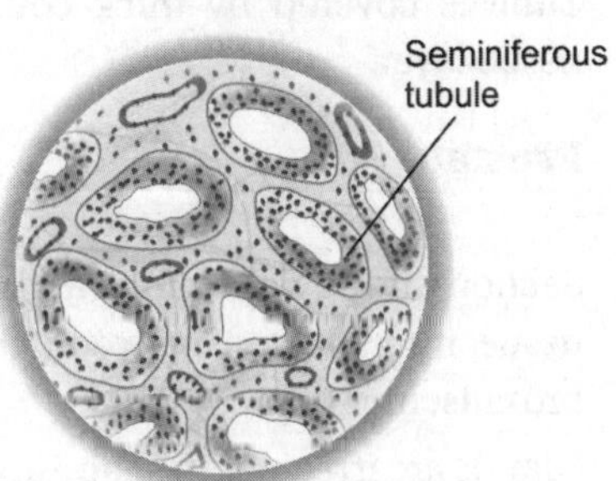

Testis

Q. Epididymis

Ans.

- Slide shows cut sections of convoluted duct

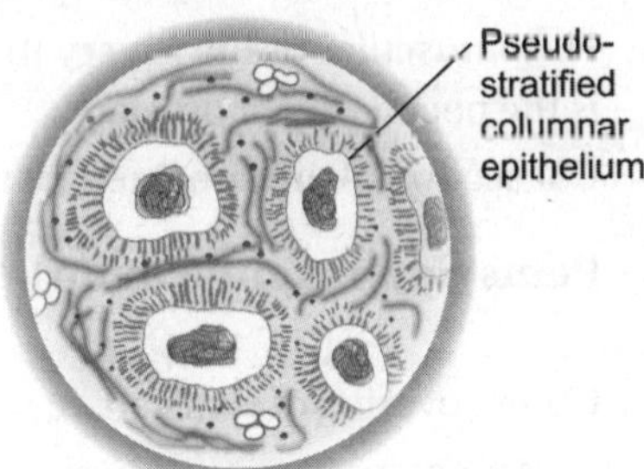

Epididymis

- Duct is lined by pseudostratified columnar epithelium
- Spermatozoa groups can be identified within the lumen of the duct
- Smooth muscle can be identified in the wall of the duct.

Q. **Ductus deferens**

Ans.

- Mucous membrane lined by pseudostratified columnar epithelium
- Below the mucosa is lamina propria
- Thick muscle coat comprises of inner longitudinal, middle circular and outer longitudinal.

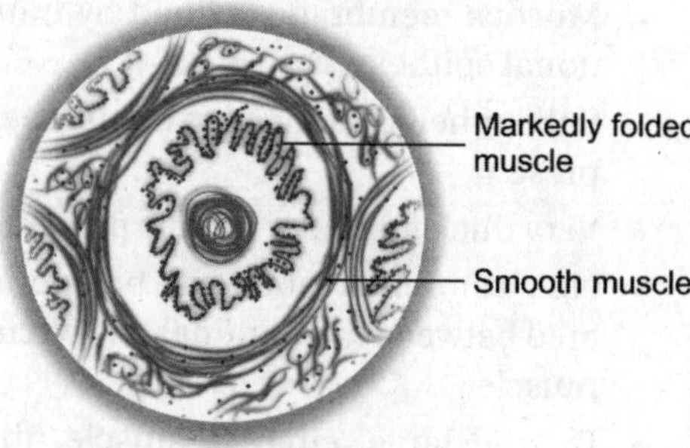

Ductus deferens

Q. **Seminal vesicle**

Ans.

- The mucosal lining of cut tubule is folded several times and branch and form a network
- Lining epithelium is simple columnar or pseudostratified
- Smooth muscle layer is very thin
- Tube is covered by thick connective tissue layer.

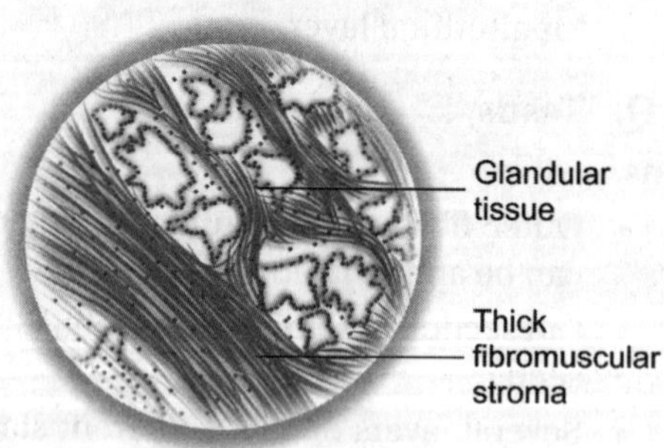

Seminal vesicle

Q. **Prostate**

Ans.

- Section shows collection of glandular tissue interspersed between thick fibromuscular tissue
- Glands are irregular in shape and lined by columnar epithelium
- Lumen may show amyloid bodies
- Fibromuscular tissue is very thick and is the peculiarity of prostate
- Cut section of urethra lined by transitional epithelium can be appreciated in low power.

Prostate

Q. **Penis (low magnification)**

Ans.

- Outer covering of skin can be seen
- Three masses of erectile tissue can be appreciated
- Masses adjacent to each other are corpora cavernosa
- Center of each corpus cavernosum shows cut section of artery

- Mass in front of corpora cavernosa is corpus spongiosum
- Corpus spongiosum is traversed by urethra
- Erectile masses are covered by thick fibrous sheath
- Urethra is lined by pseudostratified columnar epithelium
- Diverticula are seen within the urethral opening
- Outside the erectile masses, cut section of dorsal arteries can be seen within the connective tissue layer.

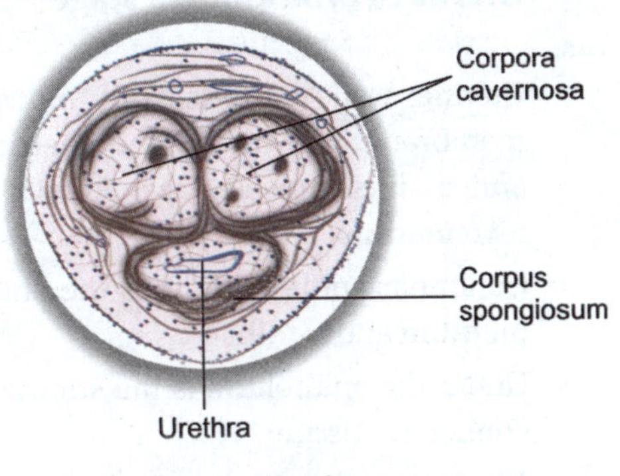

Penis

Q. Ovary

Ans.

- Surface covered by cuboidal germinal epithelium
- Below the epithelium is connective tissue layer known as tunica albuginea
- Substance of ovary divisible into outer cortex and inner medulla
- Cortex comprises of follicles, which contain developing ovum surrounded by follicular cells
- Cells surrounding the ovum form corona radiata
- Different stages of follicles can be appreciated
- Pink body corpus luteum can be seen in some slides
- The medulla comprises of connective tissue with blood vessels within.

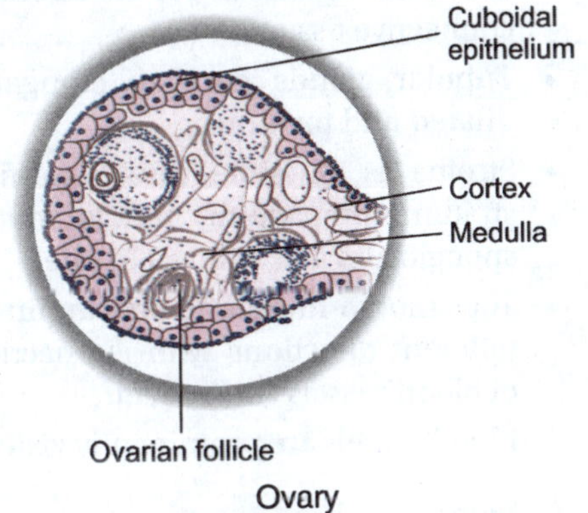

Ovary

Q. Uterine tube

Ans.

- Mucous membrane shows intricate branching pattern, which fills up the lumen of the tube
- Muscular wall of the tube is made up of outer longitudinal and inner circular layer
- Mucosa is lined by ciliated columnar epithelium.

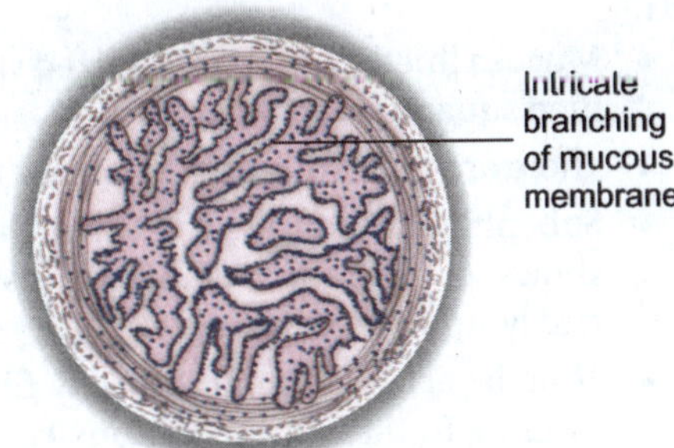

Uterine tube

Q. Uterus in proliferative stage

Ans.

- Uterine wall comprises of mucous membrane known as endometrium and a thick muscle layer known as myometrium
- Columnar epithelium lines the endometrium and is thin
- Under the epithelium is the stroma of connective tissue

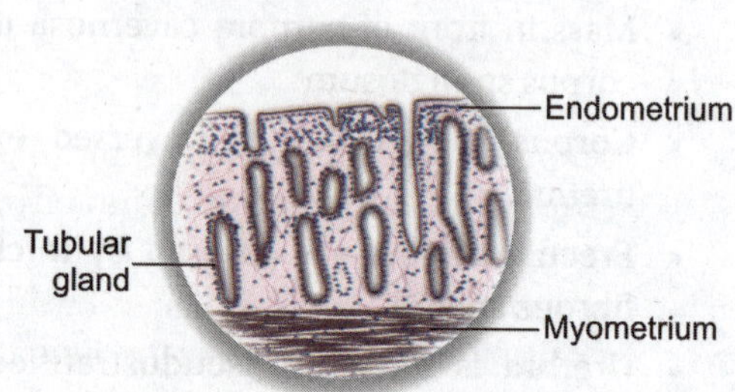

Uterus in proliferative stage

- Numerous cut sections of tubular glands, which are straight, can be seen in the stroma
- Smooth muscle fibers running in different directions with cut sections of blood vessels can be seen.

Q. Uterus in secretory phase

Ans.

- Uterine wall comprises of mucous membrane known as endometrium and a thick muscle layer known as myometrium
- Columnar epithelium lines the endometrium and is thick
- Under the epithelium is the stroma of connective tissue
- Tubular glands become elongated, dilated and tortuous
- Stroma is divisible into superficial stratum compactum, middle stratum spongiosum and stratum basale
- The smooth muscle fibers running in different directions with cut sections of blood vessels can be seen
- Blood vessels are prominently visible.

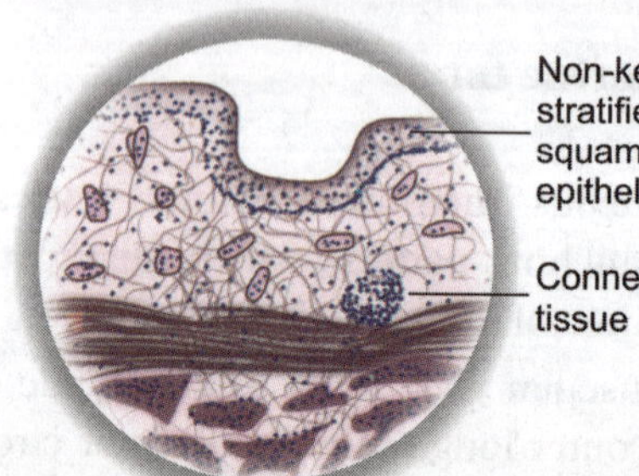

Uterus in secretory phase

Q. Vagina

Ans.

- Mucosa lined by non-keratinized stratified squamous epithelium
- There are no glands in the mucosa
- Subepithelial connective tissue layer shows cut sections of blood vessels and lymphatic follicles
- Thin layer of circular muscle fibers running in different directions can be appreciated.

Vagina

Q. Mammary gland

Ans.

- Comprises of lobules of glandular tissue with intervening connective tissue and fat
- Cut sections of glands are lined by cuboidal epithelium and have large lumen
- Within the connective tissue cut section of duct can be appreciated lined by two layers of cuboidal or squamous epithelium.

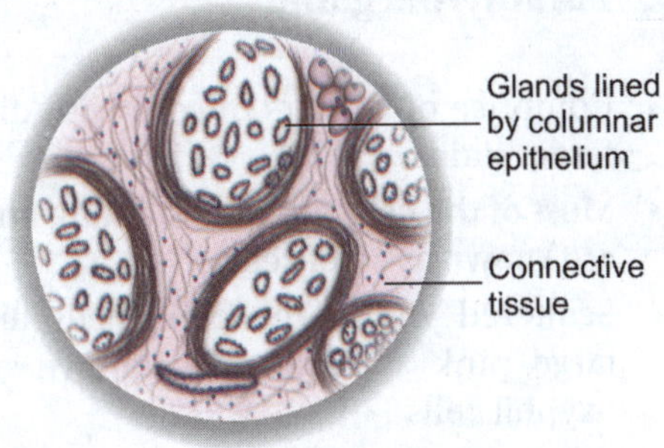

Mammary gland

Q. Pituitary gland

Ans.

- Section shows pars anterior, pars intermedia and pars posterior
- Pars anterior comprises of groups of cells (α, β and chromophobe)
- α cells or acidophils are pink
- β cells or basophils are blue
- Nuclei are closely packed and cytoplasm not distinct in chromophobe cells
- Pars intermedia comprises of colloid filled vesicle, blood vessels and few α and β cells
- Pars posterior is collection of nerve fibers and neuroglial cells.

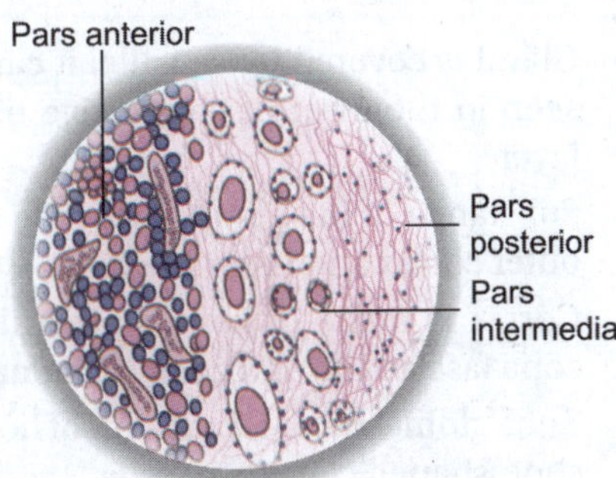

Pituitary gland

Q. Thyroid gland

Ans.

- Numerous follicles are seen in the section lined by cuboidal epithelium
- Follicles contain homogenous pink colloid within
- In between the follicles is connective tissue
- Parafollicular cells can be seen adjacent to the follicles and in the connective tissue.

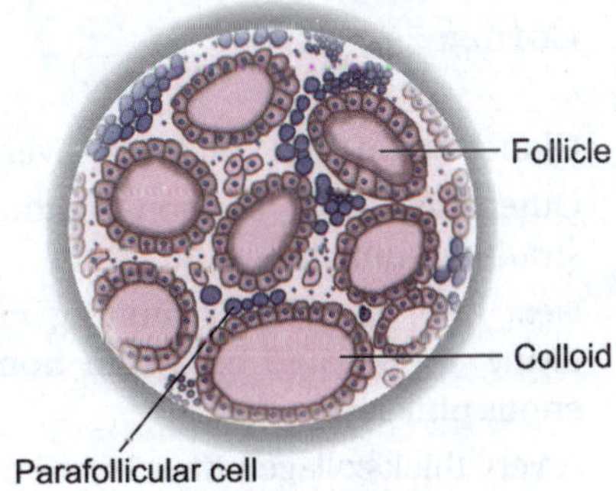

Thyroid gland

Q. Parathyroid gland

Ans.

- Comprise of clusters of cells with different stains
- Most of the cells are blue staining and are known as chief cells
- Scattered within the chief cells are large pink staining cells known as oxyphil cells
- Cut sections of blood vessels can be appreciated in the slide.

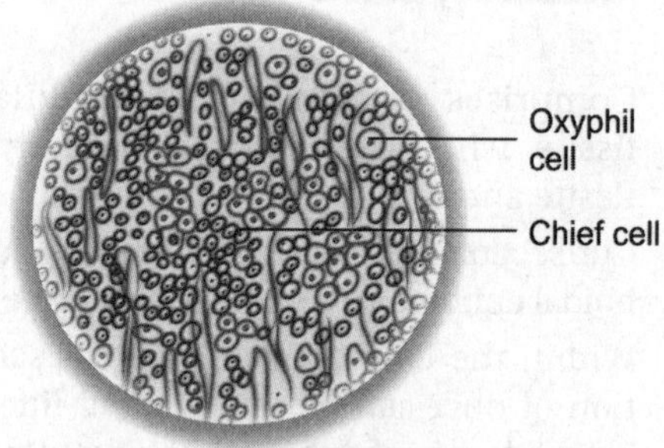

Parathyroid gland

Q. Suprarenal gland

Ans.

- Gland is covered by capsule, it can be seen in the form of connective tissue layer
- Substance of the gland is divided into outer cortex and inner medulla
- Cortex is made of zona glomerulosa, zona fasciculata and zona reticularis
- Zona glomerulosa is made up of horse-shoe-shaped clusters of cells
- Zona fasciculata is made up of vertical columns of cells with interspersed sinusoids
- Zona reticularis is made up of network of cords of cells
- Medulla is made up of groups of cells, sympathetic neurons and sinusoids between the cells.

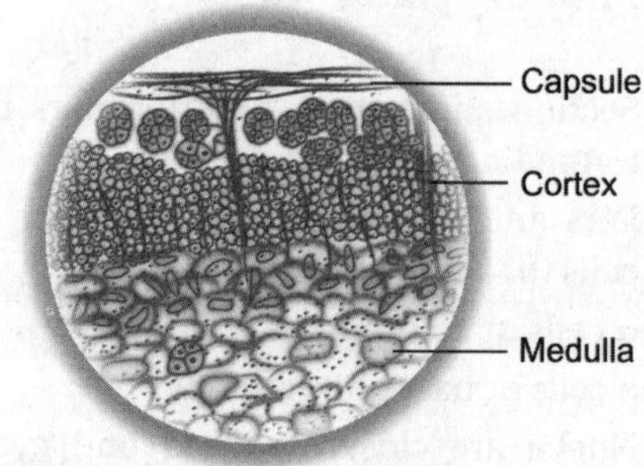

Suprarenal gland

Q. Cornea

Ans.

- Glance at the slide will show several layers
- Outermost layer is non-keratinized stratified squamous epithelium
- Next layer is anterior limiting membrane appreciated as a thin homogenous pink layer
- A very thick collagen fiber layer known as substantia propria embedded in ground substance is the peculiar feature
- Below the propria is posterior limiting lamina
- Innermost layer is a single layer of cuboidal cells.

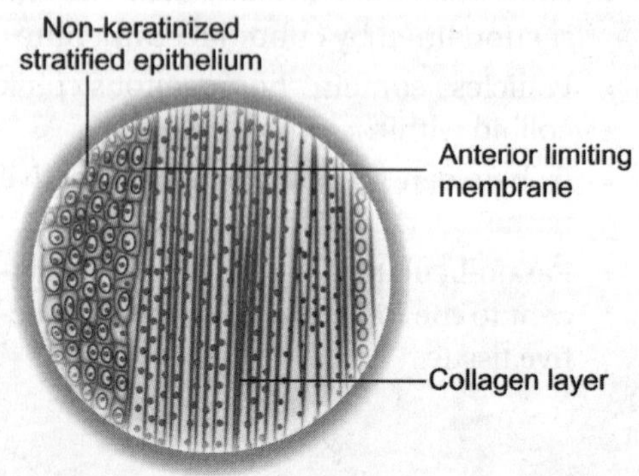

Cornea

Q. Wall of eyeball

Ans. Following layers of eyeball can be appreciated:

- Sclera in the form of collagen fibers
- Choroid made up of blood vessels and pigment cells
- Pigment cell layer of retina
- Rods and cones layer
- Outer nuclear layer
- Outer plexiform layer
- Inner nuclear layer
- Inner plexiform layer
- Ganglion cell layer
- Layer of optic nerve fibers.

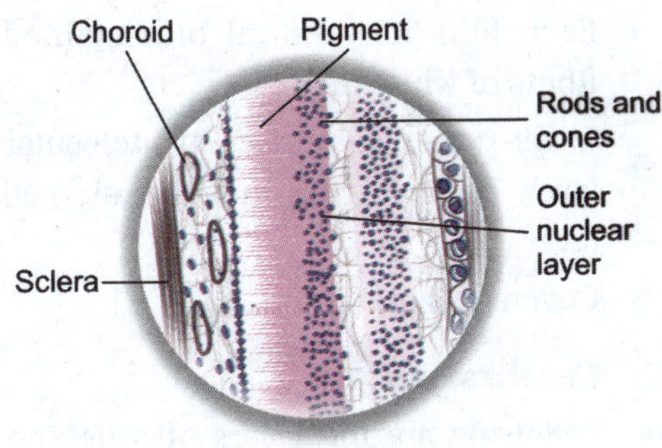

Wall of eyeball

Q. Cochlea

Ans.

- Bony tissue can be appreciated outside the cochlea
- Cochlea is in the form of spiral canal seen as six cut section
- Modiolus contains a canal through which cochlear nerve fibers pass
- Group of spiral ganglion neurons can be appreciated near the canal section
- Three parts can be identified in the cochlea namely scala vestibuli, scala tympani and cochlear duct
- Vestibular membrane lies between scala vestibuli and cochlear duct
- On the basilar membrane is organ of Corti.

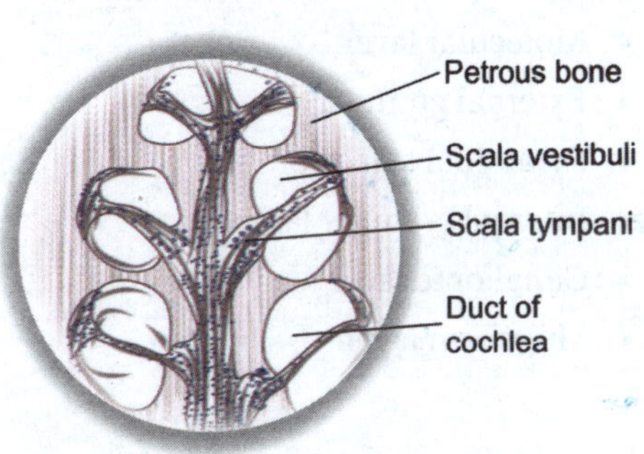

Cochlea

Q. Spinal cord (special stain)

Ans.

- H-shaped lightly stained gray matter (groups of cell bodies) can be appreciated
- Around the gray matter is densely stained myelinated fibers, which forms the white matter of spinal cord
- Central canal can be seen within the gray matter
- Vertically long and thin posterior median septum can be seen
- Wide and short anterior median sulcus can be appreciated.

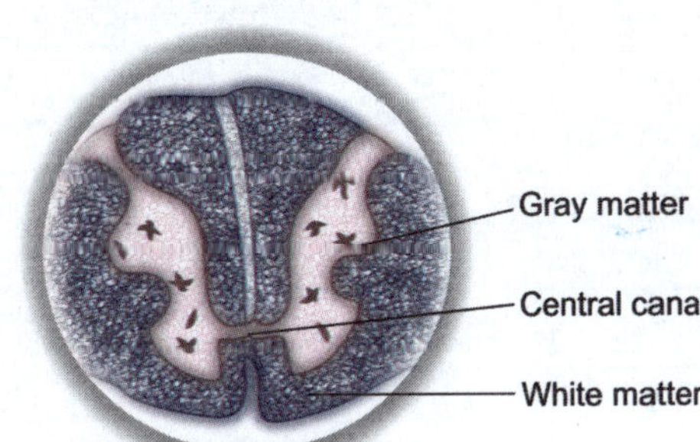

Spinal cord

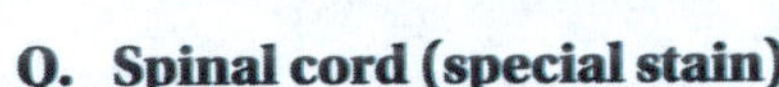

Q. Cerebellum

Ans.

- Section depicts leaf-like folia
- Each folia has central blue-stained fibers of white matter
- Outer cortex comprises of molecular layer, Purkinje cells and granule cell layer
- Covered by pia mater.

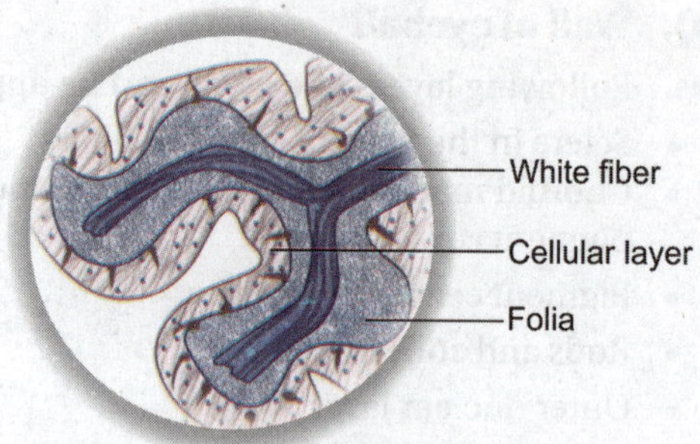

Cerebellum

Q. Cerebral cortex

Ans. Following are the layers of cells and nerve fibers, which form the cerebral cortex:

- Molecular layer
- External granular
- Pyramidal cell layer
- Internal granular layer
- Ganglionic layer
- Multiform layer.

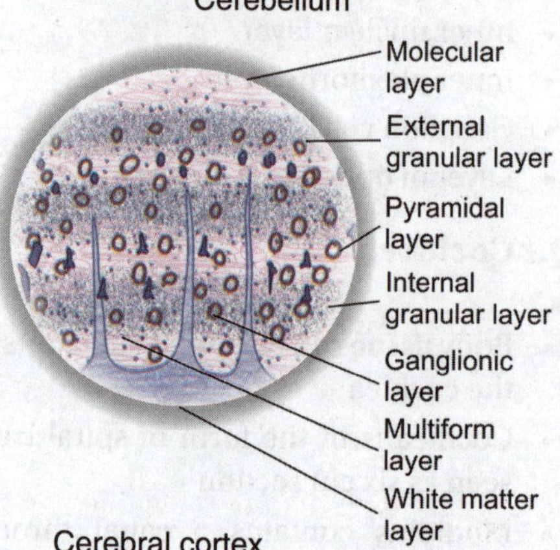

Cerebral cortex

Section - IX

ANATOMY NOMENCLATURE

Chapter 37

Literal Meanings of Anatomical Terms

TERM		DESCRIPTION
▶ A		
Acetabulum	:	Vinegar cup, Latin word, 'Acetum'—vinegar
Acoustic	:	Greek word, 'Akouein'—to hear
Adenoid	:	Greek word, 'Glandular'
Adenoids	:	Enlarged adenoid gland
Amnion	:	Greek word, 'Amnion'—lamb
Amygdaloid	:	Latin word, 'Almond'
Amyloid	:	Latin word, 'Amylum'—starch
Anatomy	:	Greek word, 'Ana'—up or through, 'Tomy'—cutting
Antrum	:	Latin word—cavity or a chamber
Aqueduct	:	Latin word, 'Aquaeductus', 'Aqua'—water, 'Ductus'—a leading pipe
Arachnoid	:	Greek word, 'Arachne'—like a spider
Arcuate	:	Latin word, 'Arcuatus'—curved like a bow
Argentaffin	:	Latin word, 'Argentum'—silver
Arytenoid	:	Shaped like a jug or pitcher
Auditory	:	Latin word, 'Auditories'—to hear
▶ B		
Bregma	:	Latin word—top of head
Brevis	:	Latin word—short
Bulla	:	Latin word—bubble/seal
Bursa	:	Latin word—purse/pouch

▶ **C**

Calamus	:	Latin word—cane, Greek word, 'Kalamos'—reed
Calcaneus	:	Latin word, 'Calx'—limestone; heel bone looked like a lump of chalk
Capitate	:	Latin word, 'Caput'—head
Carpus	:	Greek word, 'Karpos'—wrist
Caudate	:	Latin word—having a tail/tail-like appendage
Cavernous	:	Spongy
Cerebellum	:	Latin word—diminutive of cerebrum; 'Cartesian maze' (plural—cerebella)
Cerebrum	:	Latin word, 'Cerebrate'—to use the mind to think; Rome—understanding a fiery
Cervix	:	Neck
Chiasm	:	Decussation/crossing over
Chorea	:	Latin word—ceaseless occurrence of rapid, jerky movements
Cinereum	:	Latin word—ashes, ash colored
Cingulate	:	Latin word, 'Cingulum'—a belt worn by roman soldiers to protect their groin
Cingulate gyrus	:	Girdle-like marking; band or ridge zone
Claustrum	:	Latin word—barrier (plural—claustra)
Clavicle	:	Latin word, 'Clavicula'—little key
Clinoid	:	Greek word, 'Kline'—bed; 'Oid'—resemblance
Clivus	:	Latin word—slope
Coccyx	:	Greek word, 'Kokku'—cuckoo
Cochlea	:	Latin word—snail; Greek word, 'Kokhlias'—spiral, snail shell
Colliculus	:	Latin word—a small elevation
Condyloid	:	Latin word, 'Condylus'—knuckle
Corniculate	:	Shaped like a small horn
Coronal	:	Latin word—crown
Coronoid	:	Crown like
Cribriform	:	Perforated like sieve
Crura	:	Latin word—leg/leg like
Cubital	:	Latin word, 'Cubit'—elbow, unit of length
Cuboid	:	Cube like
Culmen	:	Upper ridge of bird's bill

Culmus	:	Latin word—stalk
Cuneatus	:	Latin word—tapering/pointed like a wedge
Cuneiform	:	Latin word—shaped like wedge

▶ D

Deltoid	:	Shaped like a delta, triangular
Diaphragm	:	Latin word—midriff; Greek word—partition
Diencephalon	:	Greek word—portion of brain between the cerebrum and the mesencephalon
Diploë	:	Greek word—fold
Duodenum	:	Latin word, 'Duodenum digitorum'—12 fingers' breadth
Dura	:	Hard

▶ E

Ecto	:	Outside
Emissary	:	Latin word—to send out; an agent sent on a mission to represent or advance the interests of others
Encephalon	:	En—in; Greek word, 'Kephale'—head
Epi	:	Above
Epididymis	:	Greek word, 'Epi'—on; 'Didymos'—twin
Ethmoid	:	Spongy

▶ F

Falx	:	Latin word—sickle shaped
Fastigium	:	Latin word—summit
Fibula	:	Latin word, 'Clasp'—brooch
Flexion	:	Latin word, 'Flexus'—to bend
Fontanel	:	Old French, 'Fontanel'—fountain
Foramina	:	Latin word—opening
Fornix	:	Latin word—arch-like structure
Fossa	:	Latin word—ditch
Fundus	:	Latin word—bottom

▶ G

Gaster	:	Greek word—belly
Gastrocnemius	:	Latin word—calf of leg, 'Gastro'—belly

Glabella	:	Latin word, 'Glabellus'—hairless
Glenoid	:	Saucer like
Glial	:	Greek word—glue
Globus Pallidus	:	Latin word—sphere, globe; 'Pallidus'—pale
Gluteal	:	Greek word, 'Gloutos'—buttock
Goblet	:	French word—drinking cup with a thin stem
Griseum	:	Latin word, 'Griseus'—bluish or gray

▶ H

Habenula	:	Latin word, 'Habena'—rein
Hallux	:	Latin word, 'Hallex'—big toe
Hamulus	:	A hook
Hiatus	:	Latin word, 'Hiare'—an opening, to gape or yawn
Hilum	:	Latin word—depression/pit
Hippocampus	:	Greek word, 'Hippokampus', 'Hippos'—horse, 'Kampos'—sea monster
Holo	:	Greek word—whole, entire
Hyoid	:	Greek word, 'Hyoeides'—shaped like a letter Epsilon
Hypo	:	Below

▶ I

Ileum	:	Greek word, 'Eileo'—to roll up, twist
Ilium	:	Latin word—groin
Incus	:	Anvil
Indusium	:	Latin word, 'Induere'—to put on, kind of tunic
Inguinal	:	Latin word, 'Inguin'—groin
Innominate	:	No name
Ischium	:	Greek word, 'Ishion'—hip joint

▶ J

Jejunum	:	Latin word, 'Jejunus'—fasting
Jugular	:	Latin word, 'Jugulum'—throat
Juvenile	:	Latin word, 'Juvenis'—young

▶ L

Labrum	:	Latin word—lip edge
Lamella	:	Latin word—diminutive of lamina
Lamina	:	Latin word—thin plate
Lepto	:	Greek word—thin
Limbus	:	Latin word, 'Limbus'—border
Linea aspera	:	Latin word, 'Spera'—rough or hard
Lumbricals	:	Earthworm
Lunate	:	Moon shaped

▶ M

Malleus	:	Latin word—hammer
Mammillary	:	Resembling breast or nipple
Mandible	:	Latin word, 'Mandere'—to chew
Masseter	:	Latin word—chewer
Mastoid	:	Greek word,—'Mastoeides', breast like
Mater	:	Latin word—mother (slang)
Maxilla	:	Latin word—jawbone
Meatus	:	Latin word—opening, to go
Mesencephalon	:	Greek word, 'Mesos'—middle

▶ N

Navicular	:	Latin word—boat
Nidus	:	Latin word—nest

▶ O

Obex	:	Latin word—barrier
Obturator	:	Latin word, 'Obturare'—to stop up or closing on opening
Olive	:	Latin word—symbol of piece
Ovary	:	Latin word—egg
Oxyntic	:	Greek word, 'Oxyno'—secreting acid, to make sour acid

▶ P

Parietal	:	Latin word—belonging to the wall
Patella	:	Latin word, 'Dish/Pan'—saucer like
Pectineus	:	Latin word, 'Pecten'—comb
Pellucidum	:	Per—through, 'Lucere'—to shine
Peritoneum	:	Greek word, 'Tonos'—stretching, 'Peri'—around
Peroneus	:	Greek word, 'Perone'—pin of a brooch or buckle
Petrous	:	Latin word, 'Petra'—stone
Phalanx	:	Greek word, 'Phalangos'—finger
Physis	:	Greek word—growth
Pia mater	:	Latin word—tender mother
Pilus	:	Latin word—hair
Pineal	:	Latin word—pine cone
Piriformis	:	Latin word—pear shaped
Pisiform	:	Latin word, 'Pisum'—pea shaped
Pituitary	:	'Phlegm'—gland that produces mucus
Pons	:	Latin word—bridge
Popliteus	:	Latin word, 'Poples', 'Poplit'—back of the knee
Postrema	:	Latin word—for back end area
Profunda	:	Deep
Propria	:	Latin word, 'Proprius'—proper, own
Prostate	:	Greek word, 'Prostates'—one who stands before, protector, guardian
Psoas	:	Greek word, 'Psoa'—loin region, either of muscle of the loin that rotate the hip joint and flex the spine
Pterygoid	:	Like bird's wings
Pulvinar	:	Latin word—a cushion
Putamen	:	Latin word—falls off in pruning
Putane	:	To prune/to think

▶ R

Ramus	:	Branch
Restiform	:	Latin word, 'Restis'—rope, 'Forma'—form; shaped like a rope
Rima	:	A gap or cleft between two symmetrical parts
Rostrum	:	Roused platform on which person stands

▶ S

Sacrum	:	Latin word—sacred/strong bone
Saphenous	:	Greek word—easily seen
Sartorius	:	Latin word, 'Sartor'—tailor
Scaphoid	:	Greek word—shaped like a boat
Scapula	:	Greek word, 'Scaphein'—to dig
Sciatic	:	Latin word, 'Sciaticus'—derived from Greek word, 'Ischiadikos'—pertaining to/located near ischium
Septum	:	Latin word—dividing wall, partition
Sinus	:	Space
Soleus	:	Latin word, 'Solea'—sandal
Sphenoid	:	Shaped like a wedge
Spine	:	Latin word—point
Splenium	:	Band-like structure
Stapes	:	Latin word—stirrup
Sternum	:	Breast, chest
Striae	:	Latin word—thin line or band
Stroma	:	Greek word—bed
Subiculum	:	Latin word—support
Sural	:	Latin word, 'Sura'—calf of leg

▶ T

Tapetum	:	Latin word—coverlet
Tarsus	:	Latin word—tarsus, Greek word—wicker
Tectum	:	Latin word—roof
Tegmentum	:	Latin word—covering
Tela	:	Latin word—web-like tissue
Temporal	:	Not lasting forever
Tenia	:	Greek word—headband
Tentorium	:	Latin word—tent
Teres	:	Latin word—round and long
Testis	:	Latin word—witness
Thalamus	:	Greek word, 'Thalamos'—chamber
Thyroid	:	Greek word—shield like

Tibia	:	Latin word—flute, shinbone
Tonsils	:	Check posts
Trapezoid	:	Greek word—table shaped; Latin word—shaped like a trapezium
Triceps	:	Latin word, 'Caput'—3 heads
Triquetral	:	Latin word—3 cornered
Trochanter	:	Greek word—wheel
Trochlea	:	Latin word—system of pulleys, Greek word, 'Trokhileia'—to run
Tubercle	:	Wart-like growth
Tympanic	:	Drum

▶ U

Ulna	:	Yard, 3 feet
Urethra	:	Greek word, 'Ourein'—to urinate
Uterus	:	Latin word—womb

▶ V

Vagina	:	Latin word—sheath/scabbard
Vastus	:	Latin word—vast, huge
Vertebra	:	Latin word, 'Vertere'—to turn, joint, spinal column
Vomer	:	Latin word—plowshare, ploughshare

▶ X

Xiphoid	:	Like a sword

▶ Z

Zygoma	:	Greek word, 'Zygon'—a yoke

Bibliography

1. Anne MR Agur, Arthur F Dalley. Grant's Atlas of Anatomy, 13th edition. Philadelphia: Lippincott Williams & Wilkins; 2013.
2. Chummy S Sinnatamby. Last's Anatomy: Regional and Applied, 12th edition. London: Churchill Livingstone; 2011.
3. Romanes GJ. Cunningham's Manual of Practical Anatomy, vol. 1-3, 15th edition. India: Thomson Press (India) Ltd; 2012.
4. Decker GAG, Lee McGregor. Synopsis of Surgical Anatomy, 12th edition. Bristol: John Wright & Sons Ltd; 1986.
5. Inderbir Singh. Textbook of Human Histology, 5th edition. New Delhi: Jaypee Brothers Medical Publishers; 2008.
6. Krishna Garg, Chaurasia BD. Human Anatomy, vol. 1-3, 6th edition. New Delhi: CBS Publishers & Distributors; 2013.
7. Malcolm B Carpenter. Core Textbook of Neuroanatomy, 4th edition. Philadelphia: Lippincott Williams & Wilkins; 1900.
8. Norman S Williams, Christopher JK Bulstrode, P Ronan O'Connell. Bailey and Love's Short Practice of Surgery, 25th edition. UK: Edward Arnold Publishers Ltd; 2008.
9. Susan Standring. Gray's Anatomy, 40th edition. London: Churchill Livingstone Elsevier; 2008.
10. Maran AGD. Logan Turner's Diseases of the Nose, Throat and Ear, 10th edition. UK: Butterworth-Helnemann Ltd; 1999.